Textbook of Oncofertility Research and Practice

Teresa K. Woodruff
Divya K. Shah
Wendy S. Vitek
Editors

Textbook of Oncofertility Research and Practice

A Multidisciplinary Approach

Springer

Editors
Teresa K. Woodruff
Department of Obstetrics and Gynecology
Northwestern University
Chicago, IL
USA

Divya K. Shah
Department of Obstetrics and Gynecology
University of Pennsylvania
Philadelphia, PA
USA

Wendy S. Vitek
Department of Obstetrics and Gynecology
University of Rochester
Rochester, NY
USA

ISBN 978-3-030-02867-1 ISBN 978-3-030-02868-8 (eBook)
https://doi.org/10.1007/978-3-030-02868-8

This Springer imprint is published by the registered company Springer Nature Switzerland AG
The registered company address is: Gewerbestrasse 11, 6330 Cham, Switzerland

To Megan Connolly

Preface

The field of oncofertility began with an urgent unmet need – the fertility concerns of young cancer patients. Today, due to the research and clinical interventions documented in prior books, the field of oncofertility has matured. Now, clear didactics are needed to ensure that clinicians who are new to this field of medicine can quickly come up to speed with treatment strategies. In this first ever *Textbook of Oncofertility Research and Practice*, the coeditors and coauthors met this need with two kinds of chapters. First, in the didactic chapters, questions are posed that are instructional and provide the best evidence available on each of the subjects. They may also provide a springboard toward new research or improvements in clinical care. The second chapter type is represented by case studies. Every oncofertility case differs significantly based on the age of the individual, expectations about fertility needs, timing, and the type of cancer care, and this complexity is detailed in each chapter. As a collection, they represent the best thinking of clinicians who have been on the frontline of oncofertility care since its inception. In the end, we hope these chapters and the case studies enable the kind of learning that is enduring and propels the field forward.

The coeditors on this book are Divya Shah, MD, and Wendy Vitek, MD. Both of these clinicians are extraordinary educators and have dedicated their careers to teaching oncofertility practices to residents and fellows across the multiple subspecialties that represent this diverse field. They are the founders and directors of the Oncofertility Fellow Education Day that brings students together on an annual basis to learn about the field and how to collaborate across disciplines. They also led the Oncofertility Consortium's efforts to create free online didactics that are available through the American Society of Reproductive Medicine (ASRM). Through these efforts, they are enabling the next generation of clinicians to learn either in person, online, or through this textbook. Education that has no boundaries is boundless! I am grateful to them for their partnership in each of these endeavors.

This textbook could not exist without the time and expertise of our authors; their dedication ensures this is a volume that is highly valuable to the field today and will be the foundation for updates in our collective future. These chapters and cases are built on experience, and the truths that are presented are hard-won, first-person voyages into delivery of care when intentions were good but guidelines were scarce. Our authors are on the front lines, but rarely make headlines – they are the champions of oncofertility.

It would also not exist without the expert handling of the administrative details of this and other Oncofertility Consortium educational tools by Lauren Ataman-Millhouse and Brigid Martz-Smith. These two outstanding leaders have enabled our field to flourish for more than half a decade. Their personal commitment and professional passion for oncofertility ensure that the field is coordinated so that patient treatment is optimized. Team science often moves more slowly because of coordination penalties. Oncofertility is different, and the difference is Lauren and Brigid. They make possible any idea that I imagine, and, as a consequence, we have made remarkable advances in a short period of time. Our field is made better by and is grateful to Lauren and Brigid for their expertise and partnership.

This book was also aided by the team of editors, including Tracy Marton, at Springer Nature, and, most importantly, Kristopher Spring. This is my seventh book with Kristopher, and his careful handling of our field as we coalesced our ideas over the years is remarkable. Indeed, our first book, published in 2007, was immediately after the word *oncofertility* was coined. One has only to peruse the titles of our books to know that Springer has never shied away from the needs of our field as it developed [1–6].

Most importantly, I want to thank the field of oncofertility. This will be my last preface in a book that I edit on this topic. I have been part of a global movement that created the basic science rationale, clinical investigatory opportunities, and clinical breakthroughs that we now take for granted in fertility management of the young cancer patient. My first conversations with clinicals – REIs, oncologists, and embryologists – were met with incredulity. The time was too long; the patients were too ill; the need to protect fertility was subordinate to all else. These early discussions led directly the creation of the Oncofertility Consortium, a global community of care that represents a collegial group of members across the disciplinary spectrum who are "the community of the willing." As a consequence of this groups' good work, young cancer patients now expect a fertility consult, and while not yet universal, options are available in many clinical settings providing hope for an expectant future. Today, there are five states that have enacted insurance and reimbursement legislation, ensuring access to patients from all socioeconomic backgrounds. In the end, my contribution has been as a grassroots organizer, recognizing from the beginning that for the field to reach its full potential in the shortest possible timeframe, we needed to think not just about the research breakthroughs or clinical options, but we had to think about practice management strategies and what questions the patient might have including about legal issues, ethical concerns, and faith-based crisis that could modify decisioning. By including all of the wisdom of the academy, we accelerated the work.

While this is my last chapter in oncofertility, my own work with continue in the lab, which is the best outcome for research – that a once intractable problem now has tangible solutions. Drs. Shah and Vitek will take over as coeditors of this textbook in future years, ensuring that we have the most up-to-date content so that it becomes a vibrant part of the fertility preservation movement. The Oncofertility Consortium meetings will continue because the field has problems it must continue to solve and only by convening do we understand each other's points of view.

Finally, this textbook is dedicated to all of the cancer patients who have fought this disease. Megan Connolly, to whom this book is dedicated, is my personal hero, and she represents the many heroes who have overcome the adversity of cancer to shine as a beacon on health and hope to many generations to come. She is living proof that the promise of basic science in medicine is that tomorrow's patient will be treated better than todays.

This textbook is the tangible evidence of that promise.

1. Woodruff TK, Snyder K. (Eds). Oncofertility. New York: Springer; 2007.
2. Woodruff TK, Zoloth L, Campo-Engelstein L, Rodriguez SB. (Eds). Oncofertility: ethical, legal, social, and medical perspectives. New York: Springer Publishing Company; 2010.
3. Woodruff TK, Gracia C. (Eds). Oncofertility medical practice: clinical issues and implementation. New York: Springer Publishing Company; 2012.
4. Woodruff TK, Clayman ML, Waimey KE. (Eds). Oncofertility communication: sharing information and building relationships across disciplines. New York: Springer Publishing Company; 2013.
5. Woodruff TK, Gosiengfiao YC. (Eds). Pediatric and adolescent oncofertility: best practices and emerging technologies. Cham: Springer International Publishing; 2017.
6. Goetsch A, Kimelman D, Woodruff TK. (Co-authors). Fertility preservation and restoration for patients with complex medical conditions. New York: Springer Publishing Company; 2017.

Teresa K. Woodruff, PhD
Chicago, IL, USA

The academic medical center endorses a tripartite mission: providing excellent clinical care, advancing cutting-edge medical research, and educating the next generation of physicians and leaders. Though the three goals are typically described in a single breath, medical education has frequently taken a back seat to research and clinical programs. In recent years, however, medical education is increasingly valued as an independent mission – one that requires a team of professionals who are both committed and specifically trained to advance it.

Never is this need more evident than in oncofertility, where the multidisciplinary and interprofessional nature of the field requires an as-yet-undetermined approach to education and training. Under the guidance of Dr. Teresa Woodruff, the Oncofertility Consortium has assumed this challenge. An early needs assessment identified both the desire for and the dearth of a structured, formalized, easily accessible curriculum in fertility preservation among obstetrics and gynecology fellows, with subsequent roundtable discussions clarifying the goals and structure of such an endeavor. The outcome of these efforts has been the launch of a multimodal curriculum in fertility preservation that offers a variety of learning opportunities to address the heterogeneous learning styles and personal preferences of the targeted adult learners. Part one includes a free online certificate course, representing a collaboration between the American Society for Reproductive Medicine and the Oncofertility Consortium, that is comprised of 12 modules spanning the breath of fertility preservation and survivorship. This is supplemented by an in-person one-day course at the annual Oncofertility Consortium meeting, which includes both didactic- and case-based instruction, the latter of which occurs in multidisciplinary teams. This text represents the culmination of this educational effort and is directed specifically toward trainees and independent practitioners who are new to the field of oncofertility.

The book is structured with two types of chapters: topical and case-based. The topics are selected for their relevance to the clinical practice of oncofertility and are intended to appeal to an international audience from a variety of disciplines. The authors were selected for their expertise in the field as well as their ability to distill complex evidence into a structured and easily digestible format. The case-based chapters are intended as an adjunct to the topical chapters but with a different goal. Each begins with a real clinical scenario encountered by the authors; like clinical medicine itself, the cases can be complicated, messy, multifaceted, and rely upon knowledge and judgment from a wide array of topics. The intent of the cases is to illustrate the breath and complexity of this field through the eyes of experts, providing a springboard for thoughtful discussion and reflection on one's own experience. Questions for learner self-assessment are available at the end of each chapter. If you are new to the field, we recommend that you read the topical content for foundational knowledge and the associated cases for application and self-assessment. We anticipate that you will find it helpful to return to the cases for guidance when you encounter complex cases in your own practice. If you have been providing oncofertility care in your practice, we anticipate that reading the topical content and cases will provide a concise update of the recent progress made in the field.

As faculty in Reproductive Endocrinology and Infertility as well as medical educators, we embraced the challenge of distilling the field of fertility preservation down to what we hope is a practical but also thought-provoking text. We look forward to keeping this resource up to date and relevant for years to come.

Wendy S. Vitek, MD
Rochester, NY, USA

Divya Kelath Shah, MD, MME
Philadelphia, PA, USA

Teresa does it again! I was there when Dr. Woodruff first shared her idea for a NIH Roadmap grant proposal focusing on fertility preservation for the cancer patient, with leaders of the reproductive research community. The application was successful and the discipline of oncofertility was born and now espoused worldwide. One of the original aims of this novel transdisciplinary initiative was the education and training of providers who treat cancer patients, but do not have reproduction on their radar screens. Dr. Woodruff launched the now global Oncofertility Consortium, hosted annual Oncofertility Conferences, published numerous scientific studies and now, this inspired effort culminates in the publication of the *Textbook of Oncofertility Research and Practice*. For most, if not all cancer survivors, family building is synonymous with quality of life. It all starts with basic education and awareness of the facts and what opportunities and treatment options are possible. This book, co-edited by Drs. Vitek and Shah, two up and coming reproductive medicine specialists and educators, provides all the needed information; it should be a "must read" for any healthcare provider, primary care or specialist treating pediatric cancer patients or patients of reproductive age with cancer.

Christos Coutifaris, MD, PhD
Celso-Ramon Garcia Professor
Department of Obstetrics
and Gynecology
University of Pennsylvania
President, ASRM

Contents

III Care of the Opatient

IV Oncofertility in Clinical Practice

VII Case Studies: Egg Banking

VIII Case Studies: Embryo Banking

XII Case Studies: Pediatric Female Fertility Preservation

Contributors

Teresa Almeida-Santos, MD, PhD
Center for Fertility Preservation,
Reproductive Medicine Unit
Centro Hospitalar e Universitário de Coimbra
Coimbra, Portugal

Faculty of Medicine, University of Coimbra
Coimbra, Portugal

Center for Neuroscience and Cell Biology
University of Coimbra
Coimbra, Portugal

Human Reproduction Department
Coimbra University Hospital
Coimbra, Portugal
teresaalmeidasantos@chuc.min-saude.pt
anateresasantos.tas@gmail.com

Sarah Amari, MD
Gynecology, obstetrics and Reproductive
Medicine Department
Aziza Othmana University Hospital
Tunis, Tunisia

Faculté de Médecine de Tunis
Tunis, Tunisia
dr.sarahamari@gmail.com

Antoinette Anazodo, BSc, MSc, MBBS
Department of Paediatric Oncology
Kids Cancer Centre, Sydney Children's Hospital
Sydney, NSW, Australia

Department of Adult Oncology
Nelune Cancer Centre, Prince of Wales Hospital
Sydney, NSW, Australia

School of Women's and Children's Health
University of New South Wales
Sydney, NSW, Australia
antoinette.anazodo@health.nsw.gov.au

Leslie Coker Appiah, MD
Department of Obstetrics and Gynecology
The Ohio State University College
of Medicine, The Ohio State University
Wexner Medical Center
Columbus, OH, USA

The Ohio State University Comprehensive
Cancer Center - James Cancer Hospital
and Solove Research Institute
Columbus, OH, USA

Nationwide Children's Hospital
Columbus, OH, USA
leslie.appiah@osumc.edu

Nicoleta Arva, MD, PhD
Department of Pathology and Laboratory
Medicine
Ann & Robert H. Lurie Children's Hospital
of Chicago
Chicago, IL, USA
narva@luriechildrens.org

Linda Ballard, APRN, CPNP
Aflac Cancer and Blood Disorders Center
Children's Healthcare of Atlanta
Atlanta, GA, USA
linda.ballard@choa.org

Bruna Barros, BSc
Huntington Medicina Reprodutiva
São Paulo, SP, Brazil
bbarros@huntington.com.br

Amy R. Benjamin, MD
Department of Obstetrics and Gynecology
University of Rochester School of
Medicine & Dentistry
Rochester, NY, USA
amy_benjamin@urmc.rochester.edu

Janie Benoit, MD, FRCSC
Department of Obstetrics and Gynecology
Ste-Justine Hospital, University of Montreal
Montreal, QC, Canada
janie.benoit@umontreal.ca
janiebenoit@yahoo.ca

Christina E. Boots, MD
Division of Reproductive Endocrinology
and Infertility, Northwestern University
Feinberg School of Medicine
Chicago, IL, USA
christina.boots@northwestern.edu

Hammouda Boussen, MD
Medical Oncology Department
Mahmoud Materi Hospital
Ariana, Tunisia

Faculté de Médecine de Tunis
Tunis, Tunisia
boussen2011@yahoo.fr

Meghan Bowman-Curci, MPH
Alliance for Fertility Preservation (501 ©(3))
Moffitt Cancer Center, Health Outcomes
and Behavior Program
Lafayette, CA, USA

Health Outcomes and Behavior Program
Moffitt Cancer Center
Tampa, FL, USA
meghan@allianceforfertilitypreservation.org

Andrea Bradford, PhD
Section of Gastroenterology and Hepatology
Department of Medicine
Baylor College of Medicine
Houston, TX, USA
annie@ambradford.com

Marouen Braham, MD
Gynecology, Obstetrics and Reproductive
Medicine Department
Aziza Othmana University Hospital
Tunis, Tunisia

Faculté de Médecine de Tunis
Tunis, Tunisia
marouen.braham@fmt.utm.tn

Robert E. Brannigan, MD
Division of Male Reproductive Surgery and
Men's Health, Department of Urology
Northwestern University Feinberg
School of Medicine
Chicago, IL, USA
r-brannigan@northwestern.edu

Mats Brännström, MD, PhD
Department of Obstetrics and Gynecology
Sahlgrenska University Hospital
Gothenburg, Sweden

Department of Obstetrics and Gynecology
Sahlgrenska Academy, University of Gothenburg
Gothenburg and Stockholm IVF
Stockholm, Sweden
mats.brannstrom@obgyn.gu.se

Lesley Breech, MD
Cincinnati Children's Hospital Medical Center
Cancer and Blood Diseases Institute
Cincinnati, OH, USA
gynecology@cchmc.org

Margarida Brito, MD
Instituto Português de Oncologia
Francisco Gentil Lisboa
Lisbon, Portugal
mbgoncalves@ipolisboa.min-saude.pt

Karen Burns, MD, MS
Cincinnati Children's Hospital Medical Center,
Cancer and Blood Diseases Institute
Cincinnati, OH, USA
karen.burns@cchmc.org

Sukhkamal Campbell, MD
Department of Obstetrics and Gynecology
Division of Reproductive Endocrinology
and Infertility, Baylor College of Medicine
Houston, TX, USA
sukhkamal.campbell@bcm.edu

Lisa Campo-Engelstein, PhD
Alden March Bioethics Institute
and Department of Obstetrics and Gynecology
Albany Medical College
Albany, NY, USA
campoel@amc.edu

Glenn M. Cannon, MD
Department of Urology
University of Pittsburgh School of Medicine,
Children's Hospital of Pittsburgh of UPMC
Pittsburgh, PA, USA
cannongm@upmc.edu

Mollie Rose Canzona, MA, PhD
Assistant Professor
Department of Communication
Wake Forest University
Winston-Salem, NC, USA

Department of Social Sciences
and Health Policy
Wake Forest School of Medicine
Winston-Salem, NC, USA
canzonmr@wfu.edu

R. Cardoso, MD
Pediatric Endocrinology Unit
Hospital Pediátrico, Centro Hospitalar e Universitário de Coimbra
Coimbra, Portugal
ritacfc@hotmail.com

A. Carvalho, BS, MS
Center for Fertility Preservation
Reproductive Medicine Unit, Centro Hospitalar e Universitário de Coimbra
Coimbra, Portugal

Center for Neuroscience and Cell Biology
University of Coimbra
Coimbra, Portugal
alexandra.fernandes.carvalho@gmail.com

Rajeev Chaudhry, MD
Department of Urology
University of Pittsburgh School of Medicine
Children's Hospital of Pittsburgh of UPMC
Pittsburgh, PA, USA
rajeev.chaudhry@chp.edu

Mauricio Barbour Chehin, MD, PhD
Huntington Medicina Reprodutiva
São Paulo, SP, Brazil

Gynecology Department
Universidade de Santo Amaro – UNISA
São Paulo, SP, Brazil
mchehin@huntington.com.br

Diane Chen, PhD
Assistant Professor, Division of Adolescent Medicine, Departments of Child & Adolescent Psychiatry and Pediatrics
Ann & Robert H. Lurie Children's Hospital of Chicago, Northwestern University Feinberg School of Medicine
Chicago, IL, USA
dichen@luriechildrens.org

Brooke Cherven, MPH, RN, CPON
Aflac Cancer and Blood Disorders Center
Children's Healthcare of Atlanta
Atlanta, GA, USA
Brooke.Cherven@choa.org

Tulin D. Cil, MD, MEd, FRCSC
Department of Surgery, University of Toronto
Breast Surgical Oncology, Princess Margaret Cancer Centre and Women's College Hospital
Toronto, ON, Canada
tulin.cil@uhn.ca

Marla L. Clayman, PhD, MPH
Department of Health Care Research and Evaluation, American Institutes for Research
Chicago, IL, USA
mclayman@air.org
marla.clayman@gmail.com

Allison G. Close, MD
Division of Pediatric Hematology/Oncology
Department of Pediatrics, University of Pittsburgh School of Medicine, Children's Hospital of Pittsburgh of UPMC
Pittsburgh, PA, USA
closeag@upmc.edu

Pierre Comizzoli, DVM, PhD
Center for Species Survival, Smithsonian Conservation Biology Institute
Front Royal, VA, USA
comizzolip@si.edu

Kristine S. Corkum, MD
Division of Pediatric Surgery
Ann and Robert H. Lurie Children's Hospital of Chicago
Chicago, IL, USA

Department of Surgery
Northwestern University Feinberg School of Medicine
Chicago, IL, USA
Kristine.corkum@northwestern.edu

Susan L. Crockin, JD
Georgetown U. Law Center, O'Neill Center for National & Global Health Law
Washington, DC, USA
slcrockin@crockinlaw.com

Aarati Didwania, MD, MSCI
Division of General Internal Medicine
Northwestern University Feinberg School of Medicine
Chicago, IL, USA
Aarati.Didwania@nm.org

Jeffrey S. Dungan, MD
Division of Clinical Genetics, Department of Obstetrics and Gynecology, Feinberg School of Medicine, Northwestern University
Chicago, IL, USA
jdungan@nm.org

Adam S. DuVall, MD, MPH
Oregon Health & Science University
Knight Cancer Institute
Portland, OR, USA
duvalad@ohsu.edu

Maxwell E. Edmonds, BS, BA, MD/PhD Candidate
Northwestern Feinberg School of Medicine, OB/GYN
Chicago, IL, USA
maxwell.edmonds@northwestern.edu

Thomas Einzmann, MD
Department of Obstetrics and Gynecology, Medical Faculty
University of Cologne
Cologne, Germany

Jason Elliott, MD, MSc, BSc, FRCSC, FRCSC
Department of Obstetrics, Gynecology & Reproductive Sciences, Heartland Fertility Clinic, University of Manitoba
Winnipeg, MB, Canada
jelliott@hsc.mb.ca

Nanette Elster, JD, MPH
Stritch School of Medicine, Neiswanger Institute for Bioethics, Loyola University Chicago
Chicago, IL, USA
nanetteelster@sbcglobal.net

Yuting Fan, MD, PhD
Infertility Center of St. Louis
St. Louis, MO, USA
sysufanyut@gmail.com

Courtney Finlayson, MD
Assistant Professor, Division of Endocrinology
Department of Pediatrics
Ann & Robert H. Lurie Children's Hospital of Chicago, Northwestern University Feinberg School of Medicine
Chicago, IL, USA
cfinlayson@luriechildrens.org

Joyce Fioravanti, BSc
Huntington Medicina Reprodutiva
São Paulo, SP, Brazil
jfioravanti@huntington.com.br

Chelsea Webb Fox, MD
Division of Reproductive Endocrinology and Infertility and Moores Cancer Center, University of California San Diego
La Jolla, CA, USA
cwfox@ucsd.edu

Patrick J. Fox, MD
Department of Urology
University of Pittsburgh School of Medicine, Children's Hospital of Pittsburgh of UPMC
Pittsburgh, PA, USA
foxpj@upmc.edu

Erika D. Friehling, MD
Division of Pediatric Hematology/Oncology
Department of Pediatrics
University of Pittsburgh School of Medicine, Children's Hospital of Pittsburgh of UPMC
Pittsburgh, PA, USA
erika.friehling@chp.edu

Kathrin Gassei, PhD
Department of Obstetrics
Gynecology and Reproductive Sciences, Magee-Womens Research Institute, University of Pittsburgh School of Medicine
Pittsburgh, PA, USA
gasseik@upmc.edu

Allison L. Goetsch, MS
Department of Pediatrics, Northwestern University Feinberg School of Medicine
Chicago, IL, USA

Division of Genetics, Birth Defects and Metabolism, Ann and Robert H. Lurie Children's Hospital of Chicago
Chicago, IL, USA
agoetsch@luriechildrens.org

Kara N. Goldman, MD
Department of Obstetrics and Gynecology
New York University Langone Medical Center
New York, NY, USA

Northwestern University Feinberg School of Medicine
Chicago, IL, USA
kara.goldman@nyumc.org

Veronica Gomez-Lobo, MD
Department of Women and Infant Services, Department of Surgery
MedStar Washington Hospital Center, Children's National Medical Center
Washington, DC, USA
veronica.gomez-lobo@medstar.net

Jessica R. Gorman, PhD, MPH
Oregon State University, College of Public Health and Human Sciences
Corvallis, OR, USA
Jessica.Gorman@oregonstate.edu

Yasmin Gosiengfiao, MD
Hematology, Oncology & Stem Cell Transplantation, Ann & Robert H. Lurie Children's Hospital of Chicago
Chicago, IL, USA
ygosiengfiao@hotmail.com

Tamas Gotz, MD
Department of Obstetrics and Gynaecology
University of Calgary
Calgary, AB, Canada
tamas.gotz2@ahs.ca
gotz@ualberta.ca

Clarisa R. Gracia, MD, MSCE
Department of Obstetrics and Gynecology
University of Pennsylvania
Philadelphia, PA, USA
cgracia@obgyn.upenn.edu

Ashley Graul, MD
Department of Gynecologic Oncology
University of Pennsylvania
Philadelphia, PA, USA
Ashley.Graul@uphs.upenn.edu

Katherine B. Greenberg, MD
Department of Pediatrics and Obstetrics and Gynecology, University of Rochester School of Medicine & Dentistry
Rochester, NY, USA
Katherine_greenberg@urmc.rochester.edu

Ellen M. Greenblatt, BSc, MDCM
Department of Obstetrics and Gynecology
Division of Reproductive Endocrinology and Infertility, Sinai Health System
Toronto, ON, Canada
egreenblatt@mtsinai.on.ca

Daniel M. Green, MD
Department Epidemiology and Cancer Control
Division of Cancer Survivorship, Department of Oncology, St. Jude Children's Research Hospital
Memphis, TN, USA
Daniel.green@stjude.org

Joshua A. Halpern, MD, MS
Department of Urology
Weill Cornell Medicine
New York, NY, USA
gro.pyn@1302haj.com

Jinglan Han, BSc, MD, FRCSC
Department of Obstetrics and Gynecology
Mount Sinai Fertility
Toronto, ON, Canada
jinglan519@gmail.com

Brandon Hayes-Lattin, MD
Oregon Health & Science University, Knight Cancer Institute
Portland, OR, USA
hayeslat@ohsu.edu

Jason C. Hedges, MD, PhD
Department of Urology
Oregon Health & Science University
Portland, OR, USA
hedgesja@ohsu.edu

Olivia Higgins, MD
Department of Obstetrics and Gynecology
University of Rochester School of Medicine & Dentistry
Rochester, NY, USA
olivia_higgins@urmc.rochester.edu

Holly R. Hoefgen, MD
Pediatric & Adolescent Gynecology
Washington University School of Medicine/ St. Louis Children's Hospital
St. Louis, MO, USA
hollyhoefgen@wustl.edu

Michael H. Hsieh, MD, PhD
Department of Surgery, Division of Urology
Children's National Medical Center
Washington, DC, USA
mhsieh@cnmc.org

I-Shen Huang, MD
Department of Urology
School of Medicine,
National Yang-Ming University
Taipei, Taiwan

Department of Urology
Taipei Veterans General Hospital
Taipei, Taiwan
sabien.tw@gmail.com

Evgenia Isachenko, PhD
Department of Obstetrics and
Gynecology, Medical Faculty
University of Cologne
Cologne, Germany

Vladimir Isachenko, PhD
Department of Obstetrics and
Gynecology, Medical Faculty
University of Cologne
Cologne, Germany

Hideyuki Iwahata, MD, PhD
Department of Obstetrics and Gynecology
Northwestern University
Chicago, IL, USA

Department of Obstetrics and Gynecology
St. Marianna University School of Medicine
Kawasaki, Kanagawa, Japan
iwahata.hideyuki@northwestern.edu

Yuriko Iwahata, MD
Department of Obstetrics and Gynecology
Northwestern University
Chicago, IL, USA

Department of Obstetrics and Gynecology
St. Marianna University School of Medicine
Kawasaki, Kanagawa, Japan
smz.yuriko@gmail.com

Thomas M. Jaffe, MD
Department of Urology
University of Pittsburgh School of Medicine,
Magee-Womens Hospital, University of
Pittsburgh Medical Center
Pittsburgh, PA, USA
JAFFETM2@UPMC.EDU

Jason Jarin, MD
Department of Obstetrics and Gynecology
University of Texas Southwestern Medical Center
Dallas, TX, USA
Jason.Jarin@UTSouthwestern.edu

Jacqueline S. Jeruss, MD, PhD, Director
Michigan Medicine, University of Michigan,
Rogel Cancer Center
Ann Arbor, MI, USA

Breast Care Center
Ann Arbor, MI, USA
jjeruss@med.umich.edu

Emilie K. Johnson, MD, MPH
Assistant Professor, Division of Urology,
Department of Surgery
Ann & Robert H. Lurie Children's Hospital of
Chicago, Northwestern University Feinberg
School of Medicine
Chicago, IL, USA

Division of Urology
Ann & Robert H. Lurie Children's Hospital
of Chicago
Chicago, IL, USA
ekjohnson@luriechildrens.org

James A. Kashanian, MD
Weill Cornell Medicine – Urology,
Weill Cornell Medical Center
New York, NY, USA
jak9111@med.cornell.edu

Anne Katz, PhD, RN, FAAN, RN, PhD
CancerCare Manitoba, Prostate Center
Winnipeg, MB, Canada
akatz2@cancercare.mb.ca

Kazuhiro Kawamura, MD, PhD
Department of Obstetrics and Gynecology
St. Marianna University School of Medicine
Kawasaki, Kanagawa, Japan
kawamurak@marianna-u.ac.jp

Mohamed Khrouf, MD
Gynecology, Obstetrics and Reproductive
Medicine Department, Aziza Othmana
University Hospital
Tunis, Tunisia

Faculté de Médecine de Tunis
Tunis, Tunisia
moh.khrouf@gmail.com

Selim Khrouf, MD
Hopital Abderrahmane Mami
Tunis, Tunisia
selimkhrouf@gmail.com

Karen E. Kinahan, DNP, APN, FNP-BC
Division of Hematology and Oncology
Robert H. Lurie Comprehensive Cancer
Center or Northwestern University
Chicago, IL, USA
k-kinahan@northwestern.edu

Michael Kinnaman, MD
Pediatric Oncology, Memorial Sloan
Kettering Cancer Center
New York, NY, USA
kinnamam@mskcc.org

Caprice Knapp, PhD
Department of Health Policy and
Administration
Pennsylvania State University
University Park, PA, USA
cxk47@psu.edu

Timothy Lautz, MD
Division of Pediatric Surgery
Department of Surgery, Ann & Robert H. Lurie
Children's Hospital of Chicago
Chicago, IL, USA

Northwestern University Feinberg
School of Medicine
Chicago, IL, USA
tlautz@luriechildrens.org

William Ledger, MD, PhD
School of Women's and Children's Health
University of New South Wales
Sydney, NSW, Australia

Fertility and Research Centre,
Royal Hospital for Women, Randwick
Sydney, NSW, Australia
w.ledger@unsw.edu.au

Jessica A. Lentscher, MD
Obstetrics and Gynecology,
Madigan Army Medical Center
Tacoma, WA, USA
jessica.a.lentscher.mil@mail.mil

Joseph Letourneau, MD
Department of OB/GYN
University of Utah
Salt Lake City, UT, USA
Joseph.letourneau@hsc.utah.edu

Jennifer Levine, MD, MSW
Pediatric Hematology and Oncology,
Weill Cornell Medicine
New York, NY, USA
jlevine@med.cornell.edu

Barbara A. Lockart, DNP, APN
Solid Tumors and Fertility Preservation
Ann & Robert H. Lurie Children's Hospital
of Chicago
Chicago, IL, USA
BLockart@luriechildrens.org

André Lopes, MD
Instituto Brasileiro de Controle do Câncer,
São Paulo, SP, Brazil

Hospital Paulistano,
São Paulo, SP, Brazil
andrelopes1002@hotmail.com

Sebastian Ludwig, MD
Department of Obstetrics and
Gynecology, Medical Faculty
University of Cologne
Cologne, Germany

Peter Mallmann, MD
Department of Obstetrics and
Gynecology, Medical Faculty
University of Cologne
Cologne, Germany

Sharrón Manuel, MD, PhD
Prentice Women's Hospital
Department of Obstetrics and Gynecology,
Feinberg School of Medicine,
Northwestern University
Chicago, IL, USA
sharronmanuel2019@u.northwestern.edu

Jeffrey H. Margolis, MD
Division of Clinical Hematology and Medical Oncology, Rose Cancer Treatment Center, William Beaumont Hospital
Royal Oak, MI, USA
Jeffmargolis@me.com

Jamie A. M. Massie, MD
Obstetrics and Gynecology, Madigan Army Medical Center
Tacoma, WA, USA
jamie.a.massie2.mil@mail.mil

Eileen McMahon, RN(EC), MN, PNC(C)
Department of Obstetrics and Gynaecology/Mount Sinai Fertility, Mount Sinai Hospital
Toronto, ON, Canada
Eileen.mcmahon@sinaihealthsystem.ca

Lillian R. Meacham, MD
Department of Pediatrics, Emory University School of Medicine, Aflac Cancer Center/Children's Healthcare of Atlanta
Atlanta, GA, USA
Lillian.meacham@emory.edu

Michael S. Mersol-Barg, MD
Michigan Reproductive Medicine
Bloomfield Hills, MI, USA
mikemb@mireproductivemedicine.com

David M. Mintzer, MD
Abramson Cancer Center at Pennsylvania Hospital
Philadelphia, PA, USA
david.mintzer@uphs.upenn.edu

Fehmi Msaddak, MD
Hematology Department, Military Hospital of Tunis, Faculté de Médecine de Tunis
Tunis, Tunisia
fehmimsadek@gmail.com

Lívia Munhoz, MD
Huntington Medicina Reprodutiva
São Paulo, SP, Brazil
lmunhoz@huntington.com.br

Devin Murphy, MSW, OMSIII
Edward Via College of Osteopathic Medicine
Auburn, AL, USA
dmurphy@auburn.vcom.edu

Seema Niphadkar, DO
Drexel University College of Medicine
Division of Hematology/Oncology
Philadelphia, PA, USA

Abington Hospital – Jefferson Health
Abington, PA, USA
seema721@gmail.com

Kyle E. Orwig, PhD
Department of Obstetrics Gynecology and Reproductive Sciences, Magee-Womens Research Institute, University of Pittsburgh School of Medicine
Pittsburgh, PA, USA
orwigke@upmc.edu

Bansari G. Patel, MD
Obstetrics and Gynecology
Reproductive Medicine
Wake Forest Baptist Health
Winston-Salem, NC, USA
bgpatel@wakehealth.edu

Mary Ellen Pavone, MD, MSCI
OB/GYN, Division of Reproductive Endocrinology and Infertility
Northwestern Memorial Hospital
Chicago, IL, USA
m-pavone@northwestern.edu
Maryellen.pavone@nm.org

Jana Pittman, MSc
School of Medicine, Western Sydney University
Sydney, NSW, Australia
jana@janapittman.com

Gwendolyn P. Quinn, PhD, MS, BS
Department of Obstetrics and Gynecology
New York University
New York, NY, USA
gwendolyn.quinn@nyumc.org

Gohar Rahimi, MD
Department of Obstetrics and Gynecology, Medical Faculty
University of Cologne
Cologne, Germany

Joyce D. Reinecke, AB, JD
Alliance for Fertility Preservation (501 ©(3))
Lafayette, CA, USA
joyce@allianceforfertilitypreservation.org
jdreinecke@live.org

Chad Ritenour, MD
Division of Men's Health/Infertility
and General Urology, Department of Urology
Emory University
Atlanta, GA, USA
criteno@emory.edu

Erin Rowell, MD
Division of Pediatric Surgery, Ann and Robert
H. Lurie Children's Hospital of Chicago
Chicago, IL, USA

Department of Surgery, Northwestern
University Feinberg School of Medicine
Chicago, IL, USA
erowell@luriechildrens.org

Mahmoud Salama, MD, PhD
Department of Obstetrics and
Gynecology, Medical Faculty
University of Cologne
Cologne, Germany

Department of Obstetrics and Gynecology
Feinberg School of Medicine,
Northwestern University
Chicago, IL, USA
Mahmoud.salama@uk-koeln.de

John M. Salsman, PhD
Associate Professor, Director of Clinical Research
in Adolescent and Young Adult Oncology
Department of Social Sciences and Health Policy
Wake Forest School of Medicine
Winston-Salem, NC, USA
jsalsman@wakehealth.edu

Amani Sampson, BA
Department of Obstetrics and Gynecology
New York University School of Medicine
New York, NY, USA
amani.sampson@nyumc.org

Matthew B. Schabath, PhD
H. Lee Moffitt Cancer Center & Research
Institute, Cancer Epidemiology,
University of South Florida
Tampa, FL, USA
matthew.schabath@moffitt.org

Dana Marie Scott, MD
Michigan Medicine, University of Michigan,
Rogel Cancer Center
Ann Arbor, MI, USA
danamarie.scott@gmail.com

Ivana Sehovic-Neff, MPH
Department of Research Integrity &
Compliance, University of South Florida
Tampa, FL, USA
isehovic@usf.edu

Divya Kelath Shah, MD, MME
Reproductive Endocrinology and Infertility,
Department of Obstetrics and Gynecology,
University of Pennsylvania
Philadelphia, PA, USA
divya.shah@uphs.upenn.edu

Nikita M. Shah, MD
Michigan Medicine, University of Michigan,
Rogel Cancer Center
Ann Arbor, MI, USA
nikitamshah@gmail.com

Jacquelyn Shaw, MD
Department of Obstetrics and Gynecology
Northwestern University, New York University
Langone Medical Center
New York, NY, USA
jacquelyn.shaw@nyumc.org

Kathleen Shea, MS, CPNP
Pediatric Hematology/Oncology/Stem Cell
Transplantation
Columbia University Medical Center
New York, NY, USA
kas10@cumc.columbia.edu

Ksenya Shliakhsitsava, MD
Division of Pediatric Hematology and Oncology
Rady Children's Hospital-San Diego
San Diego, CA, USA
kshliakhtsitsava@ucsd.edu

Lee P. Shulman
Division of Clinical Genetics,
Department of Obstetrics and Gynecology
Feinberg School of Medicine,
Northwestern University
Chicago, IL, USA
lee.shulman@nm.org

Sherman Silber, MD
Infertility Center of St. Louis
St. Louis, MO, USA
silber@infertile.com

Elizabeth Sniderman, MSN
Division of Hematology, Oncology and Stem Cell Transplant, Department of Pediatrics
Ann & Robert H. Lurie Children's Hospital of Chicago
Chicago, IL, USA
liz.sniderman@stjude.org

Nucharin Songsasen, DVM, PhD
Center for Species Survival, Smithsonian Conservation Biology Institute
Front Royal, VA, USA
songsasenn@si.edu

Ana Paula Sousa, PhD
Center for Fertility Preservation
Reproductive Medicine Unit
Centro Hospitalar e Universitário de Coimbra
Coimbra, Portugal

Center for Neuroscience and Cell Biology
University of Coimbra
Coimbra, Portugal
anapauladesousa.apms@gmail.com

H. Irene Su, MD, MSCE
Division of Reproductive Endocrinology and Infertility and Moores Cancer Center
University of California San Diego
La Jolla, CA, USA
hisu@ucsd.edu

Nao Suzuki, MD, PhD
Department of Obstetrics and Gynecology
St. Marianna University School of Medicine
Kawasaki, Kanagawa, Japan
nao@marianna-u.ac.jp

Seido Takae, MD, PhD
Department of Obstetrics and Gynecology
St. Marianna University School of Medicine
Kawasaki, Kanagawa, Japan
s2takae@marianna-u.ac.jp

Christina Tamargo, BA
University of Miami, Miller School of Medicine
Miami, FL, USA
christina.tamargo@med.miami.edu

Alexis Thompson, MD, MPH
Department of Hematology Oncology Transplantation Ann and Robert H. Lurie Children's Hospital of Chicago
Chicago, IL, USA
a-thompson@northwestern.edu

Susan Thomas Vadaparampil, PhD, MHSE, MPH, BS
Department of Health Outcomes and Behavior Program
Moffitt Cancer Center
Tampa, FL, USA

Department of Oncologic Sciences
Moffitt Cancer Center and Research Institute, Health Outcomes & Behavior Program, University of South Florida, Morsani College of Medicine
Tampa, FL, USA

H. Lee Moffitt Cancer Center & Research Institute, University of South Florida
Tampa, FL, USA
susan.vadaparampil@moffitt.org

Hanna Valli-Pulaski, PhD
Department of Obstetrics, Gynecology and Reproductive Sciences, Magee-Womens Research Institute, University of Pittsburgh School of Medicine
Pittsburgh, PA, USA
vallih2@upmc.edu

Wendy S. Vitek, MD
Department of Pediatrics and Obstetrics and Gynecology
University of Rochester School of Medicine & Dentistry
Rochester, NY, USA
wendy_vitek@urmc.rochester.edu

Andrew F. Wagner, MD
Division of Clinical Genetics, Department of Obstetrics and Gynecology, Feinberg School of Medicine, Northwestern University
Chicago, IL, USA
andrew.wagner@nm.org

Marissa Steinberg Weiss, MD
Department of Obstetrics & Gynecology
University of Pennsylvania
Philadelphia, PA, USA
marissa.weiss@uphs.upenn.edu

Lynn M. Westphal, MD
Obstetrics and Gynecology,
Stanford University School of Medicine
Stanford, CA, USA
lynnw@stanford.edu

Terri L. Woodard, MD
Department of Gynecologic Oncology
and Reproductive Medicine
The University of Texas MD Anderson
Cancer Center
Houston, TX, USA

Division of Reproductive Endocrinology and
Infertility, Baylor College of Medicine
Houston, TX, USA
tlwoodard@mdanderson.org

Carley Zeal, MD, MPH
Department of Obstetrics and Gynecology
Washington University in
St. Louis – Barnes Jewish Hospital
St. Louis, MO, USA
cjzeal@wustl.edu

Fethi Zhioua, MD
Gynecology, Obstetrics and Reproductive
Medicine Department, Aziza Othmana
University Hospital
Tunis, Tunisia

Faculté de Médecine de Tunis
Tunis, Tunisia
zhiouafethi@gmail.com

Rhonda Zwingerman,
MD, MSc, FRCSC, FRCSC
Department of Obstetrics and Gynaecology
University of Toronto
Toronto, ON, Canada
Rhonda.Zwingerman@sinaihealthsystem.ca

Abbreviations

AAP	American Academy of Pediatrics
ACOG	American College of Obstetricians and Gynecologists
AMH	Anti-Müllerian hormone
ART	Assisted reproductive technology
ASCO	American Society of Clinical Oncology
AYA	Adolescent and young adult
BPA	Bisphenol A
CDC	Centers for Disease Control and Prevention
DES	Diethylstilbestrol
DHEA	Dehydroepiandrosterone
DSDs	Disorders of sexual development
DSM	*Diagnostic and Statistical Manual of Mental Disorders*
ESHRE	European Society of Human Reproduction and Embryology
FP	Fertility preservation
FSH	Follicle-stimulating hormone
GD	Gender dysphoria
GnRH	Gonadotropin-releasing hormone
HPG	Hypothalamic-pituitary-gonadal
IOM	Institute of Medicine
LGBTQ	Lesbian, gay, bisexual, transsexual/transgender, queer/questioning
LH	Luteinizing hormone
NCCN	National Comprehensive Cancer Network
PCBs	Polychlorinated biphenyls
PCOS	Polycystic ovarian syndrome
PESA	Percutaneous sperm aspiration
QoL	Quality of life
TESA	Testicular sperm aspiration
TESE	Testicular sperm extraction
WHO	World Health Organization
WPATH	World Professional Association for Transgender Health

Fertility Implications in Oncologic and Non-oncologic Settings

Contents

Fertility Risk with Cancer Therapy

Leslie Coker Appiah and Daniel M. Green

T. K. Woodruff et al. (eds.), *Textbook of Oncofertility Research and Practice*,
https://doi.org/10.1007/978-3-030-02868-8_1

1.1 Introduction

The incidence of cancer has slowly stabilized with 1.7 million new cases estimated in 2018 [1]. Of those, 10,270 are estimated to occur in the pediatric population ages 0–14 with 70,000 in the adolescent and young adult (AYA) population ages 15–39. Advances in cancer treatments have significantly improved the outcome for pediatric cancers, with 80% of children now surviving 5 years or more. Unfortunately, 5-year survival rates for AYAs remain lower at 70%. Reasons include differences in tumor biology, fewer available clinical trials, lack of comprehensive insurance coverage, and barriers to access such as location, employment, and educational time constraints [2, 3]. With improvements in treatment, there are estimated to be 500,000 childhood cancer survivors by 2020, and 1 in 25 will be of reproductive age. Compromised fertility occurs in 12% and 66% of at-risk female and male survivors of childhood cancer [4]. Manifestations of gonadal injury include disordered puberty from hormonal deficiency, decreased reproductive and sexual function, psychosocial effects, and menopause-related health problems in female survivors such as genitourinary syndrome of menopause and cardiac, skeletal, and cognitive dysfunction [5, 6]. Standard options for fertility preservation include sperm, oocyte, and embryo banking. Investigational options include testicular, ovarian, and immature oocyte cryopreservation [7, 8]. Most options are invasive and costly, and standard options in females require an average of 10–12 days for stimulation and retrieval prior to cancer treatment. Estimating risk prior to therapy allows determination and implementation of the appropriate fertility-preserving therapies. Minimizing risk prior to therapy may mitigate the need for invasive and costly fertility-preserving therapies while preserving hormonal function after cancer treatment.

1.2 Estimating Risk

Assessment of fertility risk should be undertaken prior to the initiation of therapy to optimize fertility preservation outcomes. Surgical procedures, radiation therapy, and chemotherapy can each produce impaired fertility (■ Table 1.1). Gametogenesis and hormone production are differentially sensitive to treatment exposures in males, whereas these two functions are tightly linked in females. The risk factors for impaired fertility differ for males and females.

1.2.1 Males

Testicular surgery can affect the production of sperm and hormones or interfere with the transport of sperm [9]. Injury of the gonadotropin-releasing hormone area of the hypothalamus and/or the gonadotropin-producing anterior pituitary can also result in impaired spermatogenesis and sex steroid production [10]. Impaired transport may occur from damage to autonomic nervous system control of urethral sphincters and/or vasodilation secondary to retroperitoneal lymph node dissection or prostatectomy.

Testicular tissue is extremely radiosensitive with only small amounts of direct radiation required to cause significant impairment in spermatogenesis and hormone production [11] (■ Fig. 1.1). Direct testicular radiation has a greater effect on spermatogenesis than hormone production with immature stem cells and spermatogonia being most sensitive. Testicular irradiation markedly reduces the number of spermatocytes 2–3 weeks post-therapy with declines in ejaculated sperm counts by approximately 10 weeks. Azoospermia is typically present at 18 weeks post-therapy.

The effect of chemotherapy on spermatogenesis is dependent on the type of chemotherapeutic agent. Normal sperm count typically recovers by 12 weeks post-therapy in patients treated with non-alkylators. However, spermatogenesis is very sensitive to damage by alkylating agents including nitrogen mustard, procarbazine, cyclophosphamide, ifosfamide, chlorambucil, and busulfan, with long-lasting effects on fertility [12]. The risk of azoospermia is approximately 10% when the cyclophosphamide equivalent dose is less than 4 g/m^2, whereas approximately one-half of individuals who receive more than this dose will not retain a normal sperm concentration [13]. The duration of sperm integrity after an initial course of chemotherapy is currently unknown; therefore, fertility preservation in males should be performed prior to initiation of cancer treatments.

Table 1.1 Effects of cancer therapy on male fertility

Treatment		Effect on spermatogenesis and transport	Risk of infertility
Surgery			
	Removal of both testes	Impaired production	100%
	Removal of one testis		Low
	Damage to hypothalamic/pituitary gonadotropin producing area		Low – spermatogenesis may be stimulated with exogenous gonadotropin
	Retroperitoneal lymph node dissection	Impaired transport	Variable – retrograde ejaculation; sperm production not impaired
Radiation therapy			
	Irradiation of testes	Impaired production	Fertility very unlikely if testes dose >7.5 Gy
	Irradiation of hypothalamic/pituitary gonadotropin producing area		Dose-response relationship unclear; dose <30 Gy do not appear to produce damage
Chemotherapy	Alkylating agents	Impaired production	Cyclophosphamide equivalent dose (CED): <4 g/m^2 – risk of azoospermia <15 % >4 g/m^2 – risk of oligo- or azoospermia >50%

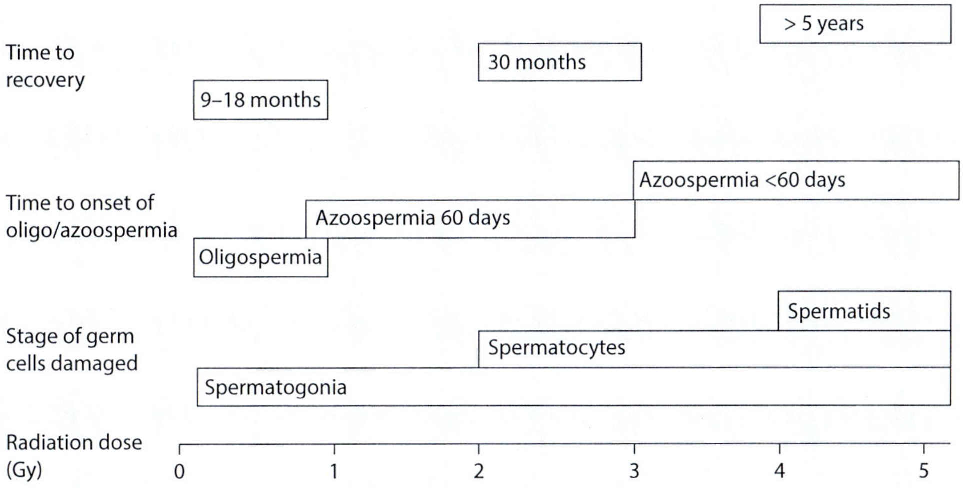

Fig. 1.1 Spermatogenesis following single-dose radiation. (Howell and Shalet [12])

1.2.2 Females

Malignancies of the ovaries require surgical interventions that impair fertility and hormone production by decreasing the number of follicles present and inciting scarring. Fertility-sparing surgery is the standard of care for the management of early-stage, low-grade tumors in women who have not completed childbearing. Fertility-sparing options include cystectomy for tumors of low malignant potential (borderline tumors) and unilateral oophorectomy for malignancies [14–16]. In the instance of cystectomy, the residual ovarian tissue is typically able to compensate if no chemotherapy or radiation is given. The impact of unilateral oophorectomy on the remaining ovarian reserve remains controversial with some authors reporting a diminished reproductive window and others observing a compensatory response from the remaining ovary [17, 18]. Pelvic surgery for nongynecologic malignancies can also have a deleterious effect on ovarian function by cytokine production and the formation of pelvic adhesions with subsequent impaired folliculogenesis, ovulation, and tubal transport [19, 20].

Alkylating agents remain highly gonadotoxic in a dose-dependent fashion. Chemotherapeutic agents affect the mature follicle through DNA damage with subsequent apoptosis and temporary amenorrhea [21]. If the primordial follicle pool is unaffected, folliculogenesis and menses resume after completion of cancer treatment. However, resumption of menses does not provide evidence that ovulatory cycles have resumed or predict long-term ovarian function. Alkylating agents such as cyclophosphamide, busulfan, and nitrogen mustard are non-cell cycle specific and thus have a deleterious effect on the primordial follicles, increasing the likelihood of acute ovarian failure and diminished ovarian reserve pool after treatment [22]. The effect of heavy metals such as cisplatin and carboplatin on ovarian reserve remains an area of debate. Historically, heavy metals have been considered highly gonadotoxic [23]. Recent studies suggest that cisplatin and carboplatin may be categorized as low risk of acute ovarian failure [24]. The effect on long-term ovarian reserve remains under investigation.

Radiation injury to the gonads is dose-dependent with younger age conferring protection. Greater than 2 Gy of ovarian irradiation results in a loss of 50% of ovarian follicles, described as the LD50 [25]. Doses greater than or equal to 15 Gy and 6 Gy in adult and prepubertal patients, respectively, result in infertility. Cortical fibrosis and irreversible damage to the uterus occur at abdominopelvic doses greater than 30 Gy [26]. Uterine injury caused by lower doses of radiation may be overcome with high-dose hormonal therapy. Radiation exposure to the hypothalamus and pituitary gland greater than 30 Gy affects the production of gonadotropins with decreased folliculogenesis, decreased production of estrogen, and infertility [27].

Risk stratification from chemotherapy is based on the cumulative dose of alkylating agents received due to the high risk of gonadotoxicity. The alkylating agent dose (AAD) and the cyclophosphamide equivalent dose (CED) risk-stratification systems allow the calculation of risk (Fig. 1.2 and Tables 1.2 and 1.3). Using the AAD, a score of 1, 2, or 3 is given for the cumulative dose of alkylating agent that falls within the first, second, or third cumulative dose tertile, respectively. The scores for individual agents are summed. Patients with a score of 3 or 4 are at an increased risk of infertility with a relative risk of pregnancy of 0.72 and 0.65, respectively [51]. The CED is calculated by summing the cyclophosphamide equivalents for cyclophosphamide, ifosfamide, procarbazine, chlorambucil, BCNU, CCNU, melphalan, thioTEPA, nitrogen mustard, and busulfan [52]. A CED >7.5 g/m^2 is associated with a relative risk of premature menopause of 4.19 (95% CI 2.18–8.08). The AAD is based on drug dose distribution from a specific cohort of patients from which the drug dose was derived, whereas the CED is derived from actual drug

Fig. 1.2 Cyclophosphamide equivalent dose calculation

CED (mg/m^2) = 1.0 (cumulative cyclophosphamide dose (mg/m^2)) + 0.244 (cumulative ifosfamide dose (mg/m^2)) + 0.857 (cumulative procarbazine dose (mg/m^2)) + 14.286 (cumulative chlorambucil dose (mg/m^2)) + 15.0 (cumulative BCNU dose (mg/m^2)) + 16.0 (cumulative CCNU dose (mg/m^2)) + 40 (cumulative melphalan dose (mg/m^2)) + 50 (cumulative Thio-TEPA dose (mg/m^2)) + 100 (cumulative nitrogen mustard dose (mg/m^2)) + 8.823 (cumulative busulfan dose (mg/m^2)).

Table 1.2 Estimating risk: alkylating agent dose (AAD) [27]

Tertile distribution of alkylating agents in cumulative dose			
	Cumulative dose by tertile		
Alkylating agent	First	Second	Third
BCNU, mg/m^2	1–300	301–529	530–3370
Busulfan, mg/m^2	1–317	318–509	510–6845
CCNU, mg/m^2	1–361	362–610	611–3139
Chlorambucil, mg/m^2	1–165	166–634	635–3349
Parenteral cyclophosphamide, mg/m^2	1–3704	3705–9200	9201–58,648
Oral cyclophosphamide, mg/m^2	1–1722	4723–10,636	10,637–143,802
Ifosfamide, mg/m^2	1–16,771	16,772–55,758	55,759–192,391
Melphalan, mg/m^2	1–39	40–137	138–574
Nitrogen mustard, mg/m^2	1–44	45–64	65–336
Procarbazine, mg/m^2	1–4200	4201–7000	7001–58,680
Intrathecal thiotepa, mg	1–80	81–320	321–914
Thiotepa, mg/m^2	1–77	78–220	221–3749

BCNU carmustine, *CCNU* lomustine
First tertile score is 1; second is 2; and third is 3

doses and therefore has applicability independent of the study population. Risk stratification by the alkylating agent is performed prior to therapy to guide implementation of fertility preservation therapies based on risk. However, treatment regimens may change during the course of therapy, and in such instances, cumulative dose and risk assessment may be recalculated post-therapy.

1.3 Minimizing Risk

As cancer survival rates improve and awareness of the effects of treatments on long-term health and fertility become widespread, consensus develops regarding the need for precision medicine and targeted therapies. Research efforts in this area include the development of cancer treatments that destroy cancer cells while also protecting the ovaries. Conversely, several agents used to manage complications of cancer treatments are also under investigation. Well-studied agents that minimize risk include apoptosis inhibitors imatinib, AS101, S1P, G-CSF, bone marrow mesenchymal stem cells, and tamoxifen. GnRHa, tamoxifen, and G-CSF are the only agents studied in humans. Other therapies have shown promise in rodent and primate studies. However, concerns remain about interference with chemotherapeutic efficacy and perpetuation of damaged DNA cell lines with resultant fetal loss and/or malformation. Further studies are required to determine efficacy and safety in humans.

1.3.1 Gonadotropin-Releasing Hormone Agonist

Gonadotropin-releasing hormone agonist (GnRHa) therapy remains the most studied fertoprotective agent. Until recently, conflicting results restricted its use in oncology to menstrual suppression and adjuvant endocrine therapy to improve long-term survival in patients with breast cancer [53–55]. Reasons include the use of various GnRHa therapies between studies and a preponderance of retrospective and prospective studies with short follow-up periods

Table 1.3 Potential fertoprotective agents during cancer treatments

Potential fertoprotective agents during cancer treatments	Mechanism of action on ovary	Studies demonstrating protective effect	Studies demonstrating no effect	Interactions with cytotoxic treatments
GnRH analog	Direct effect on ovary is unclear; suppresses hypothalamic-pituitary-ovarian axis, possible ovarian quiescence	Rodent: Meirow et al. [28], Li et al. [29] Primate: Ataya et al. [30] Human: Badawy et al. [31], Sverrisdottir et al. [48], Del Mastro et al. [32], and Demeestere et al. [33]	Human: Gerber et al. [34], Munster et al. [35], Elgindy et al. [36], and Demeestere et al. [33]	No interference with treatment drugs
Imatinib	Inhibit c-Abl kinase apoptosis pathway	Rodent: Gonfolini et al. (2009) Rodent: Kerr et al. [37]	May interfere with apoptotic action of chemotherapy drugs	
Bone marrow mesenchymal stem cells	Tissue differentiation, angiogenesis, anti-apoptosis	Rodent: Kilic et al. [38], Fu et al. [39], Rabbit: Abd-Allah et al. [40]	NTD	May cause chemotherapy drug resistance with cisplatin
S1P	Inhibit sphingomyelin apoptosis pathway	Rodent: Morita et al. [41], Jurisicova et al. [42], Hancke et al. [43], Kaya et al. [44] Primate: Zelinski et al. [45] Human xenograft: Zelinski et al. [45]	Rodent: Kaya et al. [44]	May interfere with apoptotic action of chemotherapy drugs
Potential fertoprotective agents during cancer treatments Protective agent	Mechanism of action on ovary	Studies demonstrating protective effect	Studies demonstrating no effect	Interactions with cytotoxic treatments
Tamoxifen	Anti-apoptotic activity; antioxidant activity via IGF-1 axis; possible H-P-O axis suppression	Rodent: Ting et al. [46], Mahran et al. [47]	Human: Sverrisdottir et al. [48]	Adjuvant therapy; no interference with treatment drugs
AS101	Inhibits P13K/PTEN Akt follicle activation pathway; anti-apoptosis	Rodent: Kalich-Philosoph et al. [49]	NTD	No interference w/treatment drugs May have additive/synergistic interaction w/treatment drugs
Growth-colony stimulating factor (G-CSF)	Unclear: possibly angiogenesis; anti-apoptosis	Rodent: Skaznik-Wikiel et al. [50]	NTD	No interference with treatment drugs

and less useful markers of fecundity such as return of menstrual function and FSH and estradiol levels [56–58]. Recent studies acknowledge that menses, FSH, and estradiol reflect current ovarian function but do not predict future function or likelihood of fertility and live birth. Endpoints in current literature more accurately reflect ovarian function and include pregnancy and longer follow-up periods up to 3 years [47, 59, 60]. Meta-analysis of 29 randomized controlled trials identified 10 studies that met inclusion criteria and illustrated a protective effect of GnRHa therapy on ovarian function in patients with Hodgkin lymphoma and breast cancer OR 1.83 (1.34–2.49) [47]. Updated ASCO guidelines reflect the current knowledge and state "when proven fertility preservation methods such as oocyte, embryo, or ovarian tissue cryopreservation are not feasible, and in the setting of young women with breast cancer, GnRHa may be offered to individuals in the hope of reducing the likelihood of chemotherapy-induced ovarian insufficiency" [8].

1.3.2 Anti-Mullerian Hormone

Anti-Mullerian hormone (AMH) has received significant attention over the last several years as an indirect marker of ovarian reserve. Recently investigators have assessed its role as an ovarian protective agent during gonadotoxic therapy as well as a contraceptive agent in mice [61, 62]. One of the mechanisms of chemotherapy-induced ovarian failure is accelerated recruitment of primordial follicles as a result of decreased AMH production after chemotherapy-induced follicular death of growing follicles. Kano et al. hypothesize that administration of AMH will inhibit recruitment and preserve the follicular pool. Indeed, they illustrate complete arrest of folliculogenesis, amenorrhea, and contraception after administration of superphysiological parenteral doses of AMH using either an adeno-associated virus serotype 9 (AAV9) gene therapy vector or recombinant protein. Recovery of function was evidenced with transplantation of the ovarian tissue into another mouse or with discontinuation of therapy. Further studies are needed to replicate these findings and identify dose, route of administration, and utility in the human tissue.

1.3.3 Imatinib

Imatinib is a competitive tyrosine kinase inhibitor used for cancer treatment. Chemotherapy induces c-Abl-mediated upregulation of the tumor suppressor protein p63 (a homolog of p53) with resultant apoptosis. Rodent studies show that, when given prior to cisplatin, imatinib is a potent inhibitor of c-Abl-mediated upregulation and blocks apoptosis of cells. Mice treated with imatinib prior to cisplatin show reduced primordial follicular loss and normal progeny [63, 64]. However, other studies show no protection with imatinib in two independent mouse strains [37]. Additionally, investigators show that genetic effects on the oocyte result in early embryonic mortality and marked aneuploidy. There remain concerns regarding whether imatinib and cisplatin-treated oocytes that do not undergo apoptosis harbor DNA damage that may result in miscarriage or birth defects [65, 66]. The question also remains whether imatinib reduces the efficacy of cisplatin on the primary tumor target while upregulating the effects of cisplatin in other cell types [67]. To date, there are no studies evaluating the ovarian protective effect of imatinib in human subjects.

1.3.4 Bone Marrow-Derived Mesenchymal Stem Cells

Bone marrow-derived mesenchymal stem cells (MSC) have been used to treat various diseases because of their self-renewal capacity and multipotency [68, 69]. For example, stems cells have been successful in tissue repair after spinal, renal, and myocardial injury [70, 71]. The potential benefit of stem cell therapy after acute tissue damage appears to be related to tissue integration and differentiation to replace damaged cells, angiogenesis, and anti-apoptosis. Adult MSC have not been equivocally proven to differentiate into follicles. However, several rodent studies have been conducted to assess the role of MSC as an ovarian protection agent during chemotherapy. Kilic et al. showed preservation of primordial and primary follicles in in vivo rat MSC studies, suggesting that MSC may preferentially migrate to the injured follicular cells and repair the ovarian tissue by decreased programmed cell death [38]. Similarly, Fu et al. demonstrated an increase in follicle number, as well as a normalization of FSH and estradiol levels, after several weeks in rodents treated with MSC after cyclophosphamide therapy [39]. They also illustrated in vitro production of the angiogenic and anti-apoptotic cytokines vascular endothelial growth factor (VEGF), insulin-like growth factor (IGF-1), and hepatocyte growth factor (HGF) from MSC. Effects of therapy on progeny were not assessed in either study. Abd-Allah et al. further demonstrated MSC protection of ovarian follicles in rabbit studies and were able to show in vivo cytokine production [40]. Despite the potential promise of MSC as an ovarian protection agent, studies of MSC injected intravenously in rodent models have shown MSC-mediated resistance to chemotherapeutics, specifically cisplatin [72]. More importantly, there remain no studies of the efficacy of MSC as an ovarian protective agent in human tissue.

1.3.5 Sphingosine-1-Phosphate (S1P)

Sphingosine-1-phosphate is a naturally occurring sphingolipid, which exerts anti-apoptotic effects by inhibiting ceramide-induced cell death [73]. The sphingomyelin pathway is one of several pathways that trigger apoptosis of ovarian follicles. Sphingomyelin is degraded to ceramide, a pro-apoptotic agent. Ceramide is subsequently degraded to sphingosine and then sphingosine-1-phosphate (S1P) through hydrolysis. Sphingosine-1-phosphate regulates proliferative cellular processes including cell growth and cell differentiation and inhibits apoptosis [43]. Early in vivo mouse studies of ovarian tissue xenografts treated with S1P show increased vascular density and angiogenesis with reduced follicular apoptosis. Several investigators have since provided evidence to illustrate that S1P improves the success of human ovarian tissue transplantation by enhancing and accelerating angiogenesis and stromal proliferation [74] and protects human primordial follicles from chemotherapy-induced apoptosis [75]. Recent in vitro studies in human cortical samples suggest that S1P also promotes follicle survival during culture of the human cortical tissue, which may be of benefit when processing ovarian tissue samples for cryopreservation [76, 77]. Studies of offspring in mice and primates treated with S1P prior to radiation have shown no propagation of DNA damage and no abnormalities in the offspring [78]. Limitations have been that S1P is administered systemically via tissue injection, thus limiting its clinical usefulness. There are also no clinical trials involving in vivo S1P as a therapeutic option.

1.3.6 Tamoxifen

Tamoxifen, a selective estrogen receptor modulator (SERM) with agonist–antagonist properties, is used as adjuvant treatment of hormone-sensitive breast cancer. Rodent studies have shown ovarian protection with tamoxifen administered prior to cyclophosphamide [46]. Tamoxifen has also been shown to be protective when given prior to radiation treatment in rats with a reduction in loss of primordial follicles and increase in AMH [79]. Human studies evaluating the effects of tamoxifen as an ovarian protective agent are limited and conflicting due to study design and use of different endpoints [80]. Furthermore, tamoxifen given concurrently with chemotherapy has been shown to increase the risk of thrombotic events and is not recommended [81]. The postulated mechanism of action remains unclear. However, studies suggest that the protective effects of tamoxifen may be due to the anti-apoptotic and antioxidant effects from its estrogen-agonist properties [82, 83]. Protection may also result from increased transcription and translation of IGF-1, which has been shown to augment granulosa cell FSH receptor expression in the ovary and potentiate FSH action. Antagonist effects of tamoxifen are similar to GnRHa with downregulation of the H-P-O axis and ovarian quiescence, which may also have a protective role. Human studies with tamoxifen given post-chemotherapy have shown no protection [48].

1.3.7 AS101

AS101 is a tellurium-based immunomodulator that inhibits the P13K/PTEN/Akt pathway and has anti-apoptotic and anti-inflammatory properties [84, 85]. AS101 has been shown to be protective against hematopoietic damage in mice treated with cyclophosphamide without adversely affecting treatment outcome [86–89] and conversely exhibiting synergy [86, 89–91]. Studies of gonadal protection in mice have similarly shown AS101 to protect against chemotherapy-induced follicular damage and reduce sperm DNA damage without interfering with cancer treatments [49, 92]. The proposed mechanism of action is inhibition of activation and loss of dormant primordial follicles during chemotherapy as well as reduced apoptosis in the granulosa cells of growing follicles. AS101 can be administered systemically. Phase 2 clinical trials in cancer patients to assess the role of AS101 in the management of hematologic and dermatologic side effects of chemotherapy have been inconclusive, with most studies terminating prior to conclusion (▸ www.clinicaltrials.gov). Human studies assessing the effect on gonadal protection remain lacking.

1.3.8 Granulocyte Colony-Stimulating Factor (G-CSF)

Granulocyte colony-stimulating factor (G-CSF) is a polypeptide with growth factor and cytokine properties that stimulates granulocyte and stem cell production from the bone marrow and promotes neovascularization following ischemia [93, 94]. In mice studies, G-CSF has been shown to prevent damage to microvessels and significantly reduce the destruction of primordial follicles caused by the alkylators cyclophosphamide and busulfan [50]. Additionally, next-generation breeding showed no adverse effects in the offspring. G-CSF has also been shown to be protective against the effects of cisplatin in mouse models with improvement in follicular number and AMH levels [95]. It is postulated that with neovascularization, G-CSF decreases chemotherapy-related blood vessel loss and the associated focal ischemia seen in chemotherapy-related follicle loss [22]. Potential direct effects on the follicle remain unclear. However, an anti-apoptotic mechanistic action of G-CSF has been proposed [96, 97]. The advantage of G-CSF over other agents is that it is currently used in breast cancer patients and patients undergoing autologous bone marrow transplantation for the prevention of chemotherapy-induced neutropenia and has been shown to not reduce the efficacy of chemotherapeutic agents [98]. Despite optimistic results in rodents and its current use in humans as a cancer supportive therapy, no studies evaluating the role of G-CSF as an ovarian protective agent in human subjects have been performed.

1.4 Conclusion

Improved quality of life in survivorship remains the collective goal as oncofertility specialists. No longer is it acceptable to ignore the effects of cancer treatments on fertility or to only prioritize treatment and survivorship goals for our patients. More collaborative studies and multi-site registries are needed to be better quantify risk to our patients, putting aside singular aspirations. Translation of basic science discoveries in risk mitigation from rodent and primate science to patient care is critical to improving the reproductive health of cancer survivors. In doing this, we provide our patients with a quality of reflective of the challenges they have overcome.

References

1. Siegel RL, Miller KD, Jemal A. Cancer statistics, 2018. CA Cancer J Clin. 2018;68(1):7–30.
2. Keegan TH, et al. Comparison of cancer survival trends in the United States of adolescents and young adults with those in children and older adults. Cancer. 2016;122(7):1009–16.
3. Alvarez E, et al. Adolescent and young adult oncology patients: disparities in access to specialized cancer centers. Cancer. 2017;123(13):2516–23.
4. Hudson MM, et al. Clinical ascertainment of health outcomes among adults treated for childhood cancer. JAMA. 2013;309(22):2371–81.
5. Chemaitilly W, et al. Endocrine late effects in childhood cancer survivors. J Clin Oncol. 2018;36:2153–9: p. JCO2017763268
6. Faubion SS, Loprinzi CL, Ruddy KJ. Management of hormone deprivation symptoms after cancer. Mayo Clin Proc. 2016;91(8):1133–46.
7. Practice Committees of American Society for Reproductive, M, T. Society for Assisted Reproductive. Mature oocyte cryopreservation: a guideline. Fertil Steril. 2013;99(1):37–43.
8. Oktay K, et al. Fertility preservation in patients with cancer: ASCO clinical practice guideline update. J Clin Oncol. 2018;36(19):1994–2001.
9. Djaladat H. Organ-sparing surgery for testicular tumours. Curr Opin Urol. 2015;25(2):116–20.
10. Ntali G, Karavitaki N. Efficacy and complications of pituitary irradiation. Endocrinol Metab Clin N Am. 2015;44(1):117–26.
11. Meistrich ML. Effects of chemotherapy and radiotherapy on spermatogenesis in humans. Fertil Steril. 2013;100:1180–6.
12. Howell SJ, Shalet SM. Spermatogenesis after cancer treatment: damage and recovery. J Natl Cancer Inst Monogr. 2005;34:12–7.
13. Green DM, et al. Cumulative alkylating agent exposure and semen parameters in adult survivors of childhood

cancer: a report from the St Jude Lifetime Cohort Study. Lancet Oncol. 2014;15(11):1215–23.
14. Aldrink JH, et al. Using quality improvement methodology to improve ovarian salvage for benign ovarian masses. J Pediatr Surg. 2018;53(1):67–72.
15. Luczak J, Baglaj M. Selecting treatment method for ovarian masses in children – 24 years of experience. J Ovarian Res. 2017;10(1):59.
16. Gershenson DM. Management of borderline ovarian tumours. Best Pract Res Clin Obstet Gynaecol. 2017;41:49–59.
17. Rosendahl M, Simonsen MK, Kjer JJ. The influence of unilateral oophorectomy on the age of menopause. Climacteric. 2017;20(6):540–4.
18. Bjelland EK, et al. Is unilateral oophorectomy associated with age at menopause? A population study (the HUNT2 Survey). Hum Reprod. 2014;29:835–41.
19. diZerega GS. The peritoneum and its response to surgical injury. Prog Clin Biol Res. 1990;358:1–11.
20. Practice Committee of the American Society for Reproductive Medicine. Pathogenesis, consequences, and control of peritoneal adhesions in gynecologic surgery. Fertil Steril. 2007;88(1):21–6.
21. Meirow D, Nugent D. The effects of radiotherapy and chemotherapy on female reproduction. Hum Reprod Updat. 2001;7(6):535–43.
22. Meirow D, et al. Cortical fibrosis and blood-vessels damage in human ovaries exposed to chemotherapy. Potential mechanisms of ovarian injury. Hum Reprod. 2007;22(6):1626–33.
23. Wallace WH, et al. Gonadal dysfunction due to cisplatinum. Med Pediatr Oncol. 1989;17(5):409–13.
24. van Dorp W, et al. Recommendations for premature ovarian insufficiency surveillance for female survivors of childhood, adolescent, and young adult cancer: a report from the International Late effects of Childhood Cancer Guideline Harmonization Group in Collaboration with the PanCareSurFup Consortium. J Clin Oncol. 2016;34(28):3440.
25. Wallace WH, et al. Predicting age of ovarian failure after radiation to a field that includes the ovaries. Int J Radiat Oncol Biol Phys. 2005;62(3):738–44.
26. Larsen EC, et al. Radiotherapy at a young age reduces uterine volume of childhood cancer survivors. Acta Obstet Gynecol Scand. 2004;83(1):96–102.
27. Green DM, et al. Fertility of female survivors of childhood cancer: a report from the Childhood Cancer Survivor Study. J Clin Oncol. 2009;27(16):2677–85.
28. Meirow D, et al. The GnRH antagonist cetrorelix reduces cyclophosphamide-induced ovarian follicular destruction in mice. Hum Reprod. 2004;19(6):1294–9.
29. Li X, et al. Combination of a GnRH agonist with an antagonist prevents flare-up effects and protects primordial ovarian follicles in the rat ovary from cisplatin-induced toxicity: a controlled experimental animal study. Reprod Biol Endocrinol. 2013;11(1):16.
30. Ataya K, et al. Luteinizing hormone-releasing hormone agonist inhibits cyclophosphamide-induced ovarian follicular depletion in rhesus monkeys. Biol Reprod. 1995;52(2):365–72.
31. Badawy A, et al. Gonadotropin-releasing hormone agonists for prevention of chemotherapy-induced ovarian damage: prospective randomized study. Fertil Steril. 2009;91(3):694–7.
32. Mastro D, et al. Medical approaches to preservation of fertility in female cancer patients. Expert Opin Pharmacother. 2011;12(3):387–96.
33. Demeestere I, et al. Gonadotropin-releasing hormone agonist for the prevention of chemotherapy-induced ovarian failure in patients with lymphoma: 1-year follow-up of a prospective randomized trial. J Clin Oncol. 2013;31(7):903–9.
34. Gerber B, et al. Gonadotropin-releasing hormone analogue for premenopausal women with breast cancer. JAMA. 2011;306(16):1760.
35. Munster PN, Moore AP, Ismail-Khan R, Cox CE, Lacevic M, Gross-King M, et al. Randomized trial using gonadotropin-releasing hormone agonist triptorelin for the preservation of ovarian function during (neo)adjuvant chemotherapy for breast cancer. J Clin Oncol. 2012;30(5):533–8.
36. Elgindy EA, et al. Gonadatrophin suppression to prevent chemotherapy-induced ovarian damage: a randomized controlled trial. Obstet Gynecol. 2013;121(1):78–86.
37. Kerr JB, et al. Cisplatin-induced primordial follicle oocyte killing and loss of fertility are not prevented by imatinib. Nat Med. 2012;18(8):1170–2; author reply 1172–4.
38. Kilic S, et al. Protection from cyclophosphamide-induced ovarian damage with bone marrow-derived mesenchymal stem cells during puberty. Gynecol Endocrinol. 2014;30(2):135–40.
39. Fu X, et al. Bone marrow mesenchymal stem cell transplantation improves ovarian function and structure in rats with chemotherapy-induced ovarian damage. Cytotherapy. 2008;10(4):353–63.
40. Abd-Allah SH, et al. Mechanistic action of mesenchymal stem cell injection in the treatment of chemically induced ovarian failure in rabbits. Cytotherapy. 2013;15(1):64–75.
41. Morita Y, Perez GI, Paris F, Miranda SR, Ehleiter D, Haimovitz-Friedman A, et al. Oocyte apoptosis is suppressed by disruption of the acid sphingomyelinase gene or by sphingosine-1-phosphate therapy. Nat Med. 2000;6(10):1109–14.
42. Casper RF Jurisicova A. Protecting the female germ line from cancer therapy. Nat Med 2000;6(10):1100-1.
43. Hancke K, et al. Sphingosine 1-phosphate protects ovaries from chemotherapy-induced damage in vivo. Fertil Steril. 2007;87(1):172–7.
44. Kaya H, Desdicioglu R, Sezik M, Ulukaya E, Ozkaya O, Yimaztepe A, et al. Does sphingosine-1-phosphate have a protective effect on cyclophosphamide- and irradiation-induced ovarian damage in the rat model? Fertil Steril. 2008;89(3):732–5.
45. Zelinski MB, Murphy MK, Lawson MS, Jurisicova A, Pau KYF, Toscano NP, et al. In vivo delivery of fty720 prevents radiation-induced ovarian failure and infertility in adult female nonhuman primates. Fertil Steril. 2011;95(4):1440–U289.
46. Ting AY, Petroff BK. Tamoxifen decreases ovarian follicular loss from experimental toxicant DMBA and chemotherapy agents cyclophosphamide and doxorubicin in the rat. J Assist Reprod Genet. 2010;27(11):591–7.

47. Hickman LC, et al. Preservation of gonadal function in women undergoing chemotherapy: a systematic review and meta-analysis of the potential role for gonadotropin-releasing hormone agonists. J Assist Reprod Genet. 2018;35(4):571–81.
48. Sverrisdottir A, et al. Adjuvant goserelin and ovarian preservation in chemotherapy treated patients with early breast cancer: results from a randomized trial. Breast Cancer Res Treat. 2009;117(3):561–7.
49. Kalich-Philosoph L, et al. Cyclophosphamide triggers follicle activation and "burnout"; AS101 prevents follicle loss and preserves fertility. Sci Transl Med. 2013;5(185):185ra62.
50. Skaznik-Wikiel ME, et al. Granulocyte colony-stimulating factor with or without stem cell factor extends time to premature ovarian insufficiency in female mice treated with alkylating chemotherapy. Fertil Steril. 2013;99(7):2045.
51. Green DM, et al. Quantifying alkylating agent exposure: evaluation of the cyclophosphamide equivalent dose: a report from the Childhood Cancer Survivor Study. J Clin Oncol. 2011;29(15):9547.
52. Green DM, et al. The cyclophosphamide equivalent dose as an approach for quantifying alkylating agent exposure: a report from the Childhood Cancer Survivor Study. Pediatr Blood Cancer. 2014;61(1):53–67.
53. Meirow D, et al. Prevention of severe menorrhagia in oncology patients with treatment-induced thrombocytopenia by luteinizing hormone-releasing hormone agonist and depo-medroxyprogesterone acetate. Cancer. 2006;107(7):1634–41.
54. Eifel P, et al. National Institutes of Health Consensus Development Conference Statement: adjuvant therapy for breast cancer, November 1–3, 2000. J Natl Cancer Inst. 2001;93(13):979–89.
55. Goldhirsch A, et al. Meeting highlights: International Consensus Panel on the Treatment of Primary Breast Cancer. Seventh International Conference on Adjuvant Therapy of Primary Breast Cancer. J Clin Oncol. 2001;19(18):3817–27.
56. Turner NH, et al. Utility of gonadotropin-releasing hormone agonists for fertility preservation in young breast cancer patients: the benefit remains uncertain. Ann Oncol. 2013;24(9):2224–35.
57. Del Mastro L, et al. Gonadotropin-releasing hormone analogues for the prevention of chemotherapy-induced premature ovarian failure in cancer women: systematic review and meta-analysis of randomized trials. Cancer Treat Rev. 2014;40(5):675–83.
58. Oktay K, et al. Absence of conclusive evidence for the safety and efficacy of gonadotropin-releasing hormone analogue treatment in protecting against chemotherapy-induced gonadal injury. Oncologist. 2007;12(9):1055–66.
59. Moore HC, et al. Goserelin for ovarian protection during breast-cancer adjuvant chemotherapy. N Engl J Med. 2015;372(10):923–32.
60. Lambertini M, et al. Gonadotropin-releasing hormone agonists during chemotherapy for preservation of ovarian function and fertility in premenopausal patients with early breast cancer: a systematic review and meta-analysis of individual patient-level data. J Clin Oncol. 2018;36(19):1981–90.
61. Kano M, et al. AMH/MIS as a contraceptive that protects the ovarian reserve during chemotherapy. Proc Natl Acad Sci U S A. 2017;114(9):E1688–97.
62. Woodruff TK. A win-win for women's reproductive health: a nonsteroidal contraceptive and fertoprotective neoadjuvant. Proc Natl Acad Sci U S A. 2017;114(9):2101–2.
63. Gonfloni S, et al. Inhibition of the c-Abl-TAp63 pathway protects mouse oocytes from chemotherapy-induced death. Nat Med. 2009;15(10):1179–85.
64. Morgan S, et al. Cisplatin and doxorubicin induce distinct mechanisms of ovarian follicle loss; imatinib provides selective protection only against cisplatin. PLoS One. 2013;8(7):e70117.
65. Cherry SM, Hunt PA, Hassold TJ. Cisplatin disrupts mammalian spermatogenesis, but does not affect recombination or chromosome segregation. Mutat Res Genet Toxicol Environ Mutagen. 2004;564(2):115–28.
66. Woodruff TK. Preserving fertility during cancer treatment. Nat Med. 2009;15(10):1124–5.
67. Wang-Rodriguez J, et al. STI-571 (Gleevec) potentiates the effect of cisplatin in inhibiting the proliferation of head and neck squamous cell carcinoma in vitro. Laryngoscope. 2006;116(8):1409–16.
68. Prockop DJ. Marrow stromal cells as stem cells for nonhematopoietic tissues. Science. 1997;276(5309):71–4.
69. Dawn B, et al. Cardiac stem cells delivered intravascularly traverse the vessel barrier, regenerate infarcted myocardium, and improve cardiac function. Proc Natl Acad Sci U S A. 2005;102(10):3766–71.
70. Eliopoulos N, et al. Erythropoietin gene-enhanced marrow mesenchymal stromal cells decrease cisplatin-induced kidney injury and improve survival of allogeneic mice. Mol Ther. 2011;19(11):2072–83.
71. Villanueva PD, et al. Functional multipotency of stem cells: what do we need from them in the heart? Stem Cells Int. 2012;2012:817364.
72. Roodhart JML, et al. Mesenchymal stem cells induce resistance to chemotherapy through the release of platinum-induced fatty acids. Cancer Cell. 2011;20(3):370–83.
73. Strub GM, et al. Extracellular and intracellular actions of sphingosine-1-phosphate. Adv Exp Med Biol. 2010;688:141–55.
74. Soleimani R, Heytens E, Oktay K. Enhancement of neoangiogenesis and follicle survival by sphingosine-1-phosphate in human ovarian tissue xenotransplants. PLoS One. 2011;6(4):e19475.
75. Li F, et al. Sphingosine-1-phosphate prevents chemotherapy-induced human primordial follicle death. Hum Reprod. 2014;29(1):107–13.
76. Guzel Y, Bildik G, Oktem O. Sphingosine-1-phosphate protects human ovarian follicles from apoptosis in vitro. Eur J Obstet Gynecol Reprod Biol. 2018;222:19–24.
77. Guzel Y, et al. Sphingosine-1-phosphate reduces atresia of primordial follicles occurring during slow-freez-

1

ing and thawing of human ovarian cortical strips. Mol Reprod Dev. 2018;85:858–64.
78. Paris F, et al. Sphingosine 1-phosphate preserves fertility in irradiated female mice without propagating genomic damage in offspring. Nat Med. 2002;8(9): 901–2.
79. Mahran YF, et al. Insights into the protective mechanisms of tamoxifen in radiotherapy-induced ovarian follicular loss: impact on insulin-like growth factor 1. Endocrinology. 2013;154(10):3888–99.
80. Rose DP, Davis TE. Effects of adjuvant chemohormonal therapy on the ovarian and adrenal-function of breast-cancer patients. Cancer Res. 1980;40(11):4043–7.
81. Albain KS, et al. Adjuvant chemotherapy and timing of tamoxifen in postmenopausal patients with endocrine-responsive, node-positive breast cancer: a phase 3, open-label, randomised controlled trial. Lancet. 2009;374(9707):2055–63.
82. Dubey RK, et al. Estrogen and tamoxifen metabolites protect smooth muscle cell membrane phospholipids against peroxidation and inhibit cell growth. Circ Res. 1999;84(2):229–39.
83. Nathan L, Chaudhuri G. Antioxidant and prooxidant actions of estrogens: potential physiological and clinical implications. Semin Reprod Endocrinol. 1998; 16(4):309–14.
84. Hayun M, et al. The immunomodulator AS101 induces growth arrest and apoptosis in multiple myeloma: association with the Akt/Survivin pathway. Biochem Pharmacol. 2006;72(11):1423–31.
85. Indenbaum V, et al. In vitro and in vivo activity of AS101 against West Nile virus (WNV). Virus Res. 2012;166(1–2):68–76.
86. Kalechman Y, et al. Protective and restorative role of As101 in combination with chemotherapy. Cancer Res. 1991;51(5):1499–503.
87. Kalechman Y, et al. As101 protection of bone-marrow stromal cells function from adverse-effects of cyclophosphamide treatment in-vivo or Asta-Z in-vitro. Exp Hematol Oncol. 1992;20(6):728.
88. Kalechman Y, et al. The protective role of As101 in combination with cytotoxic drugs acting by various mechanisms of action. J Immunol. 1993;150(8):A131.
89. Sredni B, et al. Ammonium trichloro (dioxoethylene-o,o′) tellurate (AS101) sensitizes tumors to chemotherapy by inhibiting the tumor interleukin 10 autocrine loop. Cancer Res. 2004;64(5):1843–52.
90. Kalechman Y, et al. Effect of the immunomodulator As101 on chemotherapy-induced multilineage myelosuppression, thrombocytopenia, and anemia in mice. Exp Hematol Oncol. 1995;23(13):1358–66.
91. Sredni B, et al. Predominance of TH1 response in tumor bearing mice and cancer patients treated with AS101. J Natl Cancer Inst. 1996;88(18):1276–84.
92. Carmely A, et al. Protective effect of the immunomodulator AS101 against cyclophosphamide-induced testicular damage in mice. Hum Reprod. 2009; 24(6):1322–9.
93. Demetri GD, Griffin JD. Granulocyte colony-stimulating factor and its receptor. Blood. 1991;78(11): 2791–808.
94. Bussolino F, et al. Granulocyte-colony and granulocyte-macrophage-colony stimulating factors induce human-endothelial cells to migrate and proliferate. Nature. 1989;337(6206):471–3.
95. Akdemir A, et al. Granulocyte-colony stimulating factor decreases the extent of ovarian damage caused by cisplatin in an experimental rat model. Gynecol Oncol. 2014;25(4):328–33.
96. Solaroglu I, et al. Anti-apoptotic effect of granulocyte-colony stimulating factor after focal cerebral ischemia in the rat. Neuroscience. 2006;143(4):965–74.
97. Harada M, et al. G-CSF prevents cardiac remodeling after myocardial infarction by activating the Jak-Stat pathway in cardiomyocytes. Nat Med. 2005;11(3): 305–11.
98. Smith TJ, et al. 2006 update of recommendations for the use of white blood cell growth factors: an evidence-based clinical practice guideline. J Clin Oncol. 2006;24(19):3187–205.

Childhood, Adolescent, and Young Adult Cancer: Fertility Implications and Clinical Practice

Karen E. Kinahan, Barbara A. Lockart, Christina E. Boots, and Aarati Didwania

T. K. Woodruff et al. (eds.), *Textbook of Oncofertility Research and Practice*,
https://doi.org/10.1007/978-3-030-02868-8_2

2

Key Points

- Gonadal toxicity from chemotherapeutic agents and gonadal radiation has been identified.
- CAYA cancer patients should be offered fertility preservation options prior to initiating therapy.
- Reproductive endocrine and urology providers can assist with fertility preservation and evaluate a patient's fertility potential.
- A multidisciplinary approach for cancer patients is optimal to address patient's medical, psychological, and fertility health.

2.1 Introduction

Each year more than 15,000 children age 19 and younger are diagnosed with cancer in the United States [46]. In recent years, adolescent and young adult (AYA) oncology has become a national and international focus as a cohort of patients with special needs at diagnosis, as well as during treatment and survivorship [7]. In general, this selection of cancer patients includes those diagnosed from 15 to 39 years of age and includes approximately 70,000 cancer diagnoses per year in the United States alone [7]. In Europe, the number of children diagnosed with cancer each year ages 0–14 is 15,000, and there is an additional 30,000 who are 15–24 years old at diagnosis [21]. Together, this group of patients are referred to as childhood, adolescent and young adult (CAYA) cancer patients and comprise a wide spectrum of malignancies, and outcomes are dependent upon histology type, disease origin and site, race, sex, and age at diagnosis [16, 63]. Fortunately, advances in treatment and supportive care have led to a significant increase in survival rates for CAYA cancer patients [21, 46]. For purposes of this chapter, we will focus on patients diagnosed at age 30 and younger, but some of the information may be applicable for older patients as well. Patients in this age group are treated on The Children's Oncology Group (COG) cancer treatment protocols as well as adult treatment protocols and clinical trials. The standard of care in CAYA oncology has now changed from prior decades of thinking primarily of cure at all cost. The standard now includes fertility preservation when possible prior to starting treatment for protocols with surgery, radiation, or chemotherapy that negatively affect any component of the hypothalamic-pituitary-gonadal axis and may adversely impact future fertility [29].

Long-term cohort studies of adult survivors of childhood cancer show significant morbidity from cancer treatment, but late mortality rates have improved with reductions of radiotherapy being delivered in treatment protocols [1–3, 6]. Recent studies demonstrate that while more CAYA cancer patients are surviving and thriving, a high percentage of survivors are encountering serious "late effects" from their therapy. These late effects include, but are not limited to, cardiac, pulmonary, and endocrine disorders including impaired fertility, increased morbidity and mortality, and moderately to severely affected status in one or more of the primary domains of health (i.e., general health, mental health, functional status, limitations in activity, fear, or anxiety) [30, 42, 43].

This chapter will not go into detail on the myriad of late effects of CAYA cancer treatment. Rather, we will focus on the fertility effects of treatment which include use of alkylating agents and newer chemotherapeutic agents, radiotherapy with potential exposure to the ovaries, and surgery that involves the reproductive organs that can lead to permanent sterilization or premature ovarian failure in female survivors. These same treatments can cause altered spermatogenesis, testosterone deficiency, and physical sexual dysfunction in male patients who have reached puberty [63]. We will cover research into the psychosocial impact of potential or lost fertility for both males and females and how providers can become their advocates. We will discuss processes for assessment and treatment of impaired fertility with adult survivors of childhood cancer and adult-onset cancer. Lastly, we will review fertility preservation practices for newly diagnosed or relapsed CAYA cancer patients.

2.2 Recent Research on Late Effects and Infertility

The 2007 Woodruff and Synder's Oncofertility book introduced early studies identifying late effects of childhood cancer treatment impacting fertility [71]. Notably, Dr. Julie Byrne, one of the pioneer investigators in this field, and her 1999 study provided some of the first data on this important complication and found that the principal risk factors for early menopause after cancer were related to treatment after the onset of puberty, treatment with radiation below the diaphragm, and the use of alkylating agent chemotherapy. Byrne found that survivors were twice as likely (RR = 2.32, $p < 0.01$) as their control siblings to reach menopause during their 20s. However, there was no excess risk during their 30s (RR = 0.78). Survivors diagnosed after puberty and treated with radiation below the diaphragm were nearly ten times more likely to reach menopause during their 20s than controls, regardless of their primary diagnosis. The RR was 9.6 for Hodgkin lymphoma survivors and 8.56 for all other cancers [9]. Advances in pediatric and adolescent research have expanded our understanding of fertility outcomes and directed clinical trials research. Recent studies from the Childhood Cancer Survivor Study (CCSS) have demonstrated a higher incidence of infertility rates and reproductive interventions in female survivors enrolled in the CCSS compared to their sibling cohort. When compared to 1366 female sibling controls, 3531 5+ year survivors who enrolled in the study between November 1992 and April 2004 had an increased risk (RR 1.48 [95% CI 1.23–1.78]; $p < 0.0001$) of clinical infertility that was most pronounced at early reproductive ages in participants less than or equal to 24 years old (RR 2.92 [95% CI 1.18–7.20]; $p = 0.020$), in survivors aged 25–29 years (RR 1.61 [95% CI 1.05–2.48]; $p = 0.029$) and in those aged 30–40 years (RR 1.37 [95% CI 1.11–1.69]; $p = 0.0035$). As other studies have demonstrated, the authors reported increasing doses of uterine radiation and alkylating agent chemotherapy were strongly associated with infertility [4].

A 2016 study from the CCSS reported on pregnancy after chemotherapy in 10,938 male and female survivors after receiving treatment with one or more of 14 alkylating and similar DNA interstrand cross-linking drugs of interest without exposure to cranial or abdominal radiation. Results were compared to 3949 sibling controls. Five thousand nine hundred and twenty-two (54%) survivors received at least one alkylating or similar DNA interstrand cross-linking drugs such as cisplatin. Results of a multivariable analysis showed survivors having a decreased likelihood of siring or having a pregnancy versus siblings (male survivors, hazard ratio [HR] 0.63; 95% CI 0.58–0.68; $p < 0.0001$; female survivors, HR 0.87; 95% CI 0.81–0.94; $p < 0.0001$). Their results showed that male survivors who received ifosfamide doses of more than 25,000 mg/m^2, procarbazine doses of more than 3000 mg/m^2, and cisplatin doses of more than 475 mg/m^2 had a significantly reduced chance of siring pregnancies and livebirth compared to survivors with no exposure [12]. For female survivors, data demonstrated that only busulfan of any dose category and lomustine ≥411 mg/m^2) were associated with significantly decreased achievement of pregnancy. Further subanalyses showed female survivors exposed to cyclophosphamide in the upper quartile (≥11,295 mg/m^2) had a lower likelihood of pregnancy than did those not exposed (HR 0.85, 95% CI 0.74–0.98; $p = 0.023$) [12].

The adverse effects of high-dose cranial radiation and direct gonadal radiation on fertility have been widely described [25, 57]. A study from St. Jude Lifetime Cohort Study (SJLIFE) assessed the effect of low doses (<26 Gy) of cranial radiation on sperm concentration of 241 adult survivors of childhood acute lymphocytic leukemia (ALL). Results show that cranial radiation doses (<26 Gy) typically used for central nervous system prophylaxis in patients with ALL had no demonstrable adverse effect on spermatogenesis although a cyclophosphamide equivalent dose (CED) exceeding 8 g/m^2 and an age at diagnosis of 5–9 years did increase the risk of oligospermia and azoospermia [26]. Other studies have demonstrated Leydig cell function being preserved after cancer treatment, but germ cell failure is common in men treated with high cumulative doses of cyclophosphamide (>7500 mg/m^2) [34, 41] and with more than 3 months of combination alkylating agent therapy [22, 27].

The ability of female survivors to carry a pregnancy to term and health of the offspring have been investigated. At-risk groups include patients treated with flank and abdominal radiation such as with patients with Wilm's tumor who have been shown to have early or threatened labor, fetal malposition, and low birth weight, all of which are increased with flank radiation dosages [11, 24]. Female CAYA cancer survivors who received flank or abdominal radiation and are fortunate enough to become pregnant should be managed by a high-risk multidisciplinary team or maternal-fetal medicine [18]. Other survivors such as those treated for leukemia and lymphoma with anthracycline therapy and/or chest irradiation need to be aware of maternal cardiopulmonary risks and should also be evaluated by a maternal-fetal medicine practice for close surveillance including echocardiograms during pregnancy and delivery and postpartum [37, 61].

A great deal of progress has been made in understanding the effects of chemotherapeutic agents and irradiation on gonadal function. As new chemotherapy agents and other therapies are discovered, research must continue with a focus on their role in not only curing cancer but also the life-altering effects such as infertility and premature menopause they may cause. These same factors and their relationship to the CAYA cancer survivor's quality of life must be investigated and addressed.

2.3 Providers Addressing Psychosocial Implications

Great importance is placed on fertility by adolescent and young adult cancer survivors themselves and by the parents of childhood cancer survivors [45, 64]. Information regarding the impact of diagnosis and treatment on fertility is one of the most cited unmet needs among adolescent and young adult survivors [39, 70, 74]. It is important for providers to recognize this need and address the concern felt by survivors even if medical treatment may not affect fertility. Fertility implications of diagnosis and treatment need to be addressed at the time of diagnosis but also after treatment has been completed as many CAYA cancer patients do not process their concerns until they are actively thinking about having children.

Reproductive concerns in survivors have been associated with depression and anxiety symptoms, grief, lowered self-esteem, and an altered sense of identity [14]. Fertility-related distress may become more acute as these survivor populations move past their treatment and consider building a family, and many survivors do not know their fertility status [48]. An exploratory study looking at the experiences of 38 survivors over time in terms of managing fertility matters following cancer treatment in their teens found that professional and social networks did not provide many opportunities for these survivors to ask questions, receive information, process feelings, or develop handling strategies. The study also found that for some survivors, fertility matters affected identity, well-being, and life planning as well as reproductive function [15].

Providers who are aware of survivors' concerns about fertility, whether founded or imagined, can have a great impact on the well-being of their patients. Secondary analyses of a qualitative study of young adult survivors of adolescent cancers by Benedict et al. concluded that females may be more at risk for distress than males, particularly in situations of uncertainty and limited knowledge regarding fertility implications of their primary disease or secondary to treatment [5]. How and when to address fertility issues may be some of the barriers to providing information to survivors. CAYA cancer survivors may still be developing cognitive and emotional abilities to manage stress and cope effectively as they mature [75]. This limitation along with parental buffering and clinicians' discomfort addressing fertility issues may result in survivors not receiving adequate information and support around fertility issues [28, 55]. Increased attention to fertility may help to alleviate CAYA's distress, facilitate engagement in decision-making about their reproductive future, and improve long-term well-being in survivorship.

Benedict et al. also found that discussing fertility elicited emotional reactions for most participants ranging from expressions of distress to feelings of hope and positivity [5]. The distress felt by participants included feeling upset, nervous, overwhelmed, and angry. Those participants who were unsure of the gonadotoxic effects of their treatment anticipated feeling devastated, hurt, and lonely if they were unable to have children. For some of the participants, this distress was associated with feeling different from their peers and excluded from normalcy in reaching parenthood [5]. Eighteen percent of participants in this study reported little to no concern about their fertility, and surprisingly, this lack of concern was not limited to those who knew that their fertility had not been affected [5]. Care providers who assume they can predict whether their survivors will have psychosocial effects from fertility concerns will miss opportunities to provide comprehensive care if they do not address the issue with their patients. Care providers will also have to build relationships with their survivors in efforts to understand the survivor's maturity and their ability to process fertility-related issues and concerns.

Survivors in the Benedict et al. study used a variety of strategies in dealing with fertility concerns including acceptance, avoidance, and taking comfort in the availability or success of assisted reproductive technology [5]. Therefore, counseling should include a balanced approach of allowing for optimism as well as setting realistic expectations. Some CAYAs may still worry about their reproductive health even if their treatment was not gonadotoxic despite provider reassurance [33]. A qualitative study by Quinn et al. found that female adolescent participants had two categories of coping styles in reaction to questions regarding loss of fertility: emotion-focused and problem-focused [56]. Wishful thinking, externalizing, and other emotion-focused coping styles are traditionally viewed as maladaptive when compared to information-seeking and other active coping styles [68]. Although these concepts are not universally held, providers aiming for successful interventions should seek to uncover CAYAs' values and presumptions about future parenthood and reproduction in hopes of assisting the psychosocial stressors and development of adaptive coping mechanisms.

The individuals within the CAYA cancer population are unique in their reaction to the gonadotoxic effects of treatment, their ability to address their concerns, and the adaptive mechanisms they employ to deal with these stressors. Practitioners should strive to become comfortable with addressing fertility effects of treatment but most importantly develop strategies to gauge their survivors' needs and limitations.

2.4 Assessment of Fertility Status in CAYA Survivors of Cancer

Many survivors of CAYA cancer are aware that their prior treatment had potentially gonadotoxic effects. However, if and when they were counseled in the past, clinicians were unlikely to have given them a definitive prediction on their future fertility status. As previously mentioned, how robustly cancer treatment affects reproductive function depends on the type and total dose of chemotherapy and if they received pelvic radiation. As female and male survivors begin to inquire more actively about their fertility status and consider building a family, they should be encouraged to consult with their primary care physicians and also consider seeking specialized consultations with a reproductive endocrinology and fertility specialist or a reproductive urologist. In the United States, there are more than 384 fertility centers in 49 states that are members of the Society for Assisted Reproductive Technology. Of these, 77 are committed members of the Oncofertility Consortium, which is a national, interdisciplinary initiative designed to explore the reproductive future of cancer survivors, and many more centers provide this care outside of the consortium.

Table 2.1 Semen analysis

Parameter	Reference value
Ejaculate volume	1.5 mL
Sperm concentration	15 million sperm/mL
Total sperm	39 million sperm/mL
Motile sperm	40%
Progressively motile sperm	32%
Normal morphology	4%

Data derived from World Health Organization [72]

For men, a clinical assessment of the current health status, reproductive history, medications, prior chemotherapy, radiation, or abdominal or genitourinary surgery should be made [53]. Symptoms of low testosterone, including low libido, erectile or ejaculatory dysfunction, inability to gain muscle mass, etc., can also be signs of poor reproductive function. Next, a semen analysis should be performed. As shown in Table 2.1, a semen analysis evaluates the volume of the ejaculate, the concentration of sperm, and the proportion of sperm that are motile and are morphologically normal [72]. At a minimum, a primary care physician can perform a medical and reproductive history and at least one semen analysis. If abnormal, the patient should be referred to a reproductive specialist, who will perform a physical exam focusing on secondary sex characteristics and the genitourinary anatomy. The etiology of abnormal sperm parameters should be further explored by an endocrinology evaluation, specifically looking at follicle-stimulating hormone (FSH) and luteinizing hormone, testosterone, and estradiol, while also excluding other etiologies for abnormal hormone levels by assessing both prolactin and thyroid-stimulating hormone. A normal semen analysis in the setting of normal hormone levels is reassuring that the survivors' fertility is minimally affected by his prior therapy.

In contrast to men, who have stem cells in their testes and create new sperm regularly, women are born with a finite number of oocytes that decrease in quantity and quality over time. While women's fertility assessment can be initiated with their primary care physician, assessing ovarian reserve is complex and prompt referral should be made to their gynecologist or reproductive endocrinology and infertility specialist. A fertility evaluation should start with a clinical history assessing overall health, prior surgeries (specifically abdominal or pelvic), prior chemotherapy, and prior radiation [52]. Focus should then be placed on her reproductive health, including prior pregnancies, pregnancy outcomes, and history of pelvic infections, and, most importantly, a careful menstrual history should be elicited. While normal menstrual cycles seem reassuring, cycling every 28 days is not a predictor of fertility. An abnormal menstrual cycle length is defined as less than 21 or greater than 35 days [51]. However, subtle changes, such as premenstrual spotting and shortening cycles, can be indicators of diminishing ovarian reserve and should not be ignored. Absence of menstrual cycles may be a sign of primary ovarian insufficiency and should be further evaluated.

Ovarian reserve is best assessed by both serum analysis and pelvic ultrasound [54, 67]. Anti-Müllerian hormone (AMH) is a protein secreted by the granulosa cells surrounding oocytes early in the process of folliculogenesis. AMH is the most sensitive assessment of the ovarian reserve, and normative values are adjusted by age; the lower the number, the smaller the pool of remaining oocytes [60]. Interestingly, the AMH value does not predict a woman's current fertility, but a lower than expected value could suggest that her reproductive time span will be shortened and her fertility will decline earlier than would be expected [65]. In addition, this value is most useful as a predictor of ovarian response to stimulation by exogenous gonadotropins, which is particularly relevant when considering fertility preservation via egg or embryo freezing or if actively seeking fertility treatment [60] (Table 2.2). Pelvic ultrasound counting the number of antral follicles is similarly sensitive and usually corroborates the interpretation of AMH. Measuring basal serum FSH early in the menstrual cycle (ideally cycle day 3) is also predictive of ovarian reserve. While less sensitive than AMH, FSH is more specific in diagnosing severely diminished ovarian reserve or primary ovarian insufficiency. FSH levels above 15 mIU/mL are suggestive of this diagnosis and, most importantly, suggest that fertility treatments have limited benefits above spontaneous conception. Even when fertility treatments are not successful, conception is possible as long as spontaneous ovulation continues to occur [50].

Table 2.2 Anti-Müllerian hormone values by age

Age (years)	Median (ng/mL)	Mean (ng/mL)	1 Standard deviation
25	3.2	4.1	4
30	2.4	3.2	3.2
35	1.3	2.1	2.5
40	0.7	1.1	1.3
45	0.3	0.5	0.9

Data derived from 17,120 women in US Fertility Centers

Ultimately, no clinical history or laboratory test is a perfect predictor of current or future fertility. Only attempting pregnancy will give patients their definitive answer. However, if patients are not yet ready to conceive but desire information, further testing is a reasonable approach and can help with family planning.

2.5 Fertility Preservation for CAYA Cancer Patients

As survival rates for CAYA cancers have risen over the last decades, many adult survivors of are left to deal with sequelae of treatment years and even decades after completion of therapy. Research shows patients are troubled by the potential of infertility during and after cancer treatment [8, 59]. In an effort to improve the health and quality of life for survivors, advances in reproductive medicine and the emergence of oncofertility as a discipline prompted the American Society of Clinical Oncology (ASCO) and the National Comprehensive Cancer Network (NCCN) to develop clinical guidelines for healthcare providers working with these patient populations [13, 38]. From 2006 to 2016, over a hundred articles were published in the field of fertility preservation alone in the childhood and adolescent cancer population, and multidisciplinary fertility preservation programs are being developed around the country [10, 32].

Fertility preservation in pediatric and adolescent patients is more complex than in young adult patients for a multitude of reasons. Prepubertal patients only have experimental fertility preservation options available to them. Children and adolescents may lack capacity to envision a future in which they want children but in adulthood regret a decision to not pursue fertility preservation when offered. There are ethical concerns regarding parents making generational choices for their children and potentially future grandchildren [40]. Additionally, the literature expresses concern that offering fertility preservation may create false hope which can be of particular concern with prepubertal patients where long-term survival and the likelihood of pregnancy in adulthood are distant and dependent on future studies and advances in available reproductive technologies and medicine [19].

Fertility preservation options available to CAYA cancer patients may be limited for several reasons. Experimental options available to prepubertal patients require Institutional Review Board (IRB) approval and are offered at a small number of pediatric institutions. Young adult patients diagnosed with a "pediatric" malignancy such as acute lymphoblastic leukemia or rhabdomyosarcoma may receive care at a pediatric institution due to pediatric oncology team's expertise treating pediatric cancers. The patient's access to fertility preservation may be limited due to the providers' lack of knowledge of fertility preservation options or due to challenges coordinating care between the pediatric institution and reproductive medicine team. Refer to ◘ Table 2.3 for a brief overview of fertility preservation options [19].

The majority of pediatric oncology physicians, advanced practice providers (APPs), and registered nurses (RNs) support educating patients and families on the risk of infertility and options for fertility preservation. Referral practices for fertility preservation in CAYAs show a discrepancy between the providers' beliefs and practices [35]. There are a multitude of factors that influence the practice of fertility preservation as identified by physicians, APPs, and RNs. Most commonly acknowledged issues are an urgency to start treatment, lack of clarity about a patient's and family's desire for the information, and concerns about cost. Lack of educational materials, unfamiliarity with options, and no relationship

◘ Table 2.3 Fertility preservation options

	Fertility preservation option	Experimental
Prepubertal males	Testicular tissue cryopreservation	Yes
Postpubertal males		
Prepubertal males	Orchiopexy	No
Postpubertal males	Testicular shielding	
Postpubertal males	Sperm banking	No
	Testicular sperm extraction	
	Post-masturbation sperm banking	
	Electroejaculation	
Prepubertal females	Ovarian tissue cryopreservation	Yes
Postpubertal females		
Postpubertal females	Oocyte cryopreservation	No
	Embryo cryopreservation	
Pre- and postpubertal females	Oophoropexy	No
	Ovarian shielding	
Pre- and postpubertal females	GnRH agonists	No consensus

Fernbach et al. [19]

with a reproductive medicine team are also identified as obstacles to fertility care in CAYA patient populations [20, 23, 69]. Two studies report non-white patients are less likely than Caucasian patients to receive fertility preservation counseling [58, 62].

Other challenges to education and access for fertility preservation include the patients' and families' culture, religion, race, language, health literacy, and cognitive level of the patient and parents. Stressors such as child care, parental relationship, and access to healthcare may all impact the individual's ability to process information and influence decision-making. Concerns regarding when a child should be included in medical decision-making and what influence the child should exert, especially regarding experimental options, impact the pursuit of fertility preservation. Adolescents are more likely than children to identify concerns about infertility make them uneasy, rather than having concerns about the procedure. Parents are shown to influence the fertility preservation decision more than physicians [73].

The burden of consent is greater when a family is considering an experimental procedure, rather than a standard treatment such as sperm banking, or when consenting for life-saving medical treatment. Neither child nor parent should feel they are coerced to make a decision. Weighing the child's ability to grasp the risk versus benefit of an experimental procedure and the parents' ability to make a decision in the child's best interest is paramount. The depth of information provided to patients is adjusted to age and cognitive level. Providing information in developmental appropriate terms may require assistance from psychologists, social workers, or child life therapists adept at sexual health discussions. Genetic counseling prior to fertility preservation should be considered if the family has a known hereditary cancer syndrome or if the patient is undergoing stem cell transplant for a condition such as sickle cell disease or thalassemia [49].

Discussions surrounding fertility preservation and consenting for procedure must be performed in the patient's and family's native language by a medical interpreter. A quiet room free of distractions is needed to improve the patient and family's understanding. Information should be free of medical speak and paced to optimize comprehension. Confidentiality is vital, and adolescents and young adults must be given the opportunity to meet privately with providers if requested.

Families of pediatric and adolescent cancer patients are concerned about the treatment's impact on fertility. Regardless of whether a family decides to pursue any fertility preservation, families do want information on risk of infertility and available fertility preservation options. Counseling and services often require coordination of care between multiple disciplines and services and possibly between pediatric and adult institutions. Reproductive health discussions in CAYA cancer patients do not end at the time of diagnosis. As the patient matures, it is imperative the medical team provides patients with developmentally appropriate information from diagnosis to survivorship.

2.6 Conclusion and Next Steps

A cancer diagnosis is an overwhelming, stressful, and life-altering time for CAYA cancer patients and their families. In an increasing number of patients, improvements in treatment and supportive care shift the cancer experience from a terminal disease to a chronic illness [17]. As a result, healthcare providers caring for survivors of CAYA cancer need to become aware of unique medical and psychosocial risks from their past treatment exposures and cancer journey experiences. Fertility implications from cancer treatment are only one adverse issue many survivors must deal with [29, 47]. As discussed, advances and details in gonadal toxicity have been discovered, and as a result, CAYA treatment protocols have been amended to promote health and quality of life of survivors [3, 66]. Nevertheless, while advances have been made in the field of oncofertility as outlined in this chapter and others, we still have an immense amount of work to do.

As providers, we need to appreciate a true understanding of the impact of infertility and sterility on our patients, as it is often an extremely difficult consequence of cancer treatment. The discussion of fertility preservation needs to occur prior to cancer treatment, but also an inquiry about patient's readiness to find out about their own fertility status needs to be brought up by providers at every encounter. This starts with oncology providers including physicians, RNs, and APPs abstracting the patient's treatment details and providing them with a Survivorship Care Plan (SCP) or treatment summary. This document serves as a conduit of information for the current medical team to understand actual or potential late effects of treatment, including fertility implications. The SCP can be shared with current and future providers such as primary care providers. As CAYA cancer patients enter into the "adult" medical world, there is a known lack of knowledge about late effects of therapy, and it becomes a barrier to care for patients and providers [31, 36, 44]. Arming our self with available resources is critical for our own knowledge and also enables us to educate our patients. An excellent resource is *The Children's Oncology Group Long-Term Follow-Up Guidelines for Survivors of Childhood, Adolescent and Young Adult Cancers* and their accompanying patient education materials called "Health Links." These are available for no cost at ▶ http://www.survivorshipguidelines.org [37]. Another useful resource for the CAYA population is ASCO's "Focus Under 40" found at ▶ http://university.asco.org/focus-under-forty which has information on male and female fertility preservation, survivorship, and supportive care. We continue to recognize the importance of quality of life for survivors, and it is our ultimate goal to have CAYA survivors a long and fulfilling life, which includes the opportunity to become a parent if desired.

Review Questions and Answers

Q1. Which class of chemotherapeutic agents is best known for their gonadal toxicity and associated infertility/sterility?

A1. Alkylating agents such as cyclophosphamide, ifosfamide, procarbazine, and busulfan are known to be associated with reduced fertility.

Q2. A 32-year-old female treated at age 15 for Hodgkin lymphoma with MOPP (nitrogen mustard (melphalan), oncovorin, procarbazine, and prednisone) without radiation arrives in your office and wants to discuss a fertility workup. She has attempted pregnancy for 9 months without success. What type of doctor would you ideally refer her to?

A2. This patient should be referred to a reproductive endocrine specialist who can counsel her on an evaluation, review results, and make appropriate referrals.

Q3. True or false? All patients who received cancer treatment are at risk for infertility/sterility.

A3. False. Many patients treated with chemotherapy and direct radiation not encompassing the abdomen or gonads may conceive or sire a pregnancy. This notion of cancer = infertility reiterates the importance for obtaining detailed cancer treatment records including cumulative dosages of alkylating agents if possible.

Q4. What are some reliable resources for physicians and advanced practice providers to access to educate themselves about advances in reproductive medicine and counseling CAYA survivors on their risk of infertility?

A4. The American Society of Clinical Oncology (ASCO) and the National Comprehensive Cancer Network (NCCN) have developed clinical guidelines and education materials for providers (▶ asco.org, ▶ NCCN.org). The ASCO website offers Focus Under 40 which includes education programs for male and female fertility preservation and survivorship at ▶ https://university.asco.org/focus-under-forty. The Children's Oncology Group Long-Term Follow-Up Guidelines available at ▶ http://www.survivorshipguidelines.org offer health links on male and female reproductive system issues.

References

1. Armstrong GT, Liu Q, Yasui Y, Neglia JP, Leisenring W, Robison LL, Mertens AC. Late mortality among 5-year survivors of childhood cancer: a summary from the Childhood Cancer Survivor Study. J Clin Oncol. 2009;27(14):2328–38. https://doi.org/10.1200/JCO.2008.21.1425.
2. Armstrong GT, Kawashima T, Leisenring W, Stratton K, Stovall M, Hudson MM, Sklar CA, Robison LL, Oeffinger KC. Aging and risk of severe, disabling, life-threatening, and fatal events in the childhood cancer survivor study. J Clin Oncol. 2014;32(12):1218–27. https://doi.org/10.1200/JCO.2013.51.1055.
3. Armstrong GT, Chen Y, Yasui Y, Leisenring W, Gibson TM, Mertens AC, Stovall M, Oeffinger KC, Bhatia S, Krull KR, Nathan PC, Neglia JP, Green DM, Hudson MM, Robison LL. Reduction in late mortality among 5-year survivors of childhood cancer. N Engl J Med. 2016;374(9):833–42. https://doi.org/10.1056/NEJMoa1510795.
4. Barton SE, Najita JS, Ginsburg ES, Leisenring WM, Stovall M, Weathers RE, Sklar CA, Robison LL, Diller L. Infertility, infertility treatment, and achievement of pregnancy in female survivors of childhood cancer: a report from the Childhood Cancer Survivor Study cohort. Lancet Oncol. 2013;14(9):873–81. https://doi.org/10.1016/s1470-2045(13)70251-1.
5. Benedict C, Shuk E, Ford JS. Fertility issues in adolescent and young adult cancer survivors. J Adolesc Young Adult Oncol. 2016;5(1):48–57. https://doi.org/10.1089/jayao.2015.0024.
6. Bhakta N, Liu Q, Ness KK, Baassiri M, Eissa H, Yeo F, Chemaitilly W, Ehrhardt MJ, Bass J, Bishop MW, Shelton K, Lu L, Huang S, Li Z, Caron E, Lanctot J, Howell C, Folse T, Joshi V, Green DM, Mulrooney DA, Armstrong GT, Krull KR, Brinkman TM, Khan RB, Srivastava DK, Hudson MM, Yasui Y, Robison LL. The cumulative burden of surviving childhood cancer: an initial report from the St Jude Lifetime Cohort Study (SJLIFE). Lancet. 2017. https://doi.org/10.1016/s0140-6736(17)31610-0.
7. Bleyer A, Ferrari A, Whelan J, Barr RD. Global assessment of cancer incidence and survival in adolescents and young adults. Pediatr Blood Cancer. 2017;64(9). https://doi.org/10.1002/pbc.26497.
8. Burns KC, Boudreau C, Panepinto JA. Attitudes regarding fertility preservation in female adolescent cancer patients. J Pediatr Hematol Oncol. 2006;28(6):350–4.
9. Byrne J. Infertility and premature menopause in childhood cancer survivors. Med Pediatr Oncol. 1999;33(1):24–8.
10. Carlson CA, Kolon TF, Mattei P, Hobbie W, Gracia CR, Ogle S, Ginsberg JP. Developing a hospital-wide fertility preservation service for pediatric and young adult patients. J Adolesc Health. 2017;61(5):571–6. https://doi.org/10.1016/j.jadohealth.2017.07.008.
11. Chiarelli AM, Marrett LD, Darlington GA. Pregnancy outcomes in females after treatment for childhood cancer. Epidemiology. 2000;11(2):161–6.
12. Chow EJ, Stratton KL, Leisenring WM, Oeffinger KC, Sklar CA, Donaldson SS, Ginsberg JP, Kenney LB, Levine JM, Robison LL, Shnorhavorian M, Stovall M, Armstrong GT, Green DM. Pregnancy after chemotherapy in male and female survivors of childhood cancer treated between 1970 and 1999: a report from the Childhood Cancer Survivor Study cohort. Lancet Oncol. 2016;17(5):567–76. https://doi.org/10.1016/s1470-2045(16)00086-3.
13. Coccia PF, Altman J, Bhatia S, Borinstein SC, Flynn J, George S, Goldsby R, Hayashi R, Huang MS, Johnson RH, Beaupin LK, Link MP, Oeffinger KC, Orr KM, Pappo AS, Reed D, Spraker HL, Thomas DA, von Mehren M, Wechsler DS, Whelan KF, Zebrack BJ, Sundar H, Shead DA. Adolescent and young adult oncology. Clinical practice guidelines in oncology. J Natl Compr Cancer Netw JNCCN. 2012;10(9):1112–50.
14. Crawshaw M. Psychosocial oncofertility issues faced by adolescents and young adults over their lifetime: a review of the research. Hum Fertil (Camb). 2013;16(1):59–63. https://doi.org/10.3109/14647273.2012.733480.
15. Crawshaw MA, Sloper P. 'Swimming against the tide' – the influence of fertility matters on the transition to adulthood or survivorship following adolescent cancer. Eur J Cancer Care (Engl). 2010;19(5):610–20. https://doi.org/10.1111/j.1365-2354.2009.01118.x.
16. Demoor-Goldschmidt C, Drui D, Doutriaux I, Michel G, Auquier P, Dumas A, Berger C, Bernier V, Bohrer S, Bondiau PY, Filhon B, Fresneau B, Freycon C, Stefan D, Helfre S, Jackson A, Kerr C, Laprie A, Leseur J, Mahe MA, Oudot C, Pluchard C, Proust S, Sudour-Bonnange H, Vigneron C, Lassau N, Schlumberger M, Conter CF, de Vathaire F. A French national breast and thyroid cancer screening programme for survivors of childhood, adolescent and young adult (CAYA) cancers – DeNaCaPST programme. BMC Cancer. 2017;17(1):326. https://doi.org/10.1186/s12885-017-3318-1.
17. Diller L, Chow EJ, Gurney JG, Hudson MM, Kadin-Lottick NS, Kawashima TI, Leisenring WM, Meacham LR, Mertens AC, Mulrooney DA, Oeffinger KC, Packer RJ, Robison LL, Sklar CA. Chronic disease in the Childhood Cancer Survivor Study cohort: a review of published findings. J Clin Oncol. 2009;27(14):2339–55. https://doi.org/10.1200/jco.2008.21.1953.
18. Edgar AB, Wallace WH. Pregnancy in women who had cancer in childhood. Eur J Cancer. 2007;43(13):1890–4. https://doi.org/10.1016/j.ejca.2007.06.011.
19. Fernbach A, Lockart B, Armus CL, Bashore LM, Levine J, Kroon L, Sylvain G, Rodgers C. Evidence-based recommendations for fertility preservation options for inclusion in treatment protocols for pediatric and adolescent patients diagnosed with cancer. J Pediatr Oncol Nurs. 2014;31(4):211–22. https://doi.org/10.1177/1043454214532025.
20. Fuchs A, Kashanian JA, Clayman ML, Gosiengfiao Y, Lockart B, Woodruff TK, Brannigan RE. Pediatric oncology providers' attitudes and practice patterns regarding fertility preservation in adolescent male cancer patients. J Pediatr Hematol Oncol. 2016;38(2):118–22. https://doi.org/10.1097/mph.0000000000000488.
21. Gatta G, Zigon G, Capocaccia R, Coebergh JW, Desandes E, Kaatsch P, Pastore G, Peris-Bonet R, Stiller CA. Survival of European children and young adults with cancer diagnosed 1995–2002. Eur J Cancer. 2009;45(6):992–1005. https://doi.org/10.1016/j.ejca.2008.11.042.

22. Gerres L, Bramswig JH, Schlegel W, Jurgens H, Schellong G. The effects of etoposide on testicular function in boys treated for Hodgkin's disease. Cancer. 1998;83(10):2217–22.
23. Goodwin T, Elizabeth Oosterhuis B, Kiernan M, Hudson MM, Dahl GV. Attitudes and practices of pediatric oncology providers regarding fertility issues. Pediatr Blood Cancer. 2007;48(1):80–5. https://doi.org/10.1002/pbc.20814.
24. Green DM, Peabody EM, Nan B, Peterson S, Kalapurakal JA, Breslow NE. Pregnancy outcome after treatment for Wilms tumor: a report from the National Wilms Tumor Study Group. J Clin Oncol. 2002;20(10):2506–13. https://doi.org/10.1200/jco.2002.07.159.
25. Green DM, Liu W, Kutteh WH, Ke RW, Shelton KC, Sklar CA, Chemaitilly W, Pui CH, Klosky JL, Spunt SL, Metzger ML, Srivastava D, Ness KK, Robison LL, Hudson MM. Cumulative alkylating agent exposure and semen parameters in adult survivors of childhood cancer: a report from the St Jude Lifetime Cohort Study. Lancet Oncol. 2014;15(11):1215–23. https://doi.org/10.1016/s1470-2045(14)70408-5.
26. Green DM, Zhu L, Wang M, Chemaitilly W, Srivastava D, Kutteh WH, Ke RW, Sklar CA, Pui CH, Kun LE, Ribeiro RC, Robison LL, Hudson MM. Effect of cranial irradiation on sperm concentration of adult survivors of childhood acute lymphoblastic leukemia: a report from the St. Jude Lifetime Cohort Studydagger. Hum Reprod. 2017;32(6):1192–201. https://doi.org/10.1093/humrep/dex082.
27. Hobbie WL, Ginsberg JP, Ogle SK, Carlson CA, Meadows AT. Fertility in males treated for Hodgkins disease with COPP/ABV hybrid. Pediatr Blood Cancer. 2005;44(2):193–6. https://doi.org/10.1002/pbc.20172.
28. Horner MJ, Ries LAG, Krapcho M, Neyman N, Aminou R, Howlader N, et al. SEER cancer statistics review, 1975–2006. Bethesda: National Cancer Institute; 2009. http://seer.cancer.gov/csr/1975_2006/.
29. Hudson MM. Reproductive outcomes for survivors of childhood cancer. Obstet Gynecol. 2010;116(5):1171–83. https://doi.org/10.1097/AOG.0b013e3181f87c4b.
30. Hudson MM, Mertens AC, Yasui Y, Hobbie W, Chen H, Gurney JG, Yeazel M, Recklitis CJ, Marina N, Robison LR, Oeffinger KC. Health status of adult long-term survivors of childhood cancer: a report from the Childhood Cancer Survivor Study. JAMA. 2003;290(12):1583–92. https://doi.org/10.1001/jama.290.12.1583.
31. Iyer NS, Mitchell HR, Zheng DJ, Ross WL, Kadan-Lottick NS. Experiences with the survivorship care plan in primary care providers of childhood cancer survivors: a mixed methods approach. Support Care Cancer. 2017;25(5):1547–55. https://doi.org/10.1007/s00520-016-3544-0.
32. Johnson EK, Finlayson C, Rowell EE, Gosiengfiao Y, Pavone ME, Lockart B, Orwig KE, Brannigan RE, Woodruff TK. Fertility preservation for pediatric patients: current state and future possibilities. J Urol. 2017;198(1):186–94. https://doi.org/10.1016/j.juro.2016.09.159.
33. Keegan TH, Lichtensztajn DY, Kato I, Kent EE, Wu XC, West MM, Hamilton AS, Zebrack B, Bellizzi KM, Smith AW. Unmet adolescent and young adult cancer survivors information and service needs: a population-based cancer registry study. J Cancer Survivorship Res Pract. 2012;6(3):239–50. https://doi.org/10.1007/s11764-012-0219-9.
34. Kenney LB, Laufer MR, Grant FD, Grier H, Diller L. High risk of infertility and long term gonadal damage in males treated with high dose cyclophosphamide for sarcoma during childhood. Cancer. 2001;91(3):613–21.
35. Kohler TS, Kondapalli LA, Shah A, Chan S, Woodruff TK, Brannigan RE. Results from the survey for preservation of adolescent reproduction (SPARE) study: gender disparity in delivery of fertility preservation message to adolescents with cancer. J Assist Reprod Genet. 2011;28(3):269–77. https://doi.org/10.1007/s10815-010-9504-6.
36. LaGrandeur W, Armin J, Howe CL, Ali-Akbarian L. Survivorship care plan outcomes for primary care physicians, cancer survivors, and systems: a scoping review. J Cancer Survivorship Res Pract. 2018. https://doi.org/10.1007/s11764-017-0673-5.
37. Landier W, Bhatia S, Eshelman DA, Forte KJ, Sweeney T, Hester AL, Darling J, Armstrong FD, Blatt J, Constine LS, Freeman CR, Friedman DL, Green DM, Marina N, Meadows AT, Neglia JP, Oeffinger KC, Robison LL, Ruccione KS, Sklar CA, Hudson MM. Development of risk-based guidelines for pediatric cancer survivors: the Children's Oncology Group Long-Term Follow-Up Guidelines from the Children's Oncology Group Late Effects Committee and Nursing Discipline. J Clin Oncol Off J Am Soc Clin Oncol. 2004;22(24):4979–90. https://doi.org/10.1200/JCO.2004.11.032.
38. Loren AW, Mangu PB, Beck LN, Brennan L, Magdalinski AJ, Partridge AH, Quinn G, Wallace WH, Oktay K. Fertility preservation for patients with cancer: American Society of Clinical Oncology clinical practice guideline update. J Clin Oncol. 2013;31(19):2500–10. https://doi.org/10.1200/jco.2013.49.2678.
39. McClellan W, Klemp JR, Krebill H, Ryan R, Nelson EL, Panicker J, Sharma M, Stegenga K. Understanding the functional late effects and informational needs of adult survivors of childhood cancer. Oncol Nurs Forum. 2013;40(3):254–62. https://doi.org/10.1188/13.onf.254-262.
40. McDougall RJ, Gillam L, Delany C, Jayasinghe Y. Ethics of fertility preservation for prepubertal children: should clinicians offer procedures where efficacy is largely unproven? J Med Ethics. 2018;44(1):27–31. https://doi.org/10.1136/medethics-2016-104042.
41. Meistrich ML, Wilson G, Brown BW, da Cunha MF, Lipshultz LI. Impact of cyclophosphamide on long-term reduction in sperm count in men treated with combination chemotherapy for Ewing and soft tissue sarcomas. Cancer. 1992;70(11):2703–12.
42. Mertens AC, Yasui Y, Neglia JP, Potter JD, Nesbit ME Jr, Ruccione K, Smithson WA, Robison LL. Late mortality experience in five-year survivors of childhood and adolescent cancer: the Childhood Cancer Survivor Study. J Clin Oncol. 2001;19(13):3163–72.
43. Mertens AC, Liu Q, Neglia JP, Wasilewski K, Leisenring W, Armstrong GT, Robison LL, Yasui Y. Cause-specific late mortality among 5-year survivors of childhood cancer: the Childhood Cancer Survivor Study. J Natl Cancer Inst. 2008;100(19):1368–79. https://doi.org/10.1093/jnci/djn310.

2

44. Morgan MA, Denlinger CS. Survivorship: tools for transitioning patients with cancer. J Natl Compr Cancer Netw JNCCN. 2014;12(12):1681–7.
45. Nieman CL, Kinahan KE, Yount SE, Rosenbloom SK, Yost KJ, Hahn EA, Volpe T, Dilley KJ, Zoloth L, Woodruff TK. Fertility preservation and adolescent cancer patients: lessons from adult survivors of childhood cancer and their parents. Cancer Treat Res. 2007; 138:201–17.
46. Noone AM, Cronin KA, Altekruse SF, Howlader N, Lewis DR, Petkov VI, Penberthy L. Cancer incidence and survival trends by subtype using data from the surveillance epidemiology and end results program, 1992–2013. Cancer Epidemiol Biomark Prev. 2017;26(4):632–41. https://doi.org/10.1158/1055-9965.epi-16-0520.
47. Oeffinger KC, Mertens AC, Sklar CA, Kawashima T, Hudson MM, Meadows AT, Friedman DL, Marina N, Hobbie W, Kadan-Lottick NS, Schwartz CL, Leisenring W, Robison LL, Childhood Cancer Survivor S. Chronic health conditions in adult survivors of childhood cancer. N Engl J Med. 2006;355(15):1572–82. https://doi.org/10.1056/NEJMsa060185.
48. Oeffinger KC, Ford JS, Moskowitz CS, Diller LR, Hudson MM, Chou JF, Smith SM, Mertens AC, Henderson TO, Friedman DL, Leisenring WM, Robison LL. Breast cancer surveillance practices among women previously treated with chest radiation for a childhood cancer. JAMA J Am Med Assoc. 2009;301(4):404–14. https://doi.org/10.1001/jama.2008.1039.
49. Peccatori FA, Mangili G, Bergamini A, Filippi F, Martinelli F, Ferrari F, Noli S, Rabaiotti E, Candiani M, Somigliana E. Fertility preservation in women harboring deleterious BRCA mutations: ready for prime time? Hum Reprod. 2018;33(2):181–7. https://doi.org/10.1093/humrep/dex356.
50. Pfeifer S, Butts S, Fossum G, Gracia C, La Barbera A, Mersereau J, Odem R, Paulson R, Penzias A, Pisarska M, Rebar R, Reindollar R, Rosen M, Sandlow J, Vernon M. Optimizing natural fertility: a committee opinion. Fertil Steril. 2017;107(1):52–8. https://doi.org/10.1016/j.fertnstert.2016.09.029.
51. Practice bulletin no. 128: diagnosis of abnormal uterine bleeding in reproductive-aged women. Obstet Gynecol. 2012;120(1):197–206. https://doi.org/10.1097/AOG.0b013e318262e320.
52. Practice Committee of the American Society for Reproductive Medicine. Diagnostic evaluation of the infertile female: a committee opinion. Fertil Steril. 2015a;103(6):e44–50. https://doi.org/10.1016/j.fertnstert.2015.03.019.
53. Practice Committee of the American Society for Reproductive Medicine. Diagnostic evaluation of the infertile male: a committee opinion. Fertil Steril. 2015b;103(3):e18–25. https://doi.org/10.1016/j.fertnstert.2014.12.103.
54. Practice Committee of the American Society for Reproductive Medicine. Testing and interpreting measures of ovarian reserve: a committee opinion. Fertil Steril. 2015c;103(3):e9–17. https://doi.org/10.1016/j.fertnstert.2014.12.093.
55. Quinn GP, Vadaparampil ST, Lee JH, Jacobsen PB, Bepler G, Lancaster J, Keefe DL, Albrecht TL. Physician referral for fertility preservation in oncology patients: a national study of practice behaviors. J Clin Oncol. 2009;27(35):5952–7. https://doi.org/10.1200/jco.2009.23.0250.
56. Quinn GP, Murphy D, Knapp CA, Christie J, Phares V, Wells KJ. Coping styles of female adolescent cancer patients with potential fertility loss. J Adolesc Young Adult Oncol. 2013;2(2):66–71. https://doi.org/10.1089/jayao.2012.0038.
57. Rowley MJ, Leach DR, Warner GA, Heller CG. Effect of graded doses of ionizing radiation on the human testis. Radiat Res. 1974;59(3):665–78.
58. Salsman JM, Yanez B, Smith KN, Beaumont JL, Snyder MA, Barnes K, Clayman ML. Documentation of fertility preservation discussions for young adults with cancer: examining compliance with treatment guidelines. J Natl Compr Cancer Netw JNCCN. 2016;14(3):301–9.
59. Schover LR. Patient attitudes toward fertility preservation. Pediatr Blood Cancer. 2009;53(2):281–4. https://doi.org/10.1002/pbc.22001.
60. Seifer DB, Baker VL, Leader B. Age-specific serum anti-Mullerian hormone values for 17,120 women presenting to fertility centers within the United States. Fertil Steril. 2011;95(2):747–50. https://doi.org/10.1016/j.fertnstert.2010.10.011.
61. Shliakhtsitsava K, Romero SAD, Dewald SR, Su HI. Pregnancy and child health outcomes in pediatric and young adult leukemia and lymphoma survivors: a systematic review. Leuk Lymphoma. 2018;59(2):381–97. https://doi.org/10.1080/10428194.2017.1352097.
62. Shnorhavorian M, Harlan LC, Smith AW, Keegan TH, Lynch CF, Prasad PK, Cress RD, Wu XC, Hamilton AS, Parsons HM, Keel G, Charlesworth SE, Schwartz SM. Fertility preservation knowledge, counseling, and actions among adolescent and young adult patients with cancer: a population-based study. Cancer. 2015;121(19):3499–506. https://doi.org/10.1002/cncr.29328.
63. Skinner R, Mulder RL, Kremer LC, Hudson MM, Constine LS, Bardi E, Boekhout A, Borgmann-Staudt A, Brown MC, Cohn R, Dirksen U, Giwercman A, Ishiguro H, Jahnukainen K, Kenney LB, Loonen JJ, Meacham L, Neggers S, Nussey S, Petersen C, Shnorhavorian M, van den Heuvel-Eibrink MM, van Santen HM, Wallace WH, Green DM. Recommendations for gonadotoxicity surveillance in male childhood, adolescent, and young adult cancer survivors: a report from the International Late Effects of Childhood Cancer Guideline Harmonization Group in collaboration with the PanCareSurFup consortium. Lancet Oncol. 2017;18(2):e75–90. https://doi.org/10.1016/s1470-2045(17)30026-8.
64. Stein DM, Victorson DE, Choy JT, Waimey KE, Pearman TP, Smith K, Dreyfuss J, Kinahan KE, Sadhwani D, Woodruff TK, Brannigan RE. Fertility preservation preferences and perspectives among adult male survivors of pediatric cancer and their parents. J Adolesc Young Adult Oncol. 2014;3(2):75–82. https://doi.org/10.1089/jayao.2014.0007.

65. Steiner AZ, Pritchard D, Stanczyk FZ, Kesner JS, Meadows JW, Herring AH, Baird DD. Association between biomarkers of ovarian reserve and infertility among older women of reproductive age. JAMA. 2017;318(14):1367–76. https://doi.org/10.1001/jama.2017.14588.
66. Stieglitz E, Dinh T, Phelps AS, Pampaloni MH, Olshen AB, Robbins E. ABVD without radiation for newly diagnosed pediatric and young adult patients with Hodgkin lymphoma: a single center retrospective analysis of 28 consecutive patients. J Pediatr Hematol Oncol. 2018. https://doi.org/10.1097/mph.0000000000001094.
67. Tal R, Seifer DB. Ovarian reserve testing: a user's guide. Am J Obstet Gynecol. 2017;217(2):129–40. https://doi.org/10.1016/j.ajog.2017.02.027.
68. Trask PC, Paterson AG, Trask CL, Bares CB, Birt J, Maan C. Parent and adolescent adjustment to pediatric cancer: associations with coping, social support, and family function. J Pediatr Oncol Nurs. 2003;20(1):36–47. https://doi.org/10.1053/jpon.2003.5.
69. Vadaparampil ST, Clayton H, Quinn GP, King LM, Nieder M, Wilson C. Pediatric oncology nurses' attitudes related to discussing fertility preservation with pediatric cancer patients and their families. J Pediatr Oncol Nurs. 2007;24(5):255–63. https://doi.org/10.1177/1043454207303878.
70. Wakefield CE, Butow P, Fleming CA, Daniel G, Cohn RJ. Family information needs at childhood cancer treatment completion. Pediatr Blood Cancer. 2012;58(4):621–6. https://doi.org/10.1002/pbc.23316.
71. Woodruff TK. The emergence of a new interdiscipline: oncofertility. Cancer Treat Res. 2007;138:3–11.
72. World Health Organization. WHO laboratory manual for the examination and processing of human semen. 2010. http://apps.who.int/iris/bitstream/10665/44261/1/9789241547789_eng.pdf. Accessed 20 Feb 2018.
73. Wyns C, Collienne C, Shenfield F, Robert A, Laurent P, Roegiers L, Brichard B. Fertility preservation in the male pediatric population: factors influencing the decision of parents and children. Hum Reprod. 2015;30(9):2022–30. https://doi.org/10.1093/humrep/dev161.
74. Zebrack B. Information and service needs for young adult cancer survivors. Support Care Cancer. 2009;17(4):349–57. https://doi.org/10.1007/s00520-008-0469-2.
75. Zebrack B, Butler M. Context for understanding psychosocial outcomes and behavior among adolescents and young adults with cancer. J Natl Compr Cancer Netw JNCCN. 2012;10(9):1151–6.

Cancer Genetics: Risks and Mechanisms of Cancer in Women with Hereditary Predisposition to Epithelial Ovarian Cancer

Andrew F. Wagner, Lee P. Shulman, and Jeffrey S. Dungan

T. K. Woodruff et al. (eds.), *Textbook of Oncofertility Research and Practice*,
https://doi.org/10.1007/978-3-030-02868-8_3

3

Key Points
- Epithelial ovarian cancer is a highly lethal gynecologic malignancy, because screening modalities are unsuccessful in identifying early-stage cancers.
- Only a small percentage of cases are associated with a hereditary predisposition due to a gene mutation, such as *BRCA1/2* or the Lynch syndrome genes.
- Identifying those women who carry the hereditary predisposition for developing epithelial ovarian cancer allows them to initiate preventive and proactive measures to reduce their risk of developing epithelial ovarian cancer.
- Knowledge of a hereditary predisposition to epithelial ovarian cancer may cause women to choose preventive measures that will temporarily reduce or permanently eliminate the ability to conceive.
- Assisted reproductive technologies may allow women to reproduce or conceive even when electing to initiate preventive measures.

3.1 Introduction

In the foreword to the first book on oncofertility by Woodruff and Snyder, the authors stated that oncofertility bridges traditional areas of basic science and medical science to provide reproductive options to young people who survive life-preserving but fertility-threatening treatments for cancer [1]. Advances in technology combined with physicians' and the general public's awareness of the hereditary predisposition to cancer have found a large cohort of reproductive-aged women potentially in need of oncofertility techniques. For many women carrying a gene mutation giving her this predisposition, she may choose to have prophylactic surgery to prevent and, essentially, treat cancer. For these mutations, there are recommendations for risk-reducing salpingo-oophorectomy (RRSO) [2]. Interventions such as RRSO can adversely affect a woman's ability to conceive and carry a pregnancy. However, women who have a hereditary predisposition to develop ovarian cancer at a higher frequency and younger age than is typically observed in the general population face not only a highly lethal malignancy but also interventions that temporarily or permanently prevent them from having children. Many women, after discovering this mutation and predisposition, identify as previvors and use this knowledge to be proactive. In the public eye, knowledge of these gene mutations and the option for preventive surgery were popularized by Academy Award-winning actress, Angelina Jolie, who had prophylactic mastectomies in 2013 and a laparoscopic bilateral salpingo-oophorectomy in 2015 after finding out that she carried a *BRCA1* mutation [3]. While preventive and therapeutic interventions for other malignancies can adversely affect the ability of affected women to reproduce, epithelial ovarian cancer (EOC) is unique in that for the highest risk women, preventive interventions usually occur during the reproductive years and that the most effective prevention involves ovarian removal, reducing the capacity to produce biologic offspring. Nonetheless, advancements described throughout this book have given promise to these women.

Epithelial ovarian cancer is associated with profound morbidity and high rates of mortality, and unfortunately, no effective or agreed-upon screening protocol has been developed for all women [4]. This is the case even with advances in ultrasound technology or years of experience using the tumor marker CA-125. Most EOCs occur in postmenopausal women without a significant family history or gene mutations. Approximately 20–25% of women with EOC carry a hereditary predisposition [5]. Although the chances are more likely, gene mutations are detected in the minority of women who develop premenopausal ovarian cancer. Nonetheless, the presence of mutations in specific genes, such as *BRCA1*, *BRCA2*, or the Lynch syndrome genes, will predispose women to develop ovarian cancer at a markedly higher frequency and younger age not commonly observed in the general population. Other lower penetrance genes have been discovered, and testing is being offered clinically, but there is little doubt that changes in other genes are responsible for the development of ovarian cancers and other solid tumors. This may often involve multiple gene aberrations and the simultaneous effect of genetic and environmental factors to explain the development of most ovarian and other malignancies. Our current knowledge of the "oncogenome" relevant to EOC has expanded and changed since the last edition of this text, but it is somewhat limited to certain genes that have been associated with the development of ovarian malignancy.

There are effective preventive approaches for reproductive-aged women at increased risk for developing epithelial ovarian cancer. These approaches are invariably associated with either fertility delay (combined oral contraceptive pills (COCPs)) or permanent infertility (tubal ligation, salpingectomy, bilateral salpingo-oophorectomy). Given this, when a reproductive-aged woman is identified at an increased risk for ovarian cancer, a discussion of these preventive approaches should be a part of family planning as well as fertility preservation for those women seeking to become pregnant now or in the future.

Our knowledge of the oncogenome continues to expand and provide important information for delineating mechanisms of tumorigenesis that are of considerable value in the development of effective preventive, screening, diagnostic, and therapeutic protocols. This can be accomplished by sequencing the tumor itself. In this way, oncofertility provides a bridge from basic science to clinical practice that can empower reproductive-aged women to conceive despite undergoing interventions chosen to prevent or treat malignancy. In order to familiarize readers with those genetic findings that increase a woman's likelihood of developing ovarian cancer, this chapter will provide a review of the disease and genomic epidemiology of EOC and the genetic mechanisms associated with a predisposition to the development of epithelial ovarian cancer.

3.2 Epithelial Ovarian Cancer

Approximately 70% of ovarian malignancies are epithelial in nature and are characterized by histological subtypes such as serous, mucinous, endometrioid, and clear-cell tumors. While cervical cancer remains the most common cause of gynecologic cancer death worldwide (265,000 per year), EOC is the leading cause of death from gynecologic malignancy in the developed world. It is estimated that EOC is diagnosed in approximately 240,000 women worldwide and results in the deaths of 150,000 women each year [6]. In the United States, there are approximately 22,000 new cases of ovarian cancer diagnosed, with more than 14,000 deaths attributed to EOC annually [7]. One reason for this difference in causes of gynecologic cancer death in the industrialized and developing world is that EOC usually does not present with unique symptoms that would indicate the presence of an early malignancy, such as endometrial cancer and abnormal uterine bleeding. Additionally, there is no effective screening algorithm to identify women with early ovarian cancer, as is available worldwide with the Papanicolaou test for cervical dysplasia and cancer [8]. While early-stage EOC is associated with generally good clinical outcomes, most ovarian cancers (approximately 70%) are unfortunately detected at a more advanced stage and are associated with generally poor survival rates despite continuing advancements in surgical techniques and chemotherapy regimens [9]. The gynecologic oncology committee of the International Federation of Gynecology and Obstetrics (FIGO) incorporated EOC, fallopian tube, and primary peritoneal cancers to one unified staging approach in 2014 [10].

In addition to the lack of unique associated symptoms and an effective screening protocol, no specific patient characteristics (e.g., obesity and endometrial cancer), lifestyle issues (multiple sexual partners or smoking and cervical cancer), or environmental factors (human papilloma virus and cervical cancer) are strongly associated with the development of EOC. Nonetheless, reproductive history does provide some information in assessing a woman's risk for developing EOC. Nulliparous women in the general population are at a higher risk for developing EOC than those women who have had children [11]. The birth of the first child reduces one's risk for developing EOC by 45%, with each additional pregnancy further reducing that risk by 15% for each pregnancy [12]. There also is a known risk reduction for ovarian cancer with a younger age at first pregnancy and birth, if under age 25, the use of COCPs, and/or breastfeeding [11]. Smoking, obesity, and assisted reproductive technologies have not been shown to increase the risks for EOC [13–15].

Outside of a known mutation in a gene imparting a hereditary predisposition to ovarian cancer, family history is the strongest risk factor associated with an increased likelihood for developing EOC. A woman who has a first-degree relative (e.g., mother, sister, daughter) with EOC will have her risk increased from the baseline 1.4% population risk to 4–5%, while two affected relatives will increase a woman's risk fivefold to 7% [16]. An additional factor in assessing risk in women with a family history of EOC is the age at diagnosis; Auranen and colleagues showed that affected relatives with a diagnosis of EOC before the age of 55 conveyed a higher risk than those relatives with EOC diagnosed after the age of 55 [17].

Despite no effective screening modality yet developed for EOC, risk reduction can be achieved by both high- and low-risk women. The use of COCPs has been shown to reduce the risk of developing EOC in all women regardless of their underlying risks. The longer the use, the greater the preventive effect there is. This is better shown with *BRCA1/2* carriers in that there can be a 33–80% risk reduction with 1 year of use in BRCA1 carriers and a 58–63% risk reduction in BRCA2 carriers [18]. In most studies, the use of COCPs in *BRCA1/2* mutation carriers does not appear to be associated with a consistently increased risk for developing breast cancer [19]. Other interventions that have been associated with risk reduction include breastfeeding, tubal ligation, bilateral salpingectomy, and RRSO. All of these interventions, including the use of COCPs, are associated with an inability to conceive, with tubal ligation, salpingectomy, and RRSO associated with permanent sterilization. For reproductive-aged women seeking future childbearing, consideration of the timing of future pregnancies is critical in the choice of a risk-reducing intervention. While the removal of the tubes and ovaries is associated with the most profound reduction in risk, RRSO is the one approach that prevents any possible future childbearing using one's own oocytes. When this is performed prior to menopause, it is associated with an increased risk for premature cardiovascular morbidity, osteoporosis, cognitive impairment, and all-cause mortality if postoperative estrogen therapy is not initiated [20, 21].

3.3 Heritable Cancer Syndromes and EOC

The majority of EOC cases occur in women without a family history indicating an increased risk. However, approximately 9–24% of EOC cases are due to the woman having inherited a mutation in a gene associated with an increased predisposition to develop EOC. A number of different genes have been associated with the hereditary predisposition to EOC including hereditary breast and ovarian cancer (HBOC) syndrome, due to mutations in *BRCA1/2*, Lynch syndrome (previously referred to as hereditary nonpolyposis colorectal cancer (HNPCC) syndrome), and other genes, such as *BRIP1*, *RAD51C*, and *RAD51D*. Other genes have been identified as having an association with a hereditary risk for EOC, and are appearing on clinical laboratory panels for testing (see ▶ Sect. 3.6). These predispositions are the result of the autosomal dominant inheritance of highly penetrant germline mutations in tumor-suppressing genes. The inheritance of a mutated copy of one of these genes not only conveys a markedly increased risk for developing EOC but also increases the likelihood of developing the malignancy at a far younger age than is usually observed in the general population. It is this characteristic of hereditary ovarian cancer that profoundly impacts the woman found to be a carrier of an inherited mutation in a tumor-suppressing gene and leads many to the consideration of risk-reducing interventions that impact the ability to conceive and may preclude the possibility of any future pregnancies.

3.4 Genetic Mechanisms

The increased risk for developing cancer in women with mutations from cancer susceptibility genes begins with the inheritance of a germline mutation from either parent. While EOC can only occur in females, genes that predispose to the development of EOC are autosomal dominant in nature and thus can be inherited from either parent. This concept is critical with regard to family history information as both parents can transmit gene mutations. Based on this, obtaining careful family histories of an individual's maternal and paternal families is key to developing an accurate risk assessment. Limited family structures, such as adoption, early ages at hysterectomy/oophorectomy in family members, and smaller numbers of women in a family can make family history interpretation more difficult.

By definition, this germline mutation is present from conception, and thus, every cell of the individual will have the gene mutation, which is a fact likely associated with the multiorgan effect of many cancer susceptibility genes. Other key genetic concepts such as penetrance and variable expressivity are present with these syndromes. Penetrance refers to the proportion of individuals with a mutation causing a particular disorder who exhibit clinical symptoms of that disorder. This is why not every individual with one of these mutations will develop cancer and some will not. Variable expressivity is the variation in the type and clinical severity of clinical features in a genetic disorder between affected individuals. In practice, this is why some women with a *BRCA1* mutation will develop only breast cancer and some will only develop ovarian cancer. This is why some women with a Lynch syndrome mutation will develop endometrial cancer and some will develop ovarian cancer.

Nonetheless, the inheritance of a cancer susceptibility allele is only the *first* step in promoting the development of EOC. Its presence does not guarantee that an individual with an inherited susceptibility gene mutation will go on to develop EOC. The development of EOC, as well as other heritable cancers, depends on the occurrence of the *second* step [22]. When an individual has inherited the first "step," this explains why such individuals have a higher risk for developing cancer than the general population and why the malignancy usually occurs at a younger age. Since the mutation is present in all cells, it also explains why cancer in multiple organs is possible or, in the case of breast cancer, why bilateral disease from two separate primary cancers is more likely.

Cancer is a disease of somatic cells; however, if two or more events are needed for the cells to become malignant, then inheriting the first step, as opposed to waiting for it to occur through environmental impact, will surely increase the likelihood of it occurring compared to those who do not inherit such mutations. The second and any subsequent step is invariably somatic (or individual to the particular cell) in nature, also explaining why not everyone who inherits a susceptibility gene develops the malignancy. Molecular studies of cancers in individuals with malignancies arising from hereditary cancer syndromes frequently show a loss of heterozygosity at the genomic position of the tumor suppressor gene in the tumor tissue. The loss in heterozygosity is the second step in the development of malignancies in individuals who have inherited mutated susceptibility genes.

It is unclear from what the second step originates. There are numerous mechanisms that likely lead to this loss of heterozygosity and, thus, inactivation of the tumor-suppressing gene. While such cellular and nuclear events are common and widespread mechanisms and are mostly random processes by which genes and chromosomes are deleted, replaced, or rearranged, in the presence of an inherited gene mutation, such events can lead to the inactivation of tumor-suppressing gene function and predispose that organ to undergo malignant transformation. In such cases, this process is known as biallelic inactivation. Inherited biallelic mutations are exceedingly rare and present with a different clinical presentation than that described with monoallelic (dominant) inheritance. These, more commonly, can cause childhood malignancies.

It is interesting to note that while most hereditary cancer syndromes, including EOC, are mostly transmitted in and present as a classic autosomal dominant inherited condition, the requirement of a second step that inactivates both alleles (biallelic inactivation) makes the cellular mechanism necessary for the promotion of tumorigenesis to be recessive in nature.

3.5 Heritable Cancer Syndromes and EOC

3.5.1 Hereditary Breast and Ovarian Cancer (HBOC)

Hereditary breast and ovarian cancer syndrome (HBOC) is characterized by families with multiple members with breast cancer and EOC, with many families having more cases of breast cancer than ovarian cancer. HBOC families, like other families with hereditary cancer predisposition syndromes, are characterized by a far earlier age of onset than is seen in the general population, as well as a higher likelihood of bilateral or multiorgan disease. In addition, HBOC families have a markedly higher frequency of family members with breast cancer and EOC occurring in the same individual and, for some gene mutations, a strikingly higher risk for breast cancer in men or possibly prostate or pancreatic cancers.

The majority of families with HBOC have inherited mutations in one of two tumoruppressing genes, *BRCA1* and *BRCA2*. The name of these genes, initially discovered by Dr. Mary-Claire King, was inspired by Paul Broca, a French pathologist, who, in the 1860s, proposed that breast cancer may run in families. The name may also come from the words breast cancer or Berkeley, California, where King attended graduate school (King MC, personal communication, 10 May 2005). Ramus and colleagues showed that 81% of families with at least two cases of EOC and one case of breast cancer had a deleterious mutation in *BRCA1* or *BRCA2*, thus confirming earlier studies and models demonstrating that the majority of cases of HBOC are associated with *BRCA1/2* mutations [23, 24].

BRCA1, discovered in 1994, is located on chromosome 17q21, contains 22 coding exons, and spans 80 kb DNA, whereas *BRCA2* is located on chromosome 13q12-13, contains 26 coding exons, and spans 70 kb DNA. Both genes are part of the DNA breakage repair pathway and appear to function as tumor suppressor genes, with mutations resulting in highly penetrant susceptibility to breast cancer and EOC. Mutations of *BRCA1/2* associated with the development of EOC and breast cancer are found throughout the coding regions and at splice sites. Most of these mutations are small insertions or deletions that lead to frameshift mutations, nonsense mutations, or splice site alterations, all of which lead to premature protein termination and altered or absent proteins [25]. In addition to these mutations and some missense mutations, large deletions and rearrangements not detectable by standard PCR have been identified and have become routinely part of the molecular testing provided to those undergoing *BRCA1/2* analysis [26]. Indeed, these large genomic alterations have been found to be relatively common in some populations from central Europe and the United States [27].

As *BRCA1/2* are autosomal genes with high penetrance, transmission can occur either maternally or paternally. Based on this, equal attention must be paid to the paternal relatives of a woman being evaluated for a possible mutation. *BRCA1* mutations do not frequently result in increased risk for cancer in men, but *BRCA2* mutations increase the risk for male breast cancer. Not seeing cancers in men in a family does not exclude the possibility that a mutation may be paternally inherited. While those families with either few members or few females pose a challenge in counseling, as affected females provide the main evidence of the existence of a deleterious *BRCA1/2* mutation, this perceived skewing of parental transmission shows that in many cases, affected females in the paternal lineage are either ignored or not considered on an equal status with affected members from the maternal lineage. This may occur because of a misperception that HBOC is a disease of women and that genetic events in paternal families do not play an important role. Both sides of the family must be considered in performing a risk assessment of family history [28].

The frequency of *BRCA1/2* mutations in the general population is estimated to be 1/300–800 [29]. *BRCA1/2* mutations are found in approximately 6–8% of EOC cases but in 80–90% of hereditary breast-ovarian cancer syndrome and in 65–85% of hereditary ovarian syndromes (see ◘ Fig. 3.1) [30, 31]. Certain populations and communities have a higher frequency of *BRCA1/2* mutations than that found in the general population. In the United States, *BRCA1/2* mutations are found in approximately 1 of every 40 individuals of Eastern European (Ashkenazi) Jewish ancestry, a frequency far higher than the general US population [32]. Specifically, three mutations (c.68_69delAG and c.5266dupC in *BRCA1* and

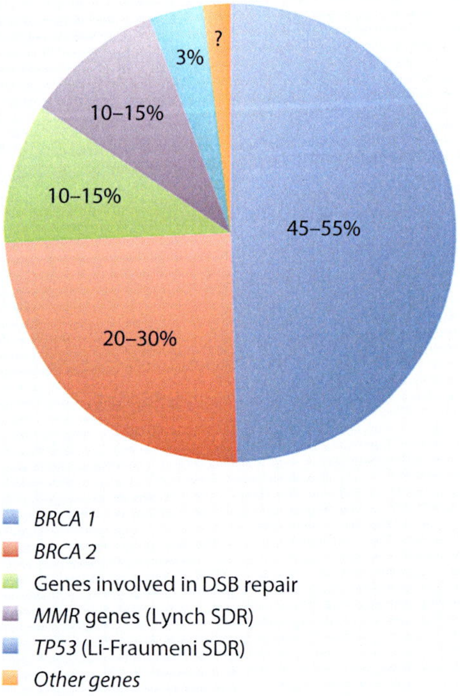

◘ **Fig. 3.1** Proportion of hereditary predisposition gene mutations associated with EOC. (With permission from Toss et al. [31])

c.5946delT in *BRCA2*) account for approximately 90% of mutations detected [33] In Iceland, the c.771_775del5 mutation in *BRCA2* accounts for approximately 8% of all cases of EOC occurring in Icelanders [34]. These mutations are known as "founder mutations," because in certain populations begun by a small ancestral group initially isolated by societal behavior, geography, or geopolitical events, certain gene variants in the original "founders" of a population can become far more common in succeeding generations than would occur in the general population.

The identification of founder mutations allows for more facile screening of individuals of those groups associated with founder mutations. As such, evaluating individuals of Ashkenazi ancestry for a *BRCA1/2* mutation can be accomplished by first determining the presence of one of these three mutations, unless previous analysis of an affected relative revealed a different (nonfounder) BRCA mutation associated with breast or ovarian cancer. However, it would be best if a "single site" analysis would be augmented with a three-site founder mutation analysis if the family history has Ashkenazi heritage on the other side of the family, due to the relatively high prevalence. If testing for a founder mutation is found to be negative, then gene sequencing and rearrangement analysis should be offered to provide a complete and thorough molecular evaluation. It is acceptable to initially proceed with sequencing and rearrangement analysis of both genes whether these two genes are the first ones tested or, now more commonly, as part of a multigene testing panel.

BRCA1 mutations appear to confer a higher risk for developing EOC than *BRCA2* mutations. Estimates of the prevalence of ovarian cancer in women with BRCA1 mutations range from 37% to 63% by the age of 70 and from 10% to 27% in BRCA2 mutation carriers [32, 35–40]. *BRCA1/2* mutations are associated with the development of serous epithelial ovarian cancers, as opposed to mucinous or borderline subtypes.

3.5.2 Lynch Syndrome

Lynch syndrome was originally described by Dr. Henry Lynch in 1966 using inspiration from a 1913 work by Dr. Aldred Scott Warthin [41]. The initial work followed families with strong family histories of nonpolyposis colorectal cancer. The name of the syndrome migrated to be known as hereditary nonpolyposis colorectal cancer (HNPCC) syndrome. As it was realized that other organ systems were also a part of the syndrome, such as endometrial, urogenital, pancreatic, and biliary tract and EOC, it is again known as Lynch syndrome. In women, the risk for colorectal cancer ranges from 18% to 53%, endometrial cancer from 16% to 60%, and EOC from 4% to 12% [42–47]. It should be noted that the risk to develop endometrial cancer may be higher in women than colorectal cancer.

Lynch syndrome mutations are seen in approximately 1:440 individuals [48]. Lynch syndrome is a result of gene mutations in the multistep mismatch repair (MMR) system. MMR genes are located on five different chromosomes and encode for proteins that recognize and repair damage in the DNA that leads to DNA mismatches. One complex of proteins consisting of the protein MSH2 combined with MSH6 or MSH3 recognizes the DNA mismatch and binds to the site. An inactivating mutation of *MSH2* blocks the ability to recognize a DNA mismatch negating the function of this complex. Mutations of either *MSH6* or *MSH3*, on the other hand, may not have a similar deleterious effect as these two proteins have overlapping functions and thus, an inactivating or adverse mutation in one may not adversely affect the function of the overall MMR system. Once the mismatch is recognized, *MLH1* (with *PMS2*) then provides the necessary steps to resynthesize the DNA strand in its original and correct sequence. A total of five MMR enzymes have been delineated, and mutations in each of these genes have been identified, namely, *MLH1*, *MSH2*, *MSH6*, *PMS2*, and *EPCAM*. Mutations in the *MLH1* and *MSH2* genes are the most common and account for approximately 90% of observed mutations, followed in frequency by mutations in MSH6 and PMS2. ◘ Table 3.1 shows genes associated with the mismatch repair system [44, 49–56].

It was surmised that the genetic mechanism for the increased risk for carcinogenesis in cases of MMR gene mutations was similar to that of BRCA mutations, Knudson's two-hit hypothesis. Dominant inheritance of a mutation provided for the germline "first-step" and that a second somatic step led to the loss of the normal or "wild-type" co-allele and that this loss of heterozygosity eventually promoted the cellular aberration that resulted in malignant transformation of the cell

3

Table 3.1 Genes associated with mismatch repair system [44, 49–56]

Gene name	Frequency in Lynch pts	Chromosome locus
MLH1	50%	3p21.3
MSH2	40%	2p22-p21
MSH6	7–10%	2p16
PMS2	<5%	7p22
EPCAM	~1–3%	2p21

and, eventually, the organ. However, Aaltonen and colleagues found no loss of heterozygosity at a locus coinciding with the MSH2 site on chromosome 2 linked to colorectal cancer in 14 cases from three families, suggesting a cellular mechanism different from the conventional mechanism attributed to biallelic inactivation and alteration of tumor-suppressing gene function in the development of tumors. Another explanation for the findings by Aaltonen and colleagues is that the MMR gene mutation, without the loss of heterozygosity, adversely affects the DNA mismatch repair mechanism, leading to a "domino-like" dysfunctional cascade on those cellular mechanisms responsible for proper growth and function [57]. Perhaps, the surprising findings of no loss of heterozygosity in Lynch colorectal cancer cases indicate that the genes being disrupted in the Lynch syndrome are those genes responsible for maintaining the proper DNA sequence and that adversely affecting their function, even with a only single allele and the maintenance of the wild-type allele, may be sufficient to initiate abnormal cellular and nuclear processes that lead to carcinogenesis.

These inactivating mutations not only prevent the repair of damaged DNA but also increase the rate of mutations at the DNA microsatellites of growth-regulating genes. Microsatellites are short, 1–5 base pair long, polymorphic DNA sequences that are repeated 15–30 times at a given locus and distributed throughout the genome. Microsatellite instability (MSI) thus serves as a marker for MMR mutations. Analysis for microsatellite instability or immunohistochemical (IHC) staining is the first diagnostic step in determining the presence of a DNA repair defect for colon and endometrial tumors [58]. IHC can evaluate tumor tissue for the presence or absence of the proteins MLH1, MSH2, MSH6, and PMS2 but cannot assess the functionality of any of these proteins. IHC cannot determine whether the protein present does not function properly because of a missense mutation or due to hypermethylation, an epigenetic effect, and thus cannot definitively identify the gene with the mutation. IHC should be combined with MSI to screen prospective tumors for MMR mutations. MSI is a common feature of Lynch-associated tumors; however, studies of MSI in the ovarian tumor tissue from EOC have not provided consistent diagnostic correlation [59].

Although *BRCA1/2* mutation accounts for the majority of cases of hereditary EOC, Lynch syndrome mutations account for a smaller proportion of EOC cases, approximately 10–15% (see Fig. 3.1) [31]. As stated, ovarian cancer associated with *BRCA1/2* mutations are mostly serous in nature. Lynch mutation-related ovarian cancer is associated with a variety of ovarian cancer histologies including endometrioid and clear-cell cancers.

Assessing a family for Lynch syndrome is accomplished by determining whether the history meets Amsterdam II criteria. If a family history is suggestive of Lynch syndrome but the criteria cannot be met because of family size or other factors, consideration of risk can be accomplished using revised Bethesda criteria. The National Comprehensive Cancer Network (NCCN) has a separate set of criteria that incorporates the above systems with updated literature reviews and is frequently updated [60]. Women with Lynch mutations do not have an associated increased risk for developing breast cancer; as such, family histories with multiple family members with ovarian cancer and no cases of breast cancer, but having family members with Lynch-associated malignancies (e.g., colorectal cancer, endometrial cancer), could first be evaluated for MMR mutations rather than *BRCA1/2* mutations if a multigene panel is not initially chosen.

The lifetime risk for developing EOC in women with a Lynch syndrome mutation is 4–12%, which is a tenfold increase over the general population risk (1–1.5%) but less than the risk associated with *BRCA1/2* mutations. Most cases of ovarian cancer in Lynch syndrome families are malignant epithelial tumors, most of which are well or moderately differentiated and are FIGO Stage I or II at the time of diagnosis. This is in sharp contradistinction to *BRCA1/2* mutation-associated tumors, which tend to present in a more advanced stage and be more poorly differentiated. As with other cancer susceptibility genes, certain mutations in particular populations may exert a different impact on cancer risk than that typically observed in the general population. However, similar to women with *BRCA1/2* mutations, women with Lynch mutations tend to develop EOC at a younger age.

3.6 Other Genes Related to EOC

At the time of this publication, three other genes have testing, screening, and management guidelines by the NCCN. These include *BRIP1*, *RAD51C*, and *RAD51D* [2]. Advances in technology, primarily utilizing multigene testing panels, have made testing for many genes outside of *BRCA1/2* and the Lynch syndrome genes much more easily clinically available.

BRIP1 is a gene in the Fanconi anemia pathway on chromosome 17q23.2. It is named for *BRCA1*-Interacting Protein 1 as it can bind to the C terminus of the BRCA1 protein. *BRIP1* mutations can alter the ability to assist in double-strand break repairs [61]. These mutations have been associated with a lifetime risk of ovarian cancer up to 5.8% [62]. Unlike *BRCA1*, *BRIP1* has not been associated with an increased risk for breast cancer [63].

RAD51C and *RAD51D* are part of the RAD51 family of genes. They code for strand-transfer proteins which are involved in the recombinational repair of DNA damage and in meiotic recombination [64]. *RAD51C* on chromosome 17q22 was first suspected to be involved in ovarian cancer in 2010, and *RAD51D* on chromosome 17q12 had its first ovarian cancer publication in 2011 [65, 66]. NCCN compared these genes' risks for ovarian cancer to the lifetime risk of a woman without a *BRCA1/2* mutation to develop ovarian cancer, 2.6%, in order to determine if there was enough evidence to assign a greater risk [67]. *RAD51C* mutations increase the risk for ovarian cancer at 60–64 years of age. *RAD51D* imparts this risk at 50–54 years of age [68]. The 2.6% figure was used to determine a mutation's excess risk in order to validate performing an RRSO.

Other genes related to ovarian cancer have been proposed. Their risks are not as well-established, but through various clinical laboratories, testing is available. These genes include *CHEK2*, *MRE11A*, *NBN*, *PALB2*, *RAD50*, and *TP53*. *TP53* is the gene, when mutated, which is responsible for Li-Fraumeni syndrome. This syndrome is characterized by a wide spectrum of cancers, especially at young ages. Soft tissue sarcomas, osteosarcomas, premenopausal breast cancer (<31 years of age), colon cancer, brain tumors, adrenocortical tumors, and others have been associated with this rare cancer predisposition syndrome (see Fig. 3.1). The lifetime rates for cancer approach 100% in men and women [69]. Current guidelines for mutations in *TP53* or *CHEK2* and *NBN* (both low penetrance breast cancer genes) mutations do not advocate for RRSO [2].

3.7 Counseling of Women at Increased Risk for Developing EOC

Even though only a small percentage of ovarian cancers can be attributed to a hereditary predisposition to cancer, identifying those women at risk for inheriting a susceptibility gene is critical in order to provide optimal care and management. Such knowledge can modify medical care for screening, chemoprophylaxis, and/or prophylactic surgery. As hereditary EOC tends to occur at an earlier age than sporadic cases, given the lack of an effective screening protocol, it is important to identify these high-risk women so that prevention and management options can be provided. These typically occur during a woman's reproductive years. While effective breast screening protocols do exist for women at increased risk for breast cancer, and while some of the preventive interventions for breast cancer can reduce fertility, such as chemoprophylaxis with a selective estrogen receptor modulator (SERM) like tamoxifen, all of the preventive measures available to reduce the risk of EOC in high-risk and low-risk women involve temporary or permanent inhibition of fertility.

Personalizing these interventions can allow a clinician to provide an optimal balance for reducing the risk of EOC and allowing a woman to maintain her reproductive capacity for as long as she wishes to conceive. This is a key goal of cancer genetics programs. Conversely, testing the entire population for susceptibility genes is not currently feasible because of economic factors and the relatively low frequency of these deleterious genes in the general population. Currently, the most effective tool for determining the risk for hereditary EOC and for providing genetic testing is genetic counseling and cancer risk assessment.

The primary care provider holds the key to the effective identification of those individuals at an increased risk for hereditable cancers. A thorough assessment of the family history is the most vital component. Individuals with a personal or family history suggestive of a hereditary predisposition or familial cancer, due to a combination of multiple genetic and environmental factors, should be referred for further counseling and cancer risk assessment. This can be performed at a genetics center, oncology center, or any facility that has trained personnel equipped to properly evaluate personal and family histories and to perform a cancer risk assessment. Such personnel are, but are not necessarily limited to, genetic counselors, clinical geneticists, oncologists, gynecologists, internists, family medicine providers, nurse practitioners, or other professionals who provide care to those who are at risk for cancer and cancer syndromes and who have the expertise and interest to do so.

Patients should never be coerced into undergoing cancer risk assessments or genetic testing. The long-standing tenet of nondirective counseling must be followed when discussing cancer risk with patients, and patient autonomy must always be respected. Counseling should be there to empower individuals to make informed decisions about their health management and not to dictate or mandate individuals to undergo or forego certain tests or management options based on the opinions of the genetic counselor or provider. Women who are identified as being at an increased risk for hereditary predisposition to EOC by their primary care provider may benefit from a thorough and detailed discussion with a specialist about their risk for developing cancer, the screening and testing that is available to define their actual risk, and the preventive interventions that are available to them, even if they ultimately choose to decline or postpone any further evaluation or risk-reducing intervention. In addition to providing information that can reduce morbidity and mortality, this counseling can also address the anxiety and the numerous psychosocial issues that a personal or family history or cancer can induce.

The process used to identify and logistics used to refer women at an increased risk for hereditary cancer syndromes may be hampered by the considerable barriers to such endeavors. Taking a family history involves time, which is something very limited in most primary care providers' daily schedules. For those clinicians who are able to develop detailed family histories, existing electronic medical record systems frequently do not easily facilitate the updating of such detailed family history information in an organized fashion. Having multiple different cancers in a family may be independent, but some combinations of cancers may indicate a higher risk for a completely different cancer syndrome. Identification of more complicated family histories and a referral to a provider more experienced in these assessments are key. A joint document between the American College of Genetics and Genomics and the National Society of Genetic Counselors was written to simplify and help guide providers in learning which genes to focus given a personal and/or family history of cancer [70]. As previously stated, the NCCN has well-delineated and frequently updated criteria for who would deserve genetic counseling and testing for many syndromes, including Lynch and HBOC [60].

When a woman is referred for further counseling, a specific cancer risk assessment can be performed. While risk models are not available for all malignancies, risk models are available for HBOC and EOC. Risk models take into account a wide spectrum of family risk factors including age of onset, number and relation of affected members, and presence of associated cancers among other personal and disease characteristics. It is again important to emphasize that cancer susceptibility genes are autosomal and thus transmissible by either one's father or one's mother. Attention must be paid to both sides of the family, with the recognition that families with relatively few females may be difficult to identify as being a family with a cancer susceptibility gene for EOC because of the relatively few individuals with a potential for ovarian cancer and the phenotypic expression of the mutated susceptibility gene.

When genetic testing is decided upon, it is optimal to test the affected family member(s), as such individuals' test results are the most informative for the family and they are most likely to possess a deleterious mutation. This is obviously not always possible, so, in such cases, testing those family members who are most closely related to those affected members is appropriate. One should be aware that such testing is not always possible and testing individuals who are neither affected nor closely related to affected members may be appropriate. These individuals' test results, especially when negative, may not be able to eliminate the possibility that there is a hereditary predisposition in the family. In some cases, family members who are either affected or closely related to affected relatives may choose not to test or choose to not release test results, requiring less closely related family members to get testing to determine their mutation status.

Genetic tests for these predisposition mutations are resulted as negative or having a sequence variant. Negative means that the genetic sequence for that gene is the wild-type as previously defined. If there is a variant in the sequence, this is further subdivided into "pathogenic," "likely pathogenic," "uncertain significance," "likely benign," and "benign" [71]. Pathogenic or likely pathogenic variants have been shown in clinical practice or by rigorous laboratory modeling to lead to a hereditary predisposition. Benign or likely benign refers to gene changes shown not to have a harmful effect or impart a hereditary predisposition. To be in the likely categories, there needs to be 90% certainty. In the middle is a variant of uncertain significance (VUS), which can be quite confusing in a clinical and counseling sense. These are sequence variants that have lack of clarity or disagreements in their definition. These variants can be reclassified with further knowledge from research and reporting of data. Caution must be made to not overcall or act on a result without a well-defined clinical meaning.

3.8 Surgical Intervention and Afterward

Given the fact that the screening options for EOC are not agreed upon nor have they been shown to be effective, surgical removal of the fallopian tubes and ovaries is the most definitive method to decrease a woman's risk for EOC. A meta-analysis has shown the decrease in EOC risk by 80% in *BRCA1/2* carriers [72]. When performed prior to menopause, there is an added decrease in breast cancer risk by 37–100% [73]. The fallopian tubes are included, as it is now believed that the tube is the origin for many ovarian and peritoneal cancers and fallopian tube cancer is a part of both the spectra of HBOC and Lynch syndromes [74]. It is felt that 60% of ovarian cancers originate in the tubes [75]. A precursor lesion in the tube, called serous tubal intraepithelial carcinoma (STIC), is being increasingly identified and is seen more often in *BRCA1/2* carriers, up to 10–15% [76]. STIC lesions and a different precursor lesion, somatic *TP53* mutant single epithelial layers, can also be seen in women without a hereditary predisposition [77].

Some women choose to have a salpingectomy prior to an oophorectomy, especially if they have completed childbearing but they are not yet ready for surgical menopause. Salpingectomy can be done to achieve female permanent sterilization. Traditional tubal ligation, in which a segment of the fallopian tubes is removed to achieve sterilization, has been shown to decrease the risk for ovarian cancer. Studies looking at salpingectomy in an unselected population showed a decrease in EOC rate of up to 65% [78]. There now are debates on the necessity of, surgical ease with, and cancer prevention related to salpingectomy as a means for sterilization or as a part of a hysterectomy for benign reasons [79].

After removal of the ovaries, the woman is no longer able to produce oocytes; however, it is not impossible for her to achieve a pregnancy through assisted reproductive technologies. She could use a donor oocyte to get pregnant, or with advance planning, she could have had an oocyte retrieval and use her own. With her own oocytes, through in vitro fertilization, the embryos could undergo preimplantation genetic testing for the known familial mutation. After these studies are completed, she could choose to only transfer back an embryo(s) which do not carry the mutation. This option is also possible when the male partner is a carrier for such a mutation or after salpingectomy when she has her ovaries intact.

3.9 Conclusions

Epithelial ovarian cancer is a highly lethal gynecologic malignancy, primarily because screening modalities are, in most cases, unable to detect early, and more treatable, stages of EOC. Most cases of EOC are not associated with a family history and appear to be sporadic in nature with some risk modification from a woman's reproductive history and exposure to COCPs. Only a small percentage of cases are associated with a hereditary predisposition due to a gene mutation, such as *BRCA1/2* or the Lynch syndrome genes. Such cases are likely to occur bilaterally and develop earlier in life than EOC in the general population, making the identification of such individuals an important priority. However, until an effective and agreed-upon screening modality is available for the general population, analysis of family history and cancer risk assessment followed by genetic testing the right individuals will remain the main tools to assess one's risk for developing EOC.

Identifying those women who carry the hereditary predisposition for developing EOC allows them to initiate preventive and proactive measures to reduce their risk of developing EOC. Because these measures either temporarily reduce or permanently eliminate the ability to conceive, appropriate counseling of these women regarding their plans and desires for reproduction is crucial. The identification of these high-risk women through family history and genetic testing also brings the consideration of reproductive technologies into the discussion. These technologies may allow women to reproduce or conceive even when electing to initiate preventive measures. They also may be able to prevent future inheritance of these gene mutations through preimplantation genetic testing. This brings oncofertility counseling and interventions for reproductive-aged women at increased risk for EOC into the primary care, gynecologic, and genetic scopes of practice. This becomes important for providing effective overall care to these women and the potential for reproduction for women seeking EOC prevention with contraceptives, elective sterilization, or risk-reducing surgical measures.

Review Questions and Answers

Q1. CA-125 levels and pelvic ultrasounds have been shown to successfully identify epithelial ovarian cancer in an early or precancerous stage. True or False?

A1. False

Q2. *BRCA1/2* mutations:
(a) Are only inherited through the maternal line
(b) Are only inherited through the paternal line
(c) Can be seen more frequently in certain ethnicities as a founder mutation
(d) Guarantee that a carrier will develop epithelial ovarian cancer
(e) Increase the risk for colon cancer in carriers

A2. (c)

Q3. Lynch syndrome gene mutations:
(a) Are associated with familial adenomatous polyposis
(b) Are responsible for more epithelial ovarian cancer cases than *BRCA1/2* mutations
(c) Do not increase the risk for urogenital cancer
(d) Have an ethnic predilection
(e) May cause more endometrial cancer than ovarian cancer

A3. (e)

Q4. 60% of ovarian cancers originate in the fallopian tubes. True or false?

A4. True

Q5. The most important element of cancer risk assessment is taking an accurate family history. True or false?

A5. True

References

1. Woodruff TK, Snyder KA, editors. Oncofertility. Chicago: Springer; 2007.
2. National Comprehensive Cancer Network. Genetic/familial high-risk assessment: breast and ovarian. Version 1.2018—October 3, 2017. 2017. https://www.nccn.org/professionals/physician_gls/pdf/genetics_screening.pdf. Accessed 18 Apr 2018.
3. Jolie Pitt A. Angelina Jolie Pitt: diary of a surgery. The New York Times [online]. 2015. p. 1. Available at: https://www.nytimes.com/2015/03/24/opinion/angelina-jolie-pitt-diary-of-a-surgery.html. Accessed 18 Apr 2018.
4. Schorge JO, Modesitt SC, Coleman RL, et al. SGO White Paper on ovarian cancer: etiology, screening and surveillance. Gynecol Oncol. 2010;119(1):7–17.
5. Walsh T, Casadei S, Lee MK, et al. Mutations in 12 genes for inherited ovarian, fallopian tube, and peritoneal carcinoma identified by massively parallel sequencing. Proc Natl Acad Sci U S A. 2011;108(44):18032–7.

6. International Agency for Research on Cancer (World Health Organization). In GLOBOCAN 2012: estimated cancer incidence mortality and prevalence worldwide in 2012. 2012. http://globocan.iarc.fr/Pages/fact_sheets_population.aspx. Accessed 19 Apr 2018.
7. American Cancer Society. In cancer facts & figures, 2018. 2018. https://www.cancer.org/content/dam/cancer-org/research/cancer-facts-and-statistics/annual-cancer-facts-and-figures/2018/cancer-facts-and-figures-2018.pdf. Accessed 20 Apr 2018.
8. Nelson HD, Fu R, Goddard K, et al. Risk assessment, genetic counseling, and genetic testing for BRCA-related cancer: systematic review to update the U.S. Preventive Services Task Force recommendation. (2014). Ann Intern Med. 2013;160(4):255–66.
9. Sopik V, Iqbal J, Rosen B, et al. Why have ovarian cancer mortality rates declined? Part I. Incidence. Gynecol Oncol. 2015;138:741–9.
10. Berek JS, Crum C, Friedlander M. Cancer of the ovary, fallopian tube, and peritoneum. Int J Gynecol Obstet. 2015;131:S111–22.
11. Fleming GF, Seidman J, Lengyel E. Epithelial ovarian cancer. In: Barakat RR, Markman M, Randall ME, editors. Principles and practice of gynecologic oncology. 6th ed. Philadelphia: Lippincott Williams & Wilkins; 2013. p. 757–847.
12. Hankinson SE, Colditz GA, Hunter DJ, et al. A prospective study of reproductive factors and risk of epithelial ovarian cancer. Cancer. 1995;76:284–90.
13. Wentzensen N, Poole EM, Trabert B, et al. Ovarian cancer risk factors by histologic subtype: an analysis from the Ovarian Cancer Cohort Consortium. J Clin Oncol. 2016;34:2888–98.
14. van Leeuwen FE, Klip H, Mooij TM, et al. Risk of borderline and invasive ovarian tumours after ovarian stimulation for in vitro fertilization in a large Dutch cohort. Hum Reprod. 2011;26:3456–65.
15. Olsen CM, Nagle CM, Whiteman DC, et al. Obesity and risk of ovarian cancer subtypes: evidence from the Ovarian Cancer Association Consortium. Endocr Relat Cancer. 2013;20:251–62.
16. Bristow R, Armstrong D, editors. Early diagnosis and treatment of cancer: ovarian. Cambridge, MA: Elsevier; 2009.
17. Auranen A, Pukkala E, Makinen J, et al. Cancer incidence in the first degree relatives of ovarian cancer patients. Br J Cancer. 1996;74:280–4.
18. Friebel TM, Domchek SM, Rebbeck TR. Modifiers of cancer risk in BRCA1 and BRCA2 mutation carriers: systematic review and meta-analysis. J Natl Cancer Inst. 2014. https://doi.org/10.1093/jnci/dju091.
19. Moorman PG, Havrilesky LJ, Gierisch JM, et al. Oral contraceptives and risk of ovarian cancer and breast cancer among high-risk women: a systematic review and meta- analysis. J Clin Oncol. 2013;31:4188–98.
20. Shuster LT, Gostout BS, Grossardt BR, et al. Prophylactic oophorectomy in premenopausal women and long-term health. Menopause Int. 2008;14:111–6.
21. Parker WH, Broder MS, Chang E, et al. Ovarian conservation at the time of hysterectomy and long-term health outcomes in the nurses' health study. Obstet Gynecol. 2009;113:1027–37.
22. Knudson AG. Two genetic hits (more or less) to cancer. Nat Rev Cancer. 2001;1:157–62.
23. Ramus SJ, Harrington PA, Pye C, et al. Contribution of BRCA1 and BRCA2 mutations to inherited ovarian cancer. Hum Mutat. 2007;28:1207–15.
24. Bewtra C, Watson P, Conway T, et al. Hereditary ovarian cancer: a clinicopathological study. Int J Gynecol Pathol. 1992;11:180–7.
25. Rebbeck TR, Mitra N, Wan F, et al. Association of type and location of *BRCA1* and *BRCA2* mutations with risk of breast and ovarian cancer. JAMA. 2015;313(13):1347–61.
26. Ewald IP, Ribeiro PL, Palmero EI, et al. Genomic rearrangements in BRCA1 and BRCA2: a literature review. Genet Mol Biol. 2009;32:437–46.
27. Walsh T, Casadei S, Coats KH, et al. Spectrum of mutations in BRCA1, BRCA2, CHEK2, and TP53 in families at high risk of breast cancer. JAMA. 2006;295:1379–88.
28. Senst N, Llacuachaqui M, Lubinski J, et al. Parental origin of mutation and the risk of breast cancer in a prospective study of women with a *BRCA1* or *BRCA2* mutation. Clin Genet. 2013;84(1):43–6.
29. Whittemore AS, Balise RR, Pharoah PD, et al. Oral contraceptive use and ovarian cancer risk among carriers of BRCA1 or BRCA2 mutations. Br J Cancer. 2004;91:1911–5.
30. Lynch HT, Casey MJ, Snyder CL, et al. Hereditary ovarian carcinoma: heterogeneity, molecular genetics, pathology, and management. Mol Oncol. 2009;3:97–137.
31. Toss A, Tomasello C, Razzaboni E, et al. Hereditary ovarian cancer: not only BRCA 1 and 2 genes. Biomed Res Int. 2015;2015:341723. https://doi.org/10.1155/2015/341723.
32. King MC, Marks JH, Mandell JB, et al. Breast and ovarian cancer risks due to inherited mutations in BRCA1 and BRCA2. Science. 2003;302:643–6.
33. Rosenthal E, Moyes K, Arnell C, et al. Incidence of *BRCA1* and *BRCA2* non-founder mutations in patients of Ashkenazi Jewish ancestry. Breast Cancer Res Treat. 2015;149:223–7.
34. Johannesdottir G, Gudmundsson J, Bergthorsson JT, et al. High prevalence of the 999del5 mutation in Icelandic breast and ovarian cancer patients. Cancer Res. 1996;56(16):3663–5.
35. Ford D, Easton DF, Stratton M, et al. Genetic heterogeneity and penetrance analysis of the BRCA1 and BRCA2 genes in breast cancer families. The Breast Cancer Linkage Consortium. Am J Hum Genet. 1998;62:676–89.
36. Antoniou A, Pharoah PD, Narod S, et al. Average risks of breast and ovarian cancer associated with BRCA1 or BRCA2 mutations detected in case series unselected for family history: a combined analysis of 22 studies. Am J Hum Genet. 2003;72:1117–30.
37. Chen S, Parmigiani G. Meta-analysis of BRCA1 and BRCA2 penetrance. J Clin Oncol. 2007;25:1329–33.
38. Easton DF, Ford D, Bishop DT. Breast and ovarian cancer incidence in BRCA1-mutation carriers. Breast Cancer Linkage Consortium. Am J Hum Genet. 1995;56:265–71.
39. Satagopan JM, Boyd J, Kauff ND, et al. Ovarian cancer risk in Ashkenazi Jewish carrier of BRCA1 and BRCA2 mutations. Clin Cancer Res. 2002;8:3776–81.

40. Mavaddat N, Peock S, Frost D, et al. Cancer risks for BRCA1 and BRCA2 mutation carriers: results from prospective analysis of EMBRACE. J Natl Cancer Inst. 2013;105:812–22.
41. Boland CR, Lynch HT. The history of Lynch syndrome. Familial Cancer. 2013;12(2):145–57.
42. Meyer LA, Broaddus RR, Lu KH. Endometrial cancer and Lynch syndrome: clinical and pathologic considerations. Cancer Control. 2009;16:14–22.
43. Barrow E, Hill J, Evans DG. Cancer risk in Lynch syndrome. Familial Cancer. 2013;12:229–40.
44. Senter L, Clendenning M, Sotamaa K, et al. The clinical phenotype of Lynch syndrome due to germline PMS2 mutations. Gastroenterology. 2008;135:419–28.
45. Baglietto L, Lindor NM, Dowty DM, et al. Risks of Lynch syndrome cancers for MSH6 mutation carriers. J Natl Cancer Inst. 2010;102:193–201.
46. Bonadona V, Bonaïti B, Olschwang S, et al. Cancer risks associated with germline mutations in MLH1, MSH2, and MSH6 genes in Lynch syndrome. JAMA. 2011;305:2304–10.
47. Giardiello FM, Allen JI, Axilbund JE, et al. Guidelines on genetic evaluation and management of Lynch syndrome: a consensus statement by the US Multi-society Task Force on colorectal cancer. Am J Gastroenterol. 2014;109:1159–79.
48. Chen S, Wang W, Lee S, et al. Prediction of germline mutations and cancer risk in the Lynch syndrome. JAMA. 2006;296:1479–87.
49. Smith MJ, Urquhart JE, Harkness EF, et al. The contribution of whole gene deletions and large rearrangements to the mutation spectrum in inherited tumor predisposing syndromes. Hum Mutat. 2016;37:250–6.
50. Miyaki M, Konishi M, Tanaka K, et al. Germline mutation of MSH6 as the cause of hereditary nonpolyposis colorectal cancer. Nat Genet. 1997;17:271–2.
51. Berends MJ, Wu Y, Sijmons RH, et al. Molecular and clinical characteristics of MSH6 variants: an analysis of 25 index carriers of a germline variant. Am J Hum Genet. 2002;70:26–37.
52. Peltomäki P. Role of DNA mismatch repair defects in the pathogenesis of human cancer. J Clin Oncol. 2003; 21:1174–9.
53. Hegde M, Ferber M, Mao R, et al. ACMG technical standards and guidelines for genetic testing for inherited colorectal cancer (Lynch syndrome, familial adenomatous polyposis, and MYH-associated polyposis). Genet Med. 2014;16:101–16.
54. Niessen RC, Hofstra RM, Westers H, et al. Germline hypermethylation of MLH1 and EPCAM deletions are a frequent cause of Lynch syndrome. Genes Chromosome Cancer. 2009;48:737–44.
55. Goel A, Nguyen TP, Leung HC, et al. De novo constitutional MLH1 epimutations confer early-onset colorectal cancer in two new sporadic Lynch syndrome cases, with derivation of the epimutation on the paternal allele in one. Int J Cancer. 2011;128:869–78.
56. Kuiper RP, Vissers LE, Venkatachalam R, et al. Recurrence and variability of germline EPCAM deletions in Lynch syndrome. Hum Mutat. 2011;32:407–14.
57. Aaltonen LA, Peltomaki P, Leach FS, et al. Clues to the pathogenesis of familial colorectal cancer. Science. 1993;260:812–6.
58. American College of Obstetricians and Gynecologists. Lynch syndrome. Practice bulletin no. 147. Obstet Gynecol. 2014;124:1042–54.
59. Lee JH, Cragun D, Thompson Z, et al. Association between IHC and MSI testing to identify mismatch repair-deficient patients with ovarian cancer. Genet Test Mol Biomark. 2014;18(4):229–35.
60. National Comprehensive Cancer Network. NCCN guidelines for detection, prevention, & risk reduction. 2018. https://www.nccn.org/professionals/physician_gls/default.aspx#detection. Accessed 2 May 2018.
61. Cantor SB, Bell DW, Ganesan S, et al. BACH1, a novel helicase-like protein, interacts directly with BRCA1 and contributes to its DNA repair function. Cell. 2001;105:149–60.
62. Ramus SJ, Song H, Dicks E, et al. Germline mutations in the BRIP1, BARD1, PALB2, and NBN genes in women with ovarian cancer. J Natl Cancer Inst. 2015. https://doi.org/10.1093/jnci/djv214.
63. Easton DF, Lesueur F, Decker B, et al. No evidence that protein truncating variants in BRIP1 are associated with breast cancer risk: implications for gene panel testing. J Med Genet. 2016;53(5):298–309.
64. Hamosh A. *602774: RAD51, S. CEREVISIAE, HOMOLOG OF, C; RAD51C. In OMIM. 2013. https://www.omim.org/entry/602774?search=rad51c&highlight=rad51c. Accessed 2 Apr 2018.
65. Meindl A, Hellebrand H, Wiek C, et al. Germline mutations in breast and ovarian cancer pedigrees establish RAD51C as a human cancer susceptibility gene. Nat Genet. 2010;42:410–4.
66. Loveday C, Turnbull C, Ramsay E, et al. Germline mutations in RAD51D confer susceptibility to ovarian cancer. Nat Genet. 2011;43:879–82.
67. Tung N, Domchek SM, Stadler Z, et al. Counselling framework for moderate-penetrance cancer-susceptibility mutations. Nat Rev Clin Oncol. 2016;13:581–8.
68. Song H, Dicks E, Ramus SJ, et al. Contribution of germline mutations in the RAD51B, RAD51C, and RAD51D genes to ovarian cancer in the population. J Clin Oncol. 2015;33:2901–7.
69. Mai PL, Best AF, Peters JA, et al. Risks of first and subsequent cancers among TP53 mutation carriers in the National Cancer Institute Li-Fraumeni syndrome cohort. Cancer. 2016;122(23):3673–81.
70. Hampel H, Bennett RL, Buchanan A, et al. A practice guideline from the American College of Medical Genetics and Genomics and the National Society of Genetic Counselors: referral indications for cancer predisposition assessment. Genet Med. 2015;17(1):70–87.
71. Richards S, Aziz N, Bale S, et al. Standards and guidelines for the interpretation of sequence variants: a joint consensus recommendation of the American College of Medical Genetics and Genomics and the Association for Molecular Pathology. Genet Med. 2015;17(5):405–24.
72. Rebbeck TR, Kauff ND, Domchek SM. Meta-analysis of risk reduction estimates associated with risk-reducing

salpingo-oophorectomy in BRCA1 or BRCA2 mutation carriers. J Natl Cancer Inst. 2009;101:80–7.
73. Segev Y, Iqbal J, Lubinski J, et al. The incidence of endometrial cancer in women with BRCA1 and BRCA2 mutations: an international prospective cohort study. Hereditary Breast Cancer Study Group. Gynecol Oncol. 2013;130:127–31.
74. Kuhn E, Kurman RJ, Shih IM. Ovarian cancer is an imported disease: fact or fiction? Curr Obstet Gynecol Rep. 2012;1:1–9.
75. Kurman RJ. Origin and molecular pathogenesis of ovarian high-grade serous carcinoma. Ann Oncol. 2013;24(10):x16–21.
76. Daly MB, Dresher CW, Yates MS, et al. Salpingectomy as a means to reduce ovarian cancer risk. Cancer Prev Res (Phila). 2015;8(5):342–8.
77. Labidi-Galy SI, Papp E, Hallberg D, et al. Nat Commun. 2017. https://doi.org/10.1038/s41467-017-00962-1.
78. Falconer H, Yin L, Gronberg H, et al. Ovarian cancer risk after salpingectomy: a nationwide population-based study. J Natl Cancer Inst. 2015. https://doi.org/10.1093/jnci/dju410.
79. American College of Obstetricians and Gynecologists. Salpingectomy for ovarian cancer prevention. Committee opinion no. 620. Obstet Gynecol. 2015;125:279–81.

Fertility Preservation in Patients with Disorders (Differences) of Sex Development

Diane Chen, Emilie K. Johnson, and Courtney Finlayson

T. K. Woodruff et al. (eds.), *Textbook of Oncofertility Research and Practice*,
https://doi.org/10.1007/978-3-030-02868-8_4

4

Key Points

- Infertility in DSD may result from abnormal gonadal development, abnormal hormone production, and/or prophylactic gonadectomy due to gonadal malignancy risk.
- Fertility potential is poorly understood in many DSD conditions and requires further study.
- Experience in fertility preservation in DSD is very limited and primarily focused on turner syndrome and Klinefelter syndrome.
- There are many ethical considerations about medical care in the DSD field in general, and these are complicated further when incorporating experimental fertility preservation techniques.

4.1 Introduction

Strides made in fertility preservation for cancer patients have inspired the expansion of the field of oncofertility to other medical conditions associated with infertility. One of the emerging areas is that of disorders of sex development (DSD).

4.1.1 DSD Conditions: An Introduction to the Current Treatment Paradigm

DSD are conditions in which there is incongruence in an individual's chromosomal, gonadal, or phenotypic sex [17]. There are three main steps in sex development: establishment of chromosomal sex, determination of gonadal sex, and differentiation to phenotypic sex. Errors in meiosis or translocation of the genetic material may result in sex chromosome DSD (e.g., Klinefelter syndrome). Abnormalities in transcription factors determining gonadal development into testes or ovaries may lead to disorders of gonadal development (e.g., ovotesticular DSD). Finally, disorders of androgen synthesis, androgen excess, or androgen action account for most of the remaining DSD (e.g., Complete Androgen Insensitivity Syndrome; Congenital Adrenal Hyperplasia) [11].

DSD are commonly thought of as conditions presenting with ambiguous genitalia in an infant, but there are many other presentations as well. Children may present with premature virilization, adolescents with primary amenorrhea or delayed pubertal development, or adults with infertility. ◘ Table 4.1 categorizes DSD conditions based on a consensus statement on intersex disorders and their management published in 2006 [11]. This landmark paper changed the approach to clinical care for this group of patients. In the preceding 50 years, the "optimal-gender policy" was followed, in which sex reassignment surgery was favored at a young age. It was thought that individuals were psychosexually neutral and that early surgery, without the knowledge of the patient, facilitated stable gender identity development and gender role behaviors that conformed to assigned sex at birth [24]. Over time, the "optimal-gender policy" approach to DSD care grew more controversial [7]. Patients treated according to this earlier approach grew up and began voicing discontent about the secrecy, the surgical outcomes, and the common terminology such as "intersex" and "hermaphrodite," which were viewed as pejorative. Molecular genetics was also advancing and changing the etiological understanding of many DSD conditions. These multitude of factors led to the 2006 Consensus Statement that acknowledged the controversial issues in DSD management and proposed recommendations about nomenclature, and evaluation, management, and care for these patients to be delivered as part of a multidisciplinary team including surgeons, endocrinologists, behavioral health experts, ethicists, and geneticists. Such programs are primarily housed within major academic centers but are becoming increasingly available for patients with DSDs around the world. In 2016, an update to the 2006 Consensus statement was published [14]. Many previous topics were reviewed, but, in addition, a small section was added to address fertility which noted that the potential for fertility may be increased with advancing assisted fertility techniques.

Nomenclature remains a controversial issue in this field. The 2006 Consensus Statement modified the overarching terms of "intersex" and "hermaphrodite" to DSD in an effort to make the term less pejorative. Other terms such as variation in sex development and difference in sex development were also considered, but ultimately, DSD was cho-

Table 4.1 Categorization of disorders of sex development

Sex chromosome DSD	46, XY DSD	46, XX DSD
	Disorders of gonadal development	
45, X, 45X/46, XX, 45, X/46, XY Turner syndrome	Complete gonadal dysgenesis	Ovotesticular DSD
47, XYY Klinefelter syndrome	Partial gonadal dysgenesis	Testicular DSD
45,X/46,XY mixed gonadal dysgenesis, ovotesticular DSD	Gonadal regression	Gonadal dysgenesis
46, XX/46, XY chimeric, ovotesticular DSD	Ovotesticular DSD	
	Disorders of androgen synthesis or action	*Disorders of androgen excess*
	Androgen biosynthesis defect (e.g., 5-alpha reductase deficiency)	Fetal androgen excess (e.g., 21-hydroxylase deficiency, congenital adrenal hyperplasia)
	Defect in androgen action (e.g., complete androgen insensitivity or partial androgen insensitivity syndrome)	Fetoplacental androgen excess (e.g., aromatase deficiency)
	LH receptor defects	Maternal (e.g., luteoma)
	Other	
	Cloacal exstrophy	Cloacal exstrophy
	Disorders of anti-Mullerian hormone	Vaginal atresia
	Severe hypospadias	Mayer-Rokitansky-Kuster-Hauser syndrome

sen. Some affected individuals continue to prefer the term "intersex," while others prefer DSD and yet others dislike both terms. Presumably, the words "disorder" and "sex" have negative connotations to some individuals, and there are a few studies addressing this topic. In 2011, Davies et al. surveyed parents of affected individuals ($N = 19$) and healthcare professionals ($N = 15$) and found that DSD was preferred to "intersex" among both patients and professionals but that only 37% of parents viewed DSD as an "acceptable term to describe an individual's overall condition when it has not been possible to assign them male or female at birth" [6]. Conclusions from this study, however, were limited by sample size. In 2015, Lin-Su et al. reported results from a survey of 589 patients with congenital adrenal hyperplasia who are members of the CARES support group. In this group, 71% disliked or strongly disliked the DSD term. This study, however, is of a very specific medical condition conducted with the membership of one particular support group; therefore, these results may not be generalized to the population of individuals with DSD. A 2017 study by Johnson et al. found that individuals with a range of DSD conditions belonging to the AIS-DSD Support Group also tended to view recommended DSD terminology negatively. This study also found that a majority of support group members who responded to a survey about DSD nomenclature had had a negative emotional experience due to the clinical use of specific DSD terms [13]. Despite the important information provided by these few studies, there have been no large-scale investigations of affected individuals and the medical community as a whole to determine whether a universally acceptable term may be identified. The term DSD is used in this chapter as it is the currently accepted medical terminology but with the understanding that this is not the preferred term for many affected individuals.

4

4.1.2 Fertility Preservation for Patients with DSD

Medical, surgical, and psychosocial care for individuals with DSD is improving, but fertility preservation has rarely been addressed despite the number of conditions associated with fertility or sterility risk. Fertility concerns among individuals with DSD are different from those faced in patients with cancer. ◘ Table 4.2 outlines fertility issues facing individuals with specific DSD conditions. First, some DSD are associated with abnormal gonadal development resulting in streak gonads or dysgenetic testes and ovaries [5]. This may result in gonadal failure from birth or progressive gonadal failure in childhood or adolescence. A pilot study to evaluate the presence of germ cells in gonads of individuals with DSD found that 68% of the individuals studied had germ cells present. It also showed that germ cells were more likely to be present at younger ages. This suggests that fertility potential may be greater than previously thought. Further studies are needed, however, to apply this to a larger population and to determine the quality of the germ cells [8].

Second, the presence of abnormal gonads, specifically in 46, XY DSD, increases risk for developing gonadal tumors [4]. Screening intraabdominal gonads using radiology techniques is not sufficient to rule out tumor growth [16]. To prevent the development of cancer, prophylactic gonadectomy has historically been recommended in most 46, XY DSD conditions at the time of diagnosis, often in infancy or early childhood. However, this practice is changing, and increasingly, gonadal tumor risk can be stratified by specific diagnosis. Abaci et al. estimated tumor risk for each type of DSD. High-risk conditions included gonadal dysgenesis with intraabdominal gonad (15–35% risk) and partial androgen insensitivity syndrome (PAIS) with nonscrotal gonad (50% risk). Intermediate risk included Turner syndrome with Y chromosome (12% risk), PAIS with scrotal gonad (unknown risk), and gonadal dysgenesis with scrotal gonad (unknown risk). Low-risk conditions were complete androgen insensitivity syndrome (CAIS) and ovotesticular DSD [1]. Thus, risk varies, and in some conditions, it may be safe to delay gonadectomy [22]. One reason for delaying gonadectomy may be to preserve the possibility for biological fertility. On the other hand, the above pilot study noted germ cells were more likely to be present at younger ages; thus, the greatest potential for fertility preservation may be via earlier gonadectomy [8]. The decision to pursue prophylactic gonadectomy is challenging for patients and families and is often considered in infancy through adolescence, depending on the timing of diagnosis and individual preference. So, while in the oncology patient there is a known time for surgical resection of gonads prior to the initiation of gonadotoxic chemotherapy, in DSD, the optimal timing of fertility preservation is less clear.

Third, due to the nature of DSD, an individual's gonads and germ cells may not align with their gender identity, thus leading to an assumption that the individual would not be interested in fertility with a gamete that does not match their gender identity. In CAIS, for example, patients have a 46, XY karyotype and their gonads develop into functional testicles, but due to mutations in the gene encoding in the androgen receptor, the body is unable to respond to androgen. Thus, internally individuals with CAIS have testes, Wolffian structures, and no Mullerian structures, but externally the genitalia appear typically female with a blind-ending vagina. The vast majority of individuals with CAIS have a female gender identity. There is a risk of gonadoblastoma; thus, many undergo gonadectomy, which may be done at any age but increasingly is performed after puberty. If fertility preservation options were to be considered, this would involve preserving sperm for an individual who identifies as a woman. If we expand our thinking about fertility potential, however, these individuals may have biological fertility potential.

Fertility preservation has begun to gain momentum in two particular DSD conditions: Turner syndrome and Klinefelter syndrome. Spontaneous fertility in Turner syndrome is rare, estimated at about 2–5% [12]. There is an accelerated loss of oocytes from the ovaries beginning after the 18th week of fetal development through the first few postnatal months or years such that most girls with Turner syndrome have lost all of their germ cells before completing puberty [12]. Parenting options for women with Turner syndrome have historically focused on adoption, but increasingly there is emphasis on expanding biological options. These options have included heterologous in vitro fertilization (IVF) with ovum donation or homologous IVF with embryo transfer resulting in live births in women with

Table 4.2 Fertility issues by DSD diagnosis

Category	Disorder	Karyotype	Fertility issues	Malignancy concern	Common discordance between gender identity and gonadal type
Sex chromosome DSD					
	Turner syndrome	45, X 45, X/46, XX 45, X/46, XY	Premature ovarian failure, streak gonads	Yes, if Y chromosome material	No
	Klinefelter syndrome	47, XXY	Testicular failure	No	No
	Mixed gonadal dysgenesis	45, X/46, XY	Gonadal failure	Yes	Yes
46, XY DSD					
	Complete or partial gonadal dysgenesis (e.g., SRY, SOX9)	46, XY	Potential streak gonads or gonadal failure	Yes	Yes
	Ovotesticular DSD	46, XY	Potential streak gonads or gonadal failure	Yes	Yes
	LH receptor mutations	46, XY	Testes slightly reduced in size but mature Leydig cells absent/scarce (Leydig cell hypoplasia)	No	No
	5alpha-reductase deficiency	46, XY	Oligospermia, azoospermia	No	Yes
	Complete androgen insensitivity syndrome	46, XY	Not much evidence, suspect azoospermia or oligospermia	Yes	Yes
	Partial androgen insensitivity syndrome	46, XY	Not much evidence, suspect azoospermia or oligospermia	Yes	Yes
	Persistent Mullerian duct syndrome	46, XY	Maybe (if prolonged cryptorchidism or anatomic obstruction) but likely normal sperm production	Possibly (cryptorchidism or of Mullerian remnants)	No

(continued)

Table 4.2 (continued)

Category	Disorder	Karyotype	Fertility issues	Malignancy concern	Common discordance between gender identity and gonadal type
46, XX DSD					
	Gonadal dysgenesis	46, XX	Potential streak gonads or gonadal failure	Yes	Yes
	Ovotesticular DSD	46, XX	Potential streak gonads or gonadal failure	Possibly	Yes
	Testicular DSD (SRY+, dup SOX9)	46, XX	Potential infertility	Possibly	No
	Congenital adrenal hyperplasia	46, XX	Often due to anovulation, but treated medically with success	No	No
	Aromatase deficiency	46, XX	Hypergonadotropic hypogonadism	No	Yes

Turner syndrome. Other modalities have been considered but have not yet resulted in live births. This includes homologous IVF with oocyte cryopreservation, which is scientifically possible at this time, and ovarian tissue cryopreservation from prepubertal children, which remains experimental [10]. Controversy has arisen about women with Turner syndrome carrying pregnancies because their risk of morbidity is much higher than for women without Turner syndrome [9]. Of primary concern is the increased risk of circulatory complications such as aortic dissection. The American Society for Reproductive Medicine has stated that Turner syndrome is a relative contraindication to pregnancy and that in a patient with Turner syndrome and a documented cardiac anomaly, Turner syndrome is an absolute contraindication to pregnancy [19]. Thus, patients are advised to use a gestational carrier for the term of their pregnancy. Oktay et al. recommend that all children with Turner syndrome undergo evaluation, with consideration of cryopreservation of mature oocytes or ovarian tissue [18].

Classical Klinefelter syndrome is characterized by germ cell regression, which begins in utero, accelerating during spontaneous puberty, leading to testicular fibrosis and hyalinization of the seminiferous tubules and hyperplasia of the interstitium in late adolescence and adulthood [2]. Often, pubertal development is incomplete, and testosterone production fails during this period, which typically leads to infertility. Many men with Klinefelter syndrome are azoospermic, but successful assisted reproduction in adult men has been achieved by testicular sperm extraction followed by intracytoplasmic sperm injection. It has been suggested that cryopreservation of spermatozoa might be best achieved early in adolescence. This has proven difficult as timing and rate of pubertal maturation vary, as does the ability of an adolescent boy to produce ejaculate with masturbation [2]. Studies in adolescents have shown conflicting results. One study of the testicular tissue in 13- to 16-year-old boys with Klinefelter syndrome showed massive fibrosis and hyalinization and only showed tubular spermatogonia in the youngest patients, suggesting that testicular tissue cryopreservation is most likely to be successful at younger ages [23]. Another study showed that in men with Klinefelter syndrome ages 12–25 years, sperm retrieval rates were similar to those seen in older men, suggesting that earlier preservation may not improve fertility rates [15]. Thus, further evaluation to determine the role or optimal timing of preservation is needed.

4.1.3 Fertility Preservation in DSD: Current Questions and Future Directions

Infertility or sterility is clearly a potential problem and a complicated issue for individuals with DSD and their parents, who may make decisions before a child is mature enough to participate in that process. It is presumed that fertility is an important consideration in DSD management, but there is no clear understanding of the DSD community's views of fertility, as the issue has not been comprehensively studied [3, 20, 21]. A better appreciation of the views of affected individuals is necessary to guide the field. Working on the assumption that some individuals with DSD will desire fertility preservation, there are many more questions that arise. For example, are patients with DSD conditions likely to benefit from fertility preservation. When should fertility preservation be offered for optimal chances of successful preservation? Again, there is little to no evidence about the presence and quality of germ cells in patients with DSD, and this requires evaluation. Should a surgical procedure and its associated risks be undertaken in an otherwise healthy child for the cryopreservation of tissue for fertility preservation, when this procedure remains experimental? Whereas some patients with DSD may be undergoing gonadectomy during which fertility preservation techniques can be done simultaneously, others may not. In traditional 45, X or 45, X/45, and XX mosaic Turner syndrome, for example, there is progressive loss of germ cells but no indication for gonadectomy. Should parents have the option to choose that surgery be undertaken in early childhood because more germ cells are present for preservation? In Turner syndrome, with a higher risk of pregnancy-associated morbidity, should efforts for fertility preservation be pursued at all? As gender identity may not match an individual's gonads and potential production of sperm versus ova, how does this affect considerations of fertility preservation? If a parent acts as the proxy for the child in fertility preservation decision-making, how is responsibility for preservation and ownership of the reproductive material delineated? Many DSD are caused by genetic mutations; thus, there is a risk of offspring inheriting the same condition. How should this affect decisions about fertility preservation, and how should preimplantation genetics be employed in these cases? There are many complicated questions facing the field of fertility preservation for DSD patients. Future research efforts must address these questions to better serve this patient population.

Review Questions and Answers

? Q1. How is the cause of infertility different in patients with DSD versus cancer?

✓ A1. Unlike the cancer population, in whom gonadal development and function are usually normal prior to cancer treatment, individuals with DSD often have inherent risk for infertility due to abnormal gonadal development or function.

? Q2. Do all patients with DSD conditions share the same risk of infertility?

✓ A2. No, it is highly variable among diagnoses and sometimes varies within individuals with the same diagnosis as well.

? Q3. Is fertility preservation an option in patients with DSD?

✓ A3. Fertility preservation should be considered. In some diagnoses, including Turner syndrome and Klinefelter syndrome, postpubertal preservation of eggs and sperm may be successful. In many situations, fertility preservation of immature or abnormal gonadal tissue may be considered via experimental techniques.

? Q4. How do we consider gender identity a factor when considering fertility preservation in patients with DSD?

✓ A4. Historically, it was often assumed that an individual was infertile if their gametes would not match their gender identity (e.g., in complete androgen insensitivity syndrome, immature gametes are immature sperm), but as we think more broadly, these individuals do have potential biological reproductive capability. There is little data, but anecdotally, some individuals with DSD may desire preservation of such gametes, while others may not. Further research is needed.

4

References

1. Abaci A, Catli G, Berberoglu M. Gonadal malignancy risk and prophylactic gonadectomy in disorders of sexual development. J Pediatr Endocrinol Metab. 2015. https://doi.org/10.1515/jpem-2014-0522.
2. Aksglaede L, Juul A. Testicular function and fertility in men with Klinefelter syndrome: a review. Eur J Endocrinol. 2013;168(4):R67–76. https://doi.org/10.1530/EJE-12-0934.
3. Campo-Engelstein L, Chen D, Baratz AB, Johnson EK, Finlayson C. The ethics of fertility preservation for pediatric patients with differences (disorders) of sex development. J Endocr Soc. 2017;1(6):638–45. https://doi.org/10.1210/js.2017-00110.
4. Cools M, Looijenga LH, Wolffenbuttel KP, T'Sjoen G. Managing the risk of germ cell tumourigenesis in disorders of sex development patients. Endocr Dev. 2014;27:185–96. https://doi.org/10.1159/000363642.
5. Cools M, van Aerde K, Kersemaekers AM, Boter M, Drop SL, Wolffenbuttel KP, Steyerberg EW, Oosterhuis JW, Looijenga LH. Morphological and immunohistochemical differences between gonadal maturation delay and early germ cell neoplasia in patients with undervirilization syndromes. J Clin Endocrinol Metab. 2005;90(9):5295–303. https://doi.org/10.1210/jc.2005-0139.
6. Davies JH, Knight EJ, Savage A, Brown J, Malone PS. Evaluation of terminology used to describe disorders of sex development. J Pediatr Urol. 2011;7(4):412–5. https://doi.org/10.1016/j.jpurol.2010.07.004.
7. Diamond M, Sigmundson HK. Sex reassignment at birth. Long-term review and clinical implications. Arch Pediatr Adolesc Med. 1997;151(3):298–304.
8. Finlayson C, Fritsch MK, Johnson EK, Rosoklija I, Gosiengfiao Y, Yerkes E, Madonna MB, Woodruff TK, Cheng E. Presence of germ cells in disorders of sex development: implications for fertility potential and preservation. J Urol. 2016. https://doi.org/10.1016/j.juro.2016.08.108.
9. Hagman A, Kallen K, Bryman I, Landin-Wilhelmsen K, Barrenas ML, Wennerholm UB. Morbidity and mortality after childbirth in women with turner karyotype. Hum Reprod. 2013;28(7):1961–73. https://doi.org/10.1093/humrep/det113.
10. Hewitt JK, Jayasinghe Y, Amor DJ, Gillam LH, Warne GL, Grover S, Zacharin MR. Fertility in Turner syndrome. Clin Endocrinol. 2013;79(5):606–14. https://doi.org/10.1111/cen.12288.
11. Houk CP, Hughes IA, Ahmed SF, Lee PA, Writing Committee for the International Intersex Consensus Conference P. Summary of consensus statement on intersex disorders and their management. International intersex consensus conference. Pediatrics. 2006;118(2):753–7. https://doi.org/10.1542/peds.2006-0737.
12. Hovatta O. Pregnancies in women with Turner's syndrome. Ann Med. 1999;31(2):106–10.
13. Johnson EK, Rosoklija I, Finlayson C, Chen D, Yerkes EB, Madonna MB, Holl JL, Baratz AB, Davis G, Cheng EY. Attitudes towards "disorders of sex development" nomenclature among affected individuals. J Pediatr Urol. 2017;13(6):608 e601–8. https://doi.org/10.1016/j.jpurol.2017.03.035.
14. Lee PA, Nordenstrom A, Houk CP, Ahmed SF, Auchus R, Baratz A, Baratz Dalke K, Liao LM, Lin-Su K, Looijenga LH 3rd, Mazur T, Meyer-Bahlburg HF, Mouriquand P, Quigley CA, Sandberg DE, Vilain E, Witchel S, Global DSDUC. Global disorders of sex development update since 2006: perceptions, approach and care. Horm Res Paediatr. 2016;85(3):158–80. https://doi.org/10.1159/000442975.
15. Nahata L, Yu RN, Paltiel HJ, Chow JS, Logvinenko T, Rosoklija I, Cohen LE. Sperm retrieval in adolescents and young adults with Klinefelter syndrome: a prospective, pilot study. J Pediatr. 2016;170:260–5. e261–262. https://doi.org/10.1016/j.jpeds.2015.12.028.
16. Nakhal RS, Hall-Craggs M, Freeman A, Kirkham A, Conway GS, Arora R, Woodhouse CR, Wood DN, Creighton SM. Evaluation of retained testes in adolescent girls and women with complete androgen insensitivity syndrome. Radiology. 2013;268(1):153–60. https://doi.org/10.1148/radiol.13121068.
17. Ohnesorg T, Vilain E, Sinclair AH. The genetics of disorders of sex development in humans. Sexual development: genetics, molecular biology, evolution, endocrinology, embryology, and pathology of sex determination and. Differentiation. 2014;8(5):262–72. https://doi.org/10.1159/000357956.
18. Oktay K, Bedoschi G, Berkowitz K, Bronson R, Kashani B, McGovern P, Pal L, Quinn G, Rubin K. Fertility preservation in women with turner syndrome: a comprehensive review and practical guidelines. J Pediatr Adolesc Gynecol. 2016;29(5):409–16. https://doi.org/10.1016/j.jpag.2015.10.011.
19. Practice Committee of American Society For Reproductive M. Increased maternal cardiovascular mortality associated with pregnancy in women with Turner syndrome. Fertil Steril. 2012;97(2):282–4. https://doi.org/10.1016/j.fertnstert.2011.11.049.
20. Rives N, Milazzo JP, Perdrix A, Castanet M, Joly-Helas G, Sibert L, Bironneau A, Way A, Mace B. The feasibility of fertility preservation in adolescents with Klinefelter syndrome. Hum Reprod. 2013;28(6):1468–79. https://doi.org/10.1093/humrep/det084.

21. Sanders C, Carter B, Lwin R. Young women with a disorder of sex development: learning to share information with health professionals, friends and intimate partners about bodily differences and infertility. J Adv Nurs. 2015. https://doi.org/10.1111/jan.12661.
22. van der Zwan YG, Biermann K, Wolffenbuttel KP, Cools M, Looijenga LH. Gonadal maldevelopment as risk factor for germ cell cancer: towards a clinical decision model. Eur Urol. 2015;67(4):692–701. https://doi.org/10.1016/j.eururo.2014.07.011.
23. Van Saen D, Gies I, De Schepper J, Tournaye H, Goossens E. Can pubertal boys with Klinefelter syndrome benefit from spermatogonial stem cell banking? Hum Reprod. 2012;27(2):323–30. https://doi.org/10.1093/humrep/der425.
24. Wiesemann C, Ude-Koeller S, Sinnecker GH, Thyen U. Ethical principles and recommendations for the medical management of differences of sex development (DSD)/intersex in children and adolescents. Eur J Pediatr. 2010;169(6):671–9. https://doi.org/10.1007/s00431-009-1086-x.

Fertility Preservation in Patients with Gender Dysphoria

Jason Jarin, Emilie K. Johnson, and Veronica Gomez-Lobo

T. K. Woodruff et al. (eds.), *Textbook of Oncofertility Research and Practice*,
https://doi.org/10.1007/978-3-030-02868-8_5

Key Points

- Gender-affirming hormonal and surgical treatments can affect the future fertility of individuals with gender dysphoria.
- Use of gender-affirming hormones does not appear to render most individuals completely infertile, and hormonal effects on the gonads appear to be at least partially reversible.
- Options for biological parenthood among transgender individuals include several different assisted reproductive technologies; spontaneous pregnancies have also been reported.
- Procedures necessary to obtain oocytes or sperm for cryopreservation can exacerbate gender dysphoria in some individuals.
- Uptake of fertility preservation has been very low among adolescents with gender dysphoria, despite counseling prior to initiation of gender-affirming hormones.

5.1 Introduction

Recent events have demonstrated increasing media attention to transgender individuals. The *Diagnostic and Statistical Manual of Mental Disorders, Fifth Edition* (DSM-5), changed the nomenclature for transgender individuals from gender identity disorder to gender dysphoria (GD) in 2013. GD refers to the psychological distress encountered in persons for whom sex assigned at birth is incongruent with their gender identity. The psychiatric focus is on the distress experienced due to the incongruence between assigned and affirmed gender, and current evidence supports that gender-affirming therapy greatly improves psychological outcomes [1]. The American Psychiatric Association further states that such individuals should be able to obtain care without fear of discrimination and that treatment options for this condition include counseling, gender-affirming hormones (previously referred to as cross-sex hormones), gender-affirming surgery, and social and legal transition to the desired sex [1]. In 2009, the Endocrine Society along with the Pediatric Endocrine Society, World Professional Association for Transgender Health (WPATH), European Society of Endocrinology, and the European Society for Pediatric Endocrinology first published the "Endocrine treatment of transsexual persons: an Endocrine Society clinical practice guideline" [2]. These guidelines, which were reaffirmed in 2017, support the use of hormones to further the gender-affirming process and recommend counseling regarding fertility and options for fertility preservation (FP), as gender-affirming hormone therapy may impair future fertility.

5.2 Nomenclature

Although this chapter is titled "Fertility Preservation in Patients with Gender Dysphoria," the information and concepts presented herein apply to the spectrum of individuals who exhibit gender variance and desire medical interventions to facilitate transition to a gender other than the one assigned at birth. These medical interventions include pubertal suppression, gender-affirming hormone therapy, and gonadectomy, all of which have the potential to affect future fertility. For consistency in this chapter, the authors have chosen to use the terms "trans," "trans-woman," and "trans-man." However, a much larger range of terminology is applicable and relevant to the mental and physical health of individuals with gender variance, many of whom may pursue medical interventions which have the potential to affect fertility in the future.

The authors recognize that terminology related to the transgender experience is in evolution and aim to provide some basic information about relevant nomenclature. It is important to note that some of the terms used may be preferable to some individuals, while offensive to others. Additionally, there have been recent shifts in language use that may not be fully reflected in the terms defined in this chapter. However, assembling the nonexhaustive list below was thought to be important to provide clarity and context for the remainder of the chapter:

Sex Versus Gender

- *Sex* – Anatomy of a person's reproductive system and secondary sex characteristics.
- *Gender* – Social roles based on sex, typically culturally based.

Gender-Related Terms

- *Biological sex/natal sex* – Sex assigned at birth, generally based on anatomy and (sometimes) chromosomes.
- *Gender identity/affirmed gender* – An individual's internal sense of their[1] own gender, may it be male, female, or another gender. It may not be aligned with biological/natal sex.
- *Gender expression* – Physical manifestation of an individual's gender identity (e.g., clothing, mannerisms, pronouns, chosen name).
- *Gender role* – Societal norms regarding how men and women should think, behave, speak, and dress.
- *Gender variance, gender nonconforming* – Closely related terms describing behavior not conforming to socially defined male or female norms (e.g., dress, activities) based on sex.

Gender Identity

- *Cisgender* – Individuals for whom internal gender identity agrees with their anatomy and the sex they were assigned at birth.
- *Genderqueer* – Individuals who identify with both male and female genders or who identify with neither gender.
- *Gender fluid* – A dynamic mix between male and female gender identities.
- *Gender nonconforming* – A person whose gender role or gender expression does not conform to societal norms of typical male or typical female.
- *Transgender, trans* – A person whose gender identity does not match their anatomy and gender assigned at birth. Often also abbreviated as *trans** to emphasize the range of individuals who do not identify as a traditional cisgender man or woman.
- *Transsexual* – A person who has the strong desire to assume the physical characteristics and gender role of the opposite sex. This term has a more binary connotation than transgender and has been viewed somewhat negatively in recent years and thus is being used less often than terms such as transgender and trans.
- *Trans-woman, male-to-female (MTF) transgender* – Individuals with a male natal gender but female gender identity. For this chapter, the authors have chosen the term trans-woman, as it affirms the individual's gender identity.
- *Trans-man, female-to-male (FTM) transgender* – Individuals with a female natal gender but male gender identity. For this chapter, the authors have chosen the term trans-man, as it affirms the individual's gender identity.

Other Helpful Terminologies

- *Gender dysphoria* – The DSM-5 diagnosis used by medical and mental health professionals to describe psychological distress caused by discontent with one's natal sex. *Gender identity disorder* (*GID*) was the terminology previously used by the DSM-IV and has largely been abandoned.
- *Sexual orientation* – Pattern of romantic or sexual attraction; separate from gender identity and gender expression. For example, a trans-man is not necessarily romantically attracted only to women. Traditional categories include heterosexual, homosexual, and bisexual. Newer classifications include asexual, polysexual, and pansexual.
- *Transitioning* – The process of physically changing external gender presentation to align with one's internal gender identity. Genital surgery is not a requirement.

5.3 Current Treatment Guidelines

5.3.1 Psychological Evaluation

It is essential that individuals with GD be evaluated and managed by an experienced mental health provider in order to assess whether they meet criteria for the diagnosis and to evaluate for confounding psychological factors. The mental health provider may also provide psychotherapy and evaluate for psychological readiness for medical interventions such as puberty blockers and/or gender-affirming hormones. Persons with GD are at high risk of adverse mental health including anxiety, depression, self-harm and suicide, poor school performance, and drug and alcohol abuse.

1 Intentionally grammatically incorrect to avoid using binary gender-based terminology.

Thus, ideally, a mental health provider will continue to evaluate and support the individual during social and biological transition.

5.3.2 Pubertal Suppression

Some children with GD experience increasing distress during puberty as their body begins to change. The Endocrine Society Guidelines support the use of puberty blockers starting when the child reaches Tanner 2 stage (breast budding in natal girls and testicular volume of 4 cc in natal boys) [2]. WPATH guidelines recommend that a mental health provider assesses each adolescent prior to the initiation of pubertal suppression, to confirm understanding of the goals, risks, and benefits [3]. Pubertal suppression addresses the mental distress of the child from developing unwanted changes that are not congruent with gender identity. Suppression also prevents secondary sexual characteristics from developing, which may later be difficult to alter, such as the Adam's apple or large breasts. In general, pubertal suppression is usually achieved with gonadotropin-releasing hormone (GnRH) agonists such as a histrelin rod or Depot-Lupron.

5.3.3 Gender-Affirming Hormones

Regardless of whether pubertal suppression was undertaken, the Endocrine Society Guidelines support the initiation of gender-affirming hormones around the age of 16 years. Furthermore, recent data have shown that gender-affirming hormones may be started as early as 14 years of age in appropriate clinical settings [4]. Individuals considering gender-affirming hormones need to be counseled extensively regarding expected results of treatment and possible adverse health effects. Such a discussion should include the effects on fertility and options for FP, as gender-affirming hormone therapy may impair future fertility. In addition, prior to the initiation of gender-affirming hormone therapy, the WPATH recommends that a qualified mental health professional should provide documentation (such as a referral letter) of the patient's personal and treatment history, eligibility, and need for gender-affirming hormones? [3].

5.3.4 Gender-Affirming Surgery

Gender-affirming surgery is also an option for individuals with GD who desire changes to align their physical appearance with gender identity. Patients who choose oophorectomy, orchiectomy, and/or hysterectomy as part of their treatment plan should also be counseled about their options for fertility and future reproduction prior to surgery.

5.4 Estrogen Treatment for Trans-girls and Trans-women

Hormone therapy for adolescents desiring feminizing therapy is complex, with most clinical studies reporting the concurrent use of antiandrogens with estrogen therapy if the patient has not undergone pubertal suppression [5]. Puberty induction, in suppressed individuals, may be undertaken with oral estrogen, transdermal (patch), or parenteral formulations. While the inherent risk of venous thromboembolism in the adolescent population is less than that in adults, transdermal preparations may offer an advantage by lowering these risks [6]. Following puberty induction, serum estradiol should be maintained at premenopausal levels (<200 pg/ml), and testosterone should be in the physiologic female range (<55 ng/dl). For individuals who have experienced puberty, this treatment may require high doses of estradiol (2–6 mg) along with androgen blockers such as spironolactone. As with testosterone therapy, regular clinical and laboratory assessment should be performed to monitor for adverse effects.

5.5 Testosterone Treatment for Trans-boys and Trans-men

Testosterone is recommended to achieve the desired masculinization of a natal female with GD. In cases where an adolescent has received pubertal suppression, testosterone is given in low doses and increased slowly (as done with induction of puberty). In both prepubertal and postpubertal individuals, testosterone is generally administered subcutaneously or intramuscularly every 1–2 weeks at the lowest dose needed to maintain the desired clinical result and levels within normal male physiologic levels (320–1000 ng/dl) [7]. Prior to initiating therapy, patients should be aware of the risks of masculinizing hormone therapy, and timing of development of the desired effects, so that the patient has reasonable expectations. Monitoring for adverse effects includes both clinical and laboratory evaluation specific to the risks of hormone therapy and the patient's individual risks/comorbidities [8]. The most concerning morbidity noted in trans-men is polycythemia which can be treated with reduction of the testosterone and/or phlebotomy with blood donation.

5.6 Gender-Affirming Hormones: Effect on Fertility

5.6.1 Estrogen and Fertility in Trans-women

Although some estrogen is necessary for spermatogenesis, an overabundance of estrogen can be detrimental to fertility. Limited data exists regarding the effect of exogenous estrogen on sperm production in trans-women. Data from animal studies, human epidemiologic studies, and studies related to the effect of obesity on human male reproductive function are relevant also may be relevant to trans-women who may desire biological children in the future.

5.6.1.1 Animal Data

There is a large body of literature demonstrating reduced fertility parameters and alterations in genital anatomy in male rodents exposed to estrogenic compounds in utero. Of more relevance to the trans-women who may begin estrogen supplementation during adolescence or adulthood, several studies of adult rodents have explored the impact of exogenous estrogens on multiple measures of fertility potential. For example, increasing doses of exogenous estrogens have been associated with alteration in sperm counts and motility [9], testicular histology [10], and epididymal sperm content [11] in adult male rats. High doses of exogenous estrogens administered to adult male rats have also been associated with lower fertility rates, as measured by litter size [9–11]; one study even demonstrated a complete loss of potency at the highest dose of an estrogen receptor-α agonist [10]. Reversibility of the effects of estrogen on testicular histology has been demonstrated, suggesting that the effects of estrogen on fertility potential may not be permanent [11].

5.6.1.2 Evidence in Humans

Environmental Estrogens

In addition to the animal data, concern has existed for many years that environmental estrogens may be contributing impairments in male reproductive health and functioning, including an increase in male factor infertility [12]. To a great extent, concern regarding the effects of environmental estrogens on male fertility is a result of studies evaluating the link between in utero diethylstilbestrol (DES) exposure and adult male infertility. Although there have been several studies suggesting a link between fetal DES exposure and reduced adult semen parameters, the data are far from definitive [13]. Similarly, concern exists that exposure to endocrine disruptors with estrogenic properties such as phthalates, polychlorinated biphenyls (PCBs), and bisphenol A (BPA) may be associated with male infertility [14], although clear causality has not been established.

A few studies have attempted to link environmental endocrine disrupters to male factor infertility. For example, one Argentinian study demonstrated an association between exposure to pesticides and solvents (as measured by self-report) and lower semen parameters [15]. In that study, pesticide exposure was also associated with higher serum estrogen concentrations and lower luteinizing hormone concentrations compared with men not exposed to pesticides [15]. This suggests that any effect of chemical exposure on fertility may be at least partially hormonally mediated.

In a study of men presenting to an infertility clinic in India, infertile men were found to have detectable PCBs in their seminal plasma, whereas normal controls were not [16]. Seminal plasma phthalates were also found to be higher in infertile men compared with controls [16]. Not surprisingly, total motile sperm count was also lower in the infertile men, although a causal relationship between estrogenic chemicals and fertility was only suggested, not proven, by this investigation.

Elevated Estrogen in Obese Men

Obesity has been associated with male infertility, and the mechanisms are likely multifactorial. In addition to hormonal abnormalities, obesity is also associated with erectile dysfunction and increased intrascrotal temperatures, all of which can cause difficulties with fertility [17]. From an endocrine standpoint, increasing BMI is associated with both infertility and hormonal derangements including low testosterone, elevated estradiol, and low inhibin B levels [18]. Additionally, semen parameters have been found to be altered in some studies of infertile obese men, although results have been inconsistent [17, 19, 20].

The exact relationship between hormonal profiles and semen parameters and paternity among obese men remains to be fully elucidated. A decreased serum testosterone-to-estradiol ratio has also been associated with infertility in a subset of men presenting with this complaint regardless of BMI, again suggesting that elevated estradiol can have a detrimental effect on fertility [21]. However, the relative contribution of elevated estrogen to fertility has not been determined.

Effects of Estrogen Exposure in Trans-women

A few recent studies in trans-women related to the effects of estrogen exposure on testicular function and histology are available. A study of orchiectomy specimens from trans-women with GD who were treated with estrogen demonstrated unpredictable negative effects on testicular histology [22]. Histologic changes generally were unassociated with serum and intratesticular testosterone levels, and 24% of patients actually had normal spermatogenesis [22]. Furthermore, a recent series of trans-women who chose to bank sperm prior to gender-affirming hormones demonstrated multiple impaired semen parameters, even without medically prescribed hormonal therapy [23]. One possible reason for poor sperm quality includes nondisclosed hormone use [23]. Other possible explanations include young patient age or changes in testicular function due to self-induced high positioning of the testes or tight underwear use [23].

5.6.1.3 Summary

- Although low levels of estrogen are necessary for male fertility, higher levels of exogenous estrogen administration appear to have a detrimental effect on the fertility potential of male gametes, as supported by both rodent data and human epidemiologic and clinical studies.
- The negative effects of estrogen on the testis appear to be at least partially reversible.
- Threshold levels for the amount and duration of exogenous estrogen exposure necessary to have a negative effect on fertility have yet to be established.

5.6.2 Testosterone and Fertility in Trans-men

Analogous to the role estrogen plays in male fertility, some testosterone is necessary for normal reproductive functioning in women. Also similar to the effect of estrogen on testicular function, exogenous testosterone can cause negative effects on ovarian function leading to fertility problems. However, there is relatively little data specifically examining the effects of testosterone on future fertility on trans-men. In addition to the small amount of data regarding trans-men directly, relevant animal data do exist, and information regarding the effects of elevated testosterone in women with polycystic ovarian syndrome (PCOS) may also be extrapolated to trans-men who use exogenous testosterone.

5.6.2.1 Animal Data

Data from animal studies has established that supraphysiological androgen levels have a negative effect on the ovary. For example, exogenous testosterone administration has been associated with reduced ovarian weight in both adult female rats [18] and homing pigeons [24]. Suggested mechanisms include delayed follicular maturation [24] and follicular atresia potentially due to an antiestrogenic effect of testosterone [18]. Administration of a potent androgen, dehydroepiandrosterone (DHEA), to adult female rats has also been associated with follicular atresia [25]. Additionally, DHEA administration may cause local ovarian testosterone production and inflammation, leading to reductions in fertility potential [25].

5.6.2.2 Evidence in Humans

Polycystic Ovarian Syndrome Data

PCOS is characterized by endocrine and reproductive dysfunction. Women with PCOS have manifestations of hyperandrogenism including challenges with fertility. In addition to elevated androgens, other endocrine abnormalities are also present, including elevated levels of insulin, inhibin B, and luteinizing hormone [26]. Through a multifactorial pathway, folliculogenesis is impaired, potentially due to a delay or arrest in follicular maturation [26, 27]. Although androgens certainly play a role in PCOS-related ovarian dysfunction, infertility related to PCOS is not solely due to androgen effects. One key factor associated with infertility in women with PCOS may be the estradiol-to-testosterone ratio, with lower ratios being associated with anovulation [28].

Effects of Testosterone Exposure in Trans-men

From available data, effects of testosterone (at doses typically used by trans-men) on ovarian function appear to be incomplete and/or at least partially reversible. One recent study of trans-men undergoing oophorectomy as part of surgical transition demonstrated a surprisingly normal distribution of follicle types, despite a >1-year average duration of testosterone treatment [29]. Oocytes were also able to be matured in vitro after surgical removal [29], indicating that FP at the time of oophorectomy may be a viable option for some trans-men. Pregnancy (as documented by a self-report) has been also reported in trans-men who have previously used testosterone, including some who were still amenorrheic from testosterone use [30, 31]. There also are cases of pregnancy occurring while trans-men were still taking testosterone [32].

5.6.2.3 Summary

- Low levels of testosterone are necessary for female fertility, although higher levels are associated with changes in ovarian histology and function that can lead to infertility.
- The effects of exogenous testosterone on the ovaries do not cause sterility, as pregnancies have been reported in trans-men with current and previous testosterone use.
- Threshold levels for the amount and duration of exogenous testosterone exposure necessary to have a negative effect on fertility have yet to be established.

5.7 Ethics of Fertility Preservation Options for Trans-individuals

Because of the potential effects of treatment on fertility, loss of reproductive potential has long been viewed as an inexorable consequence to transition [33]. It was not until 2001 that the Endocrine Society explicitly stated that reproductive issues need to be discussed prior to the initiation of treatment. Furthermore, the American Academy of Child and Adolescent Psychiatry has maintained that there has been no credible evidence that shows that a parent's sexual orientation or gender identity will adversely affect the development of offspring, further supporting an ethical obligation to discuss the reproductive needs of transgender individuals and their potential as parents [34].

Current established methods of FP include sperm, oocyte, and embryo cryopreservation, all of which have been considered standard of care for patients receiving gonadotoxic therapy [35]. It is reasonable to extend this standard to trans-men and trans-women receiving gender-affirming hormones. Informed consent to access assisted reproductive technology poses further ethical questions in the adolescent population, as they are still considered minors. However, research on cognition and capacity suggests that adolescents show significant ability to provide informed consent, suggesting that content and wording of informed consent forms for adolescents should resemble those used with adults [36]. The American Academy of Pediatrics state that children and adolescents need to be involved in decisions involving their health care in a developmentally appropriate manner [37]. This includes obtaining parental consent in matters involving adolescents as well as obtaining assent in minors who are able to understand the choices presented prior to treatment.

Experimental procedures such as ovarian or testicular tissue cryopreservation may be reasonable to perform in adult trans-individuals in research settings with institutional review board (IRB) oversight [35]. Their use in the transgender adolescent population, however, is precluded by current WPATH recommendations not to perform irreversible surgery (i.e., orchiectomy or oophorectomy) in trans-adolescents, the lack of data regarding the success of these procedures (especially testicular tissue cryopreservation), and the current paucity of data regarding the actual risk of gonadotoxicity of hormonal treatments.

5.8 Fertility Preservation Options Prior to Initiation of Gender-Affirming Hormones

5.8.1 Trans-women

Trans-women who have undergone male puberty prior to initiating estrogen therapy may opt for FP through sperm cryopreservation. Sperm cryopreservation was first reported in 1953 by Bunge and Sherman and has since become the most widely used method of FP for men faced with fertility challenges [38]. This can be accomplished at sperm-banking facilities, with sperm classically obtained through masturbation [39]. The physical act of obtaining a semen specimen through masturbation may exacerbate GD in trans-women [40]. In these cases, and others in which sperm is not possible to be obtained through ejaculation, surgical techniques exist that may retrieve sperm for cryopreservation including testicular sperm aspiration (TESA), percutaneous sperm aspiration (PESA), and testicular sperm extraction (TESE). Experimental testicular tissue cryopreservation has been reported for prepubertal patients with cancer [41] but is not currently considered an option for children with GD.

5.8.2 Trans-men

Trans-men who have undergone female puberty can choose to preserve fertility through embryo cryopreservation or oocyte cryopreservation. The success of embryo cryopreservation in achieving viable pregnancies has long been documented. Furthermore, oocyte cryopreservation has improved dramatically over the past decade so much so that it is currently recommended by the American Society for Reproductive Medicine for patients undergoing chemotherapy or other potentially gonadotoxic therapies [42]. Pregnancies resulting from assisted reproductive technology have been reported in trans-men undergoing testosterone therapy [30]. Successful pregnancies have also been documented in trans-men that were achieved using cryopreserved oocytes obtained prior to initiating testosterone; these pregnancies were carried by their sexually intimate partners [43]. As with trans-women, the procedures necessary (i.e., ovulation induction, transvaginal ultrasounds) to obtain oocytes in trans-men may also exacerbate GD [44].

Ovarian tissue cryopreservation is currently an experimental option but one that possibly carries the most potential and has been offered to women undergoing chemotherapy [45]. All currently reported pregnancies after ovarian tissue cryopreservation have transpired through autotransplantation of the thawed tissue. Given that the effects of testosterone on ovarian function may be reversible and the damage inflicted on the ovarian tissue in the process of surgical removal, cryopreservation, and thawing, this option is not yet currently justified. In the future, if in vitro oocyte maturation yields pregnancies, ovarian tissue cryopreservation may become more widely utilized for trans-men who desire FP, as it does not require hormonal stimulation. However, as previously discussed, ovarian tissue cryopreservation is not currently recommended for transgender adolescents given the irreversibility of oophorectomy.

Fertility in trans-men can be achieved through in vitro fertilization of an individual's oocytes with implantation in a partner or surrogate or through spontaneous or assisted reproductive technologies. As stated before, pregnancies in trans-men have been reported. It is important to note that trans-men must stop testosterone therapy before and during pregnancy and that pregnancy and delivery may be associated with higher rates of depression and suicidality than in cis-women [30, 31].

5.9 Special Considerations

5.9.1 Fertility Preservation After Pubertal Suppression

FP after pubertal suppression presents unique issues as the gonads (both testes and ovary) have not fully matured at Tanner stage 2, which is when the Endocrine Society recommends starting suppression. There have been reports of successful sperm retrieval either by electroejaculation or testicular sperm extraction in adolescents scheduled to undergo gonadotoxic therapy for malignancy; however, successful extraction was documented only in adolescents with at least Tanner stage 3 development [46]. Ovulation induction in adolescents also presents a similar challenge, with only one case report of successful ovarian stimulation and oocyte retrieval on a premenarcheal natal female with Tanner stage 3 breast development and Tanner stage 1 pubic hair [47].

To circumvent this, the Endocrine Society Guidelines recommend fertility-preserving measures to be performed after cessation of gonadotropin suppression but prior to gender-affirming hormone treatment [2]. Pubertal suppression with GnRH analogues is reversible and should not prevent resumption of pubertal development upon cessation of treatment; however, patients need to be counseled that there is no data in this population concerning the time required for sufficient spermatogenesis or for resumption of ovulation following pubertal suppression [48]. Furthermore, cessation of suppression without subsequent gender-affirming hormone therapy may result in irreversible and undesirable sex characteristics, depending on the length treatment to be withheld [2]. Currently, no experimental protocols exist for pre- or peri-pubertal gonadal tissue cryopreservation, given that it would require an otherwise medically unnecessary surgical procedure.

5.9.2 Fertility Preservation Options at Time of Gonadectomy

Currently in the United States, there are several investigational protocols for ovarian or testicular tissue freezing in young men and women whose fertility is threatened by needed cancer therapy. These involve removal of a portion or the entire gonad with cryopreservation of the tissue for possible thawing and future use. The American Society of Clinical Oncology currently recommends that these procedures be performed under institutional review board oversight as they are experimental [48]. As discussed above the Endocrine Society Guidelines state that it is reasonable to perform gonadectomy after age 18 as part of gender-affirming surgery in transgender adolescents and adults, and at this time, tissue freezing under IRB protocol could be considered [2]. Most patients undergo surgery after they have initiated hormonal therapy, and thus, their gonadal function may already be affected. This highlights the need for all transgender individuals to be informed and counseled regarding options for fertility prior to medical or surgical treatment.

5.10 Attitudes Toward and Utilization of Fertility Preservation in Patients with Gender Dysphoria

As mentioned above, the WPATH recommends discussing fertility effects of pubertal suppression and gender-affirming hormones prior to initiation of these therapies. Furthermore, it is recommended that healthcare professionals discuss fertility options for future reproduction needs prior to patients with GD undergoing medical or surgical treatments that could impact their ability to have a biological child in the future [3]. Despite these WPATH recommendations about fertility counseling, and a stated desired of many transgender individuals to have biological children [49–51], relatively few individuals with GD currently pursue FP.

Two recent series of adolescents with GD demonstrate a 3–4% rate of attempted FP prior to the initiation of hormonal treatments [40, 52]. Sperm cryopreservation is currently more common than oocyte cryopreservation, at least in part due to perceived discomfort associated with the procedures required to harvest oocytes [52]. Other identified barriers to FP among individuals with GD include cost [40, 52], perceived misgendering/poor treatment by sperm bank technician [52], and concerns about the delay of hormonal treatments [40, 44].

Although the uptake of FP among individuals with GD has been historically low, several recent studies provide reasons for a more positive view of future fertility and FP for transgender individuals. A recent qualitative study of transgender men found that while procedures to harvest oocytes can be potentially distressing, the FP process was less distressing to some trans-men than expected and that coping strategies (including the use of cognitive behavioral techniques and reliance on a support system) were helpful to many [44]. Cases of transgender individuals using previously preserved oocytes and sperm to have biological children are emerging in the literature [43, 53], demonstrating concrete utility of the WPATH recommendations to discuss future fertility and FP for individuals with GD. The use of gender-neutral terminology (e.g., gametes instead of oocytes or bleeding instead of menstruation) [44, 54] and development of trans-inclusive clinic forms [54] may facilitate the uptake of FP and use of assisted reproductive technologies by more transgender individuals in the future.

5.11 Future Research Priorities

The field of oncofertility has heightened awareness about fertility concerns in patients with cancer; however, the application of FP in transgender medicine is emerging. While prolonged use of gender-affirming hormones can have negative effects on both ovarian and testicular function, there is no data examining the amount and duration of exposure that guarantees infertility (or fertility) in either trans-men or trans-women. Establishing the extent of gonadotoxicity of gender-affirming hormone therapy would allow clinicians to better inform their patients about their options for FP and future. Furthermore, pubertal suppression raises the possibility of (1) ovulation induction and sperm extraction in adolescents who may be in mid- or late adolescence but relatively early in their pubertal development [46, 47] and (2) development of research protocols whereby children who are in Tanner stages 2–3 could choose to undergo gonadal biopsy and experimental cryopreservation. Further research is needed to ascertain the safety and acceptability of these possible interventions in children who are in Tanner stages 2–3. Finally, patient-centered outcomes research related to family planning and fertility has been established as priority for future transgender healthcare research [55].

5.12 Conclusion

Advances in the field of oncofertility have opened doors to FP in other populations, including transgender children and adolescents. However, this population presents its own unique set of challenges because of the early timing of pubertal suppression and the unknown extent of gonadotoxicity of gender-affirming hormones. Furthermore, while there is available data on the views of both parents and children regarding FP in the setting of cancer, there is a paucity of literature describing the attitudes of transgender children and adolescents regarding potential future childbearing [56]. Nevertheless, all transgender individuals should be informed and counseled regarding their options for future fertility prior to the initiation of pubertal suppression or gender-affirming hormones.

Review Questions and Answers

Q1. What types of hormonal therapies cause subfertility in individuals with gender dysphoria?

A1. Pubertal suppression and gender-affirming hormones (testosterone for trans-men and estrogen for trans-women) can both cause subfertility. Both are thought to be at least partially reversible once stopped.

Q2. True or false: Trans-men who have used testosterone cannot carry a pregnancy.

A2. False – Trans-men who have previously used testosterone *can* carry a pregnancy, although testosterone must be stopped before attempting pregnancy.

Q3. Which fertility preservation options are not recommended for adolescents with gender dysphoria, according to WPATH?

A3. Ovarian or testicular tissue cryopreservation is currently considered experimental and is not recommended for adolescents due to (1) the need to potentially perform irreversible procedures (gonadectomy), (2) lack of data regarding potential success of the procedures, and (3) unclear data regarding exact gonadotoxicity of gender-affirming hormones.

Q4. Approximately what percentage of transgender adolescents attempt fertility preservation prior to the initiation of gender-affirming hormones?

5

A4. Approximately 3–4%, with sperm banking being more commonly reported than oocyte cryopreservation.

References

1. Association AP. Diagnostic and statistical manual of mental disorders. 5th ed. Arlington: American Psychiatric Association; 2013.
2. Hembree WC, et al. Endocrine treatment of transsexual persons: an Endocrine Society clinical practice guideline. J Clin Endocrinol Metab. 2009;94(9):3132–54.
3. Coleman E, et al. Standards of care for the health of transsexual, transgender, and gender-nonconforming people, version 7. Int J Transgenderism. 2012;13(4): 165–232.
4. de Vries AL, et al. Young adult psychological outcome after puberty suppression and gender reassignment. Pediatrics. 2014;134(4):696–704.
5. Gooren L. Hormone treatment of the adult transsexual patient. Horm Res. 2005;64(Suppl 2):31–6.
6. Coleman E, Bockting W, Botzer M, Cohen-Kettenis P, DeCuypere G, Feldman J, et al. The world professional association for transgender health standards of care for the health of transsexual, transgender, and gender-nonconforming people, version 7. Int J Transgenderism. 2012;13:165–232.
7. Delemarre-Van de Waal HA, Cohen-Kettenis P. Clinical management of gender identity disorder in adolescents. Eur J Endocrinol. 2006;155(Suppl 1):S131–7.
8. Feldman J. Hormone therapy in adults: suggested revisions to the sixth version of the standards of care. Int J Transgenderism. 2009;11(3):146–82.
9. Dumasia K, et al. Effect of estrogen receptor-subtype-specific ligands on fertility in adult male rats. J Endocrinol. 2015;225(3):169–80.
10. Gill-Sharma MK, et al. Antifertility effects of estradiol in adult male rats. J Endocrinol Investig. 2001;24(8): 598–607.
11. Robaire B, Duron J, Hales BF. Effect of estradiol-filled polydimethylsiloxane subdermal implants in adult male rats on the reproductive system, fertility, and progeny outcome. Biol Reprod. 1987;37(2):327–34.
12. Sharpe RM, Skakkebaek NE. Are oestrogens involved in falling sperm counts and disorders of the male reproductive tract? Lancet. 1993;341(8857):1392–5.
13. Fisch H, Hyun G, Golden R. The possible effects of environmental estrogen disrupters on reproductive health. Curr Urol Rep. 2000;1(4):253–61.
14. Skakkebaek NE, et al. Is human fecundity declining? Int J Androl. 2006;29(1):2–11.
15. Oliva A, Spira A, Multigner L. Contribution of environmental factors to the risk of male infertility. Hum Reprod. 2001;16(8):1768–76.
16. Rozati R, et al. Role of environmental estrogens in the deterioration of male factor fertility. Fertil Steril. 2002;78(6):1187–94.
17. Du Plessis SS, et al. The effect of obesity on sperm disorders and male infertility. Nat Rev Urol. 2010;7(3):153–61.
18. Hillier SG, Ross GT. Effects of exogenous testosterone on ovarian weight, follicular morphology and intraovarian progesterone concentration in estrogen-primed hypophysectomized immature female rats. Biol Reprod. 1979;20(2):261–8.
19. Pauli EM, et al. Diminished paternity and gonadal function with increasing obesity in men. Fertil Steril. 2008;90(2):346–51.
20. Palmer NO, et al. Impact of obesity on male fertility, sperm function and molecular composition. Spermatogenesis. 2012;2(4):253–63.
21. Pavlovich CP, et al. Evidence of a treatable endocrinopathy in infertile men. J Urol. 2001;165(3):837–41.
22. Schneider F, et al. Testicular functions and clinical characterization of patients with gender dysphoria (GD) undergoing sex reassignment surgery (SRS). J Sex Med. 2015;12(11):2190–200.
23. Hamada A, et al. Semen characteristics of transwomen referred for sperm banking before sex transition: a case series. Andrologia. 2015;47(7):832–8.
24. Goerlich VC, Dijkstra C, Groothuis TG. Effects of in vivo testosterone manipulation on ovarian morphology, follicular development, and follicle yolk testosterone in the homing pigeon. J Exp Zool A Ecol Genet Physiol. 2010;313(6):328–38.
25. Velez LM, et al. Effect of hyperandrogenism on ovarian function. Reproduction. 2015;149(6):577–85.
26. van der Spuy ZM, Dyer SJ. The pathogenesis of infertility and early pregnancy loss in polycystic ovary syndrome. Best Pract Res Clin Obstet Gynaecol. 2004;18(5):755–71.
27. Dumesic DA, Padmanabhan V, Abbott DH. Polycystic ovary syndrome and oocyte developmental competence. Obstet Gynecol Surv. 2008;63(1):39–48.
28. Amato MC, et al. Low estradiol-to-testosterone ratio is associated with oligo-anovulatory cycles and atherogenic lipidic pattern in women with polycystic ovary syndrome. Gynecol Endocrinol. 2011;27(8):579–86.
29. De Roo C, et al. Ovarian tissue cryopreservation in female-to-male transgender people: insights into ovarian histology and physiology after prolonged androgen treatment. Reprod BioMed Online. 2017;34(6):557–66.

30. Light AD, et al. Transgender men who experienced pregnancy after female-to-male gender transitioning. Obstet Gynecol. 2014;124(6):1120–7.
31. Ellis SA, Wojnar DM, Pettinato M. Conception, pregnancy, and birth experiences of male and gender variant gestational parents: it's how we could have a family. J Midwifery Womens Health. 2015;60(1):62–9.
32. Light A, et al. Family planning and contraception use in transgender men. Contraception. 2018;98:266–9.
33. Lawrence AA, et al. Health care needs of transgendered patients. JAMA. 1996;276(11):874.
34. American Academy of Child and Adolescent Psychiatry. Facts for families: children with lesbian, gay, bisexual, and transgender parents. Washington, DC: American Academy of Child and Adolescent Psychiatry; 2013.
35. Ethics Committee of American Society for Reproductive, M. Fertility preservation and reproduction in patients facing gonadotoxic therapies: a committee opinion. Fertil Steril. 2013;100(5):1224–31.
36. Santelli JS, et al. Guidelines for adolescent health research: a position paper of the society for adolescent medicine. J Adolesc Health. 1995;17(5):270–6.
37. Fallat ME, et al. Preservation of fertility in pediatric and adolescent patients with cancer. Pediatrics. 2008; 121(5):e1461–9.
38. Bunge RG, Sherman JK. Fertilizing capacity of frozen human spermatozoa. Nature. 1953;172(4382):767–8.
39. Wang JH, Muller CH, Lin K. Optimizing fertility preservation for pre- and postpubertal males with cancer. Semin Reprod Med. 2013;31(4):274–85.
40. Nahata L, et al. Low fertility preservation utilization among transgender youth. J Adolesc Health. 2017;61(1): 40–4.
41. Ginsberg JP, et al. Testicular tissue cryopreservation in prepubertal male children: an analysis of parental decision-making. Pediatr Blood Cancer. 2014;61(9):1673–8.
42. Practice Committees of American Society for Reproductive, M. and T. Society for Assisted Reproductive. Mature oocyte cryopreservation: a guideline. Fertil Steril. 2013;99(1):37–43.
43. Maxwell S, et al. Pregnancy outcomes after fertility preservation in transgender men. Obstet Gynecol. 2017;129(6):1031–4.
44. Armuand G, et al. Transgender men's experiences of fertility preservation: a qualitative study. Hum Reprod. 2017;32(2):383–90.
45. De Sutter P. Gender reassignment and assisted reproduction: present and future reproductive options for transsexual people. Hum Reprod. 2001;16(4):612–4.
46. Berookhim BM, Mulhall JP. Outcomes of operative sperm retrieval strategies for fertility preservation among males scheduled to undergo cancer treatment. Fertil Steril. 2014;101(3):805–11.
47. Reichman DE, et al. Fertility preservation using controlled ovarian hyperstimulation and oocyte cryopreservation in a premenarcheal female with myelodysplastic syndrome. Fertil Steril. 2012; 98(5):1225–8.
48. Loren AW, et al. Fertility preservation for patients with cancer: American Society of Clinical Oncology clinical practice guideline update. J Clin Oncol. 2013; 31(19):2500–10.
49. De Sutter P, et al. The desire to have children and the preservation of fertility in transsexual women: a survey. Int J Transgenderism. 2003;6(3):1.
50. Wierckx K, et al. Reproductive wish in transsexual men. Hum Reprod. 2012;27(2):483–7.
51. Chen D, et al. Attitudes toward fertility and reproductive health among transgender and gender-nonconforming adolescents. J Adolesc Health. 2018; 63:62–8.
52. Chen D, et al. Fertility preservation for transgender adolescents. J Adolesc Health. 2017;61(1):120–3.
53. Broughton D, Omurtag K. Care of the transgender or gender-nonconforming patient undergoing in vitro fertilization. Int J Transgenderism. 2017;18(4):372–5.
54. James-Abra S, et al. Trans people's experiences with assisted reproduction services: a qualitative study. Hum Reprod. 2015;30(6):1365–74.
55. Feldman J, et al. Priorities for transgender medical and healthcare research. Curr Opin Endocrinol Diabetes Obes. 2016;23(2):180–7.
56. Schover LR. Patient attitudes toward fertility preservation. Pediatr Blood Cancer. 2009;53(2):281–4.

Options for Preserving Fertility

Contents

Embryo and Oocyte Banking

Lynn M. Westphal, Jamie A. M. Massie, and Jessica A. Lentscher

T. K. Woodruff et al. (eds.), *Textbook of Oncofertility Research and Practice*,
https://doi.org/10.1007/978-3-030-02868-8_6

Key Points

- Significant improvements in treatments in oncologic conditions have increased survival rates in reproductive-age women, and as a result, a woman's fertility potential is an important counseling area for pre-cancer treatment.
- Embryo cryopreservation before chemotherapy is the most well-established and widely available method of fertility preservation for women; oocyte cryopreservation gives women the most reproductive autonomy.
- Oocyte or embryo banking require controlled ovarian hyperstimulation and oocyte retrieval procedures and take approximately 12–14 days to complete. Patients must carefully consult with their gynecologic oncologist or oncologist prior to determine if this modest delay in treatment will significantly impact their treatment and prognosis.
- The majority of reproductive-age women who are diagnosed with cancer are candidates for fertility preservation and should receive counseling prior to the initiation of cancer treatments.

6.1 Introduction

Due to significant improvements in cancer treatments, patients affected by oncologic disease are living longer, fuller lives. As a result, the fertility potential of reproductive-age women affected by cancer has become an increasing focus for those who counsel and treat such patients. Indeed, patients who have undergone fertility preservation procedures prior to oncological treatment report that fertility preservation positively impacted their quality of life during treatment [1].

Advances in reproductive medicine now allow patients diagnosed with cancer during their reproductive years to undergo various fertility preservation techniques, maintaining the potential for childbearing following successful cancer treatment [2–4]. In addition, fertility preservation options, such as oocyte cryopreservation, are now available for those patients with ethical, religious, or social concerns that may prohibit the creation and storage of embryos.

In this chapter, we will focus on the use of embryo and oocyte banking for fertility preservation.

6.2 Candidates for Fertility Preservation

Women of reproductive age who are scheduled to undergo medical treatment that could lead to premature decline of ovarian function should be counseled regarding the possibility of oocyte or embryo cryopreservation [3, 5]. Prior to initiating treatment in a patient who desires fertility preservation, a screening examination should be performed in order to confirm that the patient is a good candidate. A baseline fertility assessment, such as an antral follicle count (AFC) and measurement of anti-Müllerian hormone (AMH) and/or day 3 follicle-stimulating hormone (FSH) levels, should be part of the evaluation. In addition, tumor type and stage, timing and gonadotoxicity of chemotherapy, and overall health of the patient should be taken into consideration before initiating fertility treatment. Information collected in this baseline assessment not only aids the physician in selecting appropriate medication doses but also allows for appropriate counseling regarding expected success rates following the procedure.

The standard procedure for embryo and oocyte cryopreservation requires controlled ovarian hyperstimulation and oocyte retrieval, a process that requires approximately 12–14 days. If chemotherapy cannot be postponed for this period of time without potential compromise to the patient's immediate or long-term treatment outcomes, other fertility preservation options should be explored.

Patients should be counseled regarding all fertility preservation methods that are applicable to their specific circumstance [6, 7]. Ideally, this counseling should be performed by a physician specializing in reproductive endocrinology and infertility who has experience working with cancer patients. During the counseling session, potential complications of these treatments, such as ovarian hyperstimulation syndrome and intra-abdominal bleeding, should be discussed in detail. Although the incidence of such complications is low, occurring in approximately 5% of cycles, the potential impact of these complications on the patient's current health status and/or plans to move forward with cancer treatment may be significant [8, 9].

6.3 Embryo Banking

Since the first reported birth in 1983, several hundred thousand children have been born from cryopreserved embryos created during in vitro fertilization (IVF) cycles. For women with a committed male partner, or who are prepared to use donor sperm, embryo cryopreservation before chemotherapy is the most well-established and widely available method of fertility preservation [10–12]. This technique involves the collection of oocytes followed by fertilization in the laboratory and subsequent freezing of viable embryos.

6.3.1 Procedure

The embryo banking procedure begins with controlled ovarian hyperstimulation with injectable gonadotropins. The stimulation has traditionally started the second or third day of full menstrual flow; however, success can be achieved with initiation of ovarian stimulation during any phase of the menstrual cycle [13–15].

A classic GnRH antagonist protocol is most often employed as it can be completed quickly and has been associated with a lower risk of ovarian hyperstimulation syndrome [16]. A typical cycle is as follows:

- Daily injections with gonadotropins begin on cycle day 2 or 3 and continue daily for an average of 10–12 days.
- GnRH antagonist is added to the medication schedule when the largest ovarian follicle measures 14 mm on transvaginal ultrasound.
- Ovulation is triggered with a single injection of human chorionic gonadotropin (hCG).
- Oocyte retrieval is performed 34–36 h following hCG injection.
- Retrieved oocytes are fertilized in the laboratory. Intracytoplasmic sperm injection (ICSI) is recommended when sperm parameters are abnormal and may be chosen even when semen analysis is normal in order to reduce the risk of fertilization failure [17].
- Successful fertilization is assessed on the day following oocyte retrieval, and the embryos are monitored in the laboratory until the time of cryopreservation.
- Embryos may be cryopreserved at the 2PN (i.e., prezygote), day 3 (i.e., 8 cell), or day 5 (i.e., blastocyst) stage. The timing of cryopreservation should be individualized and based upon the wishes of the patient and the recommendation of the treating physician.

When beginning stimulation later in the cycle, a modified GnRH antagonist protocol can be utilized, as follows [5, 13–15]:

- GnRH antagonist is administered as a single 3-mg dose or daily (0.25-mg dose) for 2–3 days to induce menses within 5–7 days, at which time ovarian stimulation can begin [5].
- Alternatively, gonadotropins and GnRH antagonist can be started at the same time and continued throughout the cycle, or antagonist can be added when the leading follicle reaches 13–14 mm.
- Ovulation triggering, fertilization, and embryo cryopreservation are carried out in the same fashion as with the traditional GnRH antagonist protocol.

Ovulation induction with leuprolide acetate (single 0.4-mL (2-mg) injection) can be administered in lieu of the traditional hCG ovulation trigger to reduce the risk of ovarian hyperstimulation syndrome in those patients at risk [18].

6.3.2 Cost

The average cost of an embryo cryopreservation (i.e., IVF) cycle ranges from $9286 to $12,513 [19, 20]. In addition, the initial cost of freezing and storage may add several hundred dollars to the total charge, and there will be additional fees at the time the embryos are thawed and transferred. Costs vary from one center to another, and specifics regarding cost should be addressed with the treating physician. Insurance coverage of fertility-preserving treatments is also widely variable, and questions regarding fertility benefits should be directed toward the patient's insurance provider.

There are some nonprofit organizations dedicated to providing support for patients whose medical treatments present the risk of infertility. These organizations, such as Fertile Hope®, a national LIVE*STRONG* initiative, and the Fertile Action Program, may be able to assist patients with the financial burden associated with undergoing fertility preservation procedures. Information about these organizations may be found online or provided by the treating physician.

6.3.3 Timing

6

The duration of treatment, from stimulation start to oocyte retrieval, is approximately 12–14 days. Chemotherapy can be started 1–2 days after oocyte retrieval. In one study, the effect of beginning chemotherapy before complete recovery of the ovaries after stimulation did not show any increase in ovarian damage [21].

6.3.4 Risks

Ovarian stimulation with oocyte retrieval is a relatively low-risk process. However, a small proportion of patients will experience complications such as mild-to-severe ovarian hyperstimulation syndrome or intra-abdominal bleeding. In addition, patients may experience a delay in the initiation of cancer treatment and may have an increased risk of thromboembolic events and theoretic stimulation of estrogen-sensitive cancers [22]. In the long term, the procedure may fail to produce retrievable eggs, produce embryos, or result in a pregnancy or live birth.

6.3.5 Success Rates

Published data suggest that women opting for embryo cryopreservation prior to initiation of cancer treatment can expect success rates similar to those of women undergoing IVF for male factor infertility [23, 24]. Parameters to define success, such as oocyte yield, number of embryos cryopreserved, pregnancy rates, and live birth rates, are highly dependent upon the patient's age and baseline fertility evaluation. ◘ Table 6.1 shows national success rates for thawed embryo cycles by age.

◘ **Table 6.1** Thawed embryo success rates

Age (years)	<35	35–37	38–40	41–42
Number of thaw procedures	14,756	7733	5342	1693
Live birth/egg retrieval cycle	42.5%	39.5%	33.5%	27.8%

Data from 2014 SART statistics (Final Subsequent Outcome (Frozen Cycles), filtered for "frozen embryo")
SART Society for Assisted Reproductive Technology

6.4 Oocyte Banking

Advances in oocyte cryopreservation have allowed more women to pursue fertility preservation. Because a sperm source is not needed before oocyte cryopreservation, women without a male partner may consider this option. In addition, oocyte cryopreservation presents those patients who have ethical or religious objections to the creation of embryos for storage with an alternative treatment choice. This option gives women the most reproductive autonomy and should be offered to all women.

When first introduced in the 1980s, the ability of a cryopreserved oocyte to be fertilized and result in a live birth was compromised by poor oocyte survival and poor fertilization rates [25–29]. However, improvements in cryopreservation techniques have resulted in significantly improved outcomes in patients opting for this method [30–32]. In 2013, the American Society for Reproductive Medicine (ASRM) and the Society for Assisted Reproductive Technology (SART) published a joint document which cited the improvements in pregnancy success using cryopreserved oocytes and stated that oocyte cryopreservation should no longer be considered experimental [33]. Further, ASRM recommends that patients facing infertility due to treatment with gonadotoxic therapies undergo oocyte cryopreservation with appropriate counseling.

6.4.1 Procedure

The oocyte banking procedure follows the same ovarian stimulation protocols as outlined above for embryo banking. As in the case of embryo cryopreservation, the stimulation start date is traditionally the 2nd or 3rd day of full menstrual flow but can be performed at any time during the menstrual cycle [13–15].

Following oocyte retrieval, oocytes are prepared for cryopreservation. Two methods of oocyte cryopreservation are available: slow freezing and vitrification [34]. With the slow-freezing method, the oocyte is placed in a low concentration of cryoprotective solution that acts as "antifreeze" by disrupting hydrogen bonds between water, and the oocyte is then slowly frozen in a programmable freezer. In vitrification, the oocyte is placed in a high concentration of cryoprotective agents and then rapidly cooled using liquid nitrogen. The thawing process is also ultrarapid in order to avoid ice nucleation.

Current evidence suggests that vitrification results in higher survival, fertilization, implantation, and pregnancy rates than slow freezing [29, 35, 36]. Therefore, the vitrification technique is the preferred method for oocyte cryopreservation, although a number of pregnancies have been reported using oocytes that were cryopreserved using the slow-freezing method [34, 35, 37, 38].

6.4.2 Cost

The average cost of an oocyte cryopreservation cycle is approximately $7791 [19]. In addition, the initial cost of freezing and storage may add several hundred dollars to the total charge, and there are additional fees at the time of thawing and transfer. Costs vary from center to center, and specifics should be addressed by the treating physician. As with embryo cryopreservation, insurance coverage is widely variable and questions regarding fertility benefits should be directed toward the patient's insurance provider. Patients may also look into financial assistance programs for cancer survivors as described earlier.

6.4.3 Timing

The duration of treatment, from stimulation start to oocyte retrieval, is approximately 12–14 days. Chemotherapy can be started 1–2 days after oocyte retrieval. In one study, the effect of beginning chemotherapy before complete recovery of the ovaries after stimulation showed no increase in ovarian damage [21].

6.4.4 Risks

Medical risks are similar to that for embryo cryopreservation. In addition, there is a risk that the oocytes may not survive thawing, not fertilize, or not result in a pregnancy in the future. Although short-term data are reassuring with regard to the incidence of chromosomal abnormalities and congenital anomalies in pregnancies achieved with cryopreserved oocytes, long-term data on developmental outcomes are lacking [33, 39].

6.4.5 Success Rates

There is compelling evidence that pregnancy rates in patients using cryopreserved oocytes are similar to those achieved with IVF utilizing fresh oocytes in young patients [33, 40, 41]. ◘ Table 6.2 shows national success rates for thawed oocyte cycles by age.

The success of an oocyte cryopreservation cycle (i.e., oocyte yield) is highly dependent upon the patients' age and baseline fertility evaluation. It is important to provide individualized counseling, taking into account the above factors as well as clinic-specific success rates, when discussing likelihood of live birth following oocyte cryopreservation [33].

◘ Table 6.2 Thawed oocyte success rates

Age (years)	<35	35–37	38–40	41–42
Number of thaw procedures	109	52	47	61
Live birth/ egg retrieval cycle	34.9%	25.0%	17.0%	19.7%

Data from 2014 SART statistics (Final Subsequent Outcome (Frozen Cycles), filtered for "frozen embryo")
SART Society for Assisted Reproductive Technology

6.5 Tumor-Specific Considerations

6.5.1 Breast Cancer

Breast cancer is the most common neoplasm diagnosed during the reproductive years, with more than 15% of all new breast cancer diagnoses occurring under the age of 40 years [42–44]. The treatment of invasive breast cancer often includes gonadotoxic agents. As a result, a significant proportion of cancer survivors suffer from premature ovarian insufficiency, making this population an important target for fertility preservation counseling and treatment.

6

Historically, women with breast cancer have not been offered embryo or oocyte cryopreservation to preserve fertility due to the theoretical risk of tumor progression with the high estradiol levels that often occur during ovarian stimulation. However, standard stimulation protocols can be modified to include the selective estrogen modulator tamoxifen or the aromatase inhibitor letrozole. In one protocol, letrozole (5 mg/day) can be administered at the same time as gonadotropins and continued for 7 days after oocyte retrieval. The addition of an aromatase inhibitor allows for ovarian stimulation without significant increases in estradiol levels [45]. As a result, breast cancer patients should be offered the option of embryo or oocyte cryopreservation.

The timing of ovarian stimulation is of particular importance in patients with invasive breast cancer. In general, the initiation of ovarian stimulation is preferred after surgical excision, especially in those patients with hormone receptor-positive tumors. Instead, ovarian stimulation is best started in the hiatus between surgical excision and chemotherapy. In most cases, surgical excision precedes the initiation of chemotherapy by 4–6 weeks, allowing for sufficient time to undergo ovarian stimulation for fertility preservation. Retrospective studies have shown no significant delay in breast cancer treatment in patients who decide to undergo ovarian stimulation [46, 47]. Furthermore, ovarian stimulation in patients with both hormone receptor-positive and hormone receptor-negative tumors has not been associated with any difference in disease-free survival and overall survival rates compared with those not undergoing fertility preservation procedures [48, 49].

6.5.2 Ovarian Cancer

In the past, the options for fertility preservation in patients with ovarian cancer were severely limited due to the extensive surgical management that treatment of such malignancies involved. The standard of care for ovarian cancer treatment in most cases included total abdominal hysterectomy, bilateral salpingo-oophorectomy, and comprehensive surgical staging. However, less radical surgical management, such as unilateral salpingo-oophorectomy, can be considered in carefully selected cases [50]. Studies examining the 5-year survival rate of patients with early-stage disease showed no difference in survival between those who underwent fertility-sparing procedures and those who did not [51]. Generally speaking, women with early-stage ovarian cancer may be candidates for fertility preservation via embryo or oocyte cryopreservation.

6.5.3 Hematologic Malignancies

The treatment of hematologic malignancies is frequently associated with significant gonadal toxicity, making fertility preservation counseling and treatment of utmost importance in this population [52, 53]. Complicating the treatment of such patients is the urgency to begin cancer therapy as early as possible after diagnosis. Patients due to undergo immediate cancer treatment are not candidates for embryo or oocyte cryopreservation and should, instead, be offered alternative methods of fertility preservation. For those patients in whom a 2-week treatment delay is acceptable, one can proceed with embryo and/or oocyte cryopreservation using the routine protocol. As patients usually begin chemotherapy shortly after oocyte retrieval, the use of leuprolide acetate for ovulation induction can speed the interval from oocyte retrieval to next menses and minimize the symptoms of ovarian stimulation.

6.5.4 Endometrial Cancer

In reproductive-age women, endometrial cancer tends to be associated with prolonged unopposed estrogen exposure. This may be the result of obesity, anovulation, and/or polycystic ovary syndrome. As these conditions are often associated with infertility, approximately 15% of young patients found to have endometrial cancer are actually identified during the course of infertility workup [54].

Traditionally, the treatment for endometrial cancer has included total hysterectomy and bilateral salpingo-oophorectomy. Alternative treatments that may allow for fertility conservation are available for patients who meet certain criteria. Women with low-grade endometrial cancer may choose to treat their disease with hormonal therapy rather than surgery. In these cases, oral progestational agents may be used in an attempt to convert the endometrium back to a benign state [55–58]. Conservative surgical management with ovarian preservation may also be an option for those patients who are considering the use of a gestational carrier for childbearing.

In those patients who are not felt to be candidates for conservative therapy, ovarian stimulation with embryo and/or oocyte cryopreservation followed by definitive surgical treatment may be employed. A progestin-containing IUD can be placed during the stimulation [58]. It should be noted that there is a significant risk of disease recurrence and/or progression when conservative treatments for endometrial cancer are employed [59]. The decision to proceed with these types of therapy should be done only with the recommendation and guidance of a trained gynecologic oncologist.

6.5.5 Cervical Cancer

Cervical cancer is most commonly diagnosed during the reproductive years and frequently affects women who have not completed childbearing. Conventional treatment for cervical cancer may include radical hysterectomy with or without postoperative pelvic radiation and chemotherapy; however, women with early-stage disease (1A2 and 1B1) may be candidates for more conservative surgical therapy. Radical trachelectomy (surgical removal of the uterine cervix) in carefully selected patients allows for fertility preservation without a significant difference in survival rates compared with those undergoing radical hysterectomy [60, 61].

In patients undergoing hysterectomy, ovarian stimulation can be performed either pre- or postoperatively. When embryo and/or oocyte cryopreservation is pursued postoperatively, the starting point for stimulation can be made serologically, as menses cannot be used as the starting point, or a random start can be used. In addition, if oophoropexy is performed at the time of hysterectomy, ovarian monitoring and retrieval may need to be done transabdominally. Furthermore, manipulation of the ovaries may affect blood supply and decrease responsiveness to stimulation.

6.6 Conclusions

As earlier detection and treatment allow cancer patients to live longer, fuller lives, the need for timely and comprehensive counseling regarding fertility preservation in these women has become an important quality of life issue. Fortunately, the majority of reproductive-age women who are diagnosed with cancer are candidates for fertility preservation, often by embryo and/or oocyte cryopreservation. All women should be made aware of their options for fertility preservation, allowing them the potential to fulfill their reproductive goals.

Acknowledgment This work was supported by the Oncofertility Consortium NIH/NICHD 5UL1DE019587.

Review Questions and Answers

Q1. What evaluation is included prior to initiation of oocyte/embryo preservation?

A1. An antral follicle count, anti-Mullerian hormone level, and/or day 3 FSH level.

Q2. Which freezing method results in higher survival, fertilization, implantation, and pregnancy rates?

A2. Vitrification is the preferred method for oocyte or embryo preservation.

Q3. In carefully selected patients with early-stage ovarian cancer, does fertility-sparing treatment change survival rate?

A3. Studies have not shown a difference in 5-year survival rates between those who underwent fertility-sparing procedures and those who did not.

Q4. In an effort to decrease estrogen levels in a controlled ovarian stimulation cycle in patients with hormone-sensitive breast cancer, what modifications can be made to allow patients to proceed with fertility preservation?

A4. The addition of an aromatase inhibitor such as letrozole allows for ovarian stimulation without significant increase in serum estradiol levels.

References

1. Assi J, Santos J, Bonetti T, Serafini PC, Motta ELA, Chehin MB. Psychosocial benefits of fertility preservation for young cancer patients. J Assist Reprod Genet. 2018;35(4):601–6. [Epub ahead of print].
2. Lee SJ, American Society of Clinical Oncology, et al. American Society of Clinical Oncology recommendations on fertility preservation in cancer patients. J Clin Oncol. 2006;24:2917–31.
3. von Wolff M, et al. Fertility preservation in women-a practical guide to preservation techniques and therapeutic strategies in breast cancer, Hodgkin's lymphoma and borderline ovarian tumours by the fertility preservation network FertiPROTEKT. Arch Gynecol Obstet. 2011;284:427–35.
4. Wright J, et al. Fertility preservation in young women with epithelial ovarian cancer. Cancer. 2009;115: 4118–26.
5. Noyes N, et al. Oocyte cryopreservation as a fertility preservation measure for cancer patients. Reprod Biomed Online. 2011;23:323–33.
6. Kesic V, et al. Fertility preserving management in gynecologic cancer patients: the need for centralization. Int J Gynecol Cancer. 2010;20:1613–9.
7. Patel A, et al. Reproductive health assessment for women with cancer: a pilot study. Reproductive health assessment for women with cancer: a pilot study. Am J Obstet Gynecol. 2009;201:191.e1–4.
8. Forman RG, et al. Severe ovarian hyperstimulation syndrome using agonists of gonadotrophin releasing hormone for in vitro fertilization: a European series and a proposal for prevention. Fertil Steril. 1990;53:502–9.
9. MacDougall MJ, Tan SL, Jacobs HS. In vitro fertilization and the ovarian hyperstimulation syndrome. Hum Reprod. 1992;7:579–600.
10. Diedrich K, Fauser BC, Devroey P, Evian Annual Reproduction (EVAR) Workshop Group 2009. Cancer and fertility: strategies to preserve fertility. Reprod Biomed Online. 2011;22:232–48.
11. Maltaris T, et al. The effect of cancer treatment on female fertility and strategies for preserving fertility. Eur J Obstet Gynecol Reprod Biol. 2007;130:148–55.
12. Roberts JE, Oktay K. Fertility preservation: a comprehensive approach to the young woman with cancer. J Natl Cancer Inst Monogr. 2005;34:57–9.
13. von Wolff M, Thaler CJ, Frambach T, Zeeb C, Lawrenz B, Popovici RM, et al. Ovarian stimulation to cryopreserve fertilized oocytes in cancer patients can be started in the luteal phase. Fertil Steril. 2009;92:1360–5.
14. Ozkaya E, San Roman G, Oktay K. Luteal phase GnRHa trigger in random start fertility preservation cycles. J Assist Reprod Genet. 2012;29:503–5.
15. Cakmak H, Rosen M. Random-start ovarian stimulation in patient with cancer. Curr Opin Obstet Gynecol. 2015;27:215–21.
16. Al-Inany HG, Abou-Setta AM, Aboulghar M. Gonadotrophin-releasing hormone antagonists for assisted conception: a Cochrane review. Reprod Biomed Online. 2007;14:640–9.
17. Mahutte NG, Arici A. Failed fertilization: is it predictable? Curr Opin Obstet Gynecol. 2003;15:211–8.
18. Bodri D, et al. Triggering with human chorionic gonadotropin or a gonadotropin-releasing hormone agonist in gonadotropin-releasing hormone antagonist-treated oocyte donor cycles: findings of a large retrospective cohort study. Fertil Steril. 2009;91:365–71.
19. Beck LN. The average cost of fertility preservation for female cancer patients. Poster presented at 66th annual meeting of the American Society for Reproductive Medicine (ASRM), Denver. 2010.
20. Chambers GM, et al. The economic impact of assisted reproductive technology: a review of selected developed countries. Fertil Steril. 2009;91:2281–94.
21. Maman E, et al. Does controlled ovarian stimulation prior to chemotherapy increase primordial follicle loss and diminish ovarian reserve? An animal study. Hum Reprod. 2009;24:206–10.
22. The Practice Committee of the American Society for Reproductive Medicine. Fertility preservation in patients undergoing gonadotoxic therapy or gonadectomy: a committee opinion. Fertil Steril. 2013;100: 1214–23.
23. Robertson AD, Missmer SA, Ginsburg ES. Embryo yield after in vitro fertilization in women undergoing embryo banking for fertility preservation before chemotherapy. Fertil Steril. 2011;95:588–91.
24. Knopman JM, et al. Women with cancer undergoing ART for fertility preservation: a cohort study of their response to exogenous gonadotropins. Fertil Steril. 2009;91:1476–8.
25. Chen C. Pregnancy after human oocyte cryopreservation. Lancet. 1986;1:884–6.
26. Sonmezer M, Oktay K. Fertility preservation in female patients. Hum Reprod Update. 2004;10:251–66.
27. Porcu E. Oocyte freezing. Semin Reprod Med. 2001;19: 221–30.
28. Van der Elst J. Oocyte freezing: here to stay? Hum Reprod Update. 2003;9:463–70.
29. Oktay K, Cil AP, Bang H. Efficiency of oocyte cryopreservation: a meta-analysis. Fertil Steril. 2006;86: 70–80.

30. Grifo JA, Noyes N. Delivery rate using cryopreserved oocytes is comparable to conventional in vitro fertilization using fresh oocytes: potential fertility preservation for female cancer patients. Fertil Steril. 2010;93:391–6.
31. Barritt J, et al. Report of four donor-recipient oocyte cryopreservation cycles resulting in high pregnancy and implantation rates. Fertil Steril. 2007;87:189.e13–7.
32. Cobo A, et al. Comparison of concomitant outcome achieved with fresh and cryopreserved donor oocytes vitrified by the Cryotop method. Fertil Steril. 2008;89:1657–64.
33. Practice Committees of American Society for Reproductive Medicine, Society for Assisted Reproductive Technology. Mature oocyte cryopreservation: a guideline. Fertil Steril. 2013;99:37–43.
34. Fadini R, et al. Human oocyte cryopreservation: comparison between slow and ultrarapid methods. Reprod Biomed Online. 2009;19:171–80.
35. Smith GD, et al. Prospective randomized comparison of human oocyte cryopreservation with slow-rate freezing or vitrification. Fertil Steril. 2010;94:2088–95.
36. Gook DA, Edgar DH. Human oocyte cryopreservation. Hum Reprod Updat. 2007;13:591–605.
37. Cao YX, et al. Comparison of survival and embryonic development in human oocytes cryopreserved by slow-freezing and vitrification. Fertil Steril. 2009;92:1306–11.
38. Martínez-Burgos M, et al. Vitrification versus slow freezing of oocytes: effects on morphologic appearance, meiotic spindle configuration, and DNA damage. Fertil Steril. 2011;95:374–7.
39. Noyes N, Porcu E, Borini A. Over 900 oocyte cryopreservation babies born with no apparent increase in congenital anomalies. Reprod Biomed Online. 2009;18:769–76.
40. Cobo A, et al. Use of cryo-banked oocytes in an ovum donation programme: a prospective, randomized, controlled, clinical trial. Hum Reprod. 2010;25:2239–46.
41. Nagy ZP, et al. Clinical evaluation of the efficiency of an oocyte donation program using egg cryo-banking. Fertil Steril. 2009;92:520–6.
42. Hankey BF, et al. Trends in breast cancer in younger women in contrast to older women. J Natl Cancer Inst Monogr. 1994;16:7–14.
43. Higgins S, Haffty BG. Pregnancy and lactation after breast-conserving therapy for early stage breast cancer. Cancer. 1994;73:2175–80.
44. Goodwin PJ, et al. Risk of menopause during the first year after breast cancer diagnosis. J Clin Oncol. 1999;17:2365–70.
45. Oktay K, et al. Letrozole reduces estrogen and gonadotropin exposure in women with breast cancer undergoing ovarian stimulation before chemotherapy. J Clin Endocrinol Metab. 2006;91:3885–90.
46. Baynosa J, et al. Timing of breast cancer treatments with oocyte retrieval and embryo cryopreservation. J Am Coll Surg. 2009;5:603–7.
47. Madrigrano A, Westphal L, Wapnir I. Egg retrieval with cryopreservation does not delay breast cancer treatment. Am J Surg. 2007;194:477–81.
48. Azim A, Constantini-Ferando M, Oktay K. Safety of fertility preservation by ovarian stimulation with letrozole and gonadotropins in patients with breast cancer: a prospective controlled study. J Clin Oncol. 2008;26:2630–5.
49. Hashimoto T, Nakamura Y, Obata R, Doshida M, Toya M, Takeuchi T, Kyono K. Effects of fertility preservation in patients with breast cancer: a retrospective two-centers study. Reprod Med Biol. 2017;16(4):374–9.
50. Morice P, et al. Recommendations of the fertility task force of the European society of gynecologic oncology about the conservative management of ovarian malignant tumors. Int J Gynecol Cancer. 2011;21:951–63.
51. Wright JD, et al. Fertility preservation in young women with epithelial ovarian cancer. Cancer. 2009;1(15):4118–26.
52. Grigg AP, et al. Reproductive status in long-term bone marrow transplant survivors receiving busulfan-cyclophosphamide (120 mg/kg). Bone Marrow Transplant. 2000;26:1089–95.
53. Meirow D, et al. Searching for evidence of disease and malignant cell contamination in ovarian tissue stored from hematologic cancer patients. Hum Reprod. 2008;23:1007–13.
54. Kempson R, Pokorny G. Adenocarcinoma of the endometrium in women aged forty and younger. Cancer. 1968;21:650–62.
55. Ramirez PT, et al. Hormonal therapy for the management of grade 1 endometrial adenocarcinoma: a literature review. Gynecol Oncol. 2004;95:133–8.
56. Randall TC, Kurman RJ. Progestin treatment of atypical hyperplasia and well-differentiated carcinoma of the endometrium in women under age 40. Obstet Gynecol. 1997;90:434–40.
57. Yang YC, et al. Reevaluating the safety of fertility-sparing hormonal therapy for early endometrial cancer. Gynecol Oncol. 2005;99:287–93.
58. Juretzka MM, et al. Embryo cryopreservation after diagnosis of stage IIB endometrial cancer and subsequent pregnancy in a gestational carrier. Fertil Steril. 2005;83:1041.
59. Chiya L, et al. Sparing fertility in young patients with endometrial cancer. Gynecol Oncol. 2008;111:S101–4.
60. Diaz JP, et al. Oncologic outcome of fertility-sparing radical trachelectomy versus radical hysterectomy for stage IB1 cervical carcinoma. Gynecol Oncol. 2008;111:255–60.
61. Plante M, et al. Vaginal radical trachelectomy: an oncologically safe fertility-preserving surgery. An updated series of 72 cases and review of the literature. Gynecol Oncol. 2004;94:614–23.

Ovarian Tissue Cryopreservation and Transplantation

Yuting Fan, and Sherman Silber

T. K. Woodruff et al. (eds.), *Textbook of Oncofertility Research and Practice*,
https://doi.org/10.1007/978-3-030-02868-8_7

Key Points

- Ovarian cortex can be successfully cryopreserved and transplanted in young women with cancer who are risk for gonadotoxicity.
- Cortical pressure is a strong inhibitor of resting oocyte development and its decrease at the time of ovarian tissue transplantation may result in follicle depletion from over-recruitment.
- The only single-center series of frozen ovarian tissue transplantations in the United States reports a robust live birth rate.

7

7.1 Fresh Ovary Tissue Transplant

Successful fresh human ovary tissue transplantation was first reported between monozygotic twins discordant for premature ovarian failure (POF) using a cortical grafting technique [1, 2]. Normal menstrual cycles resumed after 4 months, and spontaneous pregnancy occurred 1 month later, ultimately resulting in live birth. Subsequently, a series of eight more consecutive successful cases was reported, all demonstrating resumption of normal ovulatory cycles [3, 4]. A ninth successful case was reported using a different technique, microvascular intact whole ovary transplantation, again with return of normal ovulatory cycles, spontaneous pregnancy, and delivery of a healthy child [5] (◘ Fig. 7.1).

Each of the cases in this series included primary ovarian insufficiency (POI) in one twin and proven fertility with completed childbearing in the other. In each case, careful consideration was given to alternate treatment options such as donor egg IVF and adoption. Seven of the 9 homograft patients have conceived unassisted, resulting in a total of 11 live births. Additional ovarian cortical tissue was frozen for potential future grafting should the transplanted ovary cease to function [6]. This series of fresh transplants afforded the opportunity to study the effect of transplant ischemia on the success of ovarian grafts without the concern of immunosuppression. Fresh cortical ovarian grafting results in minimal ischemic oocyte loss when performed using microsurgical techniques. The observed follicular depletion rather appears to be due to reduced cortical tissue pressure after the transplant, resulting in over-recruitment of primordial follicles. Despite representing only a small proportion of the total ovarian tissue, the

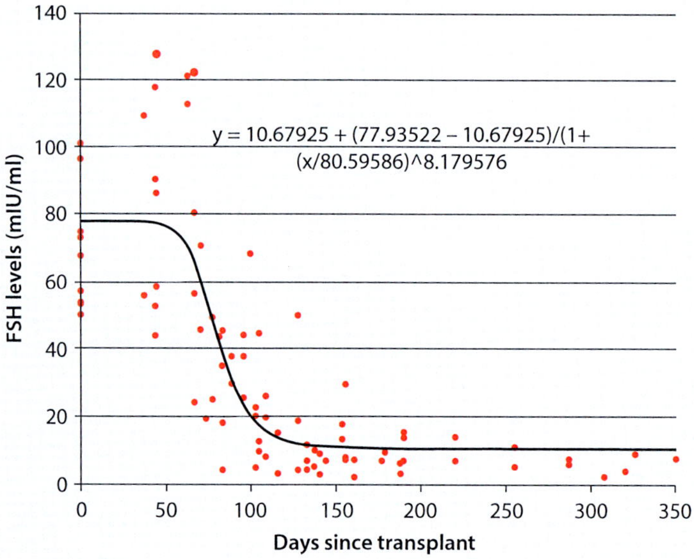

◘ **Fig. 7.1** Return of FSH levels to normal after fresh ovary transplant. Normalization of FSH following fresh ovarian tissue cortical transplant. FSH appears to normalize more rapidly after fresh (1–2 months) versus frozen (4–5 months) ovarian tissue transplant due to preservation of the primary follicle pool grafts last for 4–8 years due to a subsequent reduction in the rate of primordial follicle recruitment. The techniques pioneered in these fresh transplants have subsequently been applied to preserve fertility in patients facing sterilizing cancer treatment.

7.2 Frozen Ovary Tissue Transplant

Successful cryopreserved ovarian cortex transplants in humans were first reported in 2005, and many other case reports have subsequently followed [2, 4–22]. The first human applications were preceded by a long history of animal experimentation. Ovarian tissue was first shown to be successfully frozen and autografted in rats and mice in the 1950s–1960s, resulting in live births [23, 24]. Candy et al. then showed these mice had a normal reproductive lifespan [25]. Interest in human applications began in the 1990s after Gosdens' report of successful pregnancies following ovarian cortical transplantation in sheep [1]. While interest in cryopreserved ovarian cortical transplantation continues to grow, the current data originates from only a few centers, thus limiting its generalizability [11, 26–28].

One of the initial questions in human application of cryopreserved ovarian tissue transplantation was how to minimize oocyte loss from ischemia and/or cryopreservation. Ischemic damage can be avoided with intact whole ovary microsurgical transplantation, but the complexity and risk associated with this technique limits its utilization as compared with cortical grafting [5]. Animal data regarding the risk of oocyte loss after cortical grafting is conflicting. A significant loss of oocytes had been noted in some studies [29], while normal lifetime graft survival has been observed in others [25]. An initial human study demonstrated a maximum graft survival of only 2 years, but its generalizability was limited by the study population which included older women undergoing hysterectomy and oophorectomy [17]. It therefore remains unclear whether the modest outcomes after cryopreserved cortical grafting were limited by cryopreservation damage, ischemia time, or prior damage from chemotherapy [30].

7.2.1 Freezing Technique

The technique for slow freeze and thaw has not changed since the original description by Gosden et al. in 1994 [1, 19]. Slow freezing is the most established method of ovarian cortical cryopreservation. The cortex is removed from the medulla; divided into multiple strips measuring 1.0 × 1.5 × 0.5 cm each; incubated in 1.5 mol/L 1,2-propanedial ethylene glycol or DMSO, 0.1 mol/L sucrose with 10% SSS at 37 °C for 30 min, and then 0.2 mol/L sucrose for 5 min; and finally transferred to cryovials and cooled by computerized lowering of temperature [31]. Cooling is first done at 2 °C/min to −9 °C and then seeded. Thereafter, the cooling rate is −0.3 °C/min down to −40 °C and then −10 °C / min down to −140 °C and then plunged into liquid nitrogen. Thawing is performed rapidly (37 °C/min) in a warm water bath, and the tissue is trimmed under an operating microscope before transplantation [1, 2, 6, 31]. This slow freeze method is well established and has resulted in most of the reported pregnancies and live births to date.

However, in vitro viability analysis studies show that vitrification may be preferred due to its negligible oocyte loss rate as compared to the 50% oocyte loss with slow freezing [12, 18, 32]. For vitrification, the ovarian cortex is cut into slices measuring 10 × 10 × 1 mm. The tissue slices are initially equilibrated in 7.5% ethylene glycol (EG) and 7.5% dimethyl sulfoxide (DMSO) in HEPES-buffered handling media supplemented with 20% synthetic serum substitute (SSM) for 25 min. Then a second equilibration is performed in 20% EG and 20% DMSO with 0.5 M sucrose for 15 min or until the slices descend to the bottom of a 50 ml centrifuge tube indicating complete absorption of the cryoprotectants. The tissues are then placed on a thin metal strip (Kitayzato Bio Pharma, Japan) which are then plunged directly into sterile liquid nitrogen and inserted into a "closed" tube which contains liquid nitrogen for storage. For thawing, the metal strip is immersed swiftly into 40 ml of 37 °C HEPES-buffered handling media supplemented with 1.0 mol sucrose for 1 min and then 40 ml of 0.5 mol sucrose for 5 min at room temperature and washed twice for 10 min in standard handling media. Standard H+E histology and dye exclusion are performed to check for viability and presence of cancer cells (Figs. 7.2, 7.3, and 7.4).

7.2.2 Surgical Transplant Technique

The transplant technique has not substantially changed since the first fresh transplant in 2004 and is well described [2]. After thawing, the ovarian cortical strip is treated as though it were a full-thickness skin graft (1 × 1 cm pieces approximately 1–1.5 mm in thickness). The thawed strips are quilted together into a single graft with a 9-0 nylon sutures in vitro before the patient was anesthetized (Figs. 7.5 and 7.6). All procedures were performed with minilaparotomy and an operating microscope. Meticulous micro-bipolar cautery with pulsatile heparinized saline irrigation and multiple micro-pressure interrupted stitches of 9-0 nylon are used to minimize the formation of micro-hematomas under the graft. Constant pulsatile irrigation is used to prevent adhesions, and all transplants are performed in an orthotopic location on the denuded ovarian medulla of the remaining intact ovary in order to facilitate unassisted conception.

7

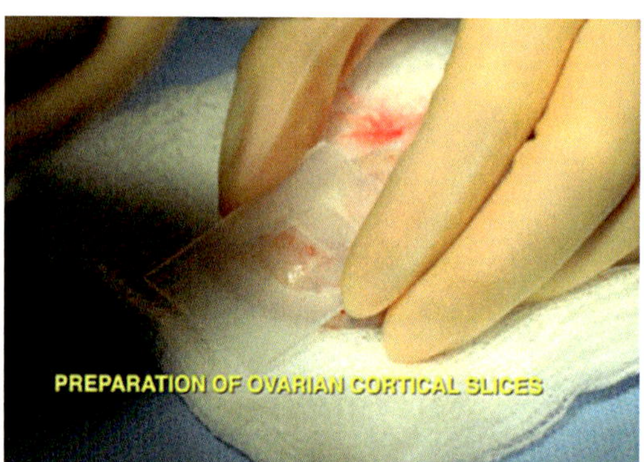

Fig. 7.2 Thin slices of ovarian cortical tissue preserve the resting follicle pool

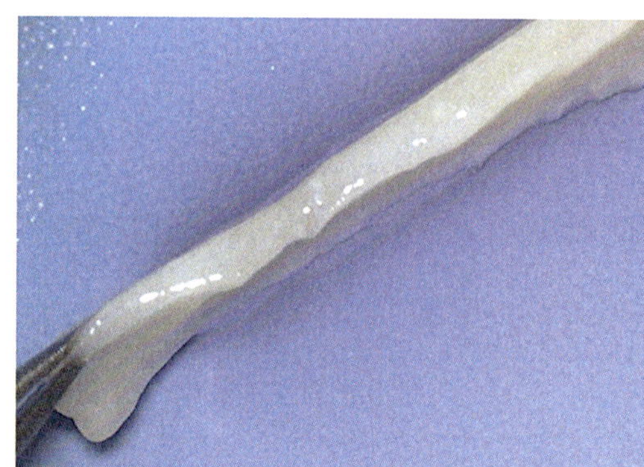

Fig. 7.3 A thin (1.5 mm) slice of ovarian cortex

Fig. 7.4 Histology of thinly sliced ovarian cortex containing primordial follicles

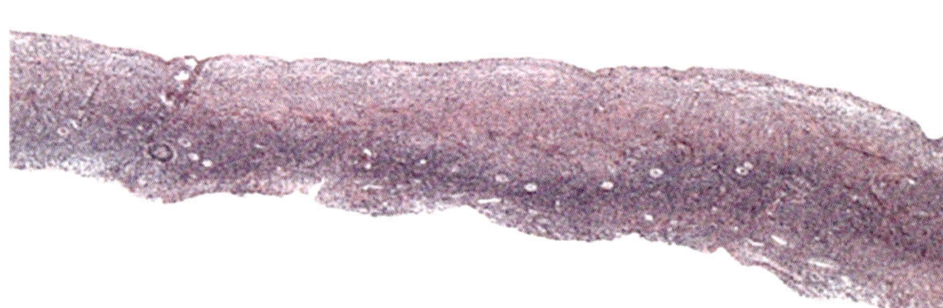

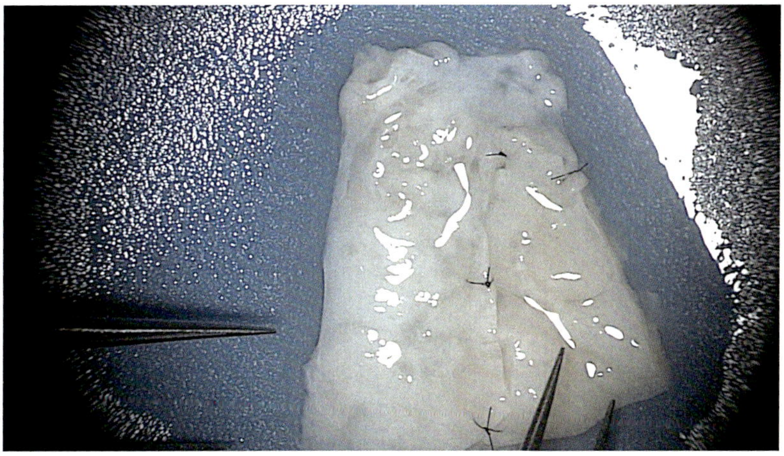

Fig. 7.5 Tissue quilting of ovarian cortical slices in vitro

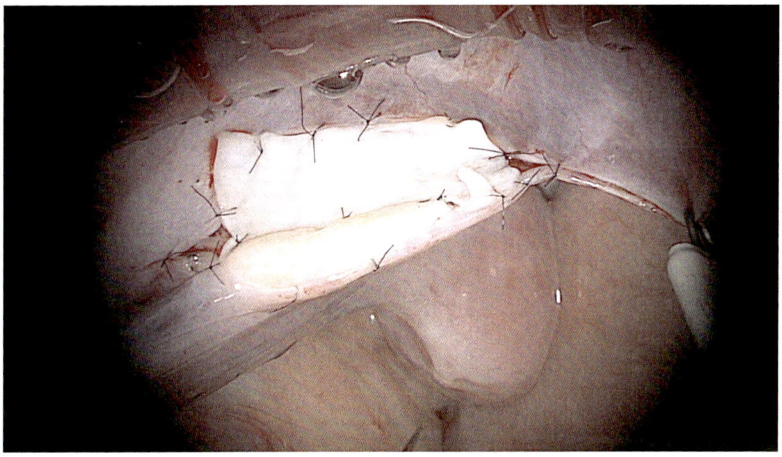

Fig. 7.6 Surgical transplantation of quilted ovarian cortical slices in vivo

7.2.3 Reproductive Outcomes

The return of FSH levels to near normal at 4–5 months following cryopreserved ovarian tissue transplantation indicates that this is the period of time required for the recruitment of primordial follicles to develop the antral and ovulatory stage (Fig. 7.7). The concomitant rise of AMH followed by a drop to very low levels suggests a massive over-recruitment of follicles and subsequent oocyte depletion [33] that has been attributed to reduced cortical tissue pressure after the transplant. Interestingly, the ovarian transplant continues to function for 4–8 years despite the low AMH, presumptively due to a decreased rate of primordial follicle recruitment in the presence of diminished ovarian reserve [34–37]. In a series of 13 women undergoing orthotopic cryopreserved ovarian cortical transplantation, 10 women have conceived unassisted, with a total of 13 live births [38]. The role of assisted reproductive technology is limited in this setting given the known diminished ovarian reserve. Cortical graft lifespan ranged between 4 and 8 years, and additional cortical slices remain frozen should additional transplant be desired.

7.2.4 Risk of Reseeding Malignancy

A carefully guarded clinical decision is necessary before transplanting the ovarian tissue back to cancer patients. Nonetheless, for patients in whom there is no significant risk of ovarian metastasis, ovary tissue transplant may remain a favorable option. In all cases, patholo-

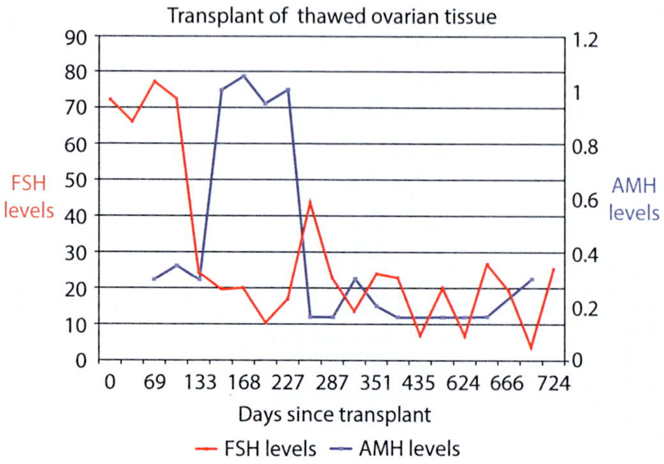

Fig. 7.7 FSH and AMH levels following transplant of cryopreserved ovarian tissue. FSH levels normalize in 4–5 months. AMH initially rises and falls to low levels by 9 months

7

gists and oncologists review samples via histology, histochemistry, and/or polymerase chain reaction testing [38]. There have now been over 100 babies born around the world from ovary tissue transplantation in cancer survivors, with no reports of reseeding malignancy to date [26–28, 39].

7.3 Conclusion and Future Directions

Fertility preservation remains a paramount concern for young women or prepubertal girls who may lose gonadal function as a result of cancer treatment [40–43]. Since the initial report by Gosden et al. of frozen ovary tissue transplantation in sheep, and the first reported cases in 2005 in humans, there has been intense interest in utilizing ovarian tissue cryopreservation and transplant for fertility preservation in cancer survivors [1, 2, 6, 13]. Due to the myriad medical and social parameters that dictate an individual patient's desire to return for utilization of cryopreserved ovarian tissue [44], long-term follow-up data after ovarian tissue transplantation is still limited to a few centers.

Although the primary impetus for ovarian tissue transplantation has been for fertility preservation prior to gonadotropic cancer therapy, it is also possible that grafts could be used in the future to delay menopause [21, 41–43], [45]. This latter application of prolonging ovarian hormonal and reproductive function against the natural aging process has even been speculated as a possible indication for ovarian tissue cryopreservation in healthy young women [46–49]. At the time of this publication, however, ovarian tissue cryopreservation remains an "experimental" therapy as defined by the American Society of Reproductive Medicine [50].

Review Questions and Answers

Q1. Who first reported (and when) successful transplantation of frozen ovarian tissue in sheep?

A1. Roger Gosden (1994).

Q2. Who reported the first successful (fresh and frozen) transplantation in humans?

A2. Jacques Donnez – Frozen, Sherman Silber – Fresh

Q3. What is the live birth rate after frozen ovary tissue transplant in the only series in the United States?

A3. 76%

Q4. What regulates primordial follicle recruitment and fetal oocyte arrest?

A4. Tissue pressure gradient.

References

1. Gosden RG, Baird DT, et al. Restoration of fertility to oophorectomized sheep by ovarian autografts stored at −196 degrees C. Hum Reprod. 1994;9(4):597–603.
2. Silber SJ, Lenahan KM, et al. Ovarian transplantation between monozygotic twins discordant for premature ovarian failure. N Engl J Med. 2005;353(1):58–63.
3. Silber SJ, Gosden RG. Ovarian transplantation in a series of monozygotic twins discordant for ovarian failure. N Engl J Med. 2007;356(13):1382–4.
4. Silber SJ, DeRosa M, et al. A series of monozygotic twins discordant for ovarian failure: ovary transplantation (cortical versus microvascular) and cryopreservation. Hum Reprod. 2008a;23(7):1531–7.
5. Silber SJ, Grudzinskas G, et al. Successful pregnancy after microsurgical transplantation of an intact ovary. N Engl J Med. 2008b;359(24):2617–8.
6. Donnez J, Dolmans MM, et al. Livebirth after orthotopic transplantation of cryopreserved ovarian tissue. Lancet. 2004;364(9443):1405–10.
7. Andersen CY, Rosendahl M, Byskov AG, Loft A, Ottosen C, Dueholm M, Schmidt KL, Andersen AN, Ernst E. Two successful pregnancies following autotransplantation of frozen/thawed ovarian tissue. Hum Reprod. 2008;23:2266–72.
8. Demeestere I, Simon P, Englert Y, Delbaere A. Preliminary experience of ovarian tissue cryopreservation procedure: alternatives, perspectives and feasibility. Reprod Biomed Online. 2003;7:572–9.
9. Dittrich R, Lotz L, Keck G, Hoffmann I, Mueller A, Beckmann MW, Van Der Ven H, Montag M. Live birth after ovarian tissue autotransplantation following overnight transportation before cryopreservation. Fertil Steril. 2012;97:387–90.
10. Donnez J, Silber S, Andersen CY, Demeestere I, Piver P, Meirow D, Pellicer A, Dolmans MM. Children born after autotransplantation of cryopreserved ovarian tissue. A review of 13 live births. Ann Med. 2011;43:437–50.
11. Donnez J, Dolmans MM, Pellicer A, Diaz-Garcia C, Sanchez Serrano M, Schmidt KT, Ernst E, Luyckx V, Andersen CY. Restoration of ovarian activity and pregnancy after trans- plantation of cryopreserved ovarian tissue: a review of 60 cases of reimplantation. Fertil Steril. 2013;99:1503–13.
12. Kagawa N, Silber S, et al. Successful vitrification of bovine and human ovarian tissue. Reprod Biomed Online. 2009;18(4):568–77.
13. Meirow D, Levron J, Eldar-Geva T, Hardan I, Fridman E, Zalel Y, Schiff E, Dor J. Pregnancy after transplantation of cryopreserved ovarian tissue in a patient with ovarian failure after chemotherapy. N Engl J Med. 2005;353:318–21.
14. Poirot C, Abirached F, Prades M, Coussieu C, Bernaudin F, Piver P. Induction of puberty by autograft of cryopreserved ovarian tissue. Lancet. 2012;379:588.
15. Revel A, Laufner N, Ben Meir A, Lebovich M, Mitrani E. Micro-organ ovarian transplantation enables pregnancy: a case report. Hum Reprod. 2011;26:1097–103.
16. Revelli A, Marchino G, Dolfin E, Molinari E, Delle Piane L, Salvagno F, Benedetto C. Live birth after orthotopic grafting of autologous cryopreserved ovarian tissue and spontaneous conception in Italy. Fertil Steril. 2013;99:227–30.
17. Sanchez M, Alama P, et al. Fresh human orthotopic ovarian cortex transplantation: long-term results. Hum Reprod. 2007;22(3):786–91.
18. Silber S, Kagawa N, Kuwayama M, Gosden R. Duration of fertility after fresh and frozen ovary transplantation. Fertil Steril. 2010;94:2191–6.
19. Silber S, Silber D, Barbey N. Long-term function of ovarian tissue transplants. Middle East Fertil Soc J. 2012;17:215–20.
20. Stern CJ, Gook D, Hale LG, Agresta F, Oldham J, Rozen G, Jobling T. First reported clinical pregnancy following heterotopic grafting of cryopreserved ovarian tissue in a woman after a bilateral oophorectomy. Hum Reprod. 2013;28:2996–9.
21. Stoop D, Cobo A, Silber SJ. Fertility preservation for age related fertility decline. Lancet. 2014;384:1311–9.
22. Silber SJ, Cossen RG. Overian transplantation in a series of monozygotic twins discordant for overian failure. N Engl J Med. 2007;356:1387–94.
23. Deanesly R. Immature rat ovaries grafted after freezing and thawing. J Endocrinol. 1954;11:197–200.
24. Mussett MV, Parrott DM. Factors affecting the fertility of mice with orthotopic ovarian grafts. J Reprod Fertil. 1961;2:80–97.
25. Candy CJ, Wood MJ, et al. Restoration of a normal reproductive lifespan after grafting of cryopreserved mouse ovaries. Hum Reprod. 2000;15(6):1300–4.
26. Donnez J, Dolmans MM. Fertility preservation in women. N Engl J Med. 2017;377:1657–65.
27. Meirow D, Ra'anani H, Shapira M, et al. Transplantations of frozen-thawed ovarian tissue demonstrate high reproductive performance and the need to revise restrictive criteria. Fertil Steril. 2016;106:467–74.
28. Shapira M, Raanani H, Barshack I, et al. First delivery in a leukemia survivor after transplantation of cryopreserved ovarian tissue, evaluated for leukemia cells contamination. Fertil Steril. 2017;109:48–53.
29. Baird DT, Webb R, et al. Long-term ovarian function in sheep after ovariectomy and transplantation of autografts stored at −196 C. Endocrinology. 1999; 140(1):462–71.
30. Donnez J, Martinez-Madrid B, et al. Ovarian tissue cryopreservation and transplantation: a review. Hum Reprod Update. 2006;12(5):519–35.
31. Newton H, Aubard Y, Rutherford A, Sharma V, Gosden R. Low temperature storage and grafting of human ovarian tissue. Hum Reprod. 1996;11:1487–91.
32. Keros V, Xella S, Hultenby K, et al. Vitrification versus controlled-rate freezing in cryopreservation of human ovarian tissue. Hum Reprod. 2009;24:1670–83.
33. Winkler-Crepaz, et al. Follicular growth after xenotransplantation of cryopreserved/thawed human ovarian tissue in SCID mice: dynamic and molecular aspects. J Assist Reprod Genet. 2016. https://doi.org/10.1007/s10815-016-0769-2.
34. Thomas-Teinturier C, El Fayech C, Oberlin O, et al. Age at menopause and its influencing factors in a cohort of survivors of childhood cancer: earlier but rarely premature. Hum Reprod. 2013;28:488–95.

35. Wallace WH, Kelsey TW. Human ovarian reserve from conception to the menopause. PLoS One. 2010;5: e8772.
36. Yasui T, Hayashi K, Mizunuma H, Kubota T, Aso T, Matsumura Y, Lee JS, Suzuki S. Factors associated with premature ovarian failure, early menopause and earlier onset of menopause in Japanese women. Maturitas. 2012;72:249–55.
37. Zhai A, Axt J, Hamilton EC, Koehler E, Lovvorn HN 3rd. Assessing gonadal function after childhood ovarian surgery. J Pediatr Surg. 2012;47:1272–9.
38. Silber S. Ovarian tissue cryopreservation and transplantation: scientific implications. J Assist Reprod Genet. 2016;33(12):1595–603.
39. Greve T, Clasen-Linde E, Andersen MT, et al. Cryopreserved ovarian cortex from patients with leukemia n complete remission contains no apparent viable malignant cells. Blood. 2012;120:4311–6.
40. Bleyer WA. The impact of childhood cancer on the United States and the world. CA Cancer J Clin. 1990;40(6):355–67.
41. Anderson RA, Cameron DA. Assessment of the effect of chemotherapy on ovarian function in women with breast cancer. J Clin Oncol. 2007;25:1630–1; author reply 2.
42. Lee SJ, Schover LR, Partridge AH, et al. American Society of Clinical Oncology recommendations on fertility preservation in cancer patients. J Clin Oncol. 2006;24:2917–31.
43. Young JL Jr, Ries LG, Silverberg E, Horm JW, Miller RW. Cancer incidence, survival, and mortality for children younger than age 15 years. Cancer. 1986;58: 598–602.
44. Maheshwari A, Porter M, Shetty A, Bhattacharya S. Women's awareness and perceptions of delay in childbearing. Fertil Steril. 2008;90:1036–42.
45. Bleyer WA. The impact of childwood cancer on the united states and the world. CA Cancer J Clin. 1990;40:355–67.
46. Andersen CY, Silber SJ, Bergholdt SH, Jorgensen JS, Ernst E. Long-term duration of function of ovarian tissue transplants: case reports. Reprod Biomed Online. 2012;25:128–32.
47. Cobo A, Domingo J, Perez S, Crespo J, Remohi J, Pellicer A. Vitrification: an effective new approach to oocyte banking and preserving fertility in cancer patients. Clin Transl Oncol. 2008;10:268–73.
48. Homburg R, Van der Veen F, Silber SJ. Oocyte vitrification – women's emancipation set in stone. Fertil Steril. 2009;91:1319–20.
49. Nagy ZP, Chang CC, Shapiro DB, Bernal DP, Kort HI, Vajta G. The efficacy and safety of human oocyte vitrification. Semin Reprod Med. 2009;27:450–5.
50. Practice Committee of American Society for Reproductive Medicine. Ovarian tissue cryopreservation: a committee opinion. Fertil Steril. 2014;101(5): 1237–43.

Surgical and Pharmacologic Fertility Preservation: The Role of Ovarian Transposition and Medical Suppression

Kara N. Goldman

T. K. Woodruff et al. (eds.), *Textbook of Oncofertility Research and Practice*,
https://doi.org/10.1007/978-3-030-02868-8_8

Key Points
- Ovarian transposition (OT), or oophoropexy, involves the surgical repositioning of the ovary outside of the planned radiation field.
- OT reduces the rate of radiation exposure to the ovary and may reduce the risk of postradiation primary ovarian insufficiency (POI), but insufficient data exist to recommend OT as a fertility preservation measure.
- Gonadotropin-releasing hormone agonists (GnRHa) administered alongside chemotherapy can be offered as a means of menstrual suppression.
- GnRHa *may* prevent or prolong the onset of POI, but GnRHa therapy is not a proven method of fertility preservation.
- Novel pharmacologic fertility preservation options target early stages of folliculogenesis, prioritizing the maintenance of follicles in a dormant primordial state during chemotherapy.

8.1 Introduction

Reproductive-age women with cancer face an imminent threat to fertility, and novel techniques offer women hope for future fertility. However, proven fertility preservation methods such as oocyte and embryo cryopreservation are not universally available. These techniques are costly, require accessibility to a fertility center, may be medically contraindicated, and require a brief delay in cancer treatment that may not be medically appropriate. In contrast, surgical techniques such as ovarian transposition or medical treatments including gonadotropin-releasing hormone (GnRH) agonists can be used in parallel with gonadotoxic chemotherapy. These techniques are relatively simple and inexpensive, but success rates have limited their clinical applicability. In this chapter, we present up-to-date information on these surgical and medical measures for fertility preservation, as well as additional surgical and medical options on the horizon.

8.2 Ovarian Transposition (OT)

High doses of local pelvic radiation compromise ovarian function, with injury more likely to occur with advancing patient age. Permanent ovarian compromise occurs with radiation doses of 30 Gy in women younger than 26 years of age, 20 Gy in patients 26–40 years, and 5–6 Gy in patients over the age of 40 [1–3]. Radiation doses frequently used to treat pelvic malignancies customarily exceed these thresholds, rendering reproductive-age women vulnerable to permanent ovarian dysfunction. Ovarian transposition, or oophoropexy, was thus first described in 1958 to reposition and protect ovaries prior to pelvic radiotherapy for cervical cancer [4].

8.2.1 Technique

OT can be performed via laparotomy, laparoscopy, robot-assisted laparoscopy, and with advanced laparoscopic techniques including single-port laparoscopy [5–8]. Regardless of the approach, OT surgical technique involves incising the utero-ovarian ligament(s) and peritoneum adjacent to the infundibulopelvic ligament(s) to mobilize the ovary outside of the radiation field. Fallopian tube transection may also be necessary to further mobilize the ovary. The ovary can be transposed laterally within the pelvis, to the paracolic gutters, anterior to the psoas muscle, or to a high antero-lateral position [9]. The location of transposed ovaries is significantly associated with preservation of ovarian function. A distance of ≥3 cm from the border of the intended radiation field is considered a common goal, and in cases of lateral ovarian transposition, a location >1.5 cm above the iliac crest is the only independent factor predicting post-treatment ovarian function [10, 11]. Clips may be placed on the transposed ovary to allow identification in future imaging studies [12].

Laparoscopic modifications have been described in both adults and children whereby the ovary is temporarily affixed to the anterior abdominal wall using a nonabsorbable suture through a small abdominal incision [13, 14]. Following completion of radiotherapy, the suture can be cut and the ovary easily returned to its pelvic location. It is not known whether returning the ovary to the pelvis impacts future fertility, but the majority of pregnancies achieved following ovarian transposition have occurred without surgical repositioning [15].

Surgical complications following OT are uncommon but include bleeding, ischemia, postoperative pelvic discomfort requiring procedure reversal, and ovarian torsion [16, 17]. While rare, metastasis to the ovary or to the abdominal wall at the site of laparoscopic trocar insertion have been described [18, 19]. Injury or early ischemia to the ovary could occur due to surgical technique. Care must be taken to limit the use of electrocoagulation and to avoid twisting or undue stretch on the ovarian pedicle during laparoscopic transposition. To avoid impaired ovarian blood supply and unintended ischemia, Arian et al. describe a technique in which the ovary is laparoscopically tunneled through the peritoneum to maintain the retroperitoneal location of the ovarian vessels and avoid alterations in blood flow [20]. One study reported that 57% of patients experienced ovarian failure when the ovary was transposed >3 cm above the umbilical line, suggesting a careful balance between the benefit of OT and the risk of insufficient vascularization and injury to ovarian vessels [9].

8.2.2 Candidates

While initially performed in the 1950s in combination with radical pelvic surgery for the treatment of cervical cancer in reproductive-age women, OT is now available to children, adolescents, and reproductive-age women with a variety of malignancies requiring pelvic radiotherapy [4, 13, 21, 22]. Cervical cancer is the fourth most common cancer in women worldwide, affecting women at a significantly younger age than most malignancies [23]. Treatment of cervical cancer often involves external beam radiation therapy (EBRT) or internal radiation therapy (Brachytherapy), with commonly achieved doses exceeding 80 Gy [24]. Two-thirds of all OT procedures are performed for cervical malignancy, and fertility preservation has become even more relevant in this population as the annual number of cervical cancer-related deaths continues to decline [25, 26].

Concerning trends have been identified in colorectal cancer, where incidence rates increased by 1–2.4% annually since the mid-1980s in adults aged 20–39 years [27]. Colorectal cancer treatment may require EBRT or brachytherapy at dosages of 45–50 Gy over 5–6 weeks, a regimen that would result in ovarian failure in addition to significant uterine damage [28]. OT has been shown to reduce the radiation dose to approximately 5–10% of the dose of nontransposed ovaries [29].

Women with Hodgkin's lymphoma may require pelvic node irradiation, with doses often leading to ovarian insufficiency; oophoropexy has thus been applied in this population with mixed results [21, 30]. OT has also been described for other pelvic malignancies requiring radiotherapy, including vaginal cancers, pelvic sarcomas, or tumors of the central nervous system (CNS) [31–33].

Within the pediatric population, OT represents one of the few available options for fertility preservation. De Lambert et al. describe 16 prepubertal patients who underwent temporary OT, by laparotomy or laparoscopy, prior to brachytherapy. Children's age ranged from 2 to 9 years old, with a median age of 3 years; the children tolerated the procedure well, and fallopian tube integrity was maintained in all children, but the long-term impact on ovarian function remains unknown [13]. The most common indications for OT among children are rhabdomyosarcomas (bladder, vagina, uterus) or soft tissue or pelvic bone sarcomas such as Ewing's sarcoma [34, 35]. Additional indications include high-risk neuroblastomas and Hodgkin's lymphoma, but fortunately, for patients with Hodgkin's lymphoma, radiation to the initially involved region has generally replaced large nodal irradiation [36, 37].

Selecting appropriate candidates for OT can be challenging. From an oncologic standpoint, the procedure is generally limited to young patients (<40 years) with early-staged, small, operable tumors requiring adjuvant radiotherapy [38]. Those with locally advanced disease or poor prognoses are considered poor candidates. While the goal of OT is to preserve ovarian endocrine function and reproductive potential, success rates for both are inconsistent. The procedure is not without surgical morbidity (as described above) as well as the possibility of unintended consequences further compromising fertility. The OT surgical technique may require that the fallopian tube be cut or damaged to allow sufficient mobilization of the ovary; in these cases, patients must be counseled that in vitro fertilization (IVF) may be necessary to achieve future pregnancy.

8.2.3 Ovarian Function and Fertility Following OT

Studies investigating the impact of OT prior to radiation therapy have produced mixed results. OT has been shown to reduce the rate of radiation exposure to the ovary from 50% to 90%, but available studies are heterogeneous regarding patient characteristics, diagnosis, and surgical approach [3, 5, 14, 18, 31, 32, 39]. Morice et al. describe 24 patients who underwent OT prior to radiotherapy for pelvic malignancies; approximately 80% maintained ovarian function [40]. In another report, 23 patients underwent laparoscopic OT for cervical cancer (n = 15), rectal cancer (n = 4), Ewing Sarcoma (n = 3), or Hodgkin lymphoma (n = 1) and 65% maintained their ovarian function; however, the authors defined ovarian function as follicle-stimulating hormone (FSH) levels ≤25 IU/L, levels far exceeding "normal" in young healthy women [5]. Clough et al. evaluated 20 women who underwent laparoscopic OT for cervical cancer, CNS tumor, and Hodgkin lymphoma whose ovaries had received a mean 1.55 Gy; no patients in this group experienced primary ovarian insufficiency (POI) [41].

Among 122 women who underwent OT, 21% subsequently received radiation therapy and 50% of these women experienced early menopause following radiotherapy (RR 17.3; 95% CI 5.3–56.1) [18]. Salih et al. describe 16 patients who underwent OT prior to pelvic radiation; 94% maintained regular menstrual cycles 3 years after OT. These studies used follicle-stimulating hormone (FSH) and resumption of menses as markers for ovarian function, but more accurate markers are now clinically available. Anti-mullerian hormone (AMH), released by the granulosa cells of growing follicles, is now the best available measure of ovarian reserve and correlates with age at natural menopause [42, 43]. Future studies are needed to assess AMH following OT. However, menstrual function and serum markers cannot be extrapolated to assume normal reproductive potential. While OT can be used as a means to preserve menstrual function, providers should be cautious when recommending OT for fertility preservation.

Few reports describe pregnancy outcomes following OT. In a study of 37 women (mean age 20.7 ± 5.7 years) who underwent OT prior to pelvic radiation, success rates varied by tumor type and location [15]. Fifteen percent became pregnant after brachytherapy with or without external radiation for vaginal or cervical clear cell carcinoma, and 80% became pregnant after external radiation for dysgerminomas and pelvic sarcomas. The variability in success rates was likely secondary to the higher dose of radiation required in clear-cell carcinomas, leading to greater ovarian radiation exposure despite transposition, as well as higher degrees of uterine radiation. Interestingly, the majority of these pregnancies were achieved without repositioning the ovaries following OT although 17% required IVF.

Among women receiving pelvic radiotherapy for vaginal, cervical, and colorectal cancer, the uterus will be contained within the radiation field. Direct uterine radiation lowers fecundity and increases the risk of adverse pregnancy outcomes [44]. Among female adult survivors of childhood cancers, radiation-induced uterine damage accounts for the majority of poor obstetrical outcomes including miscarriages, stillbirths, intrauterine fetal growth restriction, pre-eclampsia, abnormal placentation, and preterm delivery [45]. While pregnancy may be possible and has been described after high-dose direct uterine radiation, patients should be counseled that pregnancy following significant uterine radiation may require the use of a gestational carrier (GC) [28]. Ribeiro et al. describe a novel uterine transposition technique in which the uterus and adnexa are transposed to the upper abdomen during pelvic radiotherapy, but more work is needed to understand the feasibility, safety, and efficacy of this technique [46].

8.2.4 Combining OT with Other Fertility Preservation Modalities

Understanding that oocyte and embryo cryopreservation are established first-line methods of fertility preservation, patients who are offered OT should also be counseled toward gamete or embryo cryopreservation where possible [47]. If possible, OT should be performed after completion of ovarian stimulation and oocyte retrieval to facilitate ease and optimization of transvaginal oocyte retrieval. While oocyte or embryo cryopreservation can successfully occur following OT, oocyte retrieval requires abdominal retrieval which could complicate the procedure and compromise oocyte yield [48].

Ovarian tissue cryopreservation, discussed in great detail in ▶ Chap. 7, can be combined with ovarian transposition to optimize a patient's future reproductive options [49]. One surgical group described a patient with rectal cancer who underwent laparoscopic ovarian transposition accompanied by ovarian decortication of the contralateral ovary for ovarian tissue freezing [20]. While limited data exist, the combination of gamete, embryo, or ovarian tissue cryopreservation with OT has the potential to further improve a patient's future reproductive success.

Treatment planning requires thoughtful consideration of the patient's reproductive goals, resources, and time. Selecting the appropriate fertility preservation approach requires multidisciplinary planning involving the patient's medical and surgical oncologists, radiation oncologist, and reproductive endocrinologist. Prompt referral to a reproductive endocrinologist upon diagnosis can increase the likelihood that patients have an opportunity to identify the most appropriate approach.

8.3 Pharmacologic Fertility Preservation

8.3.1 Background

Among women facing systemic gonadotoxic chemotherapy, established methods of fertility preservation such as oocyte and embryo cryopreservation may not be available to all patients given time, access to a reproductive endocrinologist, medical contraindications, or financial barriers. The pediatric population is particularly limited by available options, as premenarchal females without a functional hypothalamic-pituitary-ovarian axis are not candidates for ovarian stimulation with oocyte cryopreservation. Ovarian tissue cryopreservation (described in detail in ▶ Chap. 7) has expanded options for young girls, but the technique remains experimental, requires multiple surgeries, and may not be medically appropriate based on a patient's diagnosis. The possibility of a pharmacologic agent administered alongside gonadotoxic chemotherapy is thus particularly attractive.

The promise of pharmacologic fertility preservation has led to decades of research with mixed results [50]. In the early 1980s, Glade et al. proposed the administration of gonadotropin-releasing hormone agonists (GnRHa) to preserve fertility. GnRHa had previously been administered during chemotherapy with the goal of preventing heavy menstrual bleeding and anemia, but murine models suggested that GnRHa protected male mice from cyclophosphamide-induced damage [51]. Subsequent work in female rats suggested that GnRHa attenuated chemotherapy-induced follicular depletion [52]. Investigators hypothesized that GnRHa exerted a protective effect by attenuating recruitment of primordial follicles into the growing follicle pool, decreasing utero-ovarian perfusion, resulting in lower cumulative exposure to gonadotoxic chemotherapy and decreased follicular apoptosis, or enhancing anti-apoptotic pathways [52–55].

8.3.2 Clinical Studies of Gonadotropin-Releasing Hormone Agonists

Based on early data showing possible efficacy in mice, the agents were introduced into clinical practice. In a small trial of women with Hodgkin's disease treated with the GnRHa Buserelin, 3-year follow-up showed failure to protect ovarian function or fertility [56]. In contrast, a larger prospective trial of 60 women exposed to chemotherapeutic agents for lymphoma ($n = 40$), leukemia ($n = 10$), and benign conditions ($n = 10$), and co-treated with GnRHa, showed that GnRHa preserved spontaneous ovulation and menses in a majority of treated women [57]. Another study randomized lymphoma patients to treatment with GnRHa with norethisterone or norethisterone alone alongside alkylating agents. AMH levels were significantly higher in the GnRHa group compared to control (1.4 ± 0.4 vs. 0.5 ± 0.2 ng/mL, $p = 0.04$), but there was no decreased risk of primary ovarian insufficiency (POI) following GnRHa treatment [58].

The use of GnRHa use has been widely studied and disputed in the treatment of breast cancer. In a small RCT of patients exposed to chemotherapy for breast cancer, women co-treated with GnRHa more likely had resumption of menses and had lower median FSH levels 6 months post-treatment [59]. In an RCT of 124 premenopausal breast cancer patients (<44 years) treated with chemotherapy with or without the GnRHa Triptorelin, post-treatment amenorrhea rates were comparable between treated and untreated groups [60]. In contrast, a multicenter RCT demonstrated that Triptorelin-induced ovarian suppression during chemotherapy in premenopausal women with early-stage breast cancer decreased the likelihood of POI with an odds ratio of 0.28 (95% CI 0.14–0.59; $p < 0.001$) [61]. In another large multicenter RCT, the 5-year estimate of menstrual resumption was 72.6% among the GnRHa group compared to 64% among the control group (age-adjusted HR, 1.48 [95% CI, 1.12–1.95], $p = 0.006$) [62]. In this study, there was no significant difference in pregnancy rate.

The Prevention of Early Menopause Study (POEMS) was an RCT randomizing 218 patients to chemotherapy with or without goserelin, with a primary endpoint of ovarian failure rate at 2 years [63]. The ovarian failure rate was 8% in the goserelin group and 22% in the chemotherapy-alone group (OR 0.30; 95% CI 0.09–0.97, $p = 0.04$). Pregnancy occurred in more women in the goserelin group compared to chemotherapy-alone (21% vs. 11%, $p = 0.03$), and notably women in the goserelin group had improved disease-free survival ($p = 0.04$).

The OPTION trial similarly assessed GnRHa for protection against ovarian toxicity during chemotherapy [64]. Two hundred twenty-seven patients were randomized to receive goserelin or placebo with chemotherapy. Goserelin reduced the risk of POI in women <40 years but with no efficacy in women >40 years; levels of the ovarian reserve marker anti-mullerian hormone (AMH) fell markedly and equally in both groups. The group cautioned providers regarding the limited degree of ovarian protection and unknown significance for fertility and long-term ovarian function.

A number of systematic reviews and meta-analyses have been published in an attempt to consolidate the large quantity of available data. In one such meta-analysis including data from 7 clinical trials and 1047 randomized patients, the use of GnRHa was associated with a higher rate of recovery of menses after at least 12 months (OR 1.85, 95% CI 1.33–2.59; $p < 0.001$). GnRHa were associated with more pregnancies (OR 1.85; 95% CI, 1.02–3.36, $p = 0.04$), but pregnancy was not the primary outcome in any of the trials, and this should thus be interpreted with caution [65]. Others concluded that GnRHa conferred no benefit to women with breast cancer [66]. A systematic review performed from 1960 to 2017 assessed 29 RCTs with ten meeting criteria for inclusion; the meta-analysis concluded that GnRHa may have a protective effect against the development of POI with an unclear duration of benefit [67]. Importantly, most studies focus on *menstrual function* as the primary endpoint rather than fertility. Resumption of menses is a poor proxy for reproductive potential. Some studies assessed hormonal levels in an attempt to assess ovarian reserve and function, but testing was at times performed at random, or "normal" ovarian function was defined as serum FSH levels up to 24 pg/mL or even 40 pg/mL. As pregnancy is the only way to adequately assess the impact of GnRHa on fertility, studies are needed to assess long-term *fertility outcomes* following GnRHa treatment.

8.3.3 Preclinical Studies of Gonadotropin-Releasing Hormone Agonists

Inconsistent results from clinical trials of GnRHa have led to a reemergence of investigation into the molecular mechanism. Using a murine model, Horicks et al. showed that cyclophosphamide, the alkylating chemotherapy agent considered most gonadotoxic, induces follicle loss of >50% even in the absence of FSH, suggesting that inhibition of the pituitary-ovarian axis is not one of the mechanisms of ovarian protection during GnRH agonist treatment [68]. The same group evaluated the efficacy of GnRHa in a mouse model of cyclophosphamide-induced follicular depletion; they found that GnRHa disrupted estrus cyclicity but failed to inhibit follicular recruitment and did not prevent cyclophosphamide-induced follicular damage [69]. Hasky et al. studied ovarian reserve in mice following treatment with GnRHa with various chemotherapy regimens; the authors found that co-treatment with GnRHa during cyclophosphamide therapy attenuated the decrease in AMH, and GnRHa attenuated doxorubicin-induced vascular injury as demonstrated by decreased VEGF [70].

In a translational study using ex vivo and in vitro models of human ovary and granulosa cells, ovarian cortex and granulosa cells were treated with chemotherapy with and without the GnRHa leuprolide acetate [71]. GnRHa failed to activate antiapoptotic pathways, and importantly the agents failed to prevent follicle loss, DNA damage, or apoptosis. Preclinical and in vitro data, much like the previously described clinical data, has resulted in an abundance of conflicting results.

8.3.4 Summary of GnRHa Data

Proposed molecular mechanisms for GnRHa-induced ovarian protection remain unproven, and preclinical and clinical studies of GnRHa have shown inconsistent results.

Due to unclear benefit, the American Society of Clinical Oncology (ASCO) issued a statement that GnRHa is not an effective method of fertility preservation [72]. They suggest that patients can consider GnRHa for menstrual suppression during chemotherapy or as an unproven option where other fertility preservation options are not available.

GnRHa treatment is often accompanied by side effects including vasomotor symptoms and bone loss, and thus the potential benefits must be weighed against risks. The decision to treat with GnRHa during chemotherapy requires thoughtful discussion between the patient, oncologist, and reproductive endocrinologist.

8.3.5 Novel Pharmacologic Approaches to Fertility Preservation

Ovarian physiology explains the mixed results seen with both GnRHa as fertility preservation agents, and an improved understanding of the molecular mechanisms underlying folliculogenesis and chemotherapy-induced gonadotoxicity has led to promising targeted therapies in preclinical studies. Chemotherapy targets rapidly dividing cells including the growing follicles of the ovary. Growing follicles make up a very small fraction of the follicle pool, with primordial follicles comprising a majority of the ovarian reserve. Primordial follicles lie dormant and until recruitment remain relatively protected from the antimitotic and genotoxic effects of chemotherapy. Thus, any intervention designed to protect only *growing* follicles, such as GnRHa, does not protect the bulk of the ovarian reserve.

Anti-mullerian hormone (AMH), produced by the granulosa cells of growing follicles, is a key negative regulator of primordial follicle activation. In a murine study of supraphysiological doses of AMH, AMH resulted in arrest of folliculogenesis, and co-administration with cyclophosphamide, doxorubicin, or carboplatin significantly protected murine ovarian reserve [73].

The PI3K/AKT/mTOR pathway is now known to be critically important to the recruitment and activation of primordial follicles. Kalish-Philosoph et al. demonstrated in a murine model that cyclophosphamide induces upregulation of this pathway, leading to activation of the quiescent primordial follicle pool. They observed that *follicular burnout,* rather than apoptosis, was responsible for the massive loss of primordial follicles and that administration of the immunomodulator AS101 attenuated primordial follicle activation [74]. Di Emidio et al. similarly demonstrated that AS101 protects murine ovarian reserve, further proposing that the agent may be acting upstream to the PI3K/AKT pathway [75].

Understanding the critical impact of the PI3K/AKT/mTOR pathway on primordial folliculogenesis, our group evaluated the role of mTOR inhibitors as a pharmacologic fertoprotective agent [76]. Mice were treated with cyclophosphamide alongside the mTOR1 inhibitor everolimus (RAD001) or dual mTOR1/2 inhibitor INK128 (MLN0128). Co-treatment with mTOR inhibitors downregulated the PI3K/AKT/mTOR pathway, thus preventing follicular burnout and resulting in maintenance of the primordial follicle pool, normal AMH levels, and importantly normal fertility. Everolimus is FDA approved and used for a number of conditions including in the treatment of certain malignancies, thus representing a clinically available fertility preservation option with possible antitumor activity. More work is needed to translate this work from animals to humans.

The chemotherapeutic agent cisplatin has also been shown in a murine model to induce overactivation of the primordial follicle pool through the PTEN/AKT pathway; loss of PTEN suppression leads to upregulation of the key molecules in the pathway and thus primordial follicle depletion [77]. Jang et al. observed that the melatonin and to a greater extent melatonin combined with ghrelin decreased cisplatin-mediated PTEN inhibition thus preserving ovarian reserve in mice [78, 79].

The c-Abl-Tap63 pathway is activated by DNA-damaging agents such as cisplatin, leading to Tap63 accumulation and cell death. Gonfloni et al. showed that the c-Abl kinase inhibitor imatinib counteracts these cisplatin-induced effects in human cell lines and mouse oocytes, thus preventing chemotherapy-induced cell death [80]. The mechanism was further investigated by Kim et al. who found that imatinib inhibits cisplatin-induced nuclear accumulation of c-Abl/Tap73 and thus inhibits oocyte apoptosis within primordial follicles [81]. Kerr et al. since published that imatinib did not protect primordial follicles from cisplatin-induced apoptosis or protect fertility, suggesting that more work is needed in this area [82].

Using an inhibitor of checkpoint kinase 2 (CHK2) to inhibit a key element of the oocyte DNA damage checkpoint response, investigators preserved ovarian function and normal fertility among mice exposed to sterilizing doses of radiation [83].

8.3.6 Summary of Medical Options

The most compelling benefit of GnRHa alongside chemotherapy is menstrual suppression, particularly in patients at risk for thrombocytopenia and/or anemia. GnRHa *may* preserve ovarian hormonal function and decrease the risk of POI in young women treated with chemotherapy, but the duration of benefit remains unclear and oocyte quality and quantity are likely still impaired. Data are insufficient to recommend GnRHa for the preservation of fertility. Patients should be carefully counseled that GnRHa should not be relied upon to preserve fertility but can be considered alongside established fertility preservation methods.

Novel pharmacologic approaches aim to prevent primordial follicle activation during chemotherapy. Agents such as mTOR inhibitors, AS101, and AMH show great promise in animal models, but more work is needed to translate this work to humans. The continued discovery of molecular mechanisms responsible for chemotherapy-induced ovarian injury will open doors to future targeted therapies.

8.4 Conclusions

Surgical and pharmacological approaches to fertility preservation continue to evolve. Success rates of OT are variable and depend on the patient's age, diagnosis, and treatment regimen. The practice requires thoughtful counseling but may be an acceptable option for appropriately selected patients. The use of GnRHa for medical suppression remains controversial. The benefit may be limited to menstrual suppression, with a possible benefit in the reduction of POI; however, data are inconclusive to recommend these agents to preserve fertility. Novel pharmacologic approaches target the molecular mechanisms underlying ovarian folliculogenesis to maintain primordial follicle quiescence. Future studies are needed to translate this work in humans. There exists an urgent need to identify personalized fertility preservation approaches based on a patient's unique diagnosis and treatment regimen, and multidisciplinary efforts will be required to ensure that all fertility preservation candidates achieve their reproductive goals.

Acknowledgments The author would like to acknowledge Jaime Knopman, MD, and Nicole Noyes, MD, who authored a previous version of this chapter.

Review Questions and Answers

Q1. Ovarian transposition was first introduced to preserve fertility in patients with the following malignancy
(a) Hodgkin's disease
(b) Cervical cancer
(c) Colorectal cancer
(d) Uterine cancer

A1. (b)

Q2. Following OT, ovaries must be repositioned to the pelvis for pregnancy to occur.
(a) True
(b) False

A2. (b)

Q3. In univariate analysis of factors associated with normal ovarian function following OT, the following variable was the only independent predictor of intact ovarian function:
(a) Age <40 years
(b) BMI <25
(c) Radiation dose <5040 cGy
(d) Location of transposed ovary higher than 1.5 cm above the iliac crest

A3. (d)

Q4. Gonadotropin-releasing hormone agonists (GnRHa) administered alongside chemotherapy have definitively been shown to:
(a) Reduce the quantity of menstrual bleeding
(b) Preserve ovarian function
(c) Preserve fertility

A4. (a)

Q5. Novel pharmacologic fertility preservation approaches should ensure preservation of the following follicle type:
(a) Primordial
(b) Primary
(c) Secondary
(d) Antral

A5. (a)

References

1. Donnez J, Bassil S. Indications for cryopreservation of ovarian tissue. Hum Reprod Updat. 1998;4(3): 248–59.
2. Lushbaugh CC, Casarett GW. The effects of gonadal irradiation in clinical radiation therapy: a review. Cancer. 1976;37(2 Suppl):1111–25.
3. Wo JY, Viswanathan AN. Impact of radiotherapy on fertility, pregnancy, and neonatal outcomes in female cancer patients. Int J Radiat Oncol Biol Phys. 2009;73(5):1304–12. https://doi.org/10.1016/j.ijrobp.2008.12.016.
4. McCall ML, Keaty EC, Thompson JD. Conservation of ovarian tissue in the treatment of carcinoma of the cervix with radical surgery. Am J Obstet Gynecol. 1958;75(3):590–600; discussion 600–595.
5. Al-Badawi IA, AlOmar O, Albadawi N, Abu-Zaid A. Single-port laparoscopic surgery for benign salpingo-ovarian pathology: a single-center experience from Saudi Arabia. Ann Saudi Med. 2016;36(1):64–9. https://doi.org/10.5144/0256-4947.2016.26.1.1200.
6. Molpus KL, Wedergren JS, Carlson MA. Robotically assisted endoscopic ovarian transposition. JSLS. 2003;7(1):59–62.
7. Sioulas VD, Jorge S, Chern JY, Schiavone MB, Weiser MR, Kelvin JF, Gardner GJ, Sonoda Y, Abu-Rustum NR, Goodman KA, Leitao MM Jr. Robotically assisted laparoscopic ovarian transposition in women with lower gastrointestinal cancer undergoing pelvic radiotherapy. Ann Surg Oncol. 2017;24(1):251–6. https://doi.org/10.1245/s10434-016-5650-0.
8. Williams RS, Littell RD, Mendenhall NP. Laparoscopic oophoropexy and ovarian function in the treatment of Hodgkin disease. Cancer. 1999;86(10):2138–42.
9. Huang KG, Lee CL, Tsai CS, Han CM, Hwang LL. A new approach for laparoscopic ovarian transposition before pelvic irradiation. Gynecol Oncol. 2007;105(1):234–7. https://doi.org/10.1016/j.ygyno.2006.12.001.
10. Bidzinski M, Lemieszczuk B, Zielinski J. Evaluation of the hormonal function and features of the ultrasound picture of transposed ovary in cervical cancer patients after surgery and pelvic irradiation. Eur J Gynaecol Oncol. 1993;14(Suppl):77–80.
11. Hwang JH, Yoo HJ, Park SH, Lim MC, Seo SS, Kang S, Kim JY, Park SY. Association between the location of transposed ovary and ovarian function in patients with uterine cervical cancer treated with (postoperative or primary) pelvic radiotherapy. Fertil Steril. 2012;97(6):1387–93 e1381–1382. https://doi.org/10.1016/j.fertnstert.2012.02.052.
12. Sella T, Mironov S, Hricak H. Imaging of transposed ovaries in patients with cervical carcinoma. AJR Am J Roentgenol. 2005;184(5):1602–10. https://doi.org/10.2214/ajr.184.5.01841602.
13. de Lambert G, Haie-Meder C, Guerin F, Boubnova J, Martelli H. A new surgical approach of temporary ovarian transposition for children undergoing brachytherapy: technical assessment and dose evaluation. J Pediatr Surg. 2014;49(7):1177–80. https://doi.org/10.1016/j.jpedsurg.2014.03.018.
14. Gareer W, Gad Z, Gareer H. Needle oophoropexy: a new simple technique for ovarian transposition prior to pelvic irradiation. Surg Endosc. 2011;25(7):2241–6. https://doi.org/10.1007/s00464-010-1541-9.
15. Morice P, Thiam-Ba R, Castaigne D, Haie-Meder C, Gerbaulet A, Pautier P, Duvillard P, Michel G. Fertility results after ovarian transposition for pelvic malignancies treated by external irradiation or brachytherapy. Hum Reprod. 1998b;13(3):660–3.

16. Anderson B, LaPolla J, Turner D, Chapman G, Buller R. Ovarian transposition in cervical cancer. Gynecol Oncol. 1993;49(2):206–14. https://doi.org/10.1006/gyno.1993.1109.
17. Gomez-Hidalgo NR, Darin MC, Dalton H, Jhingran A, Fleming N, Brown J, Ramirez PT. Ovarian torsion after laparoscopic ovarian transposition in patients with gynecologic cancer: a report of two cases. J Minim Invasive Gynecol. 2015;22(4):687–90. https://doi.org/10.1016/j.jmig.2015.02.009.
18. Feeney DD, Moore DH, Look KY, Stehman FB, Sutton GP. The fate of the ovaries after radical hysterectomy and ovarian transposition. Gynecol Oncol. 1995;56(1):3–7. https://doi.org/10.1006/gyno.1995.1002.
19. Picone O, Aucouturier JS, Louboutin A, Coscas Y, Camus E. Abdominal wall metastasis of a cervical adenocarcinoma at the laparoscopic trocar insertion site after ovarian transposition: case report and review of the literature. Gynecol Oncol. 2003;90(2):446–9.
20. Arian SE, Goodman L, Flyckt RL, Falcone T. Ovarian transposition: a surgical option for fertility preservation. Fertil Steril. 2017;107(4):e15. https://doi.org/10.1016/j.fertnstert.2017.01.010.
21. Baker JW, Morgan RL, Peckham MJ, Smithers DW. Preservation of ovarian function in patients requiring radiotherapy for para-aortic and pelvic Hodgkin's disease. Lancet. 1972;1(7764):1307–8.
22. Thibaud E, Ramirez M, Brauner R, Flamant F, Zucker JM, Fekete C, Rappaport R. Preservation of ovarian function by ovarian transposition performed before pelvic irradiation during childhood. J Pediatr. 1992;121(6):880–4.
23. Ferlay J, Soerjomataram I, Dikshit R, Eser S, Mathers C, Rebelo M, Parkin DM, Forman D, Bray F. Cancer incidence and mortality worldwide: sources, methods and major patterns in GLOBOCAN 2012. Int J Cancer. 2015;136(5):E359–86. https://doi.org/10.1002/ijc.29210.
24. Banerjee R, Kamrava M. Brachytherapy in the treatment of cervical cancer: a review. Int J Womens Health. 2014;6:555–64. https://doi.org/10.2147/IJWH.S46247.
25. Han SS, Kim YH, Lee SH, Kim GJ, Kim HJ, Kim JW, Park NH, Song YS, Kang SB. Underuse of ovarian transposition in reproductive-aged cancer patients treated by primary or adjuvant pelvic irradiation. J Obstet Gynaecol Res. 2011;37(7):825–9. https://doi.org/10.1111/j.1447-0756.2010.01443.x.
26. SEER. Cervical cancer stat facts. 2014. https://seer.cancer.gov/statfacts/html/cervix.html. https://seer.cancer.gov/statfacts/html/cervix.html. Accessed 21 Feb 2018.
27. Siegel RL, Fedewa SA, Anderson WF, Miller KD, Ma J, Rosenberg PS, Jemal A. Colorectal cancer incidence patterns in the United States, 1974–2013. J Natl Cancer Inst. 2017;109(8):djw322. https://doi.org/10.1093/jnci/djw322.
28. Kurt M, Uncu G, Cetintas SK, Kucuk N, Guler S, Ozkan L. Successful spontaneous pregnancy in a patient with rectal carcinoma treated with pelvic radiotherapy and concurrent chemotherapy: the unique role of laparoscopic lateral ovary transposition. Eur J Gynaecol Oncol. 2007;28(5):408–10.
29. O'Neill MT, Ni Dhonnchu T, Brannigan AE. Topic update: effects of colorectal cancer treatments on female fertility and potential methods for fertility preservation. Dis Colon Rectum. 2011;54(3):363–9. https://doi.org/10.1007/DCR.0b013e31820240b3.
30. Thomas PR, Winstanly D, Peckham MJ, Austin DE, Murray MA, Jacobs HS. Reproductive and endocrine function in patients with Hodgkin's disease: effects of oophoropexy and irradiation. Br J Cancer. 1976;33(2):226–31.
31. Cutillo G, Cignini P, Pizzi G, Vizza E, Micheli A, Arcangeli G, Sbiroli C. Conservative treatment of reproductive and sexual function in young woman with squamous carcinoma of the vagina. Gynecol Oncol. 2006;103(1):234–7. https://doi.org/10.1016/j.ygyno.2006.02.032.
32. Gubbala K, Laios A, Gallos I, Pathiraja P, Haldar K, Ind T. Outcomes of ovarian transposition in gynaecological cancers; a systematic review and meta-analysis. J Ovarian Res. 2014;7:69. https://doi.org/10.1186/1757-2215-7-69.
33. Kung FT, Chen HC, Huang CC, Ho JT, Cheng BH. Preservation of ovarian germinal follicles by temporary laparoscopic ovarian transposition in teenaged girls undergoing craniospinal irradiation for radiosensitive central nervous system tumors. Taiwan J Obstet Gynecol. 2008;47(3):300–4. https://doi.org/10.1016/S1028-4559(08)60128-X.
34. Potratz J, Dirksen U, Jurgens H, Craft A. Ewing sarcoma: clinical state-of-the-art. Pediatr Hematol Oncol. 2012;29(1):1–11. https://doi.org/10.3109/08880018.2011.622034.
35. Reguerre Y, Martelli H, Rey A, Rogers T, Gaze M, Ben Arush MW, Devalck C, Oberlin O, Stevens M, Orbach D. Local therapy is critical in localised pelvic rhabdomyosarcoma: experience of the International Society of Pediatric Oncology Malignant Mesenchymal Tumor (SIOP-MMT) committee. Eur J Cancer. 2012;48(13):2020–7. https://doi.org/10.1016/j.ejca.2011.11.011.
36. Donaldson SS. Finding the balance in pediatric Hodgkin's lymphoma. J Clin Oncol. 2012;30(26):3158–9. https://doi.org/10.1200/JCO.2012.42.6890.
37. Hudson MM, Greenwald C, Thompson E, Wilimas J, Marina N, Fairclough D, Kauffman W, Bozeman P, Mackert PW, Abromowitch M, et al. Efficacy and toxicity of multiagent chemotherapy and low-dose involved-field radiotherapy in children and adolescents with Hodgkin's disease. J Clin Oncol. 1993;11(1):100–8. https://doi.org/10.1200/JCO.1993.11.1.100.
38. Sicam RV, Huang KG, Chang YC, Lee CL. Maintenance of ovarian function in end-of-life cervical cancer patient following primary surgico-radiotherapy and ovarian transposition. J Gynecol Oncol. 2013;24(2):204–7. https://doi.org/10.3802/jgo.2013.24.2.204.
39. Clough KB, Goffinet F, Labib A, Renolleau C, Campana F, de la Rochefordiere A, Durand JC. Laparoscopic unilateral ovarian transposition prior to irradiation: prospective study of 20 cases. Cancer. 1996;77(12):2638–45. https://doi.org/10.1002/(SICI)1097-0142(19960615)77:12<2638::AID-CNCR30>3.0.CO;2-R.
40. Morice P, Castaigne D, Haie-Meder C, Pautier P, El Hassan J, Duvillard P, Gerbaulet A, Michel G. Laparoscopic ovar-

ian transposition for pelvic malignancies: indications and functional outcomes. Fertil Steril. 1998a;70(5):956–60.
41. Revised minimum standards for practices offering assisted reproductive technologies. Fertil Steril. 2008. 90(5 Suppl):S165–8. https://doi.org/10.1016/j.fertnstert.2008.08.098. doi:S0015-0282(08)03722-9 [pii].
42. Broer SL, Broekmans FJ, Laven JS, Fauser BC. Anti-Mullerian hormone: ovarian reserve testing and its potential clinical implications. Hum Reprod Updat. 2014;20(5):688–701. https://doi.org/10.1093/humupd/dmu020.
43. Depmann M, Eijkemans MJ, Broer SL, Scheffer GJ, van Rooij IA, Laven JS, Broekmans FJ. Does anti-Mullerian hormone predict menopause in the general population? Results of a prospective ongoing cohort study. Hum Reprod. 2016. https://doi.org/10.1093/humrep/dew112.
44. Teh WT, Stern C, Chander S, Hickey M. The impact of uterine radiation on subsequent fertility and pregnancy outcomes. Biomed Res Int. 2014;2014:482968. https://doi.org/10.1155/2014/482968.
45. Oktem O, Kim SS, Selek U, Schatmann G, Urman B. Ovarian and uterine functions in female survivors of childhood cancers. Oncologist. 2018;23(2):214–24. https://doi.org/10.1634/theoncologist.2017-0201.
46. Ribeiro R, Rebolho JC, Tsumanuma FK, Brandalize GG, Trippia CH, Saab KA. Uterine transposition: technique and a case report. Fertil Steril. 2017;108(2):320–24 e321. https://doi.org/10.1016/j.fertnstert.2017.06.016.
47. Martinez F, International Society for Fertility Preservation E-AEWG. Update on fertility preservation from the Barcelona International Society for Fertility Preservation-ESHRE-ASRM 2015 expert meeting: indications, results and future perspectives. Fertil Steril. 2017;108(3):407–15 e411. https://doi.org/10.1016/j.fertnstert.2017.05.024.
48. Gavrilova-Jordan L, Rowe MS, Ballenger CA, Mersereau JE, Hayslip CC. Emergent oocyte cryopreservation with a novel ovarian transposition technique in a colorectal cancer patient: a combined approach for fertility preservation. A case report. J Reprod Med. 2015;60(7–8):354–8.
49. Martin JR, Kodaman P, Oktay K, Taylor HS. Ovarian cryopreservation with transposition of a contralateral ovary: a combined approach for fertility preservation in women receiving pelvic radiation. Fertil Steril. 2007;87(1):189 e185–7. https://doi.org/10.1016/j.fertnstert.2006.04.051.
50. Blumenfeld Z, von Wolff M. GnRH-analogues and oral contraceptives for fertility preservation in women during chemotherapy. Hum Reprod Updat. 2008;14(6):543–52. https://doi.org/10.1093/humupd/dmn022.
51. Glode LM, Robinson J, Gould SF. Protection from cyclophosphamide-induced testicular damage with an analogue of gonadotropin-releasing hormone. Lancet. 1981;1(8230):1132–4.
52. Kitajima Y, Endo T, Nagasawa K, Manase K, Honnma H, Baba T, Hayashi T, Chiba H, Sawada N, Saito T. Hyperstimulation and a gonadotropin-releasing hormone agonist modulate ovarian vascular permeability by altering expression of the tight junction protein claudin-5. Endocrinology. 2006;147(2):694–9. https://doi.org/10.1210/en.2005-0700.
53. Imai A, Sugiyama M, Furui T, Tamaya T, Ohno T. Direct protection by a gonadotropin-releasing hormone analog from doxorubicin-induced granulosa cell damage. Gynecol Obstet Investig. 2007;63(2):102–6. https://doi.org/10.1159/000096062.
54. Morita Y, Perez GI, Paris F, Miranda SR, Ehleiter D, Haimovitz-Friedman A, Fuks Z, Xie Z, Reed JC, Schuchman EH, Kolesnick RN, Tilly JL. Oocyte apoptosis is suppressed by disruption of the acid sphingomyelinase gene or by sphingosine-1-phosphate therapy. Nat Med. 2000;6(10):1109–14. https://doi.org/10.1038/80442.
55. Perez GI, Knudson CM, Leykin L, Korsmeyer SJ, Tilly JL. Apoptosis-associated signaling pathways are required for chemotherapy-mediated female germ cell destruction. Nat Med. 1997;3(11):1228–32.
56. Waxman JH, Ahmed R, Smith D, Wrigley PF, Gregory W, Shalet S, Crowther D, Rees LH, Besser GM, Malpas JS, et al. Failure to preserve fertility in patients with Hodgkin's disease. Cancer Chemother Pharmacol. 1987;19(2):159–62.
57. Blumenfeld Z, Dann E, Avivi I, Epelbaum R, Rowe JM. Fertility after treatment for Hodgkin's disease. Ann Oncol. 2002;13(Suppl 1):138–47.
58. Demeestere I, Brice P, Peccatori FA, Kentos A, Gaillard I, Zachee P, Casasnovas RO, Van Den Neste E, Dechene J, De Maertelaer V, Bron D, Englert Y. Gonadotropin-releasing hormone agonist for the prevention of chemotherapy-induced ovarian failure in patients with lymphoma: 1-year follow-up of a prospective randomized trial. J Clin Oncol Off J Am Soc Clin Oncol. 2013;31(7):903–9. https://doi.org/10.1200/JCO.2012.42.8185.
59. Badawy A, Elnashar A, El-Ashry M, Shahat M. Gonadotropin-releasing hormone agonists for prevention of chemotherapy-induced ovarian damage: prospective randomized study. Fertil Steril. 2009;91(3):694–7. https://doi.org/10.1016/j.fertnstert.2007.12.044.
60. Munster PN, Moore AP, Ismail-Khan R, Cox CE, Lacevic M, Gross-King M, Xu P, Carter WB, Minton SE. Randomized trial using gonadotropin-releasing hormone agonist triptorelin for the preservation of ovarian function during (neo)adjuvant chemotherapy for breast cancer. J Clin Oncol. 2012;30(5):533–8. https://doi.org/10.1200/JCO.2011.34.6890.
61. Del Mastro L, Boni L, Michelotti A, Gamucci T, Olmeo N, Gori S, Giordano M, Garrone O, Pronzato P, Bighin C, Levaggi A, Giraudi S, Cresti N, Magnolfi E, Scotto T, Vecchio C, Venturini M. Effect of the gonadotropin-releasing hormone analogue triptorelin on the occurrence of chemotherapy-induced early menopause in premenopausal women with breast cancer: a randomized trial. JAMA. 2011;306(3):269–76. https://doi.org/10.1001/jama.2011.991.
62. Lambertini M, Boni L, Michelotti A, Gamucci T, Scotto T, Gori S, Giordano M, Garrone O, Levaggi A, Poggio F, Giraudi S, Bighin C, Vecchio C, Sertoli MR, Pronzato P, Del Mastro L, Group GIMS. Ovarian suppression with triptorelin during adjuvant breast cancer chemotherapy and long-term ovarian function, pregnancies, and

disease-free survival: a randomized clinical trial. JAMA. 2015;314(24):2632–40. https://doi.org/10.1001/jama.2015.17291.
63. Moore HC, Unger JM, Phillips KA, Boyle F, Hitre E, Porter D, Francis PA, Goldstein LJ, Gomez HL, Vallejos CS, Partridge AH, Dakhil SR, Garcia AA, Gralow J, Lombard JM, Forbes JF, Martino S, Barlow WE, Fabian CJ, Minasian L, Meyskens FL Jr, Gelber RD, Hortobagyi GN, Albain KS, Investigators PS. Goserelin for ovarian protection during breast-cancer adjuvant chemotherapy. N Engl J Med. 2015;372(10):923–32. https://doi.org/10.1056/NEJMoa1413204.
64. Leonard RC, Adamson DJA, Bertelli G, Mansi J, Yellowlees A, Dunlop J, Thomas GA, Coleman RE, Anderson RA, Anglo Celtic Collaborative Oncology G, National Cancer Research Institute T. GnRH agonist for protection against ovarian toxicity during chemotherapy for early breast cancer: the Anglo Celtic Group OPTION trial. Ann Oncol. 2017;28(8):1811–6. https://doi.org/10.1093/annonc/mdx184.
65. Munhoz RR, Pereira AA, Sasse AD, Hoff PM, Traina TA, Hudis CA, Marques RJ. Gonadotropin-releasing hormone agonists for ovarian function preservation in premenopausal women undergoing chemotherapy for early-stage breast cancer: a systematic review and meta-analysis. JAMA Oncol. 2016;2(1):65–73. https://doi.org/10.1001/jamaoncol.2015.3251.
66. Vitek WS, Shayne M, Hoeger K, Han Y, Messing S, Fung C. Gonadotropin-releasing hormone agonists for the preservation of ovarian function among women with breast cancer who did not use tamoxifen after chemotherapy: a systematic review and meta-analysis. Fertil Steril. 2014;102(3):808–15 e801. https://doi.org/10.1016/j.fertnstert.2014.06.003.
67. Hickman LC, Llarena NC, Valentine LN, Liu X, Falcone T. Preservation of gonadal function in women undergoing chemotherapy: a systematic review and meta-analysis of the potential role for gonadotropin-releasing hormone agonists. J Assist Reprod Genet. 2018. https://doi.org/10.1007/s10815-018-1128-2.
68. Horicks F, Van Den Steen G, Gervy C, Clarke HJ, Demeestere I. Both in vivo FSH depletion and follicular exposure to Gonadotrophin-releasing hormone analogues in vitro are not effective to prevent follicular depletion during chemotherapy in mice. Mol Hum Reprod. 2018. https://doi.org/10.1093/molehr/gay005.
69. Horicks F, Van Den Steen G, Houben S, Englert Y, Demeestere I. Folliculogenesis is not fully inhibited during GnRH analogues treatment in mice challenging their efficiency to preserve the ovarian reserve during chemotherapy in this model. PLoS One. 2015;10(9):e0137164. https://doi.org/10.1371/journal.pone.0137164.
70. Hasky N, Uri-Belapolsky S, Goldberg K, Miller I, Grossman H, Stemmer SM, Ben-Aharon I, Shalgi R. Gonadotrophin-releasing hormone agonists for fertility preservation: unraveling the enigma? Hum Reprod. 2015;30(5):1089–101. https://doi.org/10.1093/humrep/dev037.
71. Bildik G, Akin N, Senbabaoglu F, Sahin GN, Karahuseyinoglu S, Ince U, Taskiran C, Selek U, Yakin K, Guzel Y, Ayhan C, Alper E, Cetiner M, Balaban B, Mandel NM, Esen T, Iwase A, Urman B, Oktem O. GnRH agonist leuprolide acetate does not confer any protection against ovarian damage induced by chemotherapy and radiation in vitro. Hum Reprod. 2015;30(12):2912–25. https://doi.org/10.1093/humrep/dev257.
72. Loren AW, Mangu PB, Beck LN, Brennan L, Magdalinski AJ, Partridge AH, Quinn G, Wallace WH, Oktay K. Fertility preservation for patients with cancer: American Society of Clinical Oncology clinical practice guideline update. J Clin Oncol. 2013;31(19):2500–10. https://doi.org/10.1200/JCO.2013.49.2678.
73. Kano M, Sosulski AE, Zhang L, Saatcioglu HD, Wang D, Nagykery N, Sabatini ME, Gao G, Donahoe PK, Pepin D. AMH/MIS as a contraceptive that protects the ovarian reserve during chemotherapy. Proc Natl Acad Sci U S A. 2017;114(9):E1688–97. https://doi.org/10.1073/pnas.1620729114.
74. Kalich-Philosoph L, Roness H, Carmely A, Fishel-Bartal M, Ligumsky H, Paglin S, Wolf I, Kanety H, Sredni B, Meirow D. Cyclophosphamide triggers follicle activation and "burnout"; AS101 prevents follicle loss and preserves fertility. Sci Transl Med. 2013; 5(185):185ra162. https://doi.org/10.1126/scitranslmed.3005402.
75. Di Emidio G, Rossi G, Bonomo I, Alonso GL, Sferra R, Vetuschi A, Artini PG, Provenzani A, Falone S, Carta G, D'Alessandro AM, Amicarelli F, Tatone C. The natural carotenoid crocetin and the synthetic tellurium compound AS101 protect the ovary against cyclophosphamide by modulating SIRT1 and mitochondrial markers. Oxidative Med Cell Longev. 2017;2017:8928604. https://doi.org/10.1155/2017/8928604.
76. Goldman KN, Chenette D, Arju R, Duncan FE, Keefe DL, Grifo JA, Schneider RJ. mTORC1/2 inhibition preserves ovarian function and fertility during genotoxic chemotherapy. Proc Natl Acad Sci U S A. 2017;114(12):3186–91. https://doi.org/10.1073/pnas.1617233114.
77. Chang EM, Lim E, Yoon S, Jeong K, Bae S, Lee DR, Yoon TK, Choi Y, Lee WS. Cisplatin induces overactivation of the dormant primordial follicle through PTEN/AKT/FOXO3a pathway which leads to loss of ovarian reserve in mice. PLoS One. 2015;10(12):e0144245. https://doi.org/10.1371/journal.pone.0144245.
78. Jang H, Lee OH, Lee Y, Yoon H, Chang EM, Park M, Lee JW, Hong K, Kim JO, Kim NK, Ko JJ, Lee DR, Yoon TK, Lee WS, Choi Y. Melatonin prevents cisplatin-induced primordial follicle loss via suppression of PTEN/AKT/FOXO3a pathway activation in the mouse ovary. J Pineal Res. 2016;60(3):336–47. https://doi.org/10.1111/jpi.12316.
79. Jang H, Na Y, Hong K, Lee S, Moon S, Cho M, Park M, Lee OH, Chang EM, Lee DR, Ko JJ, Lee WS, Choi Y. Synergistic effect of melatonin and ghrelin in preventing cisplatin-induced ovarian damage via regulation of FOXO3a phosphorylation and binding to the p27(Kip1) promoter in primordial follicles. J Pineal Res. 2017;63(3). https://doi.org/10.1111/jpi.12432.

80. Gonfloni S, Di Tella L, Caldarola S, Cannata SM, Klinger FG, Di Bartolomeo C, Mattei M, Candi E, De Felici M, Melino G, Cesareni G. Inhibition of the c-Abl-TAp63 pathway protects mouse oocytes from chemotherapy-induced death. Nat Med. 2009;15(10):1179–85. https://doi.org/10.1038/nm.2033.
81. Kim SY, Cordeiro MH, Serna VA, Ebbert K, Butler LM, Sinha S, Mills AA, Woodruff TK, Kurita T. Rescue of platinum-damaged oocytes from programmed cell death through inactivation of the p53 family signaling network. Cell Death Differ. 2013;20(8):987–97. https://doi.org/10.1038/cdd.2013.31.
82. Kerr JB, Hutt KJ, Cook M, Speed TP, Strasser A, Findlay JK, Scott CL. Cisplatin-induced primordial follicle oocyte killing and loss of fertility are not prevented by imatinib. Nat Med. 2012;18(8):1170–2; author reply 1172–1174. https://doi.org/10.1038/nm.2889.
83. Rinaldi VD, Hsieh K, Munroe R, Bolcun-Filas E, Schimenti JC. Pharmacological inhibition of the DNA damage checkpoint prevents radiation-induced oocyte death. Genetics. 2017;206(4):1823–8. https://doi.org/10.1534/genetics.117.203455.

Fertility Preservation Options for Female Pediatric and Adolescent Oncology Patients

Michael Kinnaman, Kathleen Shea, and Jennifer Levine

T. K. Woodruff et al. (eds.), *Textbook of Oncofertility Research and Practice*,
https://doi.org/10.1007/978-3-030-02868-8_9

Key Points

- Preservation of fertility post cancer-directed therapy is important to survivors of pediatric and adolescent cancer.
- Exposure to high doses of alkylating agents and radiation pose risks to fertility in pediatric and adolescent cancer survivors.
- Only experimental options for fertility preservation exist for prepubertal children diagnosed with cancer.

9.1 Introduction

9

Maintaining the ability to have biological children has been identified as an important component to postcancer quality of life in survivors [32, 56]. Achieving this in younger cancer patients has become more feasible secondary to improvements in reproductive technology [24]. Healthcare providers are now increasingly called upon to be familiar with the indications and options for fertility preservation in female pediatric and adolescent cancer patients [17]. Type of cancer, age, pubertal development, the severity of illness at the time of diagnosis, and type of treatment all impact decision making related to pursuing fertility preservation [1]. Patients at highest risk of gonadal toxicity include those receiving high-dose alkylating agents particularly procarbazine and pelvic radiation which leads to depletion of ovarian reserve [19, 38]. Radiation to the brain may interfere with the hypothalamic-pituitary-gonadal axis impairing the ability of the ovaries to function correctly [20]. Cancer-directed therapies that involve surgical resection of reproductive structures have clear implications for later fertility [37]. This chapter will give an overview of current options for fertility preservation for female pediatric and adolescent cancer patients.

9.2 Protection of Ovarian Function

9.2.1 Ovarian Transposition

Ovarian transposition, also known as oophoropexy, involves surgically relocating the ovaries out of the field of radiation. By decreasing exposure to radiation, transposition can reduce the incidence of premature ovarian failure [64]. Rhabdomyosarcoma of the bladder, vagina, or uterus or soft tissue or pelvic bone sarcomas, such as Ewing's sarcoma, are the main diagnostic indications for ovarian transposition in children. The procedure can be done laparoscopically or with concomitant laparotomy. The optimal timing is just prior to radiation therapy, as the ovaries can migrate back to the pelvis. If placed correctly, radiation exposure can be reduced by 90–95%. However, patients need to be made aware that due to radiation scatter, ovaries are not always protected, and this technique is not always successful. Results are dependent on other variables such as the age of the patient, dose of radiation, degree of scatter, whether ovaries were shielded, and if gonadotoxic chemotherapy was also used [30]. A review of the literature previously identified preservation of ovarian function in 88.6% of cancer patients under the age of 40 who underwent laparoscopic ovarian transposition [10].

An additional procedure to reverse the transposition may be necessary to facilitate either spontaneous pregnancy or assisted reproduction if the ovary is not in close proximity to the fallopian tube [43]. Alternatively, transabdominal monitoring and harvesting of oocytes during assisted reproduction may be utilized. Transabdominal harvesting may result in fewer oocytes obtained compared to the use of transvaginal ultrasound but equal efficacy in terms of fertilization rates, embryo number and quality, and pregnancy rates [6]. Although ovarian transposition is generally well tolerated, potential side effects include pelvic pain, necrosis, and ovarian torsion [26]. While few long-term results in adults are available, transposition has been reported to be effective at maintaining endocrine function. The American Society of Clinical Oncology (ASCO) 2013 Guidelines for adults recommend discussing the option of ovarian transposition when pelvic radiation therapy is performed as cancer treatment [39]. For children, ASCO recommends providing information on methods that are investigational, and some would recommend ovarian transposition be discussed at a multidisciplinary meeting at the time of cancer diagnosis [30].

9.2.2 Ovarian Suppression

Strategies to protect the ovaries during chemotherapy include the use of gonadotropin-releasing hormone (GnRH) analogues in postpubertal females. Though widely studied, the efficacy of this approach has been conflicting. ASCO, the American Society for Reproductive Medicine (ASRM), and the European Society for Medical Oncology (ESMO) all have found in their most recent policy position papers that there is insufficient evidence to support GnRH analogs as a means to preserve fertility [39, 45, 48]. However, after the publication of these guidelines, a retrospective review found that in a cohort of patients with a mean age of 25 years vs. 28 years in the treated vs. untreated group, respectively, retention of cyclic ovarian function and pregnancy rates were significantly higher in the treated group [11]. Following the publication of these guidelines, the use of goserelin for ovarian suppression during chemotherapy for breast cancer appeared to protect against ovarian failure, reduce the risk of early menopause, and improve prospects for fertility [42]. Well-designed studies in the adolescent population across a variety of diagnoses and exposures remain necessary to ascertain the effectiveness of this strategy in this population, as data in adult populations with smaller ovarian reserve may not be generalizable.

9.3 Assisted Reproductive Endocrinology

9.3.1 Embryo and Oocyte Cryopreservation

Embryo and oocyte cryopreservation are considered the standard of care fertility preservation options in postpubertal patients at risk of ovarian failure [39]. Oocyte cryopreservation was designated nonexperimental by ASRM in 2012 [50]. Both embryo and oocyte cryopreservation require controlled ovarian stimulation (COS) with daily injectable gonadotropins, traditionally beginning on the third day of the menstrual cycle and continuing daily for 10–12 days on average. The potential risks of COS include mild to severe ovarian hyperstimulation syndrome or intra-abdominal bleeding. It is estimated that severe hyperstimulation syndrome will occur in 0.4–2.0% of women during ovarian stimulation [47]. Ovulation is triggered by a single dose of human chorionic gonadotropin, and transvaginal oocyte retrieval is performed 34–36 h later under sedation. Newer, more flexible protocols have been developed where ovarian stimulation is not dependent on the timing of the menstrual cycle, resulting in fewer delays and shorter time to treatment initiation [13, 33, 46, 61]. The number of total and mature oocytes retrieved, oocyte maturity rate, mature oocyte yield, and fertilization rates have been reported to be similar in random and conventional-start COS cycles [13] although duration and dose of stimulation may be longer with random start protocols [46].

In those who can delay the start of treatment, oocyte cryopreservation may be preferred by younger pubertal patients, patients without partners, those who do not wish to use donor sperm, and/or those who have religious or ethical objections to embryo freezing [3, 44]. For those individuals who do wish to preserve embryos, harvested oocytes are fertilized in vitro either with partner or donor sperm and then cryopreserved. Intracytoplasmic sperm injection (ICSI) may be recommended to offset the risk of fertilization failure.

Embryo cryopreservation has live birth rates of 30–40% per embryo transferred in the general US population, with only slightly lower rates of live births from cryopreserved oocytes [48]. Furthermore, there is good evidence that fertilization and pregnancy rates are similar to in vitro fertilization/intracytoplasmic sperm injection (IVF/ICSI) with fresh oocytes when vitrified/warmed oocytes are used as part of IVF/ICSI for young women [50]. Although data are limited, no increase in chromosomal abnormalities, birth defects, and developmental deficits has been reported in the offspring born from cryopreserved oocytes when compared to pregnancies from conventional IVF/ICSI and the general population [50]. The efficacy of oocyte cryopreservation continues to be drawn primarily from the general population as the data in cancer patients is limited. This is likely due to a combination of factors including the relatively recent introduction of this technique into clinical practice. Ten case reports detailing the accounts of 16 live births in young adult cancer patients who preserved fertility through oocyte cryopreservation have been reported, with the youngest age at the time of cryopreservation being 22 [40]. It is anticipated that, with additional time, outcomes for this procedure in the adolescent population will be better elucidated.

Despite the technical availability of these procedures, barriers continue to exist in their practical clinical application. Far more medical practitioners believe that pubertal female patients should be referred to a fertility specialist at diagnosis than those that actually make such a referral [35]. Even with random start protocols, the time to complete an embryo or oocyte cryopreservation cycle may exceed the timeframe that patients and medical practitioners are willing to delay the start of therapy [12]. For many patients, the cost of oocyte or embryo cryopreservation and future IVF cycle may be prohibitive with fees in the USA between approximately $7000 and $15,000 for a cycle [29, 66]. Many insurance companies will not cover the cost of fertility preservation procedures as cancer patients do not meet the criteria of infertility, i.e., they have not been trying to achieve pregnancy for more than 1 year [7]. To combat this potential barrier, Connecticut and Rhode Island recently passed legislation requiring coverage of fertility preservation services for patients undergoing medical treatment, which may have a deleterious effect on the gonads. This mandate only applies to commercial insurance companies; however, as more states consider similar legislation, the hope is that Medicaid will also reconsider its position [16].

9.3.2 Ovarian Tissue Cryopreservation and Transplantation

An experimental option that is increasingly being performed, ovarian tissue cryopreservation, involves surgically removing all or part of the cortex of the ovary. The tissue, which contains thousands of primordial follicles, is cut into strips and cryopreserved. As the process does not require hormonal stimulation, it is the only fertility preservation technique involving the gonadal tissue that is available to prepubertal girls or pubertal girls in whom initiation of treatment cannot be delayed [27, 31]. Following completion of treatment, when fertility is desired, the ovarian tissue can be thawed and transplanted orthotopically, i.e., at the site of the ovaries, or heterotopically, i.e., at another location. Once transplanted, the follicles within the ovary have the potential to mature when appropriately stimulated. At least 86 live births have been reported utilizing orthotopic re-transplantation in individuals who were post-pubertal at the time of retrieval [31]. No live births have been reported in the scientific literature in individuals who were prepubescent at the time of tissue cryopreservation. However, a live birth has been reported after autograft of ovarian tissue in a patient who had initiated puberty but was premenarchal at the time of the cryopreservation. The patient, who had sickle cell disease, had developed primary ovarian failure after a myeloablative conditioning regimen as part of hematopoietic stem cell transplantation [22].

Re-introduction of malignant cells via autotransplantation of the ovarian tissue has been a concern with ovarian tissue cryopreservation, particularly in those with hematologic malignancies [9, 23]. A recent case report details a successful ovarian tissue autotransplantation of a 32-year-old sterile AML survivor, who had a tissue harvest performed at the age of 19, prior to her hematopoietic stem cell transplantation but while in a complete remission of her disease. Using a sophisticated approach using next-generation sequencing and xenotransplantation to confirm that the ovarian tissue did not have any evidence of disease, transplantation was performed and a healthy newborn was eventually delivered [57]. Work is also being done in patients with solid tumors as well. RT-qPCR has been described as a highly sensitive assessment of neuroblastoma minimal residual disease in cryopreserved ovarian tissue [28].

While these reports are re-assuring, it must be acknowledged that the true risk of re-introducing malignant cells is still unknown given how few ovarian tissue autotransplants have been undertaken. Because of its investigational nature, ovarian tissue cryopreservation should be performed in centers with clinical expertise under IRB-approved protocols that include follow-up for recurrent cancer and only in patients at highest risk for infertility [39]. Obtaining tissue requires a surgical procedure with anesthesia, although ideally this could be coordinated with other procedures required for evaluation or treatment [4]. Maturation of immature follicles retrieved from the ovarian tissue remains an area of critical research. The capacity for in vitro maturation would negate the need to autotransplant the ovarian tissue in vivo [60] and would prevent the risk of reintroducing cancerous cells that may be present in transplanted ovarian tissue.

9.4 Assessment of Ovarian Reserve

Discussions about reproduction should continue post treatment and during survivorship for all patients. Patients who have developed acute ovarian failure following the completion of cancer-directed therapy can be identified by lack of entry into puberty or sustained amenorrhea and sustained elevations of FSH in the menopausal range in pubertal patients. These patients should be referred to an endocrinologist for consideration of hormone replacement. Some patients may also retain ovarian function post treatment but enter menopause earlier than anticipated. Menopause occurring prior to age 40 is referred to as premature menopause (PM). Assessments from the COG Childhood Cancer Survivor Study and St. Jude Lifetime Cohort Study found PM prevalence rates of 9.1% and 10.9%, respectively, in survivors of pediatric and adolescent cancer [18, 38]. The most significant risk factors for developing PM were patients who received high-dose alkylating agents, particularly procarbazine, stem cell transplantation, and ovarian radiotherapy at any dose [38].

The Children's Oncology Group (COG) currently recommends screening patients exposed to gonadotoxic therapy for Tanner stage and pubertal, menstrual, and pregnancy history. Current guidelines recommend screening follicle-stimulating hormone (FSH), luteinizing hormone (LH), and estradiol levels beginning at age 13 [41]; however, these measures are very inexact and are likely to become abnormal only once the ovarian reserve is significantly compromised. Early follicular phase FSH, anti-Mullerian hormone (AMH) (a product of antral follicles), and ultrasound assessments of antral follicle count are utilized in the reproductive endocrinology community to evaluate fertility and potential response to fertility interventions and show promise as better surrogate measures of the remaining ovarian reserve [49]. Refining this estimate is crucial to allowing more accurate counseling of pediatric and adolescent cancer survivors about their reproductive options post therapy.

9.5 Reproductive Options Post Therapy

9.5.1 Donor Oocytes and Embryos

Patients who experience ovarian failure may consider options such as utilization of donor oocytes or embryos if their uterus has not been impaired by cancer-directed therapy such as radiation. Oocytes from another woman (either a known or anonymous donor) may be fertilized with the patient's partner's sperm or with donor sperm and placed in the patient's uterus. The oocyte donor receives the same ovarian stimulation regimen used during an IVF cycle. The recipient receives hormonal medication to modify her cycle in preparation for the embryo transfer. If pregnancy is achieved, hormonal treatment continues through at least the 12th week of pregnancy. The use of donated embryos may also be considered in couples with infertility affecting both partners, infertility in a single woman, or couples with genetic disorders. IVF cycles may result in unused embryos that may be destroyed, donated to research, or donated to another woman to achieve pregnancy. Recipients need to be counseled and informed of the complexities involved in potential relationships between donors and recipients and individual state laws regarding parentage during pregnancy and after birth [25]. Rates of success are dependent on the age of the donor woman, quality of embryos, and the number of embryos transferred.

9.5.2 Fertility Preservation Post Therapy

For patients at risk of premature menopause, it is important to conduct conversations regarding their plan for starting a family. While it remains virtually impossible to determine the remaining reproductive window for a given individual, cryopreserving oocytes or embryos post completion of therapy may be of interest to individuals who are not certain when they might want to start a family. Recent evidence also suggests that even individuals with evidence of premature menopause can achieve pregnancies with the use of assisted reproduction such as IVF/ICSI [5].

9.5.3 Gestational Carrier

A gestational carrier or gestational surrogate is an arrangement between a woman who carries and delivers a baby for another person that is the intended parent. This option may be considered by a woman who does not have a uterus, has uterine damage or scarring, or has a condition that prevents her from carrying a pregnancy to term. This option involves an IVF cycle with embryos made from donors or the intended parent and not the gestational carrier. Medical and psychological screening is required for gestational carriers. Intended parents have genetic, medical, and psychological evaluations. Intended parents need to obtain legal counsel regarding state laws and gestational carrier contracts [2].

9.5.4 Adoption

Patients not able to have biologic children may consider adoption as a means of family building. Cancer survivors may face more challenges such as additional medical documentation of their health status and a required 5-year off treatment waiting period [54]. Individuals and couples would need to explore the various scenarios surrounding adoption such as domestic or international origins, open or closed adoption, and comfort level accepting an infant or older child, siblings, or medically fragile children. Many agencies and individual countries have age, income, and marital status requirements. Birth mothers choosing adoptive parents may have ethnic and/or religious preferences. Adoption agencies and lawyers guide candidates through the adoption process. Adoption is costly with fees ranging from $29,000 to $49,000 for domestic adoption and $17,000 to $28,000 for international adoptions. The Internal Revenue Service offers a federal tax credit (maximum $13,400) for adoptive families. Some states may have programs for adoption of children from foster care systems that may be less costly.

9.6 Access to Fertility Preservation

First and foremost in ensuring access to fertility preservation procedures for pediatric and adolescent cancer patients and their families is establishing notification of risks to fertility and possible fertility preservation options as the standard of care. Multiple publications have demonstrated that this is not currently the case [8, 51, 59]. Despite ASCO guidelines advising oncologists to discuss fertility risks and preservation strategies and make referrals to reproductive endocrinologists, over half are not doing so, and only a third have even reviewed the new guidelines [14]. Often cited barriers are the cost of treatment [14] and lack of proper training and knowledge about referrals and perception that patients could not delay treatment to pursue options and patients were not interested in discussing fertility because it was not mentioned [52]. Female oncologists and those with favorable attitudes toward fertility preservation and those with patients that ask about fertility preservation are more likely to refer to reproductive specialists [53]. In 2013, ASCO updated its guidelines to include other physicians as well as nurses, psychologists, and other nonphysician providers as candidates for disseminating information to patients regarding fertility preservation [39].

Institutions are increasingly developing fertility programs that provide guidance about the elements necessary to effectively inform patients about their risks and options and create workflows and infrastructure to provide timely referrals to reproductive endocrinology. ◘ Figure 9.1 demonstrates one algorithm for providing fertility preservation in pediatric and adolescent oncology patients. The key elements include developing institutional policies that demonstrate a commitment to fertility preservation, creating a team of individuals who "champion" the provision of these services, developing educational resources for patients and families as well as clinical staff, and developing established relationships with reproductive endocrinologists [34, 37, 55]. Programs such as LIVESTRONG provide assistance to financially eligible patients with the cost of medication and contract with agencies across the USA to provide services at reduced cost for cancer patients (► http://www.livestrong.org/we-can-help/fertility-services).

9.7 Ethical Considerations

As outlined above, numerous concerns about the comprehensive provision of fertility preservation options exist. Despite significant study in the area of gonadotoxicity, it remains extremely difficult to

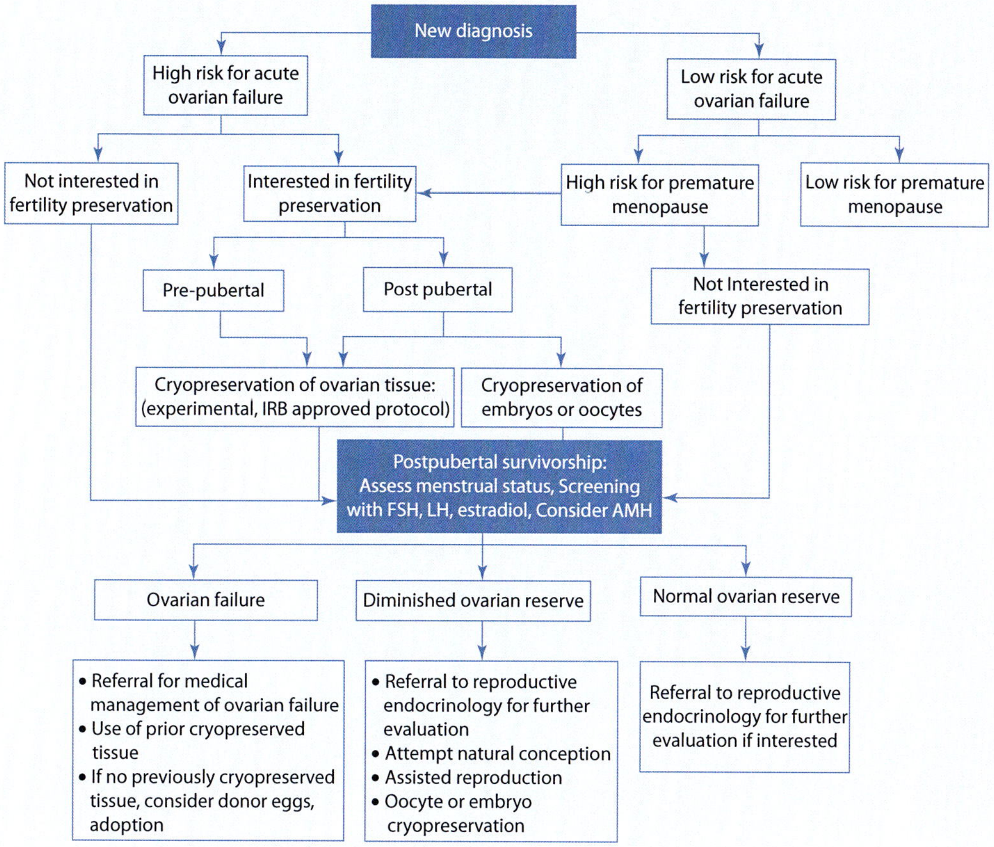

Fig. 9.1 Algorithm for fertility preservation in pediatric and adolescent oncology patients

assess the risk of acute ovarian failure or premature menopause in a given individual prior to the start of cancer-directed therapy. Because there is also limited data related to the overall efficacy of the various fertility cryopreservation techniques specifically in the pediatric oncology population clinicians, patients and parents must often make decisions about expensive, invasive procedures with limited information during an already emotional time [62]. Given that there is no standardization of coverage of these procedures by insurance companies, there is also the concern that socioeconomic disparities may exist based upon who is able to pay and therefore access interventions [3].

In the pediatric population, minors will be asked to provide their assent for procedures that are related to issues, i.e., family planning, that they may be ill-suited to consider. When specifically considering ovarian tissue cryopreservation in prepubertal girls, the question of what is in the best interest of the child remains a difficult one to answer [65].

Disposition of stored ovarian tissue, oocytes, or embryos in the setting of a patient's death remains an issue of concern, particularly in the pediatric setting where a patient is under the age of 18 and is not legally able to determine the disposition of stored tissue. While there are mechanisms by which stored tissue would not be able to be utilized unless the patient has reached maturity and consented to the use of the tissue, controversies remain [1, 65]. In the setting of embryos, the situation is further complicated by the wishes and desires of the individual who provided the sperm. Disposition of unused tissue, oocytes, or embryos can also present moral and religious conflicts if the patient is able to become pregnant via intercourse or assisted reproduction and does not require the use of the stored tissue.

9.8 Future Directions

9.8.1 Generation of Gametes from Somatic Cells

Ovarian tissue cryopreservation followed by orthotopic or heterotopic transplantation is currently the only method of fertility preservation for prepubertal girls and the only method available to pubertal girls and adolescents that cannot delay therapy to do oocyte cryopreservation. Research studying the development of ovarian follicles in vitro is underway. This presents significant challenges given the complex systems involved in oocyte development and maturation. Researchers are exploring ways to apply current culture systems to the growth and development of cryopreserved-thawed follicles for clinical use in patients who have banked ovarian tissue. This would eliminate the need for additional reimplantation surgery, eliminate the risk of reintroduction of potentially diseased ovarian tissue into a healthy recipient, and present an option when treatment cannot be delayed [21, 58, 63]. Research with the ultimate goal of creating a human bioprosthetic ovary is underway, and promising results have been published in mice using 3D printing [36].

9.8.2 Coverage of Fertility Preservation by Insurance

As noted above, fertility preservation costs are generally not covered by most insurance companies, as most cancer patients do not fit the insurance companies' definition of infertility that is being unable to achieve pregnancy after 1 year of trying. Arguments have been made that given the iatrogenic nature of infertility among patients with cancer, different eligibility criteria should be applied to these patients when considering fertility preservation interventions [15]. Increasingly bills are being introduced state by state to require coverage of fertility preservation services [16].

9.9 Conclusion

Increased knowledge about the importance of fertility preservation for pediatric and adolescent patients with cancer and improvements in assisted reproduction techniques has increased the likelihood that meeting the family planning goals for survivors of cancer has and will continue to improve over time. Fully meeting this goal means refining risk, developing the institutional infrastructure to identify patients at risk in a timely fashion, streamlining referrals to the appropriate subspecialists, advocating for insurance coverage for fertility preservation procedures, and continuing to move the research agenda forward to advance the efficacy of available options.

Review Questions and Answers

Q1. You have just diagnosed a 5-year-old girl with a rhabdomyosarcoma of the pelvis. Her treatment includes multiagent chemotherapy including cyclophosphamide and radiation to the tumor site. Which of the following would be an appropriate fertility preservation option for this patient?

(a) Embryo cryopreservation
(b) Ovarian tissue cryopreservation
(c) Use of GnRH agonist in conjunction with therapy
(d) Oocyte cryopreservation

A1. (b). Ovarian tissue cryopreservation is the only option available to prepubertal females.

Q2. A 16-year-old female who has just been diagnosed with nonmetastatic Ewing's sarcoma wishes to pursue oocyte cryopreservation. Her oncologist has agreed to a 3-week window to start therapy. Her last menstrual cycle started 10 days ago. Because the patient is mid-cycle, she cannot complete oocyte cryopreservation in the desired timeframe. True/False

A2. False. Ovarian hyperstimulation can utilize a random start protocol which, if the systems are in place to facilitate a rapid referral, should allow for stimulation and recovery of oocytes within the time frame outlined above.

Q3. An 18-year-old female survivor of Hodgkin lymphoma, off therapy for 5 years, is being seen in long-term follow-up. She was treated with four cycles of BEACOPP and four cycles of COPP/ABV. Her menstrual cycle resumed 9 months after the completion of therapy and has been regular since then. She did not undergo any fertility preservation procedures prior to the start of therapy. Appropriate interventions at the current clinic visit include:

(a) Check FSH, LH, and estradiol
(b) Discuss risk of premature menopause
(c) Discuss consideration of embryo or oocyte cryopreservation
(d) All of the above

A3. (d) Female survivors who are treated with alkylating agents, particularly procarbazine, are at increased risk of developing premature menopause and should be monitored by checking reproductive hormones. They should also have a discussion about options for family building including consideration of embryo or oocyte cryopreservation.

References

1. Anderson RA, Mitchell RT, Kelsey TW, Spears N, Telfer EE, Wallace WH. Cancer treatment and gonadal function: experimental and established strategies for fertility preservation in children and young adults. Lancet Diabetes Endocrinol. 2015;3(7):556–67. https://doi.org/10.1016/S2213-8587(15)00039-X.
2. Armour KL. An overview of surrogacy around the world: trends, questions and ethical issues. Nurs Womens Health. 2012;16(3):231–6. https://doi.org/10.1111/j.1751-486X.2012.01734.x.
3. Ayensu-Coker L, Essig E, Breech LL, Lindheim S. Ethical quandaries in gamete-embryo cryopreservation related to oncofertility. J Law Med Ethics. 2013;41(3):711–9. https://doi.org/10.1111/jlme.12081.
4. Babayev SN, Arslan E, Kogan S, Moy F, Oktay K. Evaluation of ovarian and testicular tissue cryopreservation in children undergoing gonadotoxic therapies. J Assist Reprod Genet. 2013;30(1):3–9. https://doi.org/10.1007/s10815-012-9909-5.
5. Barton SE, Najita JS, Ginsburg ES, Leisenring WM, Stovall M, Weathers RE, Sklar CA, Robison LL, Diller L. Infertility, infertility treatment, and achievement of pregnancy in female survivors of childhood cancer: a report from the Childhood Cancer Survivor Study cohort. Lancet Oncol. 2013;14(9):873–81. https://doi.org/10.1016/S1470-2045(13)70251-1.
6. Barton SE, Politch JA, Benson CB, Ginsburg ES, Gargiulo AR. Transabdominal follicular aspiration for oocyte retrieval in patients with ovaries inaccessible by transvaginal ultrasound. Fertil Steril. 2011;95(5):1773–6. https://doi.org/10.1016/j.fertnstert.2011.01.006.
7. Basco D, Campo-Engelstein L, Rodriguez S. Insuring against infertility: expanding state infertility mandates to include fertility preservation technology for cancer patients. J Law Med Ethics. 2010;38(4):832–9. https://doi.org/10.1111/j.1748-720X.2010.00536.x.
8. Bastings L, Baysal O, Beerendonk CC, Braat DD, Nelen WL. Referral for fertility preservation counselling in female cancer patients. Hum Reprod. 2014;29(10):2228–37. https://doi.org/10.1093/humrep/deu186.
9. Bastings L, Beerendonk CC, Westphal JR, Massuger LF, Kaal SE, van Leeuwen FE, Braat DD, Peek R. Autotransplantation of cryopreserved ovarian tissue in cancer survivors and the risk of reintroducing malignancy: a systematic review. Hum Reprod Update. 2013;19(5):483–506. https://doi.org/10.1093/humupd/dmt020.
10. Bisharah M, Tulandi T. Laparoscopic preservation of ovarian function: an underused procedure. Am J Obstet Gynecol. 2003;188(2):367–70.
11. Blumenfeld Z, Zur H, Dann EJ. Gonadotropin-releasing hormone agonist cotreatment during chemotherapy may increase pregnancy rate in survivors. Oncologist. 2015;20(11):1283–9. https://doi.org/10.1634/theoncologist.2015-0223.
12. Burns KC, Boudreau C, Panepinto JA. Attitudes regarding fertility preservation in female adolescent cancer patients. J Pediatr Hematol Oncol. 2006;28(6):350–4.
13. Cakmak H, Katz A, Cedars MI, Rosen MP. Effective method for emergency fertility preservation: random-start controlled ovarian stimulation. Fertil Steril. 2013;100(6):1673–80. https://doi.org/10.1016/j.fertnstert.2013.07.1992.
14. Campbell JE, Assanasen C, Robinson RD, Knudtson JF. Fertility preservation counseling for pediatric and adolescent cancer patients. J Adolesc Young Adult Oncol. 2016;5(1):58–63. https://doi.org/10.1089/jayao.2015.0040.
15. Campo-Engelstein L. Consistency in insurance coverage for iatrogenic conditions resulting from cancer treatment including fertility preservation. J Clin Oncol. 2010;28(8):1284–6. https://doi.org/10.1200/JCO.2009.25.6883.
16. Cardozo ER, Huber WJ, Stuckey AR, Alvero RJ. Mandating coverage for fertility preservation – a step in the right direction. N Engl J Med. 2017;377(17):1607–9. https://doi.org/10.1056/NEJMp1709585.
17. Caserta D, Ralli E, Matteucci E, Marci R, Moscarini M. Fertility preservation in female cancer patients: an emerging challenge for physicians. Panminerva Med. 2014;56(1):85–95.
18. Chemaitilly W, Li Z, Krasin MJ, Brooke RJ, Wilson CL, Green DM, Klosky JL, Barnes N, Clark KL, Farr JB, Fernandez-Pineda I, Bishop MW, Metzger M, Pui CH, Kaste SC, Ness

KK, Srivastava DK, Robison LL, Hudson MM, Yasui Y, Sklar CA. Premature ovarian insufficiency in childhood cancer survivors: a report from the St. Jude Lifetime Cohort. J Clin Endocrinol Metab. 2017;102(7):2242–50. https://doi.org/10.1210/jc.2016-3723.
19. Chemaitilly W, Mertens AC, Mitby P, Whitton J, Stovall M, Yasui Y, Robison LL, Sklar CA. Acute ovarian failure in the childhood cancer survivor study. J Clin Endocrinol Metab. 2006;91(5):1723–8. https://doi.org/10.1210/jc.2006-0020.
20. Crowne E, Gleeson H, Benghiat H, Sanghera P, Toogood A. Effect of cancer treatment on hypothalamic-pituitary function. Lancet Diabetes Endocrinol. 2015;3(7):568–76. https://doi.org/10.1016/S2213-8587(15)00008-X.
21. De Vos M, Smitz J, Woodruff TK. Fertility preservation in women with cancer. Lancet. 2014;384(9950):1302–10. https://doi.org/10.1016/S0140-6736(14)60834-5.
22. Demeestere I, Simon P, Dedeken L, Moffa F, Tsepelidis S, Brachet C, Delbaere A, Devreker F, Ferster A. Live birth after autograft of ovarian tissue cryopreserved during childhood. Hum Reprod. 2015;30(9):2107–9. https://doi.org/10.1093/humrep/dev128.
23. Dolmans MM, Marinescu C, Saussoy P, Van Langendonckt A, Amorim C, Donnez J. Reimplantation of cryopreserved ovarian tissue from patients with acute lymphoblastic leukemia is potentially unsafe. Blood. 2010;116(16):2908–14. https://doi.org/10.1182/blood-2010-01-265751.
24. Ginsberg JP. New advances in fertility preservation for pediatric cancer patients. Curr Opin Pediatr. 2011;23(1):9–13. https://doi.org/10.1097/MOP.0b013e3283420fb6.
25. Goedeke S, Daniels K, Thorpe M, Du Preez E. Building extended families through embryo donation: the experiences of donors and recipients. Hum Reprod. 2015;30(10):2340–50. https://doi.org/10.1093/humrep/dev189.
26. Gomez-Hidalgo NR, Darin MC, Dalton H, Jhingran A, Fleming N, Brown J, Ramirez PT. Ovarian torsion after laparoscopic ovarian transposition in patients with gynecologic cancer: a report of two cases. J Minim Invasive Gynecol. 2015;22(4):687–90. https://doi.org/10.1016/j.jmig.2015.02.009.
27. Gracia CR, Chang J, Kondapalli L, Prewitt M, Carlson CA, Mattei P, Jeffers S, Ginsberg JP. Ovarian tissue cryopreservation for fertility preservation in cancer patients: successful establishment and feasibility of a multidisciplinary collaboration. J Assist Reprod Genet. 2012;29(6):495–502. https://doi.org/10.1007/s10815-012-9753-7.
28. Greze V, Brugnon F, Chambon F, Halle P, Canis M, Amiot C, Gremeau AS, Pereira B, Yanez Peralta Y, Tchirkov A, Kanold J. Highly sensitive assessment of neuroblastoma minimal residual disease in ovarian tissue using RT-qPCR-A strategy for improving the safety of fertility restoration. Pediatr Blood Cancer. 2017;64(5). https://doi.org/10.1002/pbc.26287.
29. Hirshfeld-Cytron J, Grobman WA, Milad MP. Fertility preservation for social indications: a cost-based decision analysis. Fertil Steril. 2012;97(3):665–70. https://doi.org/10.1016/j.fertnstert.2011.12.029.
30. Irtan S, Orbach D, Helfre S, Sarnacki S. Ovarian transposition in prepubescent and adolescent girls with cancer. Lancet Oncol. 2013;14(13):e601–8. https://doi.org/10.1016/S1470-2045(13)70288-2.
31. Jensen AK, Rechnitzer C, Macklon KT, Ifversen MR, Birkebaek N, Clausen N, Sorensen K, Fedder J, Ernst E, Andersen CY. Cryopreservation of ovarian tissue for fertility preservation in a large cohort of young girls: focus on pubertal development. Hum Reprod. 2017;32(1):154–64. https://doi.org/10.1093/humrep/dew273.
32. Jeruss JS, Woodruff TK. Preservation of fertility in patients with cancer. N Engl J Med. 2009;360(9):902–11. https://doi.org/10.1056/NEJMra0801454.
33. Keskin U, Ercan CM, Yilmaz A, Babacan A, Korkmaz C, Duru NK, Ergun A. Random-start controlled ovarian hyperstimulation with letrozole for fertility preservation in cancer patients: case series and review of literature. J Pak Med Assoc. 2014;64(7):830–2.
34. Kim J, Kim KH, Mersereau JE. Building a successful fertility preservation program at a major cancer center. J Gynecol Oncol. 2014;25(2):148–54. https://doi.org/10.3802/jgo.2014.25.2.148.
35. Kohler TS, Kondapalli LA, Shah A, Chan S, Woodruff TK, Brannigan RE. Results from the survey for preservation of adolescent reproduction (SPARE) study: gender disparity in delivery of fertility preservation message to adolescents with cancer. J Assist Reprod Genet. 2011;28(3):269–77. https://doi.org/10.1007/s10815-010-9504-6.
36. Laronda MM, Rutz AL, Xiao S, Whelan KA, Duncan FE, Roth EW, Woodruff TK, Shah RN. A bioprosthetic ovary created using 3D printed microporous scaffolds restores ovarian function in sterilized mice. Nat Commun. 2017;8:15261. https://doi.org/10.1038/ncomms15261.
37. Levine JM, Kelvin JF, Quinn GP, Gracia CR. Infertility in reproductive-age female cancer survivors. Cancer. 2015;121(10):1532–9. https://doi.org/10.1002/cncr.29181.
38. Levine JM, Whitton JA, Ginsberg JP, Green DM, Leisenring WM, Stovall M, Robison LL, Armstrong GT, Sklar CA. Nonsurgical premature menopause and reproductive implications in survivors of childhood cancer: a report from the Childhood Cancer Survivor Study. Cancer. 2018;124(5):1044–52. https://doi.org/10.1002/cncr.31121.
39. Loren AW, Mangu PB, Beck LN, Brennan L, Magdalinski AJ, Partridge AH, Quinn G, Wallace WH, Oktay K, American Society of Clinical O. Fertility preservation for patients with cancer: American Society of Clinical Oncology clinical practice guideline update. J Clin Oncol. 2013;31(19):2500–10. https://doi.org/10.1200/JCO.2013.49.2678.
40. Massarotti C, Scaruffi P, Lambertini M, Remorgida V, Del Mastro L, Anserini P. State of the art on oocyte cryopreservation in female cancer patients: a critical review of the literature. Cancer Treat Rev. 2017;57:50–7. https://doi.org/10.1016/j.ctrv.2017.04.009.
41. Metzger ML, Meacham LR, Patterson B, Casillas JS, Constine LS, Hijiya N, Kenney LB, Leonard M, Lockart BA, Likes W, Green DM. Female reproductive health after childhood, adolescent, and young adult cancers: guidelines for the assessment and management of female reproductive complications. J Clin Oncol. 2013;31(9):1239–47. https://doi.org/10.1200/JCO.2012.43.5511.

42. Moore HC, Unger JM, Phillips KA, Boyle F, Hitre E, Porter D, Francis PA, Goldstein LJ, Gomez HL, Vallejos CS, Partridge AH, Dakhil SR, Garcia AA, Gralow J, Lombard JM, Forbes JF, Martino S, Barlow WE, Fabian CJ, Minasian L, Meyskens FL Jr, Gelber RD, Hortobagyi GN, Albain KS, Investigators PS. Goserelin for ovarian protection during breast-cancer adjuvant chemotherapy. N Engl J Med. 2015;372(10):923–32. https://doi.org/10.1056/NEJMoa1413204.
43. Noyes N, Knopman JM, Long K, Coletta JM, Abu-Rustum NR. Fertility considerations in the management of gynecologic malignancies. Gynecol Oncol. 2011a;120(3):326–33. https://doi.org/10.1016/j.ygyno.2010.09.012.
44. Noyes N, Knopman JM, Melzer K, Fino ME, Friedman B, Westphal LM. Oocyte cryopreservation as a fertility preservation measure for cancer patients. Reprod Biomed Online. 2011b;23(3):323–33. https://doi.org/10.1016/j.rbmo.2010.11.011.
45. Peccatori FA, Azim HA Jr, Orecchia R, Hoekstra HJ, Pavlidis N, Kesic V, Pentheroudakis G, Group EGW. Cancer, pregnancy and fertility: ESMO Clinical Practice Guidelines for diagnosis, treatment and follow-up. Ann Oncol. 2013;24(Suppl 6):vi160–70. https://doi.org/10.1093/annonc/mdt199.
46. Pereira N, Voskuilen-Gonzalez A, Hancock K, Lekovich JP, Schattman GL, Rosenwaks Z. Random-start ovarian stimulation in women desiring elective cryopreservation of oocytes. Reprod Biomed Online. 2017;35(4):400–6. https://doi.org/10.1016/j.rbmo.2017.06.002.
47. Practice Committee of American Society for Reproductive M. Ovarian hyperstimulation syndrome. Fertil Steril. 2008;90(5 Suppl):S188–93. https://doi.org/10.1016/j.fertnstert.2008.08.034.
48. Practice Committee of American Society for Reproductive M. Fertility preservation in patients undergoing gonadotoxic therapy or gonadectomy: a committee opinion. Fertil Steril. 2013;100(5):1214–23. https://doi.org/10.1016/j.fertnstert.2013.08.012.
49. Practice Committee of the American Society for Reproductive M. Testing and interpreting measures of ovarian reserve: a committee opinion. Fertil Steril. 2015; 103(3):e9–17. https://doi.org/10.1016/j.fertnstert.2014.12.093.
50. Practice Committees of American Society for Reproductive M, Society for Assisted Reproductive T. Mature oocyte cryopreservation: a guideline. Fertil Steril. 2013;99(1):37–43. https://doi.org/10.1016/j.fertnstert.2012.09.028.
51. Quinn GP, Block RG, Clayman ML, Kelvin J, Arvey SR, Lee JH, Reinecke J, Sehovic I, Jacobsen PB, Reed D, Gonzalez L, Vadaparampil ST, Laronga C, Lee MC, Pow-Sang J, Eggly S, Franklin A, Shah B, Fulp WJ, Hayes-Lattin B. If you did not document it, it did not happen: rates of documentation of discussion of infertility risk in adolescent and young adult oncology patients' medical records. J Oncol Pract. 2015a;11(2):137–44. https://doi.org/10.1200/JOP.2014.000786.
52. Quinn GP, Vadaparampil ST, King L, Miree CA, Wilson C, Raj O, Watson J, Lopez A, Albrecht TL. Impact of physicians' personal discomfort and patient prognosis on discussion of fertility preservation with young cancer patients. Patient Educ Couns. 2009a;77(3):338–43. https://doi.org/10.1016/j.pec.2009.09.007.
53. Quinn GP, Vadaparampil ST, Lee JH, Jacobsen PB, Bepler G, Lancaster J, Keefe DL, Albrecht TL. Physician referral for fertility preservation in oncology patients: a national study of practice behaviors. J Clin Oncol. 2009b;27(35):5952–7. https://doi.org/10.1200/JCO.2009.23.0250.
54. Quinn GP, Zebrack BJ, Sehovic I, Bowman ML, Vadaparampil ST. Adoption and cancer survivors: findings from a learning activity for oncology nurses. Cancer. 2015b;121(17):2993–3000. https://doi.org/10.1002/cncr.29322.
55. Reinecke JD, Kelvin JF, Arvey SR, Quinn GP, Levine J, Beck LN, Miller A. Implementing a systematic approach to meeting patients' cancer and fertility needs: a review of the Fertile Hope Centers of Excellence program. J Oncol Pract. 2012;8(5):303–8. https://doi.org/10.1200/JOP.2011.000452.
56. Schover LR. Psychosocial aspects of infertility and decisions about reproduction in young cancer survivors: a review. Med Pediatr Oncol. 1999;33(1):53–9.
57. Shapira M, Raanani H, Barshack I, Amariglio N, Derech-Haim S, Marciano MN, Schiff E, Orvieto R, Meirow D. First delivery in a leukemia survivor after transplantation of cryopreserved ovarian tissue, evaluated for leukemia cells contamination. Fertil Steril. 2018;109(1):48–53. https://doi.org/10.1016/j.fertnstert.2017.09.001.
58. Shea LD, Woodruff TK, Shikanov A. Bioengineering the ovarian follicle microenvironment. Annu Rev Biomed Eng. 2014;16:29–52. https://doi.org/10.1146/annurev-bioeng-071813-105131.
59. Shnorhavorian M, Harlan LC, Smith AW, Keegan TH, Lynch CF, Prasad PK, Cress RD, Wu XC, Hamilton AS, Parsons HM, Keel G, Charlesworth SE, Schwartz SM, Group AHSC. Fertility preservation knowledge, counseling, and actions among adolescent and young adult patients with cancer: a population-based study. Cancer. 2015;121(19):3499–506. https://doi.org/10.1002/cncr.29328.
60. Smitz J, Dolmans MM, Donnez J, Fortune JE, Hovatta O, Jewgenow K, Picton HM, Plancha C, Shea LD, Stouffer RL, Telfer EE, Woodruff TK, Zelinski MB. Current achievements and future research directions in ovarian tissue culture, in vitro follicle development and transplantation: implications for fertility preservation. Hum Reprod Updat. 2010;16(4):395–414. https://doi.org/10.1093/humupd/dmp056.
61. Sonmezer M, Turkcuoglu I, Coskun U, Oktay K. Random-start controlled ovarian hyperstimulation for emergency fertility preservation in letrozole cycles. Fertil Steril. 2011;95(6):2125 e2129–11. https://doi.org/10.1016/j.fertnstert.2011.01.030.
62. Stegmann BJ. Unique ethical and legal implications of fertility preservation research in the pediatric population. Fertil Steril. 2010;93(4):1037–9. https://doi.org/10.1016/j.fertnstert.2009.11.047.
63. Telfer EE, Zelinski MB. Ovarian follicle culture: advances and challenges for human and nonhuman primates. Fertil Steril. 2013;99(6):1523–33. https://doi.org/10.1016/j.fertnstert.2013.03.043.
64. Terenziani M, Piva L, Meazza C, Gandola L, Cefalo G, Merola M. Oophoropexy: a relevant role in preservation of ovarian function after pelvic irradiation. Fertil Steril. 2009;91(3):935 e915–36. https://doi.org/10.1016/j.fertnstert.2008.09.029.

65. Wallace WH, Kelsey TW, Anderson RA. Fertility preservation in pre-pubertal girls with cancer: the role of ovarian tissue cryopreservation. Fertil Steril. 2016;105(1):6–12. https://doi.org/10.1016/j.fertnstert.2015.11.041.

66. Walter JR, Xu S, Woodruff TK. A call for fertility preservation coverage for breast cancer patients: the cost of consistency. J Natl Cancer Inst. 2017;109(5). https://doi.org/10.1093/jnci/djx006.

9

Optimal Technique for Laparoscopic Oophorectomy for Ovarian Tissue Cryopreservation in Pediatric Girls

Kristine S. Corkum and Erin Rowell

T. K. Woodruff et al. (eds.), *Textbook of Oncofertility Research and Practice*,
https://doi.org/10.1007/978-3-030-02868-8_10

Key Points

- OTC is the only pretreatment fertility preservation option for prepubertal children at high risk for premature ovarian failure and infertility
- There is no defined standard surgical technique for the procurement of ovarian cortical children for cryopreservation in children
- Laparoscopic oophorectomy for OTC is a safe, proactive option for pediatric girls facing medical treatment with a high risk of fertility loss
- We recommend that a laparoscopic unilateral oophorectomy for OTC be carried out with minimal manipulation to the ovarian capsule, preservation of the ipsilateral fallopian tube, and division of the ovarian artery as the last step of the procedure to maintain the integrity of the ovary for cryopreservation and the presence of adnexal structures for potential future transplantation

10.1 Introduction

Ovarian tissue cryopreservation (OTC) provides children who face a fertility-threatening treatment an option to cryopreserve their ovarian tissue prior to receiving potentially sterilizing medical therapy [1]. Although OTC remains an experimental method of fertility preservation, this option has an even more powerful impact given the reported pregnancies achieved by two women who had their ovarian tissue cryopreserved in childhood prior to stem cell transplant [2, 3]. The state of the science is such that for both premenarchal and postmenarchal girls, there is more hope than ever that cryopreservation of the ovarian tissue may allow for the possibility of a natural pregnancy and biologically related child in the future.

To date, there has not been one standard operation for ovarian cortical tissue harvest. Techniques described include ovarian cortical biopsy, unilateral or bilateral hemi-oophorectomy, unilateral oophorectomy, and oophorectomy with excision of the vascular pedicle [4]. It is our institution's preference to perform a laparoscopic unilateral oophorectomy to maximize the amount of cortical tissue harvested for cryopreservation purposes while minimizing the risk of operative complications for the patient. This chapter aims to describe the preoperative, intraoperative, and postoperative considerations for laparoscopic oophorectomy for OTC.

10.2 Preoperative Considerations

For the pediatric surgeon who is asked to perform the oophorectomy, it is important to remember that treatment of the potentially life-threatening medical condition is the primary goal for both the parents and the medical team. Children who are candidates for OTC often require other procedures as part of their diagnosis or treatment, including central venous access, tumor biopsy, lumbar puncture, and/or bone marrow biopsy. Whenever possible, the oophorectomy for OTC should be coordinated under the same anesthesia with these necessary procedures. Our policy is to treat the OTC operation as an urgent case, often completed within a week of consultation, as not to delay medical therapy.

It is important to check preoperative laboratory studies, such as a complete blood count, prior to proceeding with OTC. This is crucial in children with hematologic pathology or those who have received previous chemotherapy who may have significant anemia or thrombocytopenia that requires correction preoperatively.

Laparoscopy is preferred to minimize the expected recovery time for the patient but may not be possible in some patients with intra-abdominal or intrapelvic tumors. These children may require an open incision via Pfannenstiel or midline laparotomy for OTC. Another option is to perform the oophorectomy during the initial tumor resection or debulking (Fig. 10.1). Regardless of the planned approach, the patient is asked to void just prior to entering the operating room in order to avoid the use of a Foley catheter. A decompressed bladder allows for optimal intraoperative visualization and manipulation of the adnexal structures in order to safely perform the unilateral oophorectomy.

10.3 Operative Technique

The technical details matter when removing an ovary for fertility preservation, even though the procedure itself is relatively straightforward. The ovary should be handled and treated with care as a potential organ for transplant. The laparoscopic approach typically involves a 10-mm umbilical port to accommodate the endoscopic retrieval bag, which facilitates quick removal of the ovary from the patient's body once the final ovarian arterial blood supply has been divided. Two additional 5-mm ports are needed for the dissection, which most often include left lower quadrant and suprapubic locations, for removal of the right ovary. This orientation is the same as that typically used for laparoscopic appendectomy, which is familiar to pediatric surgeons. Alternative port placements can be considered according to the child's age and abdominal size. (◘ Fig. 10.2) The procedure begins with clear visualization of the uterus and both ovaries. This requires careful lifting of the fallopian tubes to view the entire ovary for any cysts or masses (◘ Fig. 10.3). If both ovaries are normal, then dissection of the right ovary typically ensues, due to the laparoscopic orientation as described and its location away from the sigmoid colon. In patients who will receive asymmetric pelvic radiation, it is generally advisable to remove the ovary which will receive the higher

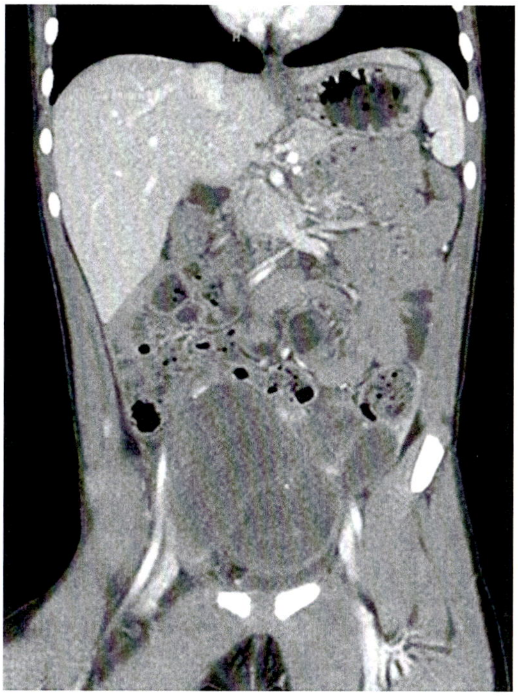

◘ **Fig. 10.1** Large rhabdomyosarcoma arising from the bladder in a 5-year-old girl who underwent an open oophorectomy for ovarian tissue cryopreservation at the time of her open tumor debulking procedure

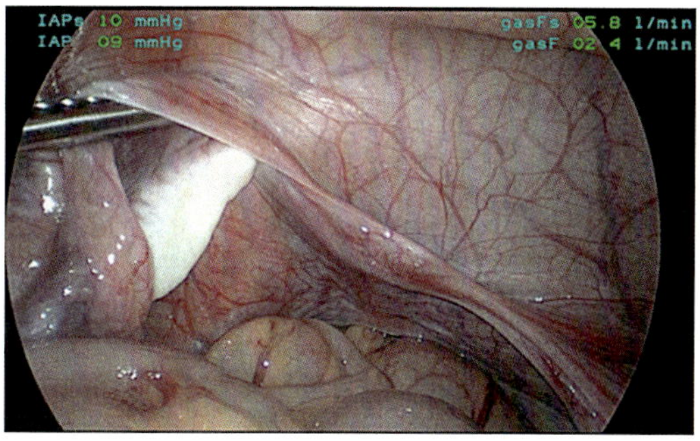

◘ **Fig. 10.3** Inspection of the uterus, fallopian tubes, and ovaries in a prepubertal girl

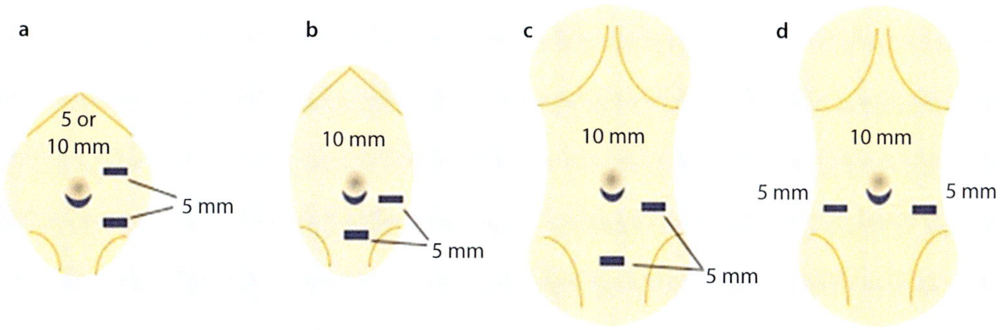

◘ **Fig. 10.2** Laparoscopic trocars for unilateral oophorectomy in **a** infant, **b** preadolescent, and **c**, **d** adolescent girls. The monitor is located at the foot of the bed for the majority of operations

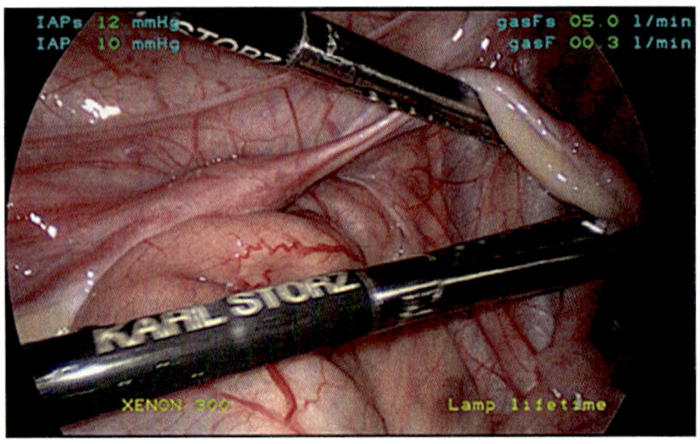

Fig. 10.4 Right ovary of a prepubertal girl with a long ovarian ligament and narrow mesovarium

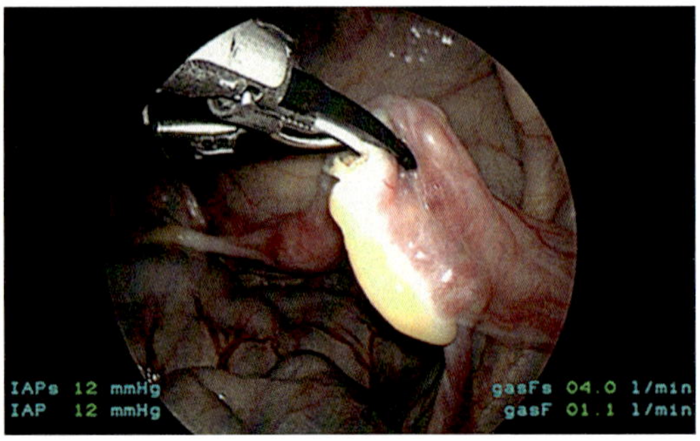

Fig. 10.5 Medial to lateral dissection of the mesovarium along the right ovary of a prepubertal girl. A small rim of tissue is used to facilitate a "no touch" dissection with minimal manipulation of the ovarian capsule

radiation dose. If the left ovary is appropriate for removal, then the suprapubic port is eliminated in favor of a right mid-abdominal 5-mm trocar. At times, both 5-mm ports are positioned in the left or right abdomen (opposite from the ovary), particularly in very young patients (Fig. 10.2).

In infants and pre-adolescent girls, the ligament of the ovary is long, the mesovarium is often narrow, and the fallopian tube is located very close to the ovary, all of which increase the possibility of burn damage if the mesovarium is divided (Fig. 10.4). The mesovarium of the broad ligament between the ovary and the fallopian tube is grasped, and the mesovarium is divided using the harmonic scalpel, at the isthmus, the location where it joins the uterus. Salpingo-oophorectomy may be required in very young girls where the mesovarium is too narrow to allow for safe tissue division using the harmonic scalpel without damaging the ovarian capsule. In peripubertal girls and teenagers, the mesovarium may be wide enough to provide a safe plane of dissection between the ovary and fallopian tube, without the need for concomitant salpingectomy. The goal is complete dissection with a no-touch technique of the ovarian capsule. The no-touch technique is achieved by creating a rim of tissue to act as a handle while dividing the mesovarium from medial to lateral (Fig. 10.5). The ovarian artery within the suspensory ligament of the ovary is divided as the final step to preserve the main arterial blood supply to the ovary during the dissection. Prior to dividing the vascular pedicle, the operating room team is alerted that the blood supply will be divided so the team is ready for specimen removal. The ovary is then quickly placed in an endoscopic retrieval bag and removed through the umbilical incision. If needed, the fascial incision is extended to minimize any crush injury to the ovary as it is being extracted. Once removed, a 4-mm biopsy punch of the ovary is obtained and submitted to the anatomic pathology lab as a routine specimen. The ovary is then placed into the cryopreservation media as quickly as possible after division of the ovarian artery.

Particularly for the youngest pediatric patients with very small ovary size, the attention to detail during the oophorectomy ensures that the maximum amount of ovarian tissue is available for preservation. Even small areas where the heat source is too close to the ovarian capsule may have catastrophic burn effects on the tissue, damaging many of the primordial follicles that lie just below the ovarian capsule. Maintaining the ovarian arterial blood supply until the very end of the dissection is crucial in all patients but particularly in younger patients with smaller vessels. In the adult literature, the Endo GIA stapler has been used to divide the ovarian blood supply and surrounding tissue, thus eliminating the need for any heat source during the dissection [5]. However, in pediatric patients, this can be problematic for several reasons: (1) need for a 12-mm trocar to accommodate the stapler and (2) small size of the pelvis in young girls which makes manipulation of the stapler difficult. Another report of laparoscopic ovarian tissue collection in the pediatric age group describes partial oophorectomy of both ovaries, using a heat source to coagulate the cut surface of the ovary [6]. We do not recommend this approach because of simultaneous damage to both ovaries and risk of hemorrhage from the raw surfaces of the ovary. Particularly in very young preadolescent patients, the ovaries are small and partial oophorectomy would risk damaging both the excised ovarian tissue and the remaining ovary left in situ.

10.4 Summary

Laparoscopic oophorectomy for OTC is a safe, proactive option for pediatric girls facing medical treatment with a high risk of fertility loss. Based on our institution's experience, we recommend that a laparoscopic unilateral oophorectomy for OTC be carried out with minimal manipulation to the ovarian capsule, preservation of the ipsilateral fallopian tube, if possible, and division of the ovarian artery as the last step of the procedure in attempt to maintain the integrity of the ovary for cryopreservation and the presence of adnexal structures for potential future transplantation.

Review Questions and Answers

Q1. Is there a defined surgical technique for the procurement of ovarian cortical tissue for OTC in children?

A1. No, there has not been one standard operation for ovarian cortical tissue harvest. Techniques described include ovarian cortical biopsy, unilateral or bilateral hemi-oophorectomy, unilateral oophorectomy, and oophorectomy with excision of the vascular pedicle.

Q2. What are important perioperative considerations before proceeding with OTC in pediatric patients?

A2. It is important to check preoperative laboratory studies, such as a complete blood count, prior to proceeding with OTC. This is crucial in children with hematologic pathology or those who have received previous chemotherapy who may have significant anemia or thrombocytopenia that requires correction preoperatively.

Q3. What are the anatomic differences between the adnexa of a prepubertal girl and a postpubertal girl?

A3. In infants and preadolescent girls, the ligament of the ovary is long, the mesovarium is often narrow, and the fallopian tube is located very close to the ovary. The average volume of a prepubertal ovary is 1 cm^3 as compared to the 5–10 cm^3 volume of a postpubertal ovary.

Q4. What are the key aspects to performing a laparoscopic unilateral oophorectomy for OTC in children?

A4. Laparoscopic unilateral oophorectomy for OTC should be carried out with minimal manipulation to the ovarian capsule, preservation of the ipsilateral fallopian tube, if possible, and division of the ovarian artery as the last step of the procedure in attempt to maintain the integrity of the ovary for cryopreservation and the presence of adnexal structures for potential future transplantation.

References

1. The Practice Committee of the American Society for Reproductive Medicine. Ovarian tissue cryopreservation: a committee opinion. Fertil Steril. 2014;101:1237–43. https://doi.org/10.1016/j.fertnstert.2014.02.052.
2. Demeestere I, Simon P, Dedeken L, Moffa F, Tsépélidis S, Brachet C, et al. Live birth after autograft of ovarian tissue cryopreserved during childhood. Hum Reprod. 2015;30:2107–9. https://doi.org/10.1093/humrep/dev128.
3. Donnelly L. Woman gives birth to baby using ovary frozen in her childhood in "world first." The Telegraph. 2016.
4. Corkum KS, Laronda MM, Rowell EE. A review of reported surgical techniques in fertility preservation for prepubertal and adolescent females facing a fertility threatening diagnosis or treatment. Am J Surg. 2017;214:695–700. https://doi.org/10.1016/j.amjsurg.2017.06.013.
5. Roux I, Grynberg M, Linehan J, Messner A, Deffieux X. Ovarian cryopreservation after laparoscopic ovariectomy using the Endo-GIA stapling device and LAPRO-clip absorbable ligating clip in a woman: a case report. J Med Case Rep. 2011;5:1–3. https://doi.org/10.1186/1752-1947-5-48.
6. Lima M, Gargano T, Fabbri R, Maffi M, Destro F. Ovarian tissue collection for cryopreservation in pediatric age: laparoscopic technical tips. J Pediatr Adolesc Gynecol. 2014;27:95–7. https://doi.org/10.1016/j.jpag.2013.11.002.

Fertility Preservation in Adult Male Cancer Patients

Joshua A. Halpern and Robert E. Brannigan

T. K. Woodruff et al. (eds.), *Textbook of Oncofertility Research and Practice*,
https://doi.org/10.1007/978-3-030-02868-8_11

Key Points
- Cancer may have negative effects upon male reproduction through multiple pathophysiologic mechanisms.
- Radiation and chemotherapy exhibit dose-dependent gonadotoxicity.
- Fertility preservation should be discussed with all male patients with a new cancer diagnosis.
- Sperm cryopreservation is the mainstay of fertility preservation, and adjunct procedures including penile vibratory stimulation, electroejaculation, and onco-TESE should be employed when appropriate.

Cancer is one of the most common disease states, with approximately 50% of men facing this diagnosis during the course of their lifetime. While the overriding focus for both health care professionals and patients has long been disease cure and survival, a number of factors have led to a significant change in this therapeutic perspective. With marked advances in early disease detection and therapy, patient survival for many cancers has increased dramatically over the last several decades. This, in turn, has provided many patients with the opportunity to live full lives beyond their diagnosis, allowing them to look past their cancer and consider life after treatment. Issues such as post-treatment marriage and parenthood are considered as important as the underlying disease by many patients. As such, measures to preserve sexual and reproductive health in the course of cancer treatment are increasingly important to many patients as they face a malignancy diagnosis.

In addition to improvements in cancer detection and treatment, there has been a growing demographic trend for both men and women to pursue efforts at initiating pregnancy later in life [1, 2]. The reasons for this are many, including initial fulfillment of educational and career goals, marriage at a later age in life, and second families started after divorce or death of a spouse. This shift has also led to a change in the traditional reproductive paradigm. Now, malignancies such as prostate, lung, and colorectal cancer are being seen in patients who may indeed wish to preserve their reproductive potential. It is specifically for these reasons that clinicians must be both vigilant and open-minded when considering the needs of patients who are facing a malignancy diagnosis. A proactive discussion with each patient regarding the possible deleterious impact of their disease state and the associated therapy must be undertaken in order to truly provide patients with comprehensive medical care. Failure to proceed in this fashion will surely lead to missed opportunities for fertility preservation in patients, some of whom may permanently lose their reproductive capability.

11.1 The Impact of Cancer on Male Reproductive Health

Cancer as a disease process can have many deleterious effects on male reproduction, even before any therapy has been initiated. These effects include disruption of the hypothalamic-pituitary-gonadal (H-P-G) axis, direct immunological or cytotoxic injury to the germinal epithelium within the testis, systemic processes such as fever and malnutrition, and psychological issues such as anxiety and depression. These pathological changes may individually or collectively lead to fertility impairment, which is sometimes present at the time of diagnosis [3, 4].

11.1.1 Endocrine Effects of Tumors

Successful spermatogenesis hinges on the normal endocrine function of the hypothalamus, pituitary gland, and testis. The delicate balance maintained by these structures is often disturbed at the time of cancer diagnosis. This is particularly true in patients with testicular cancer whose tumors may produce beta-human chorionic gonadotropin (β-hCG) and alpha-fetoprotein (AFP).

In a series of 15 patients with testicular cancer, Carroll et al. reported that two-thirds had abnormalities in key reproductive hormones. These changes included a decrease in serum follicle-stimulating hormone (FSH) levels and/or elevations in luteinizing hormone (LH) and β-hCG levels [5]. In this series, FSH was decreased in nine out of ten patients with impaired semen parameters, and four of these nine patients had elevated β-hCG levels, leading the authors to postulate a possible inhibitory effect of β-hCG on FSH in some patients. Other studies have detected markedly increased FSH levels, decreased testosterone levels, and impaired spermatogenesis in the presence of testicular tumors that produce β-hCG [6, 7]. Even in the absence of β-hCG, the presence of a testicular tumor alone may alter the H-P-G axis. In a large series of 561 patients with testicular germ cell tumors and 561 healthy controls, men with testis cancer and negative β-hCG had significantly lower serum testosterone and testosterone/LH ratio compared to healthy controls [8].

Excessive levels of AFP have also been associated with the disruption of spermatogenesis. Yazama et al. injected normal mice with AFP and found that spermatogenesis was significantly impaired relative to controls injected with bovine serum albumin [9]. Hansen et al. assessed 97 men with seminomatous and nonseminomatous germ cell tumors (NSGCT) and reported an AFP elevation in 38% of these patients [6]. In the subset of men with NSGCT, increased AFP was found on multiple regression analysis to be strongly associated with impaired semen quality.

Estrogen has also been linked to impaired spermatogenesis in men with testicular cancer. Cochran et al. noted that patients with β-hCG–producing tumors exhibited increased estradiol secretion and significantly decreased FSH production, suggesting a possible endocrinopathic pathway leading to diminished sperm production [10]. Likewise, de Bruin et al. found higher levels of estradiol and prolactin in men with elevated levels of β-hCG, which was also associated with decreased total motile sperm count [7]. Aiginger et al. suggested more broadly that increased conversion of steroid precursors to estradiol is a feature of both β-hCG-positive and β-hCG-negative testicular tumors, leading to the inhibition of the H-P-G axis and deleterious effects on spermatogenesis [11].

Much remains to be learned about the complexities of cancer-induced disruption of the H-P-G axis. Over the last decade, the numerous cytokines that are produced by immunological cells and tumor cells alike have garnered increasing interest. In addition to direct injurious effects on germinal epithelium and Leydig cells in the testis, ample evidence suggests that cytokines may also disrupt the central nervous system (CNS) endocrine processes. Cytokine receptors are present in the CNS, and studies by several investigators suggest that some cytokines may cross the blood-brain barrier to activate central kinase systems and disturb normal endocrine pathways [12, 13].

Anorexia-cachexia syndrome, which is present in 80% of patients with advanced cancer, is an example of such a cancer-related process in which cytokines have been implicated in causing disturbances in food intake and nutrition, ultimately leading to wasting, malnourishment, and death. The cytokines implicated in this process include interleukin 1, interleukin 6, tumor necrosis factor alpha, interferon gamma, leukemia inhibitory factor, ciliary neurotrophic factor, and transformation growth factor beta (TGF- β) [14–17]. Anorexia-cachexia syndrome is relevant to reproductive health in cancer patients in two regards. First, with severe depletion of nutritional reserves, processes such as reproductive function may be detrimentally affected [12]. Second, cytokine-driven CNS endocrinopathic processes such as anorexia-cachexia syndrome should prompt consideration of the existence of similar central cytokine effects on the reproductive function of the hypothalamus and pituitary gland. Further insight into the detrimental endocrine effects of cancer is needed.

11.1.2 Cytotoxic Autoimmune Response

A complicated cascade of changes in the immune system occurs in the presence of cancer. While these changes may aid in battling the neoplastic process at hand, secondary detrimental changes may result in reproductive dysfunction. Lymphocytic infiltration is associated with many testicular tumors, particularly seminomas [18]. While there is a paucity of studies examining the impact of testicular inflammation on spermatogenesis in the setting of cancer, several investigators have evaluated the effects of inflammation on spermatogenesis in normal testes.

Using models of experimentally induced orchitis, several different researchers have found that inflammatory cytokines may significantly disturb spermatogenesis. The recruitment of lymphocytic infiltrate, predominantly comprised of macrophages, is seen in a Sprague-Dawley rat model with experimentally induced orchitis [19]. Macrophage infiltrate likely mediates local inflammation via release of pro-inflammatory cytokines. Rival et al. demonstrated a link between interleukin 6 expression, germ cell sloughing, and germ cell apoptosis in the aforementioned rat model [20].

Theas et al. reported increased cytochrome *c*, caspase 8, and caspase 9 levels with associated germ cell apoptosis also using an experimentally induced orchitis rat model [21]. The same authors subsequently noted a prominent role for tumor necrosis factor-alpha in mediating macrophage-induced apoptosis of germ cells within the rat testis [22].

Reactive oxygen species (ROS) levels may also rise in the setting of testicular lymphocytic infiltrate. Spermatozoa exposure to ROS leads to sperm membrane lipid peroxidation which, in turn, may lead to fertility impairment [23]. Martinez et al. specifically evaluated the impact of several pro-inflammatory cytokines on semen samples from normospermic donors, in particular assessing ROS effects. They found interleukin 8 and tumor necrosis factor-alpha, either alone or in the presence of leukocytes, can lead to sperm plasma membrane lipid peroxidation at levels that could significantly affect sperm function and fertility potential [24].

Cytokine excess may also have direct injurious effects on the testis by disrupting the blood-testis barrier. In a rat model of experimentally induced varicocele, Oh et al. found downregulation of claudin-11, a critical element of the blood-testis barrier, was associated with upregulation of inflammatory cytokines such as tumor necrosis factor-alpha, interleukin 1, and interleukin 6 [25]. Wong et al. demonstrated that TGF-β is a key mediator in restructuring of the blood-testis barrier [26]. These findings support the hypothesis of cytokine-induced testicular injury via alterations of the blood-testis barrier.

Some authors have identified the presence of antisperm antibodies in men with testicular cancer, suggesting that autoimmune pathology and dysregulation of the blood-testis barrier may play a role in impaired spermatogenesis in these patients. Guazzieri et al. noted high levels of antisperm antibodies in men with testicular cancer, suggesting violation of the normal blood-testis barrier protecting the germinal epithelium from the immune system [27]. They found a significantly higher percentage of positivity (50%) for serum antisperm antibodies in patients with advanced disease compared with patients with low-stage disease (30%). In contrast, Paoli et al. examined 190 men with testicular cancer and found antisperm antibody positivity in just 11 (5.8%) patients 1 month following orchiectomy [28]. Further analysis revealed that among the 11 men with antibody positivity, four had no antibody bound to the sperm surface and three had IgG positivity only. Further research is needed to elucidate the relationship between malignancy, inflammation, and the blood-testis barrier.

11.1.3 Systemic Physiological Changes

Cancer is associated with a host of significant changes in normal physiology and homeostasis. As seen in many patients with chronic disease states, patients with cancer may suffer from a variety of comorbidities, including malnutrition and opportunistic infections, which may independently impair reproductive health [29, 30].

Endocrine changes are commonly associated with a number of cancer types [31–34]. The pathophysiology is not entirely understood but may arise due to inhibitory effects centrally on the hypothalamus and pituitary gland (as discussed earlier) and peripherally via impairment of the testicular Leydig cells. Low testosterone in the setting of cancer may not only impact spermatogenesis but may also decrease the desire to engage in sexual activity [35]. Anxiety, depression, and decreased overall sense of well-being may also result, either before or after treatment [36, 37].

Strasser et al. assessed men with advanced cancer who had not undergone any major intervention or treatment for 2 weeks [38]. They found that 29 out of 45 men (64%) had low free testosterone levels. LH was elevated in these men, suggesting that the low free testosterone levels were caused, at least in part, by primary testicular dysfunction. The authors acknowledged that central mechanisms may also play a role in their patients' overall hypogonadism.

Fever, a systemic effect of cancer in a variety of malignancies, has been implicated in impaired spermatogenesis. Carlsen et al. demonstrated that even among healthy men, a single febrile episode may impair sperm concentration, morphology, and motility [39]. Neoplastic fever, or tumor fever, has been associated with malignancies such as Hodgkin's lymphoma, non-Hodgkin's lymphoma, soft tissue sarcoma, leukemia, and renal cell carcinoma, among others [40]. Marmor et al. evaluated a series of 57 patients with Hodgkin's disease and found semen abnormalities in 19 (33.3%) [41].

Higher fever temperatures were associated with more severe deficits in sperm production, with severely diminished sperm concentration and even azoospermia seen in some patients. Lower temperatures were associated only with deficits in motility. Of the 19 patients with fever, only five had normal semen analyses. In a study by Viviani et al., semen analysis was performed in 92 male patients with Hodgkin's disease prior to treatment [31]. Sixty-seven percent of these men demonstrated impaired spermatogenesis independent of disease stage. Beyond fevers of neoplastic origin, fevers secondary to pharmacologic intervention or due to opportunistic infection may also impair spermatogenesis in a significant proportion of patients with malignancy.

11.1.4 Psychological Changes Associated with Cancer

Patients confronting a diagnosis of cancer often find themselves facing a number of difficult psychological issues. Anxiety and depression are common among male cancer patients, and both have the potential to negatively impact reproductive health [36, 40]. Bhongade et al. found that among male partners of infertile couples, men with psychological stress had lower serum testosterone and higher FSH levels, resulting in abnormal semen parameters [42].

Using questionnaires that addressed sexual health, fertility, and psychological issues, Arai et al. evaluated 85 men with testicular cancer who were disease-free 1 year or more after treatment [43]. Interestingly, the rates and nature of sexual dysfunction seen in the surveillance patients were similar to those seen in the other treatment groups (surgery, chemotherapy, and radiation therapy). Ejaculatory function was the only exception to this finding, with the surveillance group having better ejaculatory function than the other treatment groups. The highest rates of infertility distress were observed in chemotherapy patients. Aside from ejaculatory function, patients treated with surveillance did not have fewer sexual problems than patients in the other treatment groups. The authors concluded that sexual dysfunction and infertility distress are cancer side effects possibly attributed to psychological problems, which can persist even years after malignancy diagnosis. Likewise, van Basten et al. examined sexual dysfunction in men with testicular cancer who were treated with either orchiectomy alone or orchiectomy with chemotherapy. While the authors found substantial sexual morbidity in both groups, most patients were eugonadal and there were no differences in penile hemodynamics, suggesting a psychogenic etiology to sexual dysfunction in these men [44].

11.2 The Impact of Cancer Treatment on Male Reproductive Health

A number of treatment modalities are utilized in the management of cancer. Surgical therapy, cytotoxic drug therapy, radiation therapy, and stem cell transplantation are commonly used in the treatment of this broad disease state. Each treatment has its own associated risks and benefits, and these effects should be carefully considered and discussed with the patient prior to initiating therapy. Specific potential effects of treatment include disruption of the H-P-G axis, direct cytotoxic effects on the germinal epithelium within the testis, impairment of penile erectile function, damage to the sympathetic nervous system driving seminal emission and ejaculation, and injury to the genital ductal system required for normal sperm transport. As highlighted earlier in this chapter, many cancer patients have significantly impaired reproductive potential at the time of diagnosis. With this in mind, when fertility preservation is desired, therapeutic modalities that maximize clinical effectiveness while sparing reproductive potential should be selected.

11.2.1 Effects of Radiation Therapy

Radiation therapy causes germ cell loss in a dose-dependent fashion [46]. Damage may result from direct radiation treatment of the testis or radiation scatter from the treatment of other subdiaphragmatic organs. The testis is one of the most radiosensitive organs in the body, and the most immature cell types are the most sensitive to injury [46]. Very small doses (as low as 0.1 Gy) can affect spermatogonia, leading to histological changes in their number and shape. Exposure to

2–3 Gy of radiation leads to significant spermatocyte damage, with a resultant drop in numbers of spermatids. Doses in the 4–6 Gy range lead to significant decreases in the numbers of spermatozoa, suggesting that doses in this range lead to spermatid injury.

The timeline for radiation injury to be reflected in semen analyses is approximately 60–70 days after exposure. Radiation doses less than 0.8 Gy typically lead to oligospermia, doses 0.8–2 Gy often result in transient azoospermia, and exposure to doses greater than 2 Gy may lead to irreversible azoospermia [46].

Factors such as the fractionation schedule and the specific field of treatment determine the ultimate impact of radiation therapy on reproductive health. The larger the dose of radiation, the more precipitous the decline in sperm concentration and the longer the period of time required for recovery of spermatogenesis [46]. Hansen et al. evaluated pre-and post-radiation treatment semen parameters in 24 patients with seminomas and 24 patients with NSGCT. On Cox regression analysis, recovery of spermatogenesis depended on radiation dose, and use of adjuvant chemotherapy prolonged the patients' recovery period. Additionally, the return of spermatogenesis was impaired in men with low pretreatment total motile sperm counts and those over 25 years of age [47].

Sperm concentrations usually reach nadir by 4–6 months after the conclusion of radiation therapy. Return to pretreatment levels is typically seen within 10–24 months, with patients who receive higher doses experiencing longer recovery periods. Changes in sperm concentration over time are reflected by accompanying variations in FSH level [48].

Return of spermatogenesis following radiation therapy hinges on the survival and proliferation of surviving type-A spermatogonia. Table 11.1 details the timeline for functional recovery of the human testis after single-dose radiation treatment, based on a study by Rowley et al. [49]. Fractionated therapy tends to be associated with longer recovery times than single-dose therapy. Some patients who do ultimately regain spermatogenesis after radiation treatment may exhibit permanently diminished sperm concentration and motility. For these individuals, assisted reproductive techniques are often useful in facilitating achievement of pregnancy.

Table 11.1 Recovery of spermatogenesis after graded doses of ionizing radiation to the human testes

Radiation dosage	Time to complete recovery[a]
<1 Gy	9–18 months
2–3 Gy	30 months
≥4 Gy	≥5 years

Source: Data from Rowley et al. [49]
[a]Return to preirradiative sperm concentration

Leydig cells are much less likely to sustain functional impairment from radiotherapy than are germinal epithelial cells. However, Rowley et al. demonstrated that even doses of radiation of 0.75 Gy can lead to increases in LH levels, suggesting some degree of Leydig cell injury [49]. These authors detected no change in testosterone level at this dose, and LH levels gradually returned to normal within 30 months after radiation exposure.

Giwercman et al. evaluated men who had undergone orchiectomy and then proceeded to testicular radiation therapy for carcinoma in situ of the solitary remaining testis. These authors found that impairment in Leydig cell secretory function is generally not observed until radiation exceeds doses of 20 Gy. At this dose, not only do LH levels become elevated, but also testosterone levels decline when compared with similar patients who have not undergone radiation therapy to the remaining, solitary testis [50].

External beam radiation therapy for pelvic cancers (such as colorectal, bladder, and prostate cancer) results in testicular exposure to scatter doses of 0.4–18.7% of the administered dose [51, 52]. In particular, patients with rectal cancer treated with external beam radiation therapy have the highest doses of radiation reaching the testis. Herman et al. have shown that patients treated with 50 Gy for rectal cancer sustained an 85% increase in serum FSH levels and a 22% decline in serum testosterone levels [52].

Important questions regarding the impact of sperm DNA damage resulting from radiation therapy have yet to be answered. Stahl et al. have shown an increase in DNA fragmentation index in men with testicular carcinoma undergoing adjuvant radiation therapy compared with similar patients not treated with radiation. These transient changes were seen up to 2 years after treatment, but the clinical impact of the increases in sperm DNA fragmentation has yet to be fully clarified [53, 54]. Likewise, Smit et al. found increased sperm DNA fragmentation index in men with testicular carcinoma undergoing adjuvant radiation compared to those undergoing chemotherapy [55]. Rives et al. examined sperm aneuploidy before and after radiation therapy for testicular cancer and found that mean sperm aneuploidy returned to pretreatment baseline within 12 months [56]. Several additional small studies suggest that DNA integrity of sperm returns to levels of age-matched controls over time, but further work is needed to clarify these findings [57, 58]. A number of encouraging studies have shown no increase in congenital anomalies or other disease states in the offspring of patients treated for cancer (with radiation and/or chemotherapy) when compared with these patients' cousins and to published figures for the general population [59, 60].

11.3 Radiation Therapy for Prostate Cancer

Prostate cancer is the most common cancer in men, and approximately one third of men choose radiation therapy for treatment of their disease [61]. Men at high risk for cancer may initiate prostate-specific antigen (PSA) screening at a younger age, and as such, many men facing this diagnosis may still be interested in preserving their reproductive function. A study by Daniell et al. revealed significant differences in hormone levels between men who had received prostate external beam radiation therapy and those who had undergone radical prostatectomy [62]. Three to 8 years after completion of treatment, total testosterone levels were 27.3% less, free testosterone levels were 31.6% less, LH levels were 52.7% greater, and FSH levels were 100% greater in men who had undergone external beam radiation therapy compared with men who had undergone radical prostatectomy. No semen analysis comparison was possible as one of the groups underwent radical prostatectomy, but the significant changes in hormone levels, particularly the doubling of FSH, imply a high likelihood of significant disruption of spermatogenesis in the group treated with radiation therapy.

Brachytherapy is a common modality frequently used to treat prostate cancer. Mydlo et al. assessed semen quality in four young men (age 39–52) treated for prostate cancer with brachytherapy [63]. Assessment of semen parameters 6 months post-treatment revealed no change, and three of the four men were able to initiate pregnancies after treatment. The fourth patient, who had not yet achieved a pregnancy, was noted to have no change in sperm concentration or motility at the 6-month postoperative time point. Scatter radiation dose with brachytherapy is typically less than 20 cGy. A subsequent study by Grocela et al. found that three out of 485 men who continued to be sexually active after prostate brachytherapy achieved pregnancies with their partners. Two pregnancies were carried to term and resulted in the birth of healthy children. The third pregnancy resulted in a first trimester miscarriage. All three men had low ejaculate volume and mildly decreased total sperm count [64]. Delaunay et al. reported that four out of 270 men expressed a desire for fertility following prostate brachytherapy. All four men achieved pregnancies, though one pregnancy resulted in miscarriage [65].

11.4 Radiation Therapy for Testicular Cancer

Pelvic radiation therapy is a mainstay of treatment for some patients with testicular cancer, particularly those with seminoma. Radiation in these cases is typically delivered to the para-aortic lymph nodes and the iliac lymph nodes ipsilateral to the tumor. In this setting, the testicles receive approximately 0.3–0.5 Gy due to scatter, even if testicular shielding is used [66]. Typically, spermatogenesis will be impaired for a period of 6–8 months, followed by recovery over the next 1–2 years [56]. Despite this improvement, spermatogenesis may never return to the pretreatment baseline levels. Prognostic factors favoring more rapid or complete recovery of spermatogenesis include normal semen parameters prior to therapy and younger age at the time of treatment [67].

In comparing paternity of men with testicular cancer who underwent radiation therapy vs. those who underwent observation, Huyghe et al. found significantly lower paternity in the radiation treatment group [68]. The authors concluded that fertility in patients with testicular cancer declined by 30% after radiation treatment. They also reported that radiation therapy, when compared with chemotherapy and observation, had the most deleterious effects on reproductive potential. Huddart et al., in a study of 680 patients, did not reach similar conclusions. They found that a slightly higher percentage of patients undergoing radiation therapy were successful in conceiving when compared with patients receiving chemotherapy [69]. Nalesnik et al. examined a small group of patients who underwent radiation therapy for stage I and 2A seminoma. At a mean follow-up of 7.9 years, all patients recovered some degree of spermatogenesis [70]. However, given the clear link between even small doses of radiation exposure and impaired testicular function, several authors have recommended the use of protective gonadal shielding to decrease radiation scatter to the remaining testicle [47, 48].

11.5 Radiation Therapy for Lymphoma

Radiation therapy is often used for the treatment of Hodgkin's lymphoma, and as with other disease states, impairment of spermatogenesis occurs in a dose-dependent fashion. Kinsella et al. prospectively followed 17 men with early-stage Hodgkin's disease to assess the impact of low-dose scattered irradiation in men receiving conventional fractionated therapy. In these patients, the testicular dose ranged from 6 to 70 cGy, with follow-up ranging from 3 to 7 years after completion of radiation therapy. The authors concluded that if the scattered dose received was between 0.2 and 0.7 Gy, patients may experience a temporary rise in FSH and decline in sperm concentration. Return of normal FSH levels was seen in 12–24 months and resolution of transient oligospermia was observed within 18 months of therapy completion [71].

11.6 Radiation Therapy for Leukemia

Whole-body radiation therapy has been used to achieve myeloablation in many patients prior to stem cell transplantation [72]. Recovery of testicular function (normal FSH, LH, testosterone, and/or sperm concentration) is seen in less than 20% of men undergoing whole-body irradiation and subsequent bone marrow transplant [73]. Socie et al. in a large survey of 229 centers of the European Group for Blood and Marrow Transplantation, noted that paternity via natural means after whole-body irradiation is a rare event, with only 27 such men being identified from all of the centers surveyed. In 41 pregnancies in female partners of these same male patients, no stillbirths and only 1 miscarriage were observed. The risk for either occurrence in the normal population is approximately 10%, significantly higher than observed for these patients [74]. Given the effects of whole-body radiation on testicular function, multiple authors have described gonadal-shielding protocols on an individualized basis, when appropriate [75, 76].

11.7 Effects of Chemotherapy

Chemotherapy is a mainstay of treatment for many forms of cancer, and the aim is to kill rapidly proliferating cells. One of the most significant drawbacks for this form of therapy is the destruction of the normal, healthy tissue. A large number of chemotherapeutic agents are available, and their effects on male reproductive health are variable. Much has been learned about the impact of various cytotoxic agents since Spitz first described testicular damage in men treated with nitrogen mustard in 1948. In that report, 27 of 30 men having undergone this type of treatment were found at the time of autopsy to be azoospermic [77]. As is the case with radiation therapy, the germinal epithelium is much more sensitive to the effects of chemotherapy than are Leydig cells. While azoospermia is seen after treatment with a variety of agents, clinical hypogonadism manifest by low serum testosterone levels is less common.

The ultimate impact of chemotherapy hinges on the specific agents used, the dosage of these medications administered, and the age of the patient. The deleterious effects of chemotherapy may act in concert with injury brought about by other forms of therapy, such as radiation therapy. Below is a brief overview of the major classes of chemotherapeutic agents and their impact on male reproductive health.

11.8 Alkylating Agents (Includes Busulfan, Chlorambucil, Chlormethine, Cyclophosphamide, Ifosfamide, and Procarbazine)

Alkylating drugs are one of the most toxic classes of chemotherapeutic medications available, with a high risk of inducing post-treatment infertility. These medications disrupt DNA function via several mechanisms, including DNA base pair alkylation, formation of abnormal base cross-bridges, and mispairing of nucleotides. The end result is impaired DNA synthesis and RNA transcription leading to cellular death. These agents cause mutations in all stages of developing germinal epithelium [78].

Byrne et al. reported that severe oligospermia or azoospermia typically develop 90–120 days after alkylating agent therapy, with a significant decrease in male fertility whether or not concurrent radiation therapy was administered [79]. A number of investigators have shown that the deficits in sperm production associated with alkylating agents are often severe and irreversible. Buchanan et al. reported that even 4 years after treatment with cyclophosphamide, most patients had not yet regained spermatogenesis. Those patients that did resume sperm production did so at 31 months after treatment [80]. Kenney et al. studied 17 adult men who were treated with cyclophosphamide for childhood sarcomas and found that 58.8% had azoospermia, whereas only 11.8% had normal semen parameters [81]. Likewise, multiagent regimens that include procarbazine usually render patients irreversibly infertile, leading investigators such as Bokemeyer et al. to recommend alternative agents in its place [82].

Recently, Green et al. established the cyclophosphamide equivalent dose (CED) as a useful metric for future fertility prognosis in men who receive chemotherapy with alkylating agents [83]. The authors examined a cohort of 214 adult male survivors of childhood malignancy at a median 21 years following therapy. They found that CED was strongly associated with the degree of spermatogenesis. The majority of men (89%) with CED less than 4000 mg/m^2 had normospermia, and sperm concentration decreased with increasing CED.

11.9 Antimetabolites (Includes 5-Fluorouracil [5-FU], 6-Mercaptopurine, Gemcitabine, and Methotrexate)

The antimetabolites interfere with DNA synthesis and transcription, typically resulting in reversible, transient declines in sperm concentration. Choudhury and colleagues reported that in a rat model, 5-FU induced chromosomal aberrations in spermatogonial cells. A gradual decrease in the transmission of these cytotoxic changes from spermatogonia to sperm was noted over time, with the authors postulating that the damaged spermatogonia are gradually eliminated during the cycle of spermatogenesis [84]. D'Souza et al. reported seminiferous tubule atrophy and marked changes in sperm morphology using a rat model treated with 5-FU [85, 86]. Likewise, Sukotnik et al. used a rat model to demonstrate that methotrexate induced germ cell apoptosis and impaired spermatogenesis [87].

11.10 Platinum Analogs (Includes Cisplatin and Carboplatin)

The platinum analogs cause DNA crosslink formation, and animal studies have shown that spermatogonia and spermatocytes are the most markedly affected cell types [88]. Lampe and colleagues reported on 170 patients with testicular germ cell cancer. Approximately 25% of the men were azoospermic and approximately 25% were oligospermic prior to initiation of therapy [89]. After treatment with platinum-based chemotherapy, recovery of spermatogenesis continued over time, with approximately 50% of men with spermatogenesis 2 years and 80% of men with spermatogenesis 5 years after completion of therapy. For the subgroup of men with normal sperm concentrations prior to therapy, 64% had normal sperm concentrations at a median of 30 months after completion of platinum-based chemotherapy. These authors found a higher likelihood of recovery of spermatogenesis with carboplatin than with cisplatin therapy. Similarly, Pectasides et al. reported 90% of men had recovery of spermatogenesis after carboplatin therapy for testicular germ cell tumors [90]. In a multicenter, national trial in Norway, 80% of all men who attempted paternity following cisplatin-based chemotherapy succeeded with a 15-year actuarial paternity rate of 85% [91].

11.11 Vinca Alkaloids (Includes Vinblastine, Vincristine, Vindesine, and Vinorelbine)

The vinca alkaloids, which are derived from the periwinkle plant, exert their antineoplastic effects via inhibition of microtubule formation, which in turn inhibits mitosis. These agents have been implicated in arresting spermatogenesis and in decreasing spermatozoa motility [92]. However, other investigators, such as Sjoblom et al. and Aubier et al. have demonstrated that spermatogenesis is relatively resistant to the effects of vinblastine, in contrast to Arnon's findings [93, 94]. Meistrich et al. examined 58 men who underwent vincristine and vinblastine therapy for Hodgkin's lymphoma. While sperm concentration declined significantly within 1 month of therapy, 63% of men were normospermic after 4.5 months, and all men recovered normal spermatogenesis within 1 year [95].

11.12 Topoisomerase Inhibitor Agents (Includes Doxorubicin, Etoposide, and Bleomycin)

Topoisomerase-inhibiting agents induce damage in a variety of ways, such as DNA binding, RNA breaks, and RNA synthesis inhibition. Bleomycin, one such agent, has been shown to cause chromosomal abnormalities in spermatogonia and spermatocytes in an animal study by van Buul et al. [96] Hou et al. evaluated the effects of doxorubicin in rats of various ages and found that the initiation phase of spermatogenesis is highly susceptible to doxorubicin-induced apoptosis. They discovered that gonocytes and early spermatogonia are most vulnerable to this apoptosis, leading to a decline in the number of germline stem cells [97]. In the clinical setting, the distinct effects of these agents on spermatogenesis are difficult to discern, as they are typically administered within the context of multiagent regimens. Paoli et al. examined men treated with doxorubicin, bleomycin, vinblastine, and dacarbazine (ABVD) for Hodgkin's lymphoma and found significant impairment in sperm concentration, motility, and morphology following treatment. However, these parameters all returned to pretherapy levels within 2 years of treatment [98].

11.13 Effects of Surgery

Surgical therapy for cancer can have a wide array of deleterious effects on male reproductive health. Consideration of these effects is imperative during preoperative discussions with patients.

Men suffering from testicular cancer typically sustain a significant loss of overall testicular mass when undergoing orchiectomy, which can impair reproductive health due to lower overall germ cell mass and Leydig cell mass. This may lead to reduced sperm concentration and serum testosterone levels. Some men with testicular cancer may also undergo subsequent retroperitoneal lymphadenectomy, potentially resulting in anejaculation or retrograde ejaculation as a result of disruption of the lumbar sympathetic plexus and hypogastric plexus. Modified, nerve-sparing templates for dissection have resulted in preserved ejaculatory function in the majority of these men [99, 100]. Men who undergo surgical treatment for colorectal cancer may also experience anejaculation or retrograde ejaculation via the same mechanism [101].

Men with bladder or prostate cancer who require extirpative surgery will suffer disruption of the genital ductal system as the prostate gland and seminal vesicles are routinely removed. Patients undergoing these procedures typically still produce sperm normally – it is the transport and delivery of sperm to the prostatic urethra that are disrupted. As a result, normal ejaculatory function, and thus fertility, is destroyed.

While erectile function may be preserved in over 80% of men undergoing radical prostatectomy and radical cystectomy with nerve-sparing techniques, recovery of erections may take a year or more and may be incomplete [102]. With the advent of PDE-5 inhibitors and other therapies for erectile dysfunction, this problem is often readily treatable.

Traditional assumptions about a patient's reproductive aspirations, based on age or other demographic traits, should be carefully considered. Changes in reproductive health are a fairly common outcome of oncological surgery, and it is incumbent upon physicians to routinely discuss the potential impact of each procedure on reproductive health prior to initiating surgical therapy [103].

11.14 Effects of Opioids

Pain management is a critical component of cancer therapy. The use of opioids is often chronic and may involve high doses. Opioid-induced suppression of the H-P-G axis is well documented, and the resultant decrease in gonadotropins may lead to declines in libido, erectile function, and spermatogenesis [104]. Opioids also appear to have a direct role in regulation of male fertility via autocrine signaling [105]. All of these factors, individually or collectively, may impair fertility. Fortunately, these negative effects are typically reversible with cessation of opioid use [106].

11.15 Fertility Preservation in Male Cancer Patients

With improving diagnostic and therapeutic modalities, overall survival for most cancers has increased significantly over the last 75 years. For pediatric cancer patients, the 5-year survival rate is approximately 83% [107]. As the number of cancer survivors continues to grow, so does the number seeking fertility. Lehmann et al. found that 80% of childhood cancer survivors expressed a desire for future fertility [108]. Furthermore, many men are waiting until later in life to start their first families, and others start second families at an older age due to divorce or death of a spouse [1]. As such, an increasing number of adult male cancer survivors will be pursuing fatherhood post-treatment. The end result of this phenomenon will be an increasing pool of patients striving to achieve parenthood in the wake of fertility impairing cancer treatments.

For patients, a cancer diagnosis is often devastating and overwhelming. The immediate focus is typically on therapy and cure of the underlying disease process. Thus, it is imperative that the treating physicians actively address the issue of fertility preservation as comprehensive care is administered to the patient. While approaches such as use of donor sperm and adoption are available to facilitate paternity in cancer survivors, many patients express a strong desire to father biological children.

There is little room for communication breakdown when treating cancer patients. Diagnostic testing and therapeutic procedures in the acute care setting occupy large amounts of time, leaving very little time to address fertility preservation. However, cryopreservation of sperm in advance of cancer treatment is essential, as even one cancer treatment can reduce semen quality and induce sperm DNA damage.

Over the past decade, oncologists and professional societies have intensified efforts to improve discussions and treatment decisions pertaining to fertility preservation. An early study by Zapzalka et al. of American Society of Clinical Oncology (ASCO) members in Minnesota revealed that 100% of oncologists reported discussing fertility issues with their patients [109]. However, in a subsequent survey, Quinn et al. reported less than half of physicians referred cancer patients of childbearing age for reproductive endocrinology evaluation [110]. Likewise, in a survey of approximately 900 cancer patients, Schover et al. found that only 60% replied that they had been informed about fertility issues and only 50% had been notified about sperm banking [111]. These deficiencies ultimately led to the creation of ASCO guidelines for fertility preservation, which have substantially improved the utilization of fertility preservation over the ensuing decade [112, 113].

11.15.1 Fertility Preservation Guidelines

In 2006, ASCO published initial recommendations on fertility preservation in cancer patients [114]. The authors of this manuscript acknowledged that application of fertility preservation measures is limited by several factors, including knowledge deficits regarding fertility risks associated with cancer treatments, failure to discuss fertility-preserving options prior to treatment, lack of insurance coverage for these procedures, and the investigational status of some of the fertility preservation techniques. The expert panel recommended that oncologists discuss at the earliest opportunity the possible risk of fertility impairment associated with various cancer

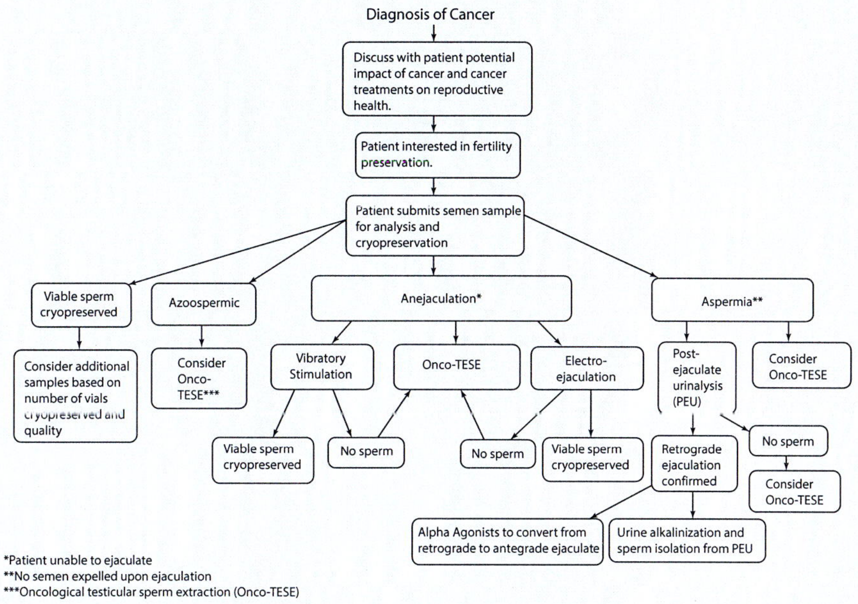

Fig. 11.1 Fertility preservation algorithm for male cancer patients

treatments. For those patients interested in pursuing fertility preservation, the prompt referral of the patient to a qualified specialist in this area was recommended. Finally, the authors advocated for the participation of patients in clinical trials to advance the state of knowledge within the field of fertility preservation. Below, several methods available for fertility preservation in men are detailed. A helpful summary algorithm is also provided (Fig. 11.1).

Since the initial publication of the 2006 ASCO guidelines, there have been subsequent iterations from ASCO, as well as formal recommendations and reports from other professional societies including the American Academy of Pediatrics, the American Society for Reproductive Medicine, and the European Society for Medical Oncology [112, 115–119]. These societies jointly recommend that health care providers should be prepared to initiate a discussion regarding infertility and fertility preservation with all patients carrying a new cancer diagnosis. Sperm cryopreservation is considered a standard of care, and men should be either offered cryopreservation or referred to a physician that can provide the necessary treatment strategies for optimal fertility preservation.

11.15.2 Fertility Preservation Program

Optimal fertility preservation requires a multidisciplinary approach and is best served by establishment of a formal fertility preservation program. The formalized program may include features such as educational seminars targeting both physicians and nurses, institutional awareness campaigns, automated triggers within the electronic medical record, and patient-directed educational tools [120]. Sheth et al. examined the utilization of fertility consultations at a single institution before and after implementation of a formalized fertility preservation program. Despite stable rates of cancer diagnoses over time, the proportion of men who received a fertility preservation consultation increased by 2.4-fold and the proportion of men who underwent sperm cryopreservation increased 2.7-fold [120]. Likewise, Lopategui et al. evaluated rates of sperm banking before and after establishment of a standardized oncofertility program in 2016. They found that sperm banking rates improved from 3.3% to 19.3% of all cancer patients after the intervention [121]. These studies suggest that all institutions providing care to patients with malignancy should consider establishment of a formal fertility preservation program in order to optimize patient care in this realm.

11.15.3 Sperm Cryopreservation

A number of articles from the "pre-in vitro fertilization" (pre-IVF) era highlighted poor outcomes of sperm cryopreservation, with a minority of semen samples provided by cancer patients being adequate to pursue intrauterine insemination [122, 123]. As such, this early literature did not advocate pretreatment sperm cryopreservation due to the low resultant pregnancy rates. Unfortunately, these historical outcomes still guide clinical decision making by some health care providers with regard to fertility preservation. With the advent of IVF and intracytoplasmic sperm injection (ICSI), literally just one sperm per oocyte is necessary to achieve possible fertilization and pregnancy [124]. Thus, even men with extremely diminished overall semen quality should be offered sperm cryopreservation, as the above assisted reproductive techniques can often overcome severe deficits in sperm production and function.

11

11.15.4 Overview of Sperm Collection Techniques

The semen collection process itself is achieved via masturbation. The patient should be provided a sterile specimen collection cup and ample time and privacy to produce the sample. Avoidance of lubricants (such as petroleum jelly and saliva) is critical, as many of these substances are spermatotoxic [125].

If no ejaculate is expelled on climax, then a post-ejaculate urinalysis should be inspected to assess for retrograde ejaculation. If retrograde ejaculation is observed, alpha agonists may be administered in an effort to convert retrograde to antegrade ejaculation. If this is not successful, then alkalinization of the urine and subsequent collection and processing of the post-ejaculate urine sample may facilitate isolation of viable sperm.

If the patient is unable to climax, care should be taken to ensure that he has had ample privacy and time. If this difficulty persists, then consideration should be given to vibratory stimulation, electro-ejaculation, or surgical testicular sperm extraction techniques, all of which have a potential role in such patients.

11.15.5 Penile Vibratory Stimulation and Electroejaculation

In patients with inadequate semen samples or those who are unable to provide a semen sample due to physiological, psychological, religious, ethical, or other barriers, penile vibratory stimulation (PVS) and electroejaculation (EEJ) may be alternative methods of obtaining a sample that is satisfactory for cryopreservation.

Due to its noninvasive nature, PVS may be preferable to EEJ in the setting of failed masturbation for cryopreservation. Schmiegelow et al. reported success of PVS in the outpatient setting, without the use of general anesthesia. In fact, the patient was able to successfully self-administer the treatment [126]. The authors recommended PVS as first-line therapy prior to EEJ for this patient population due to its ease of use and minimal morbidity.

Multiple studies have examined EEJ and cryopreservation in the setting of malignancy. Adank et al. examined 11 adolescent boys who were diagnosed with malignancy but unable to provide an adequate semen sample via masturbation prior to gonadotoxic therapy. They obtained adequate samples in 3 of the 11 boys who underwent EEJ, and they reported an overall success rate of 45% in the literature [127]. Berookhim et al. examined a cohort of adolescents and young adults with malignancy, reporting a success rate of 60% with EEJ [128].

11.15.6 Testicular Tissue Cryopreservation (Onco-TESE)

Azoospermia at the time of attempted sperm cryopreservation was noted in 13.8% of cancer patients by Lass et al. in a 1998 review of their center's data [129]. When the provided sample reveals azoospermia, surgical testicular sperm extraction prior to cancer treatment is an option [130–133]. Dubbed "Onco-TESE" (Oncological Testicular Sperm Extraction) by Schrader et al., this procedure was successful in yielding sperm retrieval in 6 of 14 men with testicular germ cell

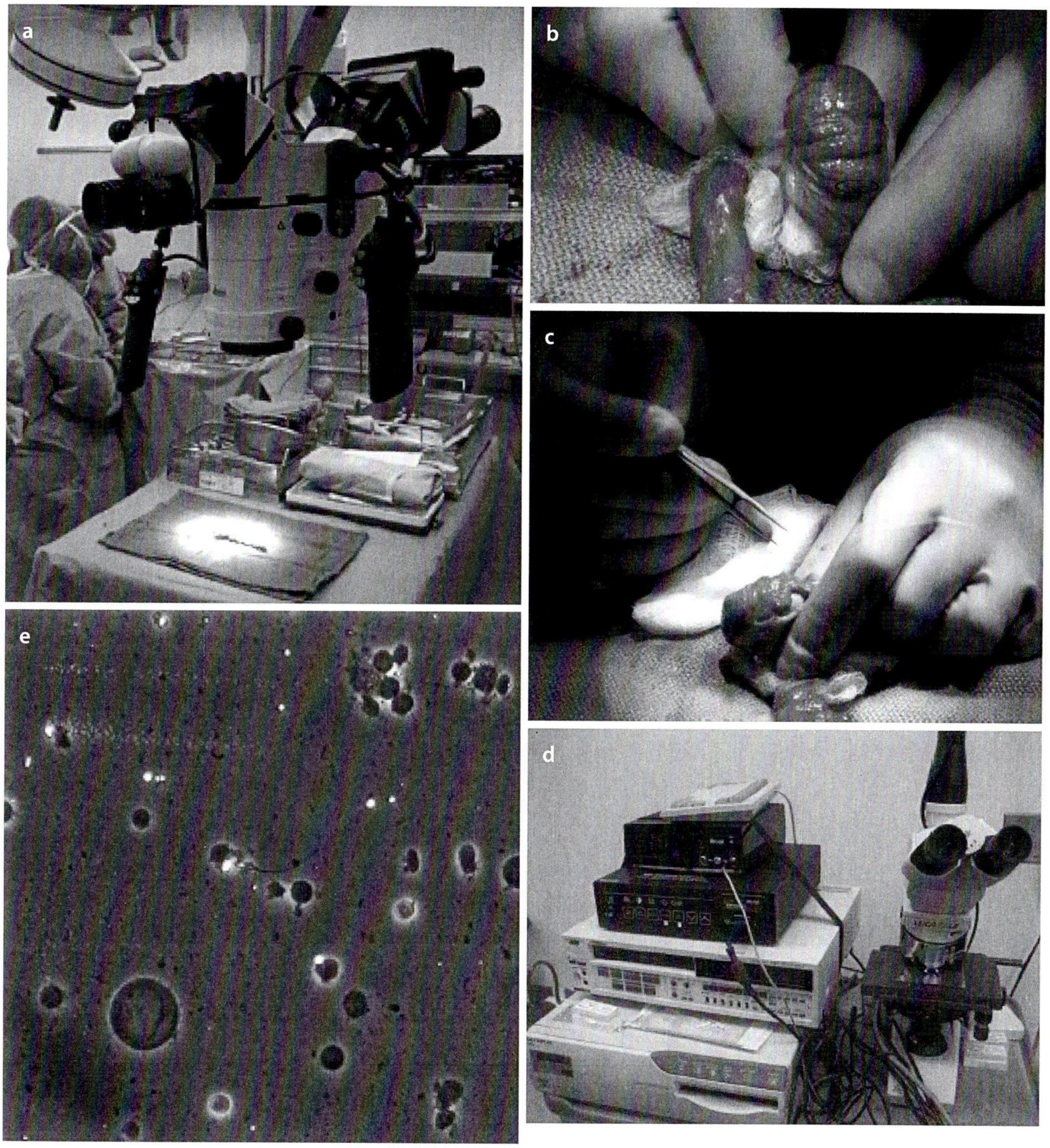

◘ **Fig. 11.2** **a** The operating microscope and sterile field where the Onco-TESE will be performed in the foreground. The radical orchiectomy is being performed in the background. **b** The radical orchiectomy specimen has been bivalved to allow microsurgical inspection and dissection of the seminiferous tubules. Seminoma with marked inflammatory change infiltrated over 90% of this testis. The postero-inferior aspect was found to be free of tumor with low levels of spermatogenesis on the wet prep slide. **c** Microsurgical inspection and dissection of the seminiferous tubules. Selected tubules are excised and teased to make a wet prep slide. **d** Phase-contrast microscope with attached video recorder and microphotograph printer for wet prep slide inspection in the operating room. **e** Wet prep slide of testicular tissue revealing the presence of viable sperm with motility. This tissue was cryopreserved

tumors and in 8 of 17 patients with malignant lymphoma [133]. Given the possible irreversible damage to germinal epithelium with cancer therapy and the good overall success rates with "Onco-TESE", Schrader et al. recommend that this procedure be considered as a means of fertility preservation in azoospermic cancer patients.

◘ Figure 11.2 illustrates the Onco-TESE procedure performed on a man with a solitary testis and azoospermia undergoing radical orchiectomy for seminoma. Critical components of this procedure include coordination of laboratory personnel with the operating room staff, availability of an operating microscope, a sterile workbench away from the operating field, and a phase-contrast microscope to inspect wet prep slides. Carrasquillo et al. have described a step-by-step approach to Onco-TESE [134].

Outcomes following Onco-TESE have been reported by multiple authors with varying success. Furuhashi et al. attempted Onco-TESE in six men with either azoospermia or severe oligospermia and retrieved sperm in four (66%) patients [135]. Two groups reported successful Onco-TESE in men with synchronous, bilateral testicular tumors [136, 137].

11.16 Future Directions in Fertility Preservation in Male Cancer Patients

Many investigational male fertility-preserving techniques are undergoing evaluation. Some have been studied more thoroughly than others, and a number of them offer hope as our understanding of male reproductive physiology grows. Several of these investigational techniques are briefly described below.

Luteinizing hormone-releasing hormone (LHRH) agonists have been used to achieve H-P-G axis suppression during chemotherapy. While early animal studies showed some evidence of gonadal protection during chemotherapy, several human studies have been less promising. This approach did not lead to fertility preservation or hasten the return of spermatogenesis in several studies in men [138–141].

Testicular tissue harvesting for future autotransplantation has also been considered by several investigators. Effects to date have focused on successful germ cell isolation and cryopreservation [142]. The hope is that after cancer treatment, the harvested germinal epithelium may be transplanted back to the patient with resumption of spermatogenesis. Alternatively, pluripotent stem cells derived from somatic tissue might be differentiated into germ cells with the same ultimate goal of autotransplantation [143, 144]. These techniques remain investigational and to date have not been effectively implemented in humans, though clinical trials are ongoing.

Testicular tissue harvesting for transplantation into immunodeficient mice is another investigational technique. Nagano and colleagues have demonstrated that this procedure is technically feasible in these mice with successful ensuing spermatogenesis, pregnancies, and live births. To date, this approach has only been successfully performed in animal models, but it may hold promise for human application, particularly in prepubescent boys [145, 146].

11.17 Conclusion

Fertility preservation in male cancer patients is an important aspect of comprehensive health care. As cancer diagnostic techniques and treatments improve, a growing number of cancer survivors will continue to look past their malignancy toward issues such as parenthood. In this chapter, we have detailed the numerous ways in which cancer itself and its associated treatments can negatively impact many aspects of normal male reproductive health. This underscores the importance of tailoring a careful discussion with each patient over the potential deleterious impact of their specific disease state and therapy prior to initiating treatment.

At the time of cancer diagnosis, patients and clinicians alike are often overwhelmed by the high volume of urgent tests and procedures that must be accomplished in a timely fashion. This situation sets the stage for a profound breakdown in communication between health care providers and patients with regard to fertility preservation. In retrospect, not only do many patients fail to recall discussions of fertility preservation, but they often harbor great disappointment and regret at the perceived oversight in this aspect of their care. Fortunately, with a proactive approach, fertility preservation in men is quite feasible and will help avoid the irreversible and permanent loss of reproductive capacity that accompanies many cancer treatments today.

Review Questions and Answers

Q1. What is the effect of radiation therapy upon spermatogenesis?

A1. Radiation therapy causes dose-dependent germ cell loss, which manifests as changes in semen analysis approximately 60–70 days following exposure. Sperm concentrations typically reach nadir at 4–6 months after therapy. Recovery of spermatogenesis is dose-dependent and typically occurs within 30 months in men receiving 2–3 Gy.

Q2. What is the best prognostic indicator for recovery of spermatogenesis after alkylating chemotherapeutic agents?

A2. The cyclophosphamide equivalent dose (CED) is strongly associated with recovery of spermatogenesis after therapy. Men with CED less than 4000 mg/m^2 are likely to have return of normal spermatogenesis.

Q3. Which male patients should be offered fertility preservation?

A3. According to multiple guidelines and recommendations, providers should discuss fertility preservation with all male patients who have a new diagnosis of malignancy. Establishment of a formal fertility preservation program can ensure optimal utilization of fertility preservation consultations and cryopreservation prior to initiation of therapy.

Q4. What is Onco-TESE?

A4. Oncological testicular sperm extraction (Onco-TESE) is the microsurgical extraction of sperm from the testis prior to initiation of therapy for malignancy. Onco-TESE should be considered in men who are unable to provide a semen sample or in whom azoospermia is present.

References

1. Khandwala YS, Zhang CA, Lu Y, Eisenberg ML. The age of fathers in the USA is rising: an analysis of 168 867 480 births from 1972 to 2015. Hum Reprod. 2017;32(10):2110–6.
2. Mathews TJ, Hamilton BE. Mean age of mothers is on the rise: United States, 2000–2014. NCHS Data Brief. 2016;232:1–8.
3. Hallak J, Kolettis PN, Sekhon VS, Thomas AJ, Agarwal A. Sperm cryopreservation in patients with testicular cancer. Urology. 1999;54(5):894–9.
4. Meirow D, Schenker JG. Cancer and male infertility. Hum Reprod. 1995;10(8):2017–22.
5. Carroll PR, Whitmore WF, Herr HW, Morse MJ, Sogani PC, Bajorunas D, et al. Endocrine and exocrine profiles of men with testicular tumors before orchiectomy. J Urol. 1987;137(3):420–3.
6. Hansen PV, Trykker H, Andersen J, Helkjaer PE. Germ cell function and hormonal status in patients with testicular cancer. Cancer. 1989;64(4):956–61.
7. de Bruin D, de Jong IJ, Arts EGJM, Nuver J, Dullaart RPF, Sluiter WJ, et al. Semen quality in men with disseminated testicular cancer: relation with human chorionic gonadotropin beta-subunit and pituitary gonadal hormones. Fertil Steril. 2009;91(6):2481–6.
8. Bandak M, Jørgensen N, Juul A, Lauritsen J, Gundgaard Kier MG, Mortensen MS, et al. Preorchiectomy leydig cell dysfunction in patients with testicular cancer. Clin Genitourin Cancer. 2017;15(1):e37–43.
9. Yazama F, Tai A. Unexpected role of α-fetoprotein in spermatogenesis. PLoS One. 2011;6(5):e19387.
10. Cochran JS, Walsh PC, Porter JC, Nicholson TC, Madden JD, Peters PC. The endocrinology of human chorionic gonadotropin-secreting testicular tumors: new methods in diagnosis. J Urol. 1975;114(4):549–55.
11. Aiginger P, Kolbe H, Kühböck J, Spona J, Geyer G. The endocrinology of testicular germinal cell tumors. Acta Endocrinol. 1981;97(3):419–26.
12. Ramos EJB, Suzuki S, Marks D, Inui A, Asakawa A, Meguid MM. Cancer anorexia-cachexia syndrome: cytokines and neuropeptides. Curr Opin Clin Nutr Metab Care. 2004;7(4):427–34.
13. Turrin NP, Ilyin SE, Gayle DA, Plata-Salamán CR, Ramos EJB, Laviano A, et al. Interleukin-1beta system in anorectic catabolic tumor-bearing rats. Curr Opin Clin Nutr Metab Care. 2004;7(4):419–26.
14. Inui A. Cancer anorexia-cachexia syndrome: are neuropeptides the key? Cancer Res. 1999;59(18):4493–501.
15. Schcolnik-Cabrera A, Chávez-Blanco A, Domínguez-Gómez G, Dueñas-González A. Understanding tumor anabolism and patient catabolism in cancer-associated cachexia. Am J Cancer Res. 2017;7(5):1107–35.
16. Campos CA, Bowen AJ, Han S, Wisse BE, Palmiter RD, Schwartz MW. Cancer-induced anorexia and malaise are mediated by CGRP neurons in the parabrachial nucleus. Nat Neurosci. 2017;20(7):934–42.
17. Tsai VW-W, Manandhar R, Jørgensen SB, Lee-Ng KKM, Zhang HP, Marquis CP, et al. The anorectic actions of the TGFβ cytokine MIC-1/GDF15 require an intact

brainstem area postrema and nucleus of the solitary tract. PLoS One. 2014;9(6):e100370.
18. Parker C, Milosevic M, Panzarella T, Banerjee D, Jewett M, Catton C, et al. The prognostic significance of the tumour infiltrating lymphocyte count in stage I testicular seminoma managed by surveillance. Eur J Cancer. 2002;38(15):2014–9.
19. Rival C, Theas MS, Suescun MO, Jacobo P, Guazzone V, van Rooijen N, et al. Functional and phenotypic characteristics of testicular macrophages in experimental autoimmune orchitis. J Pathol. 2008;215(2):108–17.
20. Rival C, Theas MS, Guazzone VA, Lustig L. Interleukin-6 and IL-6 receptor cell expression in testis of rats with autoimmune orchitis. J Reprod Immunol. 2006;70(1–2):43–58.
21. Theas MS, Rival C, Dietrich SJ, Guazzone VA, Lustig L. Death receptor and mitochondrial pathways are involved in germ cell apoptosis in an experimental model of autoimmune orchitis. Hum Reprod. 2006;21(7):1734–42.
22. Theas MS, Rival C, Jarazo-Dietrich S, Jacobo P, Guazzone VA, Lustig L. Tumour necrosis factor-alpha released by testicular macrophages induces apoptosis of germ cells in autoimmune orchitis. Hum Reprod. 2008;23(8):1865–72.
23. Aitken RJ, Sawyer D. The human spermatozoon – not waving but drowning. Adv Exp Med Biol. 2003;518:85–98.
24. Martínez P, Proverbio F, Camejo MI. Sperm lipid peroxidation and pro-inflammatory cytokines. Asian J Androl. 2007;9(1):102–7.
25. Oh YS, Jo NH, Park JK, Gye MC. Changes in inflammatory cytokines accompany deregulation of claudin-11, resulting in inter-sertoli tight junctions in varicocele rat testes. J Urol. 2016;196(4):1303–12.
26. Wong EWP, Mruk DD, Lee WM, Cheng CY. Regulation of blood-testis barrier dynamics by TGF-beta3 is a Cdc42-dependent protein trafficking event. Proc Natl Acad Sci U S A. 2010;107(25):11399–404.
27. Guazzieri S, Lembo A, Ferro G, Artibani W, Merlo F, Zanchetta R, et al. Sperm antibodies and infertility in patients with testicular cancer. Urology. 1985;26(2):139–42.
28. Paoli D, Gilio B, Piroli E, Gallo M, Lombardo F, Dondero F, et al. Testicular tumors as a possible cause of antisperm autoimmune response. Fertil Steril. 2009;91(2):414–9.
29. Baracos VE. Cancer-associated malnutrition. Eur J Clin Nutr. 2018;72(9):1255–9.
30. Heyns CF, Fisher M. The urological management of the patient with acquired immunodeficiency syndrome. BJU Int. 2005;95(5):709–16.
31. Viviani S, Ragni G, Santoro A, Perotti L, Caccamo E, Negretti E, et al. Testicular dysfunction in Hodgkin's disease before and after treatment. Eur J Cancer. 1991;27(11):1389–92.
32. Petersen PM, Giwercman A, Hansen SW, Berthelsen JG, Daugaard G, Rørth M, et al. Impaired testicular function in patients with carcinoma-in-situ of the testis. J Clin Oncol. 1999;17(1):173–9.
33. Berthelsen JG, Skakkebaek NE. Gonadal function in men with testis cancer. Fertil Steril. 1983;39(1):68–75.
34. Morrish DW, Venner PM, Siy O, Barron G, Bhardwaj D, Outhet D. Mechanisms of endocrine dysfunction in patients with testicular cancer. J Natl Cancer Inst. 1990;82(5):412–8.
35. Advani A, Johnson SJ, Nicol MR, Papacleovoulou G, Evans DB, Vaikkakara S, et al. Adult-onset hypogonadotropic hypogonadism caused by aberrant expression of aromatase in an adrenocortical adenocarcinoma. Endocr J. 2010;57(7):651–6.
36. Fosså SD, Dahl AA, Loge JH. Fatigue, anxiety, and depression in long-term survivors of testicular cancer. J Clin Oncol. 2003;21(7):1249–54.
37. Greenfield DM, Walters SJ, Coleman RE, Hancock BW, Snowden JA, Shalet SM, et al. Quality of life, self-esteem, fatigue, and sexual function in young men after cancer: a controlled cross-sectional study. Cancer. 2010;116(6):1592–601.
38. Strasser F, Palmer JL, Schover LR, Yusuf SW, Pisters K, Vassilopoulou-Sellin R, et al. The impact of hypogonadism and autonomic dysfunction on fatigue, emotional function, and sexual desire in male patients with advanced cancer: a pilot study. Cancer. 2006;107(12):2949–57.
39. Carlsen E, Andersson A-M, Petersen JH, Skakkebaek NE. History of febrile illness and variation in semen quality. Hum Reprod. 2003;18(10):2089–92.
40. Pasikhova Y, Ludlow S, Baluch A. Fever in patients with cancer. Cancer Control. 2017;24(2):193–7.
41. Marmor D, Elefant E, Dauchez C, Roux C. Semen analysis in Hodgkin's disease before the onset of treatment. Cancer. 1986;57(10):1986–7.
42. Bhongade MB, Prasad S, Jiloha RC, Ray PC, Mohapatra S, Koner BC. Effect of psychological stress on fertility hormones and seminal quality in male partners of infertile couples. Andrologia. 2015;47(3):336–42.
43. Arai Y, Kawakita M, Okada Y, Yoshida O. Sexuality and fertility in long-term survivors of testicular cancer. J Clin Oncol. 1997;15(4):1444–8.
44. van Basten JP, van Driel MF, Hoekstra HJ, Sleijfer DT, van de Wiel HB, Droste JH, et al. Objective and subjective effects of treatment for testicular cancer on sexual function. BJU Int. 1999;84(6):671–8.
45. Mazeron JJ, Gerbaulet A. The centenary of discovery of radium. Radiother Oncol. 1998;49(3):205–16.
46. Shalet SM. Effect of irradiation treatment on gonadal function in men treated for germ cell cancer. Eur Urol. 1993;23(1):148–51; discussion 152.
47. Hansen PV, Trykker H, Svennekjaer IL, Hvolby J. Long-term recovery of spermatogenesis after radiotherapy in patients with testicular cancer. Radiother Oncol. 1990;18(2):117–25.
48. Gordon W, Siegmund K, Stanisic TH, McKnight B, Harris IT, Carroll PR, et al. A study of reproductive function in patients with seminoma treated with radiotherapy and orchidectomy: (SWOG-8711). Southwest Oncology Group. Int J Radiat Oncol Biol Phys. 1997;38(1):83–94.
49. Rowley MJ, Leach DR, Warner GA, Heller CG. Effect of graded doses of ionizing radiation on the human testis. Radiat Res. 1974;59(3):665–78.
50. Giwercman A, von der Maase H, Berthelsen JG, Rørth M, Bertelsen A, Skakkebaek NE. Localized irradiation

of testes with carcinoma in situ: effects on Leydig cell function and eradication of malignant germ cells in 20 patients. J Clin Endocrinol Metab. 1991;73(3):596–603.
51. Budgell GJ, Cowan RA, Hounsell AR. Prediction of scattered dose to the testes in abdominopelvic radiotherapy. Clin Oncol (R Coll Radiol). 2001;13(2):120–5.
52. Hermann RM, Henkel K, Christiansen H, Vorwerk H, Hille A, Hess CF, et al. Testicular dose and hormonal changes after radiotherapy of rectal cancer. Radiother Oncol. 2005;75(1):83–8.
53. Ståhl O, Eberhard J, Jepson K, Spano M, Cwikiel M, Cavallin-Ståhl E, et al. The impact of testicular carcinoma and its treatment on sperm DNA integrity. Cancer. 2004;100(6):1137–44.
54. Ståhl O, Eberhard J, Jepson K, Spano M, Cwikiel M, Cavallin-Ståhl E, et al. Sperm DNA integrity in testicular cancer patients. Hum Reprod. 2006;21(12):3199–205.
55. Smit M, van Casteren NJ, Wildhagen MF, Romijn JC, Dohle GR. Sperm DNA integrity in cancer patients before and after cytotoxic treatment. Hum Reprod. 2010;25(8):1877–83.
56. Rives N, Walschaerts M, Setif V, Hennebicq S, Saias J, Brugnon F, et al. Sperm aneuploidy after testicular cancer treatment: data from a prospective multicenter study performed within the French Centre d'Étude et de Conservation des Oeufs et du Sperme network. Fertil Steril. 2017;107(3):580–588.e1.
57. Thomson AB, Campbell AJ, Irvine DC, Anderson RA, Kelnar CJH, Wallace WHB. Semen quality and spermatozoal DNA integrity in survivors of childhood cancer: a case-control study. Lancet. 2002;360(9330):361–7.
58. Chatterjee R, Haines GA, Perera DM, Goldstone A, Morris ID. Testicular and sperm DNA damage after treatment with fludarabine for chronic lymphocytic leukaemia. Hum Reprod. 2000;15(4):762–6.
59. Hawkins MM. Is there evidence of a therapy-related increase in germ cell mutation among childhood cancer survivors? J Natl Cancer Inst. 1991;83(22):1643–50.
60. Li FP, Fine W, Jaffe N, Holmes GE, Holmes FF. Offspring of patients treated for cancer in childhood. J Natl Cancer Inst. 1979;62(5):1193–7.
61. Cooperberg MR, Carroll PR. Trends in management for patients with localized prostate cancer, 1990–2013. JAMA. 2015;314(1):80–2.
62. Daniell HW, Clark JC, Pereira SE, Niazi ZA, Ferguson DW, Dunn SR, et al. Hypogonadism following prostate-bed radiation therapy for prostate carcinoma. Cancer. 2001;91(10):1889–95.
63. Mydlo JH, Lebed B. Does brachytherapy of the prostate affect sperm quality and/or fertility in younger men? Scand J Urol Nephrol. 2004;38(3):221–4.
64. Grocela J, Mauceri T, Zietman A. New life after prostate brachytherapy? Considering the fertile female partner of the brachytherapy patient. BJU Int. 2005;96(6):781–2.
65. Delaunay B, Delannes M, Bachaud JM, Bouaziz M, Salloum A, Thoulouzan M, et al. Fertility after prostate brachytherapy with Iode 125 permanent implants for localized prostate cancer. Prog Urol. 2012;22(1):53–7.
66. Jacobsen KD, Olsen DR, Fosså K, Fosså SD. External beam abdominal radiotherapy in patients with seminoma stage I: field type, testicular dose, and spermatogenesis. Int J Radiat Oncol Biol Phys. 1997;38(1):95–102.
67. Aass N, Fosså SD, Theodorsen L, Norman N. Prediction of long-term gonadal toxicity after standard treatment for testicular cancer. Eur J Cancer. 1991;27(9):1087–91.
68. Huyghe E, Matsuda T, Daudin M, Chevreau C, Bachaud J-M, Plante P, et al. Fertility after testicular cancer treatments: results of a large multicenter study. Cancer. 2004;100(4):732–7.
69. Huddart RA, Norman A, Moynihan C, Horwich A, Parker C, Nicholls E, et al. Fertility, gonadal and sexual function in survivors of testicular cancer. Br J Cancer. 2005;93(2):200–7.
70. Nalesnik JG, Sabanegh ES, Eng TY, Buchholz TA. Fertility in men after treatment for stage 1 and 2A seminoma. Am J Clin Oncol. 2004;27(6):584–8.
71. Kinsella TJ, Trivette G, Rowland J, Sorace R, Miller R, Fraass B, et al. Long-term follow-up of testicular function following radiation therapy for early-stage Hodgkin's disease. J Clin Oncol. 1989;7(6):718–24.
72. Socié G, Salooja N, Cohen A, Rovelli A, Carreras E, Locasciulli A, et al. Nonmalignant late effects after allogeneic stem cell transplantation. Blood. 2003;101(9):3373–85.
73. Sanders JE, Hawley J, Levy W, Gooley T, Buckner CD, Deeg HJ, et al. Pregnancies following high-dose cyclophosphamide with or without high-dose busulfan or total-body irradiation and bone marrow transplantation. Blood. 1996;87(7):3045–52.
74. Salooja N, Szydlo RM, Socie G, Rio B, Chatterjee R, Ljungman P, et al. Pregnancy outcomes after peripheral blood or bone marrow transplantation: a retrospective survey. Lancet. 2001;358(9278):271–6.
75. Sayan M, Cassidy RJ, Butker EE, Nanda RH, Krishnamurti L, Khan MK, et al. Gonadal shielding technique to preserve fertility in male pediatric patients treated with total body irradiation for stem cell transplantation. Bone Marrow Transplant. 2016;51(7):997–8.
76. Sanghvi PR, Kaurin DGL, McDonald TL, Holland JM. Testicular shielding in low-dose total body irradiation. Bone Marrow Transplant. 2007;39(4):247–8.
77. Spitz S. The histological effects of nitrogen mustards on human tumors and tissues. Cancer. 1948;1(3):383–98.
78. Witt KL, Bishop JB. Mutagenicity of anticancer drugs in mammalian germ cells. Mutat Res. 1996;355(1–2):209–34.
79. Byrne J, Mulvihill JJ, Myers MH, Connelly RR, Naughton MD, Krauss MR, et al. Effects of treatment on fertility in long-term survivors of childhood or adolescent cancer. N Engl J Med. 1987;317(21):1315–21.
80. Buchanan JD, Fairley KF, Barrie JU. Return of spermatogenesis after stopping cyclophosphamide therapy. Lancet. 1975;2(7926):156–7.
81. Kenney LB, Laufer MR, Grant FD, Grier H, Diller L. High risk of infertility and long term gonadal damage in males treated with high dose cyclophosphamide for sarcoma during childhood. Cancer. 2001;91(3):613–21.
82. Bokemeyer C, Schmoll HJ, van Rhee J, Kuczyk M, Schuppert F, Poliwoda H. Long-term gonadal toxicity after therapy for Hodgkin's and non-Hodgkin's lymphoma. Ann Hematol. 1994;68(3):105–10.

83. Green DM, Liu W, Kutteh WH, Ke RW, Shelton KC, Sklar CA, et al. Cumulative alkylating agent exposure and semen parameters in adult survivors of childhood cancer: a report from the St Jude Lifetime Cohort Study. Lancet Oncol. 2014;15(11):1215–23.
84. Choudhury RC, Misra S, Jagdale MB, Palo AK. Induction and transmission of cytogenetic toxic effects of 5-fluorouracil in male germline cells of Swiss mice. J Exp Clin Cancer Res. 2002;21(2):277–82.
85. D'Souza UJA. Re: 5-fluorouracil-induced sperm shape abnormalities in rats. Asian J Androl. 2003;5(4):353.
86. D'Souza UJ, Narayana K. Induction of seminiferous tubular atrophy by single dose of 5-fluorouracil (5-FU) in Wistar rats. Indian J Physiol Pharmacol. 2001;45(1):87–94.
87. Sukhotnik I, Nativ O, Roitburt A, Bejar D, Coran AG, Mogilner JG, et al. Methotrexate induces germ cell apoptosis and impairs spermatogenesis in a rat. Pediatr Surg Int. 2013;29(2):179–84.
88. Choudhury RC, Jagdale MB, Misra S. Potential transmission of the cytogenetic effects of cisplatin in the male germline cells of Swiss mice. J Chemother. 2000;12(4):352–9.
89. Lampe H, Horwich A, Norman A, Nicholls J, Dearnaley DP. Fertility after chemotherapy for testicular germ cell cancers. J Clin Oncol. 1997;15(1):239–45.
90. Pectasides D, Pectasides M, Farmakis D, Nikolaou M, Koumpou M, Kostopoulou V, et al. Testicular function in patients with testicular cancer treated with bleomycin-etoposide-carboplatin (BEC(90)) combination chemotherapy. Eur Urol. 2004;45(2):187–93.
91. Brydøy M, Fosså SD, Klepp O, Bremnes RM, Wist EA, Wentzel-Larsen T, et al. Paternity and testicular function among testicular cancer survivors treated with two to four cycles of cisplatin-based chemotherapy. Eur Urol. 2010;58(1):134–40.
92. Arnon J, Meirow D, Lewis-Roness H, Ornoy A. Genetic and teratogenic effects of cancer treatments on gametes and embryos. Hum Reprod Updat. 2001;7(4):394–403.
93. Sjöblom T, Parvinen M, Lähdetie J. Stage-specific DNA synthesis of rat spermatogenesis as an indicator of genotoxic effects of vinblastine, mitomycin C and ionizing radiation on rat spermatogonia and spermatocytes. Mutat Res. 1995;331(2):181–90.
94. Aubier F, Flamant F, Brauner R, Caillaud JM, Chaussain JM, Lemerle J. Male gonadal function after chemotherapy for solid tumors in childhood. J Clin Oncol. 1989;7(3):304–9.
95. Meistrich ML, Wilson G, Mathur K, Fuller LM, Rodriguez MA, McLaughlin P, et al. Rapid recovery of spermatogenesis after mitoxantrone, vincristine, vinblastine, and prednisone chemotherapy for Hodgkin's disease. J Clin Oncol. 1997;15(12):3488–95.
96. van Buul PP, Goudzwaard JH. Bleomycin-induced structural chromosomal aberrations in spermatogonia and bone-marrow cells of mice. Mutat Res. 1980;69(2):319–24.
97. Hou M, Chrysis D, Nurmio M, Parvinen M, Eksborg S, Söder O, et al. Doxorubicin induces apoptosis in germ line stem cells in the immature rat testis and amifostine cannot protect against this cytotoxicity. Cancer Res. 2005;65(21):9999–10005.
98. Paoli D, Rizzo F, Fiore G, Pallotti F, Pulsoni A, Annechini G, et al. Spermatogenesis in Hodgkin's lymphoma patients: a retrospective study of semen quality before and after different chemotherapy regimens. Hum Reprod. 2016;31(2):263–72.
99. Foster RS, Bennett R, Bihrle R, Donohue JP. A preliminary report: postoperative fertility assessment in nerve-sparing RPLND patients. Eur Urol. 1993;23(1):165–7; discussion 168.
100. Beck SDW, Bey AL, Bihrle R, Foster RS. Ejaculatory status and fertility rates after primary retroperitoneal lymph node dissection. J Urol. 2010;184(5):2078–80.
101. Lange MM, van de Velde CJH. Urinary and sexual dysfunction after rectal cancer treatment. Nat Rev Urol. 2011;8(1):51–7.
102. Schlegel PN, Walsh PC. Neuroanatomical approach to radical cystoprostatectomy with preservation of sexual function. J Urol. 1987;138(6):1402–6.
103. Knoester PA, Leonard M, Wood DP, Schuster TG. Fertility issues for men with newly diagnosed prostate cancer. Urology. 2007;69(1):123–5.
104. O'Rourke TK, Wosnitzer MS. Opioid-induced androgen deficiency (OPIAD): diagnosis, management, and literature review. Curr Urol Rep. 2016;17(10):76.
105. Subirán N, Casis L, Irazusta J. Regulation of male fertility by the opioid system. Mol Med. 2011;17(7–8):846–53.
106. Rajagopal A, Vassilopoulou-Sellin R, Palmer JL, Kaur G, Bruera E. Symptomatic hypogonadism in male survivors of cancer with chronic exposure to opioids. Cancer. 2004;100(4):851–8.
107. Ward E, DeSantis C, Robbins A, Kohler B, Jemal A. Childhood and adolescent cancer statistics, 2014. CA Cancer J Clin. 2014;64(2):83–103.
108. Lehmann V, Keim MC, Nahata L, Shultz EL, Klosky JL, Tuinman MA, et al. Fertility-related knowledge and reproductive goals in childhood cancer survivors: short communication. Hum Reprod. 2017;32(11):2250–3.
109. Zapzalka DM, Redmon JB, Pryor JL. A survey of oncologists regarding sperm cryopreservation and assisted reproductive techniques for male cancer patients. Cancer. 1999;86(9):1812–7.
110. Quinn GP, Vadaparampil ST, Lee J-H, Jacobsen PB, Bepler G, Lancaster J, et al. Physician referral for fertility preservation in oncology patients: a national study of practice behaviors. J Clin Oncol. 2009;27(35):5952–7.
111. Schover LR, Brey K, Lichtin A, Lipshultz LI, Jeha S. Knowledge and experience regarding cancer, infertility, and sperm banking in younger male survivors. J Clin Oncol. 2002;20(7):1880–9.
112. Oktay K, Harvey BE, Partridge AH, Quinn GP, Reinecke J, Taylor HS, et al. Fertility preservation in patients with cancer: ASCO clinical practice guideline update. J Clin Oncol. 2018;36(19):1994–2001.
113. Salsman JM, Yanez B, Smith KN, Beaumont JL, Snyder MA, Barnes K, et al. Documentation of fertility preservation discussions for young adults with cancer: examining compliance with treatment guidelines. J Natl Compr Cancer Netw. 2016;14(3):301–9.

114. Lee SJ, Schover LR, Partridge AH, Patrizio P, Wallace WH, Hagerty K, et al. American Society of Clinical Oncology recommendations on fertility preservation in cancer patients. J Clin Oncol. 2006;24(18):2917–31.
115. Loren AW, Mangu PB, Beck LN, Brennan L, Magdalinski AJ, Partridge AH, et al. Fertility preservation for patients with cancer: American Society of Clinical Oncology clinical practice guideline update. J Clin Oncol. 2013;31(19):2500–10.
116. Fallat ME, Hutter J, American Academy of Pediatrics Committee on Bioethics, American Academy of Pediatrics Section on Hematology/Oncology, American Academy of Pediatrics Section on Surgery. Preservation of fertility in pediatric and adolescent patients with cancer. Pediatrics. 2008;121(5):e1461–9.
117. Ethics Committee of the American Society for Reproductive Medicine. Electronic address: ASRM@asrm.org.Fertility preservation and reproduction in patients facing gonadotoxic therapies: an Ethics Committee opinion. Fertil Steril. 2018;110(3):380–6.
118. Martinez F. Update on fertility preservation from the Barcelona International Society for Fertility Preservation-ESHRE-ASRM 2015 expert meeting: indications, results and future perspectives. Hum Reprod. 2017;32(9):1802–11.
119. Lambertini M, Del Mastro L, Pescio MC, Andersen CY, Azim HA, Peccatori FA, et al. Cancer and fertility preservation: international recommendations from an expert meeting. BMC Med. 2016;14:1.
120. Sheth KR, Sharma V, Helfand BT, Cashy J, Smith K, Hedges JC, et al. Improved fertility preservation care for male patients with cancer after establishment of formalized oncofertility program. J Urol. 2012;187(3):979–86.
121. Lopategui DM, Ibrahim E, Aballa TC, Brackett NL, Yechieli R, Barredo JC, et al. Effect of a formal oncofertility program on fertility preservation rates-first year experience. Transl Androl Urol. 2018;7(Suppl 3):S271–5.
122. Sanger WG, Armitage JO, Schmidt MA. Feasibility of semen cryopreservation in patients with malignant disease. JAMA. 1980;244(8):789–90.
123. Bracken RB, Smith KD. Is semen cryopreservation helpful in testicular cancer? Urology. 1980;15(6):581–3.
124. Palermo G, Joris H, Devroey P, Van Steirteghem AC. Pregnancies after intracytoplasmic injection of single spermatozoon into an oocyte. Lancet. 1992;340(8810):17–8.
125. Practice Committee of the American Society for Reproductive Medicine in collaboration with the Society for Reproductive Endocrinology and Infertility. Electronic address: ASRM@asrm.org, Practice Committee of the American Society for Reproductive Medicine in collaboration with the Society for Reproductive Endocrinology and InfertilityOptimizing natural fertility: a committee opinion. Fertil Steril. 2017;107(1):52–8.
126. Schmiegelow ML, Sommer P, Carlsen E, Sønksen JO, Schmiegelow K, Müller JR. Penile vibratory stimulation and electroejaculation before anticancer therapy in two pubertal boys. J Pediatr Hematol Oncol. 1998;20(5):429–30.
127. Adank MC, van Dorp W, Smit M, van Casteren NJ, Laven JSE, Pieters R, et al. Electroejaculation as a method of fertility preservation in boys diagnosed with cancer: a single-center experience and review of the literature. Fertil Steril. 2014;102(1):199–205.e1.
128. Berookhim BM, Mulhall JP. Outcomes of operative sperm retrieval strategies for fertility preservation among males scheduled to undergo cancer treatment. Fertil Steril. 2014;101(3):805–11.
129. Lass A, Akagbosu F, Abusheikha N, Hassouneh M, Blayney M, Avery S, et al. A programme of semen cryopreservation for patients with malignant disease in a tertiary infertility centre: lessons from 8 years' experience. Hum Reprod. 1998;13(11):3256–61.
130. Rosenlund B, Westlander G, Wood M, Lundin K, Reismer E, Hillensjö T. Sperm retrieval and fertilization in repeated percutaneous epididymal sperm aspiration. Hum Reprod. 1998;13(10):2805–7.
131. Res U, Res P, Kastelic D, Stanovnik M, Kmetec A, Merlo A. Birth after treatment of a male with seminoma and azoospermia with cryopreserved-thawed testicular tissue. Hum Reprod. 2000;15(4):861–4.
132. Köhn FM, Schroeder-Printzen I, Weidner W, Montag M, van der Ven H, Schill WB. Testicular sperm extraction in a patient with metachronous bilateral testicular cancer. Hum Reprod. 2001;16(11):2343–6.
133. Schrader M, Müller M, Sofikitis N, Straub B, Krause H, Miller K. "Onco-tese": testicular sperm extraction in azoospermic cancer patients before chemotherapy-new guidelines? Urology. 2003;61(2):421–5.
134. Carrasquillo R, Sávio LF, Venkatramani V, Parekh D, Ramasamy R. Using microscope for onco-testicular sperm extraction for bilateral testis tumors. Fertil Steril. 2018;109(4):745.
135. Furuhashi K, Ishikawa T, Hashimoto H, Yamada S, Ogata S, Mizusawa Y, et al. Onco-testicular sperm extraction: testicular sperm extraction in azoospermic and very severely oligozoospermic cancer patients. Andrologia. 2013;45(2):107–10.
136. Roque M, Sampaio M, de Salles PG, Geber S. Onco-testicular sperm extraction: birth of a healthy baby after fertility preservation in synchronous bilateral testicular cancer and azoospermia. Andrologia. 2015;47(4):482–5.
137. Tsutsumi S, Kawahara T, Takeshima T, Chiba S, Uemura K, Otani M, et al. Onco-testicular sperm extraction (onco-TESE) for bilateral testicular tumors: two case reports. J Med Case Rep. 2017;11(1):139.
138. Johnson DH, Linde R, Hainsworth JD, Vale W, Rivier J, Stein R, et al. Effect of a luteinizing hormone releasing hormone agonist given during combination chemotherapy on posttherapy fertility in male patients with lymphoma: preliminary observations. Blood. 1985;65(4):832–6.
139. Waxman JH, Ahmed R, Smith D, Wrigley PF, Gregory W, Shalet S, et al. Failure to preserve fertility in patients with Hodgkin's disease. Cancer Chemother Pharmacol. 1987;19(2):159–62.
140. Brennemann W, Brensing KA, Leipner N, Boldt I, Klingmüller D. Attempted protection of spermatogenesis from irradiation in patients with seminoma

by D-Tryptophan-6 luteinizing hormone releasing hormone. Clin Investig. 1994;72(11):838–42.
141. Kreuser ED, Hetzel WD, Hautmann R, Pfeiffer EF. Reproductive toxicity with and without LHRHA administration during adjuvant chemotherapy in patients with germ cell tumors. Horm Metab Res. 1990;22(9):494–8.
142. Brook PF, Radford JA, Shalet SM, Joyce AD, Gosden RG. Isolation of germ cells from human testicular tissue for low temperature storage and autotransplantation. Fertil Steril. 2001;75(2):269–74.
143. Valli H, Phillips BT, Shetty G, Byrne JA, Clark AT, Meistrich ML, et al. Germline stem cells: toward the regeneration of spermatogenesis. Fertil Steril. 2014;101(1):3–13.
144. Gassei K, Orwig KE. Experimental methods to preserve male fertility and treat male factor infertility. Fertil Steril. 2016;105(2):256–66.
145. Nagano M, Patrizio P, Brinster RL. Long-term survival of human spermatogonial stem cells in mouse testes. Fertil Steril. 2002;78(6):1225–33.
146. Schlatt S, Honaramooz A, Ehmcke J, Goebell PJ, Rübben H, Dhir R, et al. Limited survival of adult human testicular tissue as ectopic xenograft. Hum Reprod. 2006;21(2):384–9.

Care of the Opatient

Contents

Assessing Ovarian Reserve

Yasmin Gosiengfiao and Veronica Gomez-Lobo

T. K. Woodruff et al. (eds.), *Textbook of Oncofertility Research and Practice*,
https://doi.org/10.1007/978-3-030-02868-8_12

Key Points

- Ovarian reserve testing is a surrogate marker of fertility potential developed and evaluated in women undergoing ovarian stimulation.
- Anti-Mullerian Hormone (AMH) is promising as an ovarian reserve marker in girls receiving cancer therapy, but many questions remain unanswered.
- AMH levels can be impacted by many clinical parameters including current hormonal contraception, GnRH agonist therapy, and cancer therapy.

12.1 Background

Female cancer survivors are known to be at risk for decreased fertility and early menopause. Fertility is defined as the ability to produce young [1–3]. Conversely, infertility is defined by the failure to achieve a clinical pregnancy after 12 months or more of regular unprotected sexual intercourse [4]. Having pregnancies thus would be the best measure of fertility. Using pregnancies as a measure of fertility, however, limits one to wait until a childhood cancer survivor has grown into an adult and has attempted to get pregnant. Even among adults, not all adult women attempt to get pregnant. Thus, surrogate measures of fertility are necessary to assess the effect of chemotherapy/radiation/surgery on fertility.

12

Most cancer survivors experience infertility due to direct effects of treatment on the ovary or testes. The initial number of follicles in humans is established in utero at 5 months gestation with approximately ten million primordial follicles. This number of follicles (or ovarian reserve) diminishes in utero and after birth to nearly 500,000 at menarche and continues to decline thereafter until these fall below a certain threshold and menopause appears [5]. Ovarian reserve is the concept that views reproductive potential as a function of the number and quality of oocytes. Radiation and other gonadotoxic agents are thought to affect the number of follicles by possibly accelerating this process of attrition [2, 6–8]. The effect of treatment on an individual patient's ovarian reserve depends on many factors including the age at the time of gonadotoxic treatment, the type and dose of therapy, genetic factors, previous illnesses, and prior infertility. It is important to note that even before menopause (or the cessation of menses) is noted, the number and/or quality of the follicles may preclude pregnancy [9]. Infertility may be caused by decreased ovarian reserve or sperm production, but other causes such as tubal, uterine, and cervical factors may influence fertility. Thus, surrogate measures of ovarian or testicular reserve do not fully measure fertility potential.

12.2 Assessing Ovarian Reserve

There are several markers that have been used to assess ovarian reserve (OR). It should be noted, however, that most of the research regarding these markers has been performed in healthy ovarian aging and women seeking treatment for infertility, and debate still remains regarding the ability of these markers to predict oocyte quality, quantity, and fecundity in healthy women. Furthermore, it is important to note that these tests are "screening" tests that would be helpful only if they predict ovarian reserve prior to menopause or ovarian insufficiency [6]. Thus, these markers may not be good measures of fertility for young women treated with gonadotoxic agents [10].

12.2.1 Menstrual Cycles

In 2006, the American College of Obstetrics and Gynecology (ACOG) and the American Academy of Pediatrics (AAP) issued a Committee Opinion stating that the menstrual cycle is a vital sign, thus stressing the importance of menses [11]. The average age of menarche in the western world declined rapidly in the last two centuries but has been stable since the 1950s in the developed world. Normal menstrual cycles in young females include a median age of menarche of 12 years, mean cycle interval of 32 days with a range of 21–45 days, and flow length of 7 days. Primary amenorrhea is defined as the absence of menses by age 15, and secondary amenorrhea has been defined as the absence of cycles for more than 6 months [11]. Early menopause has been defined as cessation of menses prior to age 40, and the average age of menopause in the United States is 51. Adult female survivors of childhood cancers have been noted to have earlier age of menopause and a higher rate or premature menopause than the general population [3].

The presence or absence of menses has traditionally been used as the primary measure of fertility and ovarian function in cancer survivors, but it should be noted that there are many common causes of amenorrhea including pregnancy, polycystic ovary syndrome, structural issues (scarring of the uterus), and disturbances of the central gonadotropin-releasing hormone pulse generator. These disturbances are often referred to as hypogonadotropic hypogonadism and may be caused by significant weight loss, strenuous exercise, substantial changes in sleeping or eating habits, as well as severe stressors [11]. For example, a young cancer survivor may have absence of menses due to hypothalamic disturbances caused by the stress of treatment or ovarian insufficiency due to gonadotoxic agents. In addition, women may continue to have regular menses even in the presence of diminished ovarian reserve (such as occurs in the perimenopause). Thus, the presence of menses is a poor predictor of ovarian reserve, and other markers should be used to assess OR.

12.2.2 Antral Follicle Counts and Ovarian Volume

Antral follicle counts and ovarian volume have traditionally been measured using transvaginal ultrasound in adult women. Both of these undergo an age-related decline and are good predictors of the number of eggs that can be retrieved with ovarian stimulation in women undergoing in vitro fertilization. Antral follicle count (AFC) is the number of small follicles (2–9 mm) that are observed in both ovaries during the early follicular phase of the cycle [6]. AFC is noted to have good inter-cycle and inter-observer reliability and thus is considered promising as a screening test for ovarian reserve. Again tests revealing low AFC (three to six total antral follicles) correlate with poor response to ovarian stimulation but do not reliably predict failure to conceive [6]. Ovarian volume in general correlates with a number of follicles but has been noted in some studies to have poor inter-cycle reliability [6]. Though inter-observer variability can be minimized with the use of three-dimensional sonography, this test is poor at predicting diminished ovarian reserve [6]. In children, AFC and ovarian volume can be performed transabdominally but requires a radiologist skilled in this technique and has not been well studied in this age group. Thus, antral follicle counts may help in predicting decreased ovarian reserve but deserves further study in cancer populations and children.

12.2.3 Endocrine Hormones

Biochemical tests for ovarian reserve in adult women include basal measurements such as follicle-stimulating hormone (FSH), estradiol, inhibin B, and anti-Mullerian hormone as well as stimulated tests such as the clomiphene citrate challenge test [6]. The latter cannot be performed in children, but the former should be further studied.

12.2.4 Follicle-Stimulating Hormone (FSH), Inhibin B, and Estradiol

FSH is secreted by the pituitary in order to stimulate follicular growth and varies throughout the menstrual cycle. When ovarian reserve is decreased, FSH begins to rise earlier in the cycle and lead to earlier follicular growth and increase in estradiol concentrations. As follicles further decrease in number, the FSH continues to rise and estradiol levels fall. Inhibin B is secreted by preantral follicles, and as follicles decrease, so does inhibin B, which in turn lowers central nervous system feedback and thus further increases FSH [12–14].

Serum FSH assays have significant inter- and intra-cycle variability; the absolute values differ depending on which one is used, and the sensitivity in identifying poor responders to ovarian stimulation in women varies widely [6]. In addition, children have low FSH due to hypothalamic suppression. It should be noted that in spite of these limitations, consistently high levels of FSH are predictive of diminished ovarian reserve, and repeated levels above 40 IU/L are diagnostic for premature ovarian insufficiency or menopause [6]. Estradiol assays also have poor intra- and inter-cycle variability, and basal levels do not differ between women with and without diminished ovarian reserve [6]. Furthermore, in prepubertal children, estradiol levels are also low due to hypothalamic suppression. Inhibin B has also been noted to not be a reliable measure of ovarian reserve. Thus, the use of FSH, inhibin B, and estradiol levels in assessing fertility potential of cancer patients is limited by variation with the menstrual cycles, poor sensitivity, and the low to undetectable levels in prepubertal children. Furthermore, combined ovarian reserve test models have not been shown to be superior to single tests in predicting ovarian reserve [6].

12.2.5 Anti-Mullerian Hormone (AMH)

AMH is a hormone produced by the granulosa cells, which acts as a follicular gatekeeper and is independent of FSH or gonadotropin. This marker is an indirect marker of antral follicle counts and thus ovarian reserve [15]. In childhood and adolescence, there is a complex rise in AMH level, which likely reflects the different stages of follicle development. It then peaks in a woman's early 20s before declining to menopause, correlating positively with nongrowing follicle recruitment [16].

Interest in the use of AMH as a measure of ovarian reserve to measure the gonadotoxic effect of chemotherapy/radiotherapy is growing, especially for children in whom FSH and inhibin B are not useful. When compared with other ovarian reserve markers, AMH levels reflect changes in ovarian function earlier, there is less significant fluctuation of AMH during the menstrual cycle, and it is highly predictive for the timing of menopause [17–19], suggesting that it may be the most useful marker for monitoring the decline of reproductive capacity. Moreover, serum AMH levels are detectable in healthy females from birth to menopause [16, 20], making it suitable as a marker even in prepubertal girls (Fig. 12.1).

It should be noted that though studies of AMH screening reveal an association with poor results with in vitro fertilization (IVF), levels are not necessarily predictive [6]. Low AMH cut points are associated with sensitivities in general IVF populations of 40–97% with specificities of 78–92%, and low levels of AMH are specific for poor ovarian response but not pregnancy [6]. Furthermore, there are limited data correlating AMH and natural fertility at different stages of reproductive life and especially in children and adolescents. AMH assays continue to evolve, with intra- and inter-assay variability and sample stability and storage issues [21]. Furthermore, several clinical factors may influence AMH levels: systemic illness, endometriosis, chemotherapy, current smoking, low vitamin D levels, and certain genetic factors such as BRCA1 carrier and FMR1 mutation may decrease AMH, and white race, polycystic ovary syndrome, and granulosa cell tumor may increase AMH [21]. It is also important to note that AMH decreases during cancer therapy and may recover thereafter [22, 23]. In a case series of 16 postpubertal adolescents, more than half of patients had recovery of AMH levels by 18–24 months including several with undetectable AMH immediately after therapy [23]. A review of 192 women beginning 5 years after therapy, however, did not note

12

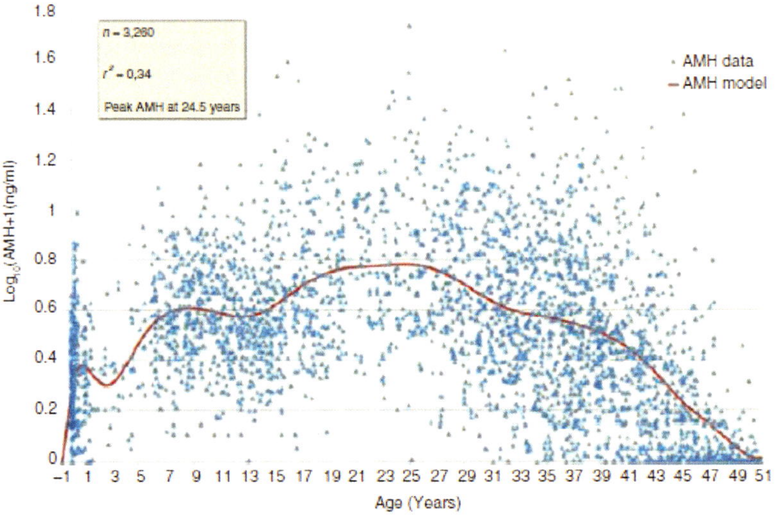

Fig. 12.1 A validated model of serum AMH from conception to menopause [16]

an accelerated decline in AMH thereafter when compared to controls [24].

Therefore, though AMH appears to be a promising tool, more long-term data is needed to ascertain the use of AMH to evaluate fertility preservation strategies as well as predict long-term ovarian function after cancer therapy.

12.2.6 Current Data on AMH in Children Receiving Cancer Therapy

In women treated with mechlorethamine, vincristine, procarbazine, and prednisone (MOPP) chemotherapy for Hodgkin lymphoma during childhood, AMH was noted to be lower compared with healthy women and women treated without MOPP [25]. In a larger series of 185 childhood cancer survivors, although the cohort's median AMH concentration was no different from controls, the AMH levels were lower than the tenth percentile of normal values in 27% of the survivors. Survivors treated with three or more procarbazine-containing chemotherapy cycles and those treated with abdominal or total body irradiation had significantly lower AMH levels than controls [26]. Recent studies have revealed low AMH in more than half of childhood cancer survivors with the lowest levels in those treated with radiation and bone marrow transplant and those treated for Hodgkin's lymphoma but effects noted even in those receiving low-risk therapies [27, 28]. As stated before, in adult women and adolescents with cancer, AMH declines during treatment followed by recovery in some patients, with the rate of recovery determined by the pretreatment AMH level [23, 29].

12.2.7 Ovarian Reserve Testing as a Predictor of Menstrual Pattern and Fertility

Ovarian reserve testing to predict the risk of acute ovarian failure and early menopause and future fertility in females prior to cancer therapy would allow us to better target patients for ovarian preservation procedures [30]. In adults, one small series in breast cancer survivors demonstrated that inhibin B and AMH prior to therapy were significantly lower in the women who went on to develop amenorrhea after treatment [31]. Similarly, in 46 adolescent and young adult women with a new cancer diagnosis requiring chemotherapy, pretreatment AMH levels were associated with the rate of recovery of AMH after treatment. Participants with a pretreatment AMH level >2 ng/mL had a faster rate of recovery of AMH after chemotherapy compared to participants with pretreatment AMH levels </= 2 ng/mL [29]. More recently, studies in breast cancer patients have provided some prognostic tools to predict the likelihood and timing of return of ovarian function after chemotherapy [21].

In addition, the ability of ovarian reserve testing to predict time to menopause and ovarian insufficiency on survivors who are menstruating would be very useful in order for them to plan post-treatment fertility preservation and other therapies [30]. In a prospective study of breast cancer survivors who were still menstruating, the patients who had cessation of menses 2 years later were more likely to have lower AMH and higher FSH at study entry [30].

Most research regarding ovarian reserve testing and prediction of ovarian function after chemotherapy have been performed in breast cancer, and thus, research in other types of cancer therapies is needed. Furthermore, to date, there is no data regarding the ability of ovarian reserve testing to predict the risk of premature menopause in prepubertal girls before therapy or in survivors of childhood cancer.

12.2.8 Effect of Female Hormones on Ovarian Reserve Testing

Many young women who receive cancer therapy are placed on birth control pills to regulate menses or estrogen replacement therapy when ovarian insufficiency is suspected. It is important to understand the effect of this treatment on ovarian reserve testing. A study evaluating ovarian reserve testing in 887 healthy women, 18–46 years old, found that AMH, antral follicle counts, and ovarian volume were all significantly decreased in oral contraception users when compared to nonusers [32]. In a small study comparing young cancer survivors on birth control pills with control women on the pills during the 3rd week of pills (while taking active pills), there were no differences noted in FSH, inhibin B, estradiol, or AMH, but the AFC was lower in the cancer survivors [33]. Furthermore, AMH levels may change with GnRH agonist administration, which is often used during cancer treatment to suppress menses or for possible ovarian protection [34].

Several studies have evaluated ovarian reserve testing during the placebo or pill-free week comparing survivors with spontaneous menses and those on birth control pills. Results from these studies are contradictory, use small samples, and compare populations exposed to cancer therapy to each other and not healthy age-matched controls [25, 35]. In addition, there are no studies which evaluate whether ovarian reserve testing in women on female hormones is predictive of menstrual function or fertility.

12.3 Conclusions

Ovarian reserve testing has been extensively studied in healthy women who seek infertility treatment but not in young girls receiving cancer therapy. This population would benefit significantly from rigorous data regarding ovarian reserve testing, which may predict their risk of early menopause and assess the risk and benefits of fertility preservation options. Research in this population is limited by the fact that the numbers of girls at individual institutions are low as well as the fact that the outcome of interest (the ability to achieve successful pregnancy) may be far in the future [33]. Future multicenter studies with collaborative efforts of reproductive specialists, oncologists, and patient advocates will need to be performed.

Review Questions and Answers

Q1. Ovarian reserve testing refers to testing to evaluate the number of follicles remaining in the ovaries. True or False?

A1. True

Q2. Menstrual history is an excellent way to assess ovarian reserve. True or False?

A2. False

Q3. Of the following markers of ovarian reserve, which is the most promising for children and adolescents?
- (a) FSH
- (b) Inhibin-B
- (c) Antral Follicle Count (AFC)
- (d) AMH
- (e) Menses

A3. (d)

Q4. AMH results are impacted as stated below except:
- (a) Current chemotherapy is associated with decreased AMH
- (b) Birth control pills are associated with increased AMH
- (c) Low vitamin D is associated with decreased AMH
- (d) Polycystic ovary syndrome (PCOS) is associated with increased AMH
- (e) White race is associated with increased AMH

A4. (b)

References

1. Byrne J, et al. Early menopause in long-term survivors of cancer during adolescence. Am J Obstet Gynecol. 1992;166(3):788–93.
2. Green DM, et al. Ovarian failure and reproductive outcomes after childhood cancer treatment: results from the Childhood Cancer Survivor Study. J Clin Oncol. 2009;27(14):2374–81.
3. Thomas-Teinturier C, et al. Age at menopause and its influencing factors in a cohort of survivors of childhood cancer: earlier but rarely premature. Hum Reprod. 2013;28(2):488–95.
4. Zegers-Hochschild F, et al. International Committee for Monitoring Assisted Reproductive Technology (ICMART) and the World Health Organization (WHO) revised glossary of ART terminology, 2009. Fertil Steril. 2009;92(5):1520–4.
5. Faddy MJ, Gosden RG. A model conforming the decline in follicle numbers to the age of menopause in women. Hum Reprod. 1996;11(7):1484–6.
6. Practice committee of the american society for reproductive medicine. Testing and interpreting measures of ovarian reserve: a committee opinion. Fertil Steril. 2015;103(3):e9–17.
7. Goodwin PJ, et al. Risk of menopause during the first year after breast cancer diagnosis. J Clin Oncol. 1999;17(8):2365–70.

8. Bines J, Oleske DM, Cobleigh MA. Ovarian function in premenopausal women treated with adjuvant chemotherapy for breast cancer. J Clin Oncol. 1996;14(5):1718–29.
9. Koyama H, et al. Cyclophosphamide-induced ovarian failure and its therapeutic significance in patients with breast cancer. Cancer. 1977;39(4):1403–9.
10. Domingues TS, Rocha AM, Serafini PC. Tests for ovarian reserve: reliability and utility. Curr Opin Obstet Gynecol. 2010;22(4):271–6.
11. ACOG Committee Opinion No. 349. November 2006: menstruation in girls and adolescents: using the menstrual cycle as a vital sign. Obstet Gynecol. 2006;108(5):1323–8.
12. Burger HG. The endocrinology of the menopause. Maturitas. 1996;23(2):129–36.
13. Richardson SJ, Senikas V, Nelson JF. Follicular depletion during the menopausal transition: evidence for accelerated loss and ultimate exhaustion. J Clin Endocrinol Metab. 1987;65(6):1231–7.
14. Burger HG, et al. The endocrinology of the menopausal transition: a cross-sectional study of a population-based sample. J Clin Endocrinol Metab. 1995;80(12):3537–45.
15. La Marca A, et al. Anti-Mullerian hormone (AMH) as a predictive marker in assisted reproductive technology (ART). Hum Reprod Update. 2010;16(2):113–30.
16. Kelsey TW, et al. A validated model of serum anti-Mullerian hormone from conception to menopause. PLoS One. 2011;6(7):e22024.
17. Tsepelidis S, et al. Stable serum levels of anti-Mullerian hormone during the menstrual cycle: a prospective study in normo-ovulatory women. Hum Reprod. 2007;22(7):1837–40.
18. van Rooij IA, et al. Serum antimullerian hormone levels best reflect the reproductive decline with age in normal women with proven fertility: a longitudinal study. Fertil Steril. 2005;83(4):979–87.
19. Broer SL, et al. Anti-mullerian hormone predicts menopause: a long-term follow-up study in normoovulatory women. J Clin Endocrinol Metab. 2011;96(8):2532–9.
20. Hagen CP, et al. Serum levels of anti-Mullerian hormone as a marker of ovarian function in 926 healthy females from birth to adulthood and in 172 Turner syndrome patients. J Clin Endocrinol Metab. 2010;95(11):5003–10.
21. Tal R, Seifer DB. Ovarian reserve testing: a user's guide. Am J Obstet Gynecol. 2017;217(2):129–40.
22. Miyoshi Y, Yasuda K, Tachibana M, Yoshida H, Miyashita E, Miyamura T, Hashii Y, Hashimoto K, Kimura T, Ozono K. Longitudinal observation of serum anti-Müllerian hormone in three girls after cancer treatment. Clin Pediatr Endocrinol. 2016;25(4):119–26.
23. Gupta AA, Lee Chong A, Deveault C, Traubici J, Maloney AM, Knight S, Lorenzo A, Allen L. Anti-Müllerian hormone in female adolescent cancer patients before, during, and after completion of therapy: a pilot feasibility study. J Pediatr Adolesc Gynecol. 2016;29(6):599–603.
24. van der Kooi AL, van den Heuvel-Eibrink MM, van Noortwijk A, Neggers SJ, Pluijm SM, van Dulmen-den Broeder E, van Dorp W, Laven JS. Longitudinal follow-up in female childhood cancer survivors: no signs of accelerated ovarian function loss. Hum Reprod. 2017;32(1):193–200.
25. van Beek RD, et al. Anti-Mullerian hormone is a sensitive serum marker for gonadal function in women treated for Hodgkin's lymphoma during childhood. J Clin Endocrinol Metab. 2007;92(10):3869–74.
26. Lie Fong S, et al. Assessment of ovarian reserve in adult childhood cancer survivors using anti-Mullerian hormone. Hum Reprod. 2009;24(4):982–90.
27. Krawczuk-Rybak M, Leszczynska E, Poznanska M, Zelazowska-Rutkowska B, Wysocka J. Anti-müllerian hormone as a sensitive marker of ovarian function in young cancer survivors. Int J Endocrinol. 2013;2013:125080.
28. Elchuri SV, Patterson BC, Brown M, Bedient C, Record E, Wasilewski-Masker K, Mertens AC, Meacham LR. Low anti-Müllerian hormone in pediatric cancer survivors in the early years after gonadotoxic therapy. J Pediatr Adolesc Gynecol. 2016;29(4):393–9.
29. Dillon KE, et al. Pretreatment antimullerian hormone levels determine rate of posttherapy ovarian reserve recovery: acute changes in ovarian reserve during and after chemotherapy. Fertil Steril. 2013;99(2):477–83.
30. Su HI. Measuring ovarian function in young cancer survivors. Minerva Endocrinol. 2010;35(4):259–70.
31. Anders C, et al. A pilot study of predictive markers of chemotherapy-related amenorrhea among premenopausal women with early stage breast cancer. Cancer Investig. 2008;26(3):286–95.
32. Birch Petersen K, et al. Ovarian reserve assessment in users of oral contraception seeking fertility advice on their reproductive lifespan. Hum Reprod. 2015;30(10):2364–75.
33. Bath LE, et al. Depletion of ovarian reserve in young women after treatment for cancer in childhood: detection by anti-Mullerian hormone, inhibin B and ovarian ultrasound. Hum Reprod. 2003;18(11):2368–74.
34. Broer SL, Broekmans FJ, Laven JS, Fauser BC. Anti-Müllerian hormone: ovarian reserve testing and its potential clinical implications. Hum Reprod Update. 2014;20(5):688–701.
35. Larsen EC, et al. Reduced ovarian function in long-term survivors of radiation- and chemotherapy-treated childhood cancer. J Clin Endocrinol Metab. 2003;88(11):5307–14.

Contraception and Menstrual Suppression for Adolescent and Young Adult Oncology Patients

Carley Zeal, Janie Benoit, and Holly R. Hoefgen

T. K. Woodruff et al. (eds.), *Textbook of Oncofertility Research and Practice*,
https://doi.org/10.1007/978-3-030-02868-8_13

Key Points

- An unintended pregnancy during cancer treatment may result in delay in therapy, teratogenic exposure, and increases in general health risks.
- A thorough discussion of indicated contraceptive methods should be undertaken with each patient, with focus placed on efficacy and safety, with an added benefit of menstrual suppression for those patients with low blood counts and those with or at risk of bone marrow suppression.
- The CDC and WHO have published Medical Eligibility Criteria for Contraceptive Use for use by healthcare providers, ranking contraceptive methods based on a four-point scale for a large number of medical conditions.
- There is special concern for increased risk of DVT/PE for patients with active cancer that is of great importance in the oncology patient population.
- Contraceptive methods are also ranked by the WHO based on efficacy, with Tier 1 most effective, long-acting methods, Tier 2 shorter-acting hormonal methods, Tier 3 barrier methods, and Tier 4 behavioral methods.

The Centers for Disease Control and Prevention adapted the World Health Organization (WHO) guidance to create the US Medical Eligibility Criteria (MEC) for Contraceptive Use, 2010 (WHO) (with updates occurring in 2011 and 2012), for use by healthcare providers. It can be found in its complete form on the CDC website in the reproductive health section (see Appendix) (▶ www.cdc.gov/reproductivehealth/UnintendedPregnancy/USMEC.htm). The US MEC ranks contraceptive methods based on a four-point scale for a large number of medical conditions [18, 60].

Categories of medical eligibility criteria for contraceptive use

1. A condition for which there is no restriction for the use of the contraceptive method
2. A condition for which the advantages of using the method generally outweigh the theoretical or proven risks
3. A condition for which the theoretical or proven risks usually outweigh the advantages of using the method
4. A condition that represents an unacceptable health risk if the contraceptive method is used

The only cancers outlined specifically are ovarian, cervical, breast, gestational trophoblastic neoplasia, and malignant hepatoma. However, there is a special designation under high risk of DVT/PE for active cancer (metastatic, on therapy, or within 6 months of clinical remission, excluding nonmelanoma skin cancer) that is also of great importance in the oncology patient population.

The WHO also classifies contraception based on efficacy into four tiers [60]:

- Tier 1: (most effective): Sterilization, implants, and intrauterine devices (IUD)
- Tier 2: Depot medroxyprogesterone acetate (DMPA) and combined hormonal methods
- Tier 3: Barrier methods
- Tier 4: Behavioral methods

Below we will outline all available methods of contraception and discuss their efficacy, safety profiles, ease of use, and common side effects. We will also note any particular concerns in the oncology population (see also ◻ Table 13.1).

Table 13.1 Contraception options

Category	Contraception	Common trade names	Failure rate[a] (%)		Continued use at 1 year (%)	ADRs	Cancer-specific issues/contraindications
			Best use	Common use			
Behavioral methods	Abstinence No method		0	0–85			Discussions should focus on counseling of more effective methods given the risk of delayed treatment and/or teratogenic concerns of oncologic treatment agents
	Coitus interruptus		4	22	46		
Barrier methods	Male condom		2	18	43	Latex or spermicide sensitivities can be seen	Also decreases the risk of STIs in this immunosuppressed patient population
	Female condom		5	21	41		
	Diaphragm		6	12	57		Diaphragm may be a viable option in hormone-sensitive cancer patients who cannot have copper IUD

Table 13.1 (continued)

Category	Contraception	Common trade names	Failure rate[a] (%)		Continued use at 1 year (%)	ADRs	Cancer-specific issues/ contraindications
			Best use	Common use			
Estrogen progestin methods	Pills	Lutera, Levora, Yaz, Sprintec, Ortho-Cyclen …	0.3	9	45–67	Increased risk of VTE Nausea/vomiting	Recommend avoidance in cancer pts if possible due to increased risk of VTE
	Transdermal patch	Xulane Ortho Evra				VTE risk similar to 35 EE COC Transient skin reactions More initial irregular VB than COC pills	Serum EE levels higher than 35 EE COC pill Not recommended for patients >90 kg
	Transvaginal ring	Nuva ring				Headache Vaginal wetness	Serum EE levels lower than most COC pills and patch
Short- or intermediate-acting progestin methods	Progestin-only pills	Norethindrone (Ortho micronor)	0.3	9	67	Uncommon: Irregular VB Headache Acne	
		DMPA (Depo-Provera)	0.2	3–6	56	Irregular VB Amenorrhea Weight gain Transient decrease in BMD	Not recommended in pts. whose treatment may/did result in decreased BMD Theoretical association with increased VTE risk; however, data limited and benefits usually outweigh risks in women with active cancer

LARC – progestin based	Progestin implant	Nexplanon	0.05	0.05	65–84	Procedural risks (rare) Bleeding, hematoma, infection Medication ADRs Unpredictable, irregular VB Headache Acne Weight gain	Irregular bleeding pattern may not be the best choice in patients with concerns for anemia
	LNG IUD	Mirena Liletta Kyleena Skyla	0.2	0.2	80	Procedural risks (minimal) Uterine perforation (1/1000), device expulsion (6%) Medication ADRs Limited irregular VB Variable rates of amenorrhea	Used for the treatment of endometrial hyperplasia and low-grade cancer May be considered for select breast cancer patients on tamoxifen Can provide effective long term contraception and menstrual lightening with minimal side effect or drug interaction Women with immunosuppression may safely use IUDs
LARC – nonhormonal	Copper IUD	ParaGard	0.8	0.6	78	Procedural risks Similar to LNG IUDs Medication ADRs May increase menstrual blood flow Irregular breakthrough VB	First line for breast cancer patients or other hormone-sensitive malignancies Less desirable if concern for anemia Provides emergency contraception and continued birth control Women with immunosuppression may safely use IUDs

ADR Adverse drug reaction, *STI* Sexually transmitted infection, *IUD* Intrauterine device, *VTE* Venous thromboembolism, *EE* Ethinyl estradiol, *COC* Combined oral contraceptive, *VB* Vaginal bleeding, *BMD* Bone mineral density, *LNG* Levonorgestrel

[a]Percentage of women experiencing unintended pregnancy within the 1st year [11]

13.1 Contraception

13.1.1 Behavioral methods

(a) Abstinence
   (i) Abstinence is a wise and safe choice at any life stage, particularly for young patients who do not feel ready for a sexual relationship. However, abstinence-only programs are ineffective in delaying sexual debut or in reducing sexual risk behaviors among teens who are already sexually active [21, 36, 57]. Comprehensive sexual education has been shown to significantly decrease teen pregnancy rates, increase age at first intercourse, and significantly increase the likelihood of contraception use at first intercourse [21, 36, 46]. Therefore, although a patient who notes abstinence as their form of contraception should be encouraged to continue, sexual health should always be part of the discussion.

(b) Noncoital sexual behaviors
   (i) Noncoital sexual behavior includes mutual masturbation, oral sex, and anal sex. It is a common expression of sexuality. The National Survey of Family Growth found that 42.4% of females aged 15–19 years have had oral sex with an opposite-sex partner [1]. Noncoital sexual behavior commonly coexists with coital behavior. Although there is little risk of pregnancy with strictly noncoital activities, given this association, contraceptive discussion is warranted. Sexually transmitted infections can be transmitted through noncoital sexual activity, and patients should be strongly counseled regarding safe sexual practices [11].

(c) Coitus interruptus/withdrawal method
   (i) This method involves the withdrawal of the penis from the vagina and away from the external genitalia prior to ejaculation. It is mentioned here as a point of discussion, as it is practiced widely, with 60% of adolescent women aged 15–19 years reporting having used the method before [1]. The failure rate of such technique is high (22% with typical use), and it does not provide protection against sexually transmitted infections [28].

13

13.1.2 Barrier methods

(a) Male condom
   (i) The male condom acts as a physical barrier, covering the penis and blocking the passage of sperm into the vagina. While it is encouraging that 97% of US teens age 15–19 report having ever used a condom for contraception, this does not speak to their consistency of use [1]. According to the 2013 youth risk behavioral surveillance system (YRBS), 41% of US high school students did not use a condom during last sexual intercourse [10]. All sexually active adolescents should be encouraged on regular condom use for the prevention of sexually transmitted infections, including HIV, as well as increased contraceptive efficacy. In typical use, the male condom alone has a failure rate of 18% [28]. For this reason, a more reliable form of contraception should be counseled as first line.

(b) Vaginal barriers/spermicides
   (i) Female condom
      1. The female condom is a soft, loose polyurethane sheath with two rings, one on either end. One ring is placed in the vagina; the other is placed outside the introitus. These devices are available over the counter. Efficacy is poor, with a typical use failure rate in the general population of 21% [28].
   (ii) Diaphragm
      1. The diaphragm is a dome-shaped flexible rubber cup. Spermicide is applied to the dome, and the device is inserted into the vagina prior to intercourse. The diaphragm must be sized and prescribed by a physician. Once in position, it can provide contraceptive protection for up to 6 h before additional spermicide is required. After intercourse, it should be left in place for at least 6 h but should not be left in place for a combined duration of longer than 24 h due to a rare risk of toxic shock syndrome. The diaphragm has a low efficacy rating with typical use

failure rates of 12%. It is not typically suggested for adolescents given lower efficacy rate and difficulty of use. However, this may be a good option in a very select subset of patients with hormone-sensitive cancers and an aversion or contraindication to the copper intrauterine device (IUD) [28].

(iii) Spermicides
   1. Spermicidal gels, creams, and foams are available for use with the diaphragm but can also be used individually for contraception. Spermicidal suppositories can be used alone or with condoms. However, efficacy is low with a typical failure rate of 28% when used alone for contraception [28]. Given the difficulty of correct usage and high failure rate, we would not commonly recommend this method for use in the adolescent population. However, it may be useful in the subset of patients for whom the diaphragm would be indicated.

13.1.3 Estrogen-containing contraceptives

The current options for combined estrogen and progestin contraceptive methods are the oral *p*ill, the transdermal *p*atch, and the vaginal *r*ing (PPR). There are many noncontraceptive benefits of using a combined regimen, including, but not limited to, the regulation of menstrual cycles and treatment of menorrhagia, dysmenorrhea, acne, and pelvic pain [2]. These regimens have been shown to decrease the risk of endometrial, ovarian, and colorectal cancers [5]. Modern formulations have minimal change in absolute breast cancer risk [45]. The basic mechanisms of action are the same for all formulations and include both inhibition of ovulation and folliculogenesis and thickening of cervical mucus. As a class, all estrogen-based contraceptives are tier 2 efficacy, with a typical use 1st-year failure rate of 9% [28]. Long-term continuation rates vary, though a large cohort study including 4708 participants reported continuation rates of 45–60% between pill, patch, and vaginal ring [22].

As a class, there is an increased risk of venous thromboembolism (VTE) that is dependent on the estrogen dose and duration and, to a lower degree, the type of synthetic progestin [27]. Although the relative risk of VTE is increased, the absolute risk for each individual user is low, as thrombosis is a rare event in the healthy young female population that commonly uses this contraceptive method. However, these combined regimens may pose a higher risk of VTE if patients are not carefully selected [28].

For the malignant diagnoses specifically listed in the MEC, PPR are noted as a category 4 (unacceptable risk) only for current breast cancer and malignant liver tumor. However, the relationship to elevated DVT/VTE risk (active cancer, or within 6 months after clinical remission, excluding nonmelanoma skin cancers), is also noted as MEC category 4. They are classified as a category 1 for ovarian cancer, endometrial cancer, and gestational trophoblastic disease and a category 2 for cervical cancer awaiting treatment. It is important to take the overall medical condition into consideration, as other conditions such as obesity, hyperlipidemia, diabetes, and liver and renal failure may be part of the medical history in chronically ill children. Similarly, it is important to note that any patient with a complicated solid organ transplant is not a candidate for estrogens (category 4), but for an uncomplicated transplant patient, estrogen-containing contraceptives are considered a category 2.

(a) Pills
   (i) Combined oral contraceptive pills (COCs) are available in a wide variety of formulations. The choice of the pill should be determined by the patient and physician based on gynecologic, sexual, and medical history, as well as patient preference. COCs are taken daily and depending on the cycling pattern chosen can be given between 21 and 90 days with a 4 to 7-day hormone-free interval for withdrawal bleeding. The use among adolescents is popular, with 56% of sexually active US teens 15–19 endorsing ever use of COCs to prevent pregnancy [1]. However, compliance and continuation may prove challenging in this age group.

(b) Patch
   (i) The contraceptive transdermal patch is a thin, flexible patch with norgestimate

and EE, which is provided at a higher dose than the standard 35 mcg COC formulations. Due to this dosage, there is a theoretical increased risk of VTE with patch, though data demonstrating the risk is conflicting [58]. The patch is applied to the buttocks, upper arm, lower abdomen, or upper torso and changed once weekly for 3 weeks, followed by a hormone-free week for withdrawal bleed. In some studies, the patch appears to enhance consistent and correct use as compared to COCs; however, their overall continuation rates and failure rates are similar. Patch users may note a transient skin reaction and more initial breakthrough bleeding than COC users; the latter effect improves with use. Patients greater than 90 kg may have a higher risk of pregnancy when using the patch [28, 56].

(c) Ring
   (i) A soft, transparent flexible ring that releases 120 mcg of etonogestrel (a major metabolite of desogestrel) and 15 mcg of EE daily. Although cases of VTE have been reported in vaginal ring users, the serum EE levels are twofold and threefold lower than those found in 35EE COCs and the birth control patch. However, there have been studies linking the progestin component of the ring to an increased risk of VTE [28, 58].

   The ring is placed vaginally once every 28 days, with the last 7 days being a ring-free timeframe to allow for withdrawal bleeding. In theory, the ease of once-monthly use should improve patient compliance and improve method success rates. However, in randomized comparative trials, the ring and COCs showed similar compliance and continuation rates. The vaginal ring has excellent cycle control, even in the first few cycles. It can be removed for up to 3 h without compromising effectiveness and is safe to use with tampons or during intercourse. The most commonly reported side effects are headache and vaginal wetness [28].

13

13.1.4 Progestin-only contraceptives

All of the progestin-only contraceptives are approved for patients at higher risk of deep venous thrombosis and pulmonary embolism (DVT/PE), such as patients with active or history of malignancy (MEC category 2) [18]. They are not associated with an increased risk of high blood pressure or cardiovascular disease. An added benefit is menstrual lightening or suppression, to different degrees depending on the formulation used. The only absolute contraindications to progestin-based medications are pregnancy and a personal history of hormone-dependent breast cancer. Progestin-only contraception may be provided as an oral medication, injectable form, or implant. Their mechanisms of action for contraception are through increased viscosity of cervical mucus, ovulatory suppression, and endometrial thinning.

(a) Progestin-only pills (norethindrone 35 mcg)
   (i) This regimen's efficacy depends on compliance with a typical use failure rate in the general population of 9% [28]. Medication should be administered at the same time or within 3 h every day, making it less than ideal for adolescents. Up to 10% of users will develop amenorrhea after 1 year of use, but 40% experience irregular cycles [63]. Side effects are uncommon but may include breakthrough bleeding, headaches, nausea, acne, and breast tenderness. The risks are minimal [28].

(b) Injectable contraceptive (depot medroxyprogesterone acetate (DMPA))
   (i) DMPA is most commonly given as a 150 mg intramuscular injection, administered every 12 weeks. It is also available in a 104 mg subcutaneous injection with identical dosing intervals [28]. Its efficacy relies on compliance with a typical use failure rate in the general population of 3–6% [28]. Up to 50% of users will develop amenorrhea after 1 year of use [63]. Side effects include initial breakthrough bleeding, weight gain, headaches, nausea, breast tenderness, acne, and mood disorder [28].

   In 2004, the FDA issued a black box warning stating that prolonged use of

DMPA may result in significant loss of bone mineral density (BMD). Following this event, the WHO collected expert reviews concluding that DMPA is associated with a risk of reversible BMD reduction during treatment, which has not been proven to increase fracture risk [15]. The American College of Obstetricians and Gynecologists (ACOG) released a Committee Opinion stating that healthcare providers should inform women and adolescents considering initiating DMPA or continuing to use the method about the benefits and the risks of DMPA and should discuss the FDA "black box" warning. However, the effect of DMPA on BMD should not prevent practitioners from prescribing DMPA or continuing use beyond 2 years [15]. The use of routine DXA scans or supplemental estrogen was not recommended in adolescent and young adult populations taking DMPA. However, discussing and recommending long-acting reversible contraception (LARC) methods that both are more efficacious and have no effect on BMD were suggested [15, 28].

DMPA has some theoretical association with a possible increased risk of deep venous thrombosis and pulmonary embolism, although benefits usually outweigh this risk in women with active cancer [17, 18, 49].

On average, patients on DMPA have a weight gain of less than 2 kg per year [8]. However, it has also been shown that certain populations, such as those that are obese or more sedentary, are more at risk for weight gain with DMPA [9, 37].

(c) Long-acting reversible contraception (LARC)

LARC methods are the most effective birth control methods with a failure rate of <1%. In September 2014, the American Academy of Pediatrics (AAP) published a new recommendation stating that the first-line contraceptive choice for adolescents who choose not to be abstinent should be a LARC method. ACOG has similarly recommended LARC for adolescents [14]. Their safety and efficacy in adolescents have been well demonstrated, and these methods are recommended for teenagers [12, 14, 20].

LARCs include intrauterine devices (IUD) and the contraceptive implant. In the Contraceptive CHOICE project, all contraceptive options were counseled and provided to participants at no cost for the duration of the 2 to 3-year project. Seventy-five percent of participants in the CHOICE project chose LARC methods; this is astounding compared to the national average of 8.5% at the time [55]. Adolescents chose LARC at similar rates to their adult counterparts (69–71%); however, the younger adolescent population appeared to favor the etonogestrel implant system [42]. A more recent analysis of the CHOICE project evaluated contraception continuation in teenagers and young women and demonstrated high rates of continuation and satisfaction with LARC, similar to that in the older adult population [24, 53]. It has also been shown that adolescents are more likely to continue LARC than non-LARC contraceptive methods [20]. The continuation rate of LARC methods in teenagers and young women has been shown to be 81% [53]. However, the use of these devices continues to be low, with only 6% of sexually active teens 15–19 years old reporting ever use of LARC methods in themselves or their partner [1].

(i) Contraceptive implants

The subdermal rod, marketed currently as Nexplanon, measures 4 cm by 2 mm and has a constant release of etonogestrel. It is currently approved for contraception at 3-year duration. The device is inserted superficially in the upper arm during a simple office procedure by a trained physician or licensed provider requiring only local anesthesia [40]. The risks of the procedure are rare but include bleeding, hematoma, and infection. The main side effects are irregular, unpredictable vaginal bleeding (50%), acne (12%), headaches

(16%), weight gain (12%), and mood disturbance (6%). About 11% of patients become amenorrheic after 1 year of use [19]. Removal requires a second small office procedure with local anesthetic and a small incision with similar risks.

Continuation rates have been shown to be higher than 80% after 1 year of use in one study [53]. Other studies have found higher discontinuation rates averaging 35%, with persistent bleeding irregularities cited as the most frequent reason for discontinuation [19].

(ii) Levonorgestrel IUDs (LNG-IUD)
This device comes in several formulations with various dosages of levonorgestrel, including Mirena (52 mg), Liletta (52 mg), Kyleena (19.5 mg), and Skyla (13.5 mg). All of these options are T-shaped and contain levonorgestrel in the barrel. They are inserted into the uterine cavity through the cervix using a speculum and indicated instruments. This is a simple office procedure in most instances.

The most commonly used LNG-IUD contains 52 mg of LNG and is marketed as Mirena with FDA approval for 5 years. Liletta has the same dose and is now also FDA approved for 5 years. Mirena releases LNG at a rate of 20 mcg/day for the first 5 years of use and gradual decrease to 10–14 mcg/day thereafter. Recent studies suggest extended efficacy to 7 years [39, 54]. Liletta releases LNG at a rate of 18.6 mcg/day for the first 3 years, with the rate decreasing to 13 mcg/day thereafter [25]. There are ongoing studies of Liletta with plans to apply for an extended approval for 7 years. The main risks are IUD expulsion (6%) [53] and uterine perforation (1/1000) [30]. It is important to clarify that overall, IUD use in teenagers is encouraged and that it does not increase the risk of PID, sexually transmitted infections (STI), or infertility [34]. Cervical screening for chlamydia and gonorrhea should be performed on all women at high risk for STIs, including all adolescents. Side effects of the LNG IUD are minimal but include limited irregular vaginal bleeding, acne, headaches, and mood disturbance. Other benefits include menstrual lightening (up to 90% of flow) or suppression (in 50% of patients at 24 months of use), alleviation of dysmenorrhea and pelvic pain, and reduction of the risk of endometrial cancer. There is limited evidence for or against IUD use in cancer-related immunocompromised patients; however, the CDC and WHO both support its use and are reassuring about its safety based on other types of immunocompromised patient data [18, 60].

A lower-dose levonorgestrel IUD became available in the United States in 2013, marketed as Skyla. This IUD contains 13.5 mg of levonorgestrel, which is initially released at a rate of 14 mcg/day that decreases to 5 mcg/day over its approved 3-year duration of use. It has a slightly smaller size and diameter, which theoretically may make it more suitable for placement in certain populations with a small uterine cavity or cervical stenosis. The low-dose levonorgestrel IUD is not currently approved for the treatment of menorrhagia and has a lower likelihood of amenorrhea (13% vs. 24%) compared with the higher-dose IUD [29, 33, 59, 62, 63].

Similarly, Kyleena contains 19.5 mg of levonorgestrel and is approved for use for pregnancy prevention for 5 years. Initially 17.5 mcg/day of levonorgestrel is released from the device, which gradually decreases to 7.4 mcg/day [33]. This is similarly marketed to a particular patient population with a smaller diameter, though with longer duration of action.

There is limited data on IUD use in patients with immunosuppression secondary to malignancy; however, there is available data from other high-risk populations (HIV positive, systemic lupus, and renal transplantation), suggesting that IUDs can be safely utilized in this population [49]. Overall, the levonorgestrel IUDs have been proven to be a highly effective birth control method that is both beneficial and safe. Nonsexually active teenagers and young adults usually tolerate insertion in the office well. Several studies have looked at pain management of office IUD insertion, and this choice is patient and provider dependent [3, 6, 47, 48]. In patients who are unable to tolerate in-office placement, such as those with special needs, the IUD can be placed under sedation or general anesthesia.

13.1.5 Nonhormonal LARC

(a) Copper IUD
The copper IUD, marketed in the United States as Copper T 380A (ParaGard), is approved for a duration of 10 years. It is the only highly effective nonhormonal contraceptive method, with a perfect and typical use failure rate of less than 1% [28]. A variety of different copper IUD types are available in other countries; in Canada, for example, the Mona Lisa N, Mona Lisa 5, and Mona Lisa 10 are each approved for 3, 5, or 10 years, respectively [7].

The Copper T 380A is a T-shaped device, with a thin copper wire wound around the stem and each arm. The copper IUD's mechanisms of action include local intrauterine inflammatory reaction, which creates an environment toxic to the sperm and ova, causing decreased sperm motility and viability and preventing fertilization primarily and implantation of the embryo secondarily and less reliably [28]. Its screening and insertion process and basic risks are similar to that of the levonorgestrel IUDs. However, common side effects are irregular breakthrough bleeding, heavier menstrual cycles (up to 50%), and dysmenorrhea, all of which should improve with time. The primary benefit is providing a reliable but rapidly reversible birth control method. It may have an additive benefit in the oncology population, as a safe and reliable form of contraception in patients with hormone-dependent malignancies.

13.2 Emergency Contraception

There is no single mechanism of action of emergency contraception (EC) [51], as it depends on the time in the menstrual cycle the medication is taken and what method is chosen. Options for emergency contraception range from high-dose combined oral contraceptive pills (the Yuzpe method), single- or multidose progestin methods (levonorgestrel or ulipristal), or placement of a copper IUD. Specific regimens can be found in ◻ Table 13.2 [35] and are most effective 0–72 h after intercourse with moderate efficacy up to 5 days [51]. According to the US MEC, given the associated complications and comorbidities of pregnancy and the short-term use of EC methods, there are absolutely no instances in which the risks outweigh the benefits of use [18]. Therefore, this option should always be considered and discussed in adolescent oncology patients. Given the urgency of timing for effective treatment following unprotected intercourse, it is imperative to begin this conversation before the need arises, such as during a general sexual health discussion. Several barriers to the use of EC have been noted in adolescents including knowledge of the option of EC in general, understanding of the use and safety of the medications, and cost barriers. Further barriers relate to difficulty of accessing medications from providers and pharmacies, where staff may not approve of or understand the laws regarding EC use in younger patients [13]. It is important to understand the exact prescribing laws for EC and adolescents as they apply in your particular state (▶ http://www.guttmacher.org/statecenter/spibs/spib_EC.pdf).

Table 13.2 Emergency contraception treatment regimens

Method	Dosing	Efficacy
Estrogen plus progestin (Yuzpe regimen)	100–120 mcg ethinyl estradiol plus 500–600 mcg levonorgestrel in each dose, given twice, 12 h apart	47–89% pregnancy prevention
[a]Levonorgestrel	0.75 mg given twice, 12 h apart, or 1.5 mg given as a single dose	59–94% pregnancy prevention
Ulipristal	30 mg dose orally ×1	98–99%
Copper intrauterine device	Inserted within 120 h after intercourse	At least 99%

EC is best used as soon as possible after unprotected intercourse
[a]Use up to 72 h after unprotected intercourse. All other methods use up to 120 h after unprotected intercourse [49]

13.3 Survivors

13

It has been shown that, in general, centers caring for adolescent and young adult (AYA) oncology patients do not routinely discuss sexual health with their patients; therefore, survivors have limited awareness of the contraceptive options available to them [49]. Even though specific data is not available for unintended pregnancy among cancer survivors, we do know that survivors in the 15 to 30-year-old range are more likely than their peers to terminate a pregnancy [26, 61]. For patients who have been cancer-free for at least 6 months and are without a history of chest wall radiation, hormonally mediated cancers, anemia, osteoporosis, or VTE, the use of all the above-noted contraception options is available. Patients with a history of chest wall radiation are at an increased risk of breast cancer and may not be candidates for exogenous hormones; therefore, the copper IUD would be first line in these patients. However, some physicians will allow modern hormone formulations, as the overall risk of breast cancer is low. In general, the important point to note is that AYA individuals with cancer need to be aware of their sexual health options during all stages of their diagnosis and treatment, and all healthcare providers should become comfortable with, at a minimum, asking the relevant questions [49].

13.4 Menstrual Regulation and Suppression

Adolescent and young adult oncology patients are at a particularly elevated risk of menorrhagia (heavy menstrual bleeding) directly from hematologic malignancy or secondarily related to treatment-induced thrombocytopenia. In other adolescent oncology patients, with normal menstrual flow and previous anemia or bothersome dysmenorrhea, providing relief of menstrual-related symptoms may also be a crucial aspect of management [16]. Gynecologists may be asked to consult on patients prophylactically prior to initiation of treatment to determine a menstrual suppression plan or in times of acute hemorrhage [16]. Options for medical management differ in these situations and are discussed below and reviewed in Table 13.3.

Certain factors should be considered in oncology patients separate from general menstrual suppression in other populations. One major issue includes a severe decrease in platelet levels, which may impair use of medications with initial breakthrough bleeding or use of intramuscular injections due to an elevated risk of hematoma formation. Clinicians should also carefully review the individual patients' VTE risk prior to consideration of hormonal therapy, especially estrogen-based medications. The overall aim of treatment is for high efficacy with minimal risk of harm [16, 43]. As discussed above, providers should be open with adolescents and young adults on their need for contraception and consider this in their choice of menstrual suppression options.

13.4.1 GnRH Agonist

GnRH agonist for the purpose of menstrual suppression is most commonly given as an injectable intramuscular (IM) medication, which offers a high amenorrhea rate (73–96%) [52]. This medication has been proven to be superior to DMPA in preventing moderate to severe bleeding in young women undergoing myelosuppressive chemotherapy with subsequent severe thrombocytopenia [41]. In patients with severe thrombocytopenia in whom IM injections are contraindicated secondary to concern

Table 13.3 Treatment of acute menstrual bleeding and menstrual suppression in oncology patients

Class	Medication	Acute vaginal bleeding management	Maintenance/menstrual suppression	Menstrual suppression amenorrhea rates	Comments
GnRH agonist	Leuprolide acetate	N/A	3.75–7.25 mg IM monthly	73–96% w/ rapid onset	GnRH treatment best started 4 weeks prior to expected thrombocytopenia to avoid BTB of flare effect
			11.25–22.5 mg IM Q3 months		Q3 months injections decrease risk of more frequent injections in thrombocytopenic patients
			Intratreatment options for patients with severe thrombocytopenia: 3.75 mg SQ month SQ formulation given 1 mg/day IV until return of platelet count to allow for safe injections		Advantages: lower risk VTE, inconclusive data shows possible advantage of ovarian protection Disadvantages: Hypoestrogenic state (vasomotor symptoms and bone density loss), risk of injection site hematoma Hormonal add-back therapy recommended, most commonly with norethindrone 5 mg PO daily
Estrogen	Conjugated estrogen (Premarin)	1.25 mg PO 2–3 times daily	N/A		[a]Evaluate patient for safety of estrogen use, risk of VTE. Consider alternative options.
	Estradiol	2 mg PO 2–3 times daily			Utilize minimum dose for the shortest duration necessary, IV therapy not commonly used >24 h
	Conjugated estrogen (IV)	25 mg IV Q6 h × 24 h			N/V common, utilize antiemetic
Estrogen/progestin	Combined oral contraceptive pills	One tablet PO 1–4 times daily (taper)	One tablet daily continuous	Great variation 88% at 12 months	[a]Evaluate patient for safety of estrogen use, risk of VTE. Consider alternative options
		35 mcg EE pill PO 3× daily × 7 days			N/V common with acute regimen, can utilize antiemetic
		50 mcg (equivalent) EE PO two pills daily			May not be as effective as E alone for the management of acute HMB
	Contraceptive patch	2 patches × 7 days, then 1 patch daily	Weekly patch continuous		Also provides a contraception method
	Contraceptive vaginal ring	N/A	Q3 week ring change continuous		Two contraceptive patches result in an estrogen level roughly equal to two 100 EE COCs, likely elevating VTE risk above other regimens

(continued)

Table 13.3 (continued)

Class	Medication	Acute vaginal bleeding management	Maintenance/menstrual suppression	Menstrual suppression amenorrhea rates	Comments
Progestin	Medroxyprogesterone acetate	20–40 mg/day PO (DD) 5 mg PO Q1–2 h × 24 h –> 20 mg/day × 10 days 20 mg PO three times daily × 3 days –> 20 mg/day for 3 weeks 20 mg PO 3 times daily × 7 days	No recommendation		Progestin-only pill regimens may not be as effective as E-based methods for the management of acute HMB Progestins can have some increased risk of VTE (not to the extent of E), but benefits are considered to outweigh risks in most patients Norethindrone 0.35 mg also provides a contraception method
	Norethindrone acetate	5–20 mg/day PO (DD)	5–15 mg/day PO (DD)		
	Megestrol acetate	40–120 mg/daily (DD)	20–40 mg/day PO (DD)		
	Norethindrone	N/A	0.35 mg/day PO	10% with continuous norethindrone	
	Depot medroxyprogesterone acetate (DMPA)	N/A	150 mg IM Q3 months 104 mg SQ Q3 months	12% at 3 months 50% at 12 months	Initial irregular vaginal bleeding may preclude use in some patients Theoretical increased VTE risk above other progestin-only regimens. Benefit usually outweighs risk Also provides a highly effective contraceptive method
	Levonorgestrel intrauterine device (LNG IUD)	N/A	52 mg LNG IUD insertion every 5 years (several other dosages noted in the chapter)	50% at 12–24 months 60% at 5 years	Initial irregular vaginal bleeding may preclude use in some patients [b]Women with immunosuppression may safely use IUDs Also provides a highly effective contraceptive method

IM Intramuscular, *SQ* Subcutaneous, *PO* By mouth, *IV* Intravenous, *VTE* Venous thromboembolism, *BTB* Breakthrough bleeding, *N/A* Not applicable, *N/V* Nausea and vomiting, *DD* In divided doses, *E* Estrogen, *HMB* Heavy menstrual bleeding, *mcg* Micrograms, *EE* Ethinyl estradiol

[a]Estrogen therapy for acute management and menstrual suppression must weigh the need for the management of vaginal bleeding and the elevated risk of thromboembolism in patients with active treatment of malignancy. Consider alternative (lower risk options) first where appropriate

[b]Based on available data from other high-risk populations (HIV positive, systemic lupus, and renal transplantation)

for hematoma, subcutaneous and intravenous regimens of leuprolide have been described and are usually given until return of platelet count to a level that is safe for regular intramuscular injection regimen. Specific regimens are listed in Table 13.3 [16].

Breakthrough bleeding for the first 2–3 weeks after initial injection is common as a result of the initial increase in FSH and LH secretion. At roughly 2 weeks, a hypogonadal effect is achieved through receptor downregulation. Due to this "flare effect," it is recommended to start GnRH agonist therapy prior to myelosuppressive therapy preferable at least 4 weeks before expected thrombocytopenia [16]. Another potential benefit to ovarian suppression with GnRH agonists that has been widely discussed is a decreased risk of premature ovarian failure in patient undergoing gonadotoxic chemotherapy, though data is mixed [31]. Due to this, current guidelines recommend patients be informed that there is insufficient evidence showing that ovarian suppression via the use of GnRH analogs protects fertility and that this should not be relied upon for this indication [38].

Possible side effects of treatment are hot flushes, insomnia, joint pain, weight gain, and mood disturbance. The main risks of GnRH agonists are a decrease in bone mineral density (BMD) and local contusion or hematoma at the injection site [16]. Consideration should be given for immediate add-back therapy to prevent vasomotor symptoms and negative impact on BMD. Options of add-back therapies include norethindrone acetate 5–10 mg daily or very low-dose estradiol with progestin. Norethindrone acetate is a progestin with estrogenic action, which has been shown to be as effective as low-dose estradiol in the prevention of decreasing BMD and vasomotor symptoms, without an increased thromboembolic risk [23].

Due to its side effect profile and potential effects on BMD with long-term use, it is recommended that menstrual suppression using GnRH agonists be limited to the duration of chemotherapy treatment and/or while patients remain at elevated risk for anemia secondary to treatment or malignancy [50].

13.4.2 Estrogens

In patients with malignancy, estrogen-based medications can increase the risk of deep venous thrombosis and pulmonary embolism. However, women with prolonged heavy menstrual bleeding and elevated risks from continued and worsening thrombocytopenia may benefit from estrogen medications for endometrial stabilization, particularly in the acute setting. Commonly used estrogen-only regimens for treatment of acute heavy menstrual bleeding are listed in Table 13.3 [16]. Due to the above-noted risks, providers should evaluate each patient's individual risk factors for VTE in conjunction with ongoing menstrual bleeding risks to determine the best management strategy. In all patients, providers should attempt to limit the duration and dose of estrogen medications to the minimum required for menstrual bleeding control with timely transition to lower risk medications.

In addition, it is important to consider that patients are likely to experience nausea and emesis during the course of their malignancy and treatment, which may be exacerbated by estrogen regimens. Therefore, regimens are often utilized in combination with an antiemetic [43].

13.4.3 Combined Hormonal Contraception (CHC) (Pill, Patch, Ring)

As noted above, the use of estrogen-based therapies for acute heavy menstrual bleeding management and preventative menstrual suppression must weigh the need for the treatment of vaginal bleeding concerns and its sequela with the elevated risk of thromboembolism in patients with active treatment of malignancy. In patients whom estrogen-based medications are deemed safe, the use of higher dose regimens of combined oral contraceptives has been shown to decrease moderate to severe vaginal bleeding within 48 h. However, this may be less effective than estrogen alone due to progestin inhibition of estrogen receptor synthesis, increased estradiol dehydrogenase, and less endometrial proliferation induction via estrogen [43].

Combined hormonal contraceptives can also be taken in extended regimens without taking the hormone-free intervals for long-term preventative menstrual suppression. About 88% of women noted light bleeding to amenorrhea after 1 year of use. There is an increased risk of breakthrough bleeding with these protocols with suggestion to stop hormonal pills for roughly 5 days when breakthrough bleeding occurs to allow for withdraw bleed

[16, 44]. Common regimens for acute and preventative CHC protocols are listed in ◘ Table 13.3.

Although data and recommendations are somewhat limited for the use of estrogen-based medications in patients with malignancy, the risk of VTE should not be understated. Given these risk-benefit considerations, CHCs are rarely used for this indication in this specific population, and data is limited regarding an ideal choice of agent. As there are other highly efficacious methods for menstrual suppression and/or contraception available, it is our practice to utilize other methods (GnRH agonists, progestin-only methods) as first line in this patient population. Careful consideration between gynecology and oncology teams is recommended on a case-specific basis.

13.4.4 Progestin-Only Pills

In patients who cannot or should not utilize estrogen-based medications, progestin-only pills (POP) can be given in various formulations and dosages for both acute menstrual bleeding and for long-term menstrual lightening or suppression. Amenorrhea is achieved in 76% of patients in 3 days compared to 88% with COCs, with less risk of VTE than estrogen-based medications [4]. Possible side effects are acne, weight gain, headache, lipid profile changes, and mood disturbance and are dose dependent. Commonly used regimens are listed in ◘ Table 13.3 [4, 16, 43]. Only norethindrone 0.35 mg is approved for use as a birth control method, and it has a documented amenorrhea rate of 10% [7].

13

13.4.5 Depot Medroxyprogesterone Acetate

This injectable hormonal contraceptive can also be used for menstrual lightening and suppression. Roughly 12% of DMPA users report being amenorrheic 3 months after their initial injection, with 50% amenorrhea rates after 1 year of use, though initial irregular vaginal bleeding is common [16, 32]. Patients with a high risk of low blood count, including anemia and thrombocytopenia, due to their malignancy or treatment regimens may not tolerate initial irregular bleeding.

13.4.6 Levonorgestrel IUD for Menstrual Suppression

The 52 mg levonorgestrel IUD can be used for menstrual lightening and suppression; however, these desired side effects develop over time in a subset of users. Menstrual lightening (up to 90% of flow) is identified in a majority of patients, with suppression noted in 50% of patients at 24 months of use [32]. There is an initial risk of light irregular menstrual bleeding for the first 3–6 months after insertion, which again may not be ideal in all patients. However, the additional benefit of highly reliable contraception with minimal to no drug-drug interaction and no further medical intervention (such as daily pills or routine injections) may outweigh this risk in selected patients. If a patient has already established menstrual lightening or suppression with a levonorgestrel IUD in place at the time of her diagnosis of malignancy, it is recommended to leave the device in place [16]. Other formulations of LNG-IUD have decreased rates of amenorrhea likely due to decreased doses of LNG. LNG-IUD 19.5 (Kyleena) results in amenorrhea in 12% at the end of 1 year, and 23% at 5 years. LNG-IUD 13.5 (Skyla) results in amenorrhea in 6% at 1 year and 12% at 2 years [29, 33]. These similarly have an initial period of bleeding irregularities [63].

One may also consider using another therapeutic option for acute menstrual suppression, such as high-dose oral progestin, in conjunction with the 52 mg levonorgestrel IUD for longer-term menstrual control and possibly contraception. These multidrug regimens are best considered in consultation with gynecology or other providers with expertise in management of these medications.

13.4.7 Other Considerations

Antifibrinolytic medications, such as tranexamic acid, prevent fibrin degradation and have been found effective for use in patients with chronic abnormal uterine bleeding and intraoperative bleeding. It is thought effective for the management of acute abnormal uterine bleeding, though it has not been specifically studied for this purpose [4]. Tranexamic acid is contraindicated in patients with active or previous history of thromboembolic disease or those with an intrinsic risk of thromboembolic disease. There is limited and contradictory evidence for its use in patients with malignancy. More data is needed on its use in the adolescent and young adult oncology population [16].

Surgical interventions in adolescent and young adult patients are considered, in close consultation with gynecology and the primary oncology team, only in the setting of severe and life-threatening hemorrhage that is unresponsive to medical management. These include dilation and curettage, uterine packing or tamponade, uterine artery embolization, or hysterectomy and are based on data extrapolated from adult women [16].

Appendix: Medical Eligibility Criteria for Contraceptive Use

Summary Chart of U.S. Medical Eligibility Criteria for Contraceptive Use

Condition	Sub-Condition	CHC	POP	Injection	Implant	LNG IUD	Cu-IUD
		I C	I C	I C	I C	I C	I C
Age		Menarche to <40=1	Menarche to <18=1	Menarche to <18=2	Menarche to <18=1	Menarche to <20=2	Menarche to <20=2
		≥40=2	18-45=1	18-45=1	18-45=1	≥20=1	≥20=1
			>45=1	>45=2	>45=1		
Anatomic abnormalities	a) Distorted uterine cavity					4	4
	b) Other abnormalities					2	2
Anemias	a) Thalassemia	1	1	1	1	1	2
	b) Sickle cell disease‡	2	1	1	1	1	2
	c) Iron-deficiency anemia	1	1	1	1	1	2
Benign ovarian tumors	*(including cysts)*	1	1	1	1	1	1
Breast disease	a) Undiagnosed mass	2*	2*	2*	2*	2	1
	b) Benign breast disease	1	1	1	1	1	1
	c) Family history of cancer	1	1	1	1	1	1
	d) Breast cancer‡						
	i) current	4	4	4	4	4	1
	ii) past and no evidence of current disease for 5 years	3	3	3	3	3	1
Breastfeeding *(see also Postpartum)*	a) <1 month postpartum	3*	2*	2*	2*		
	b) 1 month or more postpartum	2*	1*	1*	1*		
Cervical cancer	Awaiting treatment	2	1	2	2	4 2	4 2
Cervical ectropion		1	1	1	1	1	1
Cervical intraepithelial neoplasia		2	1	2	2	2	1
Cirrhosis	a) Mild *(compensated)*	1	1	1	1	1	1
	b) Severe‡ *(decompensated)*	4	3	3	3	3	1
Deep venous thrombosis (DVT)/Pulmonary embolism (PE)	a) History of DVT/PE, not on anticoagulant therapy						
	i) higher risk for recurrent DVT/PE	4	2	2	2	2	1
	ii) lower risk for recurrent DVT/PE	3	2	2	2	2	1
	b) Acute DVT/PE	4	2	2	2	2	2
	c) DVT/PE and established on anticoagulant therapy for at least 3 months						
	i) higher risk for recurrent DVT/PE	4*	2	2	2	2	2
	ii) lower risk for recurrent DVT/PE	3*	2	2	2	2	2
	d) Family history *(first-degree relatives)*	2	1	1	1	1	1
	e) Major surgery						
	i) with prolonged immobilization	4	2	2	2	2	1
	ii) without prolonged immobilization	2	1	1	1	1	1
	f) Minor surgery without immobilization	1	1	1	1	1	1
Depressive disorders		1*	1*	1*	1*	1*	1*
Diabetes mellitus (DM)	a) History of gestational DM only	1	1	1	1	1	1
	b) Non-vascular disease						
	i) non-insulin dependent	2	2	2	2	2	1
	ii) insulin dependent‡	2	2	2	2	2	1
	c) Nephropathy/retinopathy/neuropathy‡	3/4*	2	3	2	2	1
	d) Other vascular disease or diabetes of >20 years' duration‡	3/4*	2	3	2	2	1

Condition	Sub-Condition	CHC I	CHC C	POP I	POP C	Injection I	Injection C	Implant I	Implant C	LNG-IUD I	LNG-IUD C	Cu-IUD I	Cu-IUD C
Endometrial cancer‡		1		1		1		1		4	2	4	2
Endometrial hyperplasia		1		1		1		1		1		1	
Endometriosis		1		1		1		1		1		2	
Epilepsy‡	(*see also Drug Interactions*)	1*		1*		1*		1*		1		1	
Gallbladder disease	a) Symptomatic												
	i) treated by cholecystectomy	2		2		2		2		2		1	
	ii) medically treated	3		2		2		2		2		1	
	iii) current	3		2		2		2		2		1	
	b) Asymptomatic	2		2		2		2		2		1	
Gestational trophoblastic disease	a) Decreasing or undetectable ß-hCG levels	1		1		1		1		3		3	
	b) Persistently elevated ß-hCG levels or malignant disease‡	1		1		1		1		4		4	
Headaches	a) Non-migrainous	1*	2*	1*	1*	1*	1*	1*	1*	1*	1*	1*	
	b) Migraine												
	i) without aura, age <35	2*	3*	1*	2*	2*	2*	2*	2*	2*	2*	1*	
	ii) without aura, age ≥35	3*	4*	1*	2*	2*	2*	2*	2*	2*	2*	1*	
	iii) with aura, any age	4*	4*	2*	3*	2*	3*	2*	3*	2*	3*	1*	
History of bariatric surgery‡	a) Restrictive procedures	1		1		1		1		1		1	
	b) Malabsorptive procedures	COCs: 3 P/R: 1		3		1		1		1		1	
History of cholestasis	a) Pregnancy-related	2		1		1		1		1		1	
	b) Past COC-related	3		2		2		2		2		1	
History of high blood pressure during pregnancy		2		1		1		1		1		1	
History of pelvic surgery		1		1		1		1		1		1	
Human immunodeficiency virus (HIV)	High risk	1		1		1*		1		2	2	2	2
	HIV infected (*see also Drug Interactions*)‡	1*		1*		1*		1*		2	2	2	2
	AIDS (*see also Drug Interactions*)‡	1*		1*		1*		1*		3	2*	3	2*
	Clinically well on therapy	*If on treatment, see Drug Interactions*								2	2	2	2
Hyperlipidemias		2/3*		2*		2*		2*		2*		1*	
Hypertension	a) Adequately controlled hypertension	3*		1*		2*		1*		1		1	
	b) Elevated blood pressure levels (*properly taken measurements*)												
	i) systolic 140-159 or diastolic 90-99	3		1		2		1		1		1	
	ii) systolic ≥160 or diastolic ≥100‡	4		2		3		2		2		1	
	c) Vascular disease	4		2		3		2		2		1	
Inflammatory bowel disease	(*Ulcerative colitis, Crohn's disease*)	2/3*		2		2		1		1		1	

13

Abbreviations: C=continuation of contraceptive method; CHC=combined hormonal contraceptive (pill, patch, and ring); COC=combined oral contraceptive; Cu-IUD=copper-containing intrauterine device; I=initiation of contraceptive method; LNG-IUD=levonorgestrel-releasing intrauterine device; NA=not applicable; POP=progestin-only pill; P/R=patch/ring.

Legend:

1	No restriction (*method can be used*)	3	Theoretical or proven risks usually outweigh the advantages
2	Advantages generally outweigh theoretical or proven risks	4	Unacceptable health risk (*method not to be used*)

Centers for Disease Control and Prevention
National Center for Chronic Disease Prevention and Health Promotion

Summary Chart of U.S. Medical Eligibility Criteria for Contraceptive Use

Condition	Sub-Condition	CHC		POP		Injection		Implant		LNG-IUD		Cu-IUD	
		I	C	I	C	I	C	I	C	I	C	I	C
Ischemic heart disease‡	Current and history of	4		2	3	3		2	3	2	3	1	
Liver tumors	a) Benign												
	i) Focal nodular hyperplasia	2		2		2		2		2		1	
	ii) Hepatocellular adenoma‡	4		3		3		3		3		1	
	b) Malignant‡	4		3		3		3		3		1	
Malaria		1		1		1		1		1		1	
Multiple risk factors for arterial cardiovascular disease	(*such as older age, smoking, diabetes and hypertension*)	3/4*		2*		3*		2*		2		1	
Obesity	a) ≥30 kg/m² body mass index (BMI)	2		1		1		1		1		1	
	b) Menarche to <18 years and ≥30 kg/m² BMI	2		1		2		1		1		1	
Ovarian cancer‡		1		1		1		1		1		1	
Parity	a) Nulliparous	1		1		1		1		2		2	
	b) Parous	1		1		1		1		1		1	
Past ectopic pregnancy		1		2		1		1		1		1	
Pelvic inflammatory disease	a) Past, (*assuming no current risk factors of sexually transmitted infections [STIs]*)												
	i) with subsequent pregnancy	1		1		1		1		1	1	1	1
	ii) without subsequent pregnancy	1		1		1		1		2	2	2	2
	b) Current	1		1		1		1		4	2*	4	2*
Peripartum cardiomyopathy‡	a) Normal or mildly impaired cardiac function												
	i) <6 months	4		1		1		1		2		2	
	ii) ≥6 months	3		1		1		1		2		2	
	b) Moderately or severely impaired cardiac function	4		2		2		2		2		2	
Postabortion	a) First trimester	1*		1*		1*		1*		1*		1*	
	b) Second trimester	1*		1*		1*		1*		2		2	
	c) Immediately post-septic abortion	1*		1*		1*		1*		4		4	
Postpartum (*see also Breastfeeding*)	a) <21 days	4		1		1		1					
	b) 21 days to 42 days												
	i) with other risk factors for venous thromboembolism (VTE)	3*		1		1		1					
	ii) without other risk factors for VTE	2		1		1		1					
	c) >42 days	1		1		1		1					
Postpartum (*in breastfeeding or non-breastfeeding women, including post-cesarean section*)	a) <10 minutes after delivery of the placenta									2		1	
	b) 10 minutes after delivery of the placenta to <4 weeks									2		2	
	c) ≥4 weeks									1		1	
	d) Puerperal sepsis									4		4	
Pregnancy		NA*		NA*		NA*		NA*		4*		4*	
Rheumatoid arthritis	a) On immunosuppressive therapy	2		1		2/3*		1		2	1	2	1
	b) Not on immunosuppressive therapy	2		1		2		1		1		1	
Schistosomiasis	a) Uncomplicated	1		1		1		1		1		1	
	b) Fibrosis of the liver‡	1		1		1		1		1		1	
Severe dysmenorrhea		1		1		1		1		1		2	

Condition	Sub-Condition	CHC I	CHC C	POP I	POP C	Injection I	Injection C	Implant I	Implant C	LNG-IUD I	LNG-IUD C	Cu-IUD I	Cu-IUD C
Sexually Transmitted Infections (STI)	a) Current purulent cervicitis or chlamydial infection or gonorrhea	1		1		1		1		4	2*	4	2*
	b) Other STIs (*excluding HIV and hepatitis*)	1		1		1		1		2	2	2	2
	c) Vaginitis (*including trichomonas vaginalis and bacterial vaginosis*)	1		1		1		1		2	2	2	2
	d) Increased risk of STIs	1		1		1		1		2/3*	2	2/3*	2
Smoking	a) Age <35	2		1		1		1		1		1	
	b) Age ≥35, <15 cigarettes/day	3		1		1		1		1		1	
	c) Age ≥35, ≥15 cigarettes/day	4		1		1		1		1		1	
Solid organ transplantation‡	a) Complicated	4		2		2		2		3	2	3	2
	b) Uncomplicated	2*		2		2		2		2		2	
Stroke‡	History of cerebrovascular accident	4		2	3	3		2	3	2		1	
Superficial venous thrombosis	a) Varicose veins	1		1		1		1		1		1	
	b) Superficial thrombophlebitis	2		1		1		1		1		1	
Systemic lupus erythematosus‡	a) Positive (*or unknown*) antiphospholipid antibodies	4		3		3	3	3		3		1	1
	b) Severe thrombocytopenia	2		2		3	2	2		2*		3*	2*
	c) Immunosuppressive treatment	2		2		2	2	2		2		2	1
	d) None of the above	2		2		2	2	2		2		1	1
Thrombogenic mutations‡		4*		2*		2*		2*		2*		1*	
Thyroid disorders	Simple goiter/hyperthyroid/hypothyroid	1		1		1		1		1		1	
Tuberculosis‡ (*see also Drug Interactions*)	a) Non-pelvic	1*		1*		1*		1*		1		1	
	b) Pelvic	1*		1*		1*		1*		4	3	4	3
Unexplained vaginal bleeding	(*suspicious for serious condition*) before evaluation	2*		2*		3*		3*		4*	2*	4*	2*
Uterine fibroids		1		1		1		1		2		2	
Valvular heart disease	a) Uncomplicated	2		1		1		1		1		1	
	b) Complicated‡	4		1		1		1		1		1	
Vaginal bleeding patterns	a) Irregular pattern without heavy bleeding	1		2		2		2		1	1	1	
	b) Heavy or prolonged bleeding	1*		2*		2*		2*		1*	2*	2*	
Viral hepatitis	a) Acute or flare	3/4*	2	1		1		1		1		1	
	b) Carrier/Chronic	1	1	1		1		1		1		1	
Drug Interactions													
Antiretroviral therapy	a) Nucleoside reverse transcriptase inhibitors	1*		1		1		1		2/3*	2*	2/3*	2*
	b) Non-nucleoside reverse transcriptase inhibitors	2*		2*		1		2*		2/3*	2*	2/3*	2*
	c) Ritonavir-boosted protease inhibitors	3*		3*		1		2*		2/3*	2*	2/3*	2*
Anticonvulsant therapy	a) Certain anticonvulsants (*phenytoin, carbamazepine, barbiturates, primidone, topiramate, oxcarbazepine*)	3*		3*		1		2*		1		1	
	b) Lamotrigine	3*		1		1		1		1		1	
Antimicrobial therapy	a) Broad spectrum antibiotics	1		1		1		1		1		1	
	b) Antifungals	1		1		1		1		1		1	
	c) Antiparasitics	1		1		1		1		1		1	
	d) Rifampicin or rifabutin therapy	3*		3*		1		2*		1		1	

13

Please see the complete guidance for a clarification to this classification. ‡Condition that exposes a woman to increased risk as a result of unintended pregnancy. Updated June 2012.
This summary sheet only contains a subset of the recommendations from the *U.S. Medical Eligibility Criteria for Contraceptive Use*, 2010. For complete guidance, see: http://www.cdc.gov/reproductivehealth/unintendedpregnancy/USMEC.htm.

Review Questions and Answers

Q1. Which of the following describes the CDC medical eligibility criteria for contraceptive use category 2?
(a) A condition for which there is no restriction for the use of the contraceptive method
(b) A condition that represents an unacceptable health risk if the contraceptive method is used
(c) A condition for which the advantages of using the method generally outweigh the theoretical or proven risks
(d) A condition for which the theoretical or proven risks usually outweigh the advantages of using the method

A1. (c)

Q2. When weighing the risks of administration of estrogen or estrogen-containing contraceptives to control acute heavy vaginal bleeding in a patient with chemotherapy-induced thrombocytopenia, we should consider…
(a) Volume of bleeding and hemodynamic stability
(b) Thromboembolic risks
(c) Relative medical risks of alternative therapies
(d) All of the above

A2. (d)

Q3. According to American Academy of Pediatrics (AAP) published recommendation, what is the first-line contraceptive choice for adolescents who choose not to be abstinent?
(a) Barrier methods
(b) Injectable contraceptive (depot medroxyprogesterone acetate – DMPA)
(c) Long-acting reversible contraceptive (LARC)
(d) Combined hormonal contraceptives (pill, patch, ring)

A3. (c)

Q4. Which of the following clinical scenarios would be a contraindication to the use of emergency contraception 1 day following unprotected intercourse?
(a) An adolescent girl in active treatment for leukemia
(b) A young adult woman with known liver disease
(c) A teenage female, 2 months after BMT for sickle cell disease
(d) There are no instances in which the risks outweigh the benefits of use

A4. (d)

References

1. Abma JC, Martinez GM. Sexual activity and contraceptive use among teenagers in the United States, 2011–2015. Natl Health Stat Report. 2017;104:1–23.
2. ACOG Practice Bulletin No. 110: noncontraceptive uses of hormonal contraceptives (2010). Obstet Gynecol. 115 (1):206–18. https://doi.org/10.1097/AOG.0b013e3181cb50b5
3. Akers AY, Steinway C, Sonalkar S, Perriera LK, Schreiber C, Harding J, Garcia-Espana JF. Reducing pain during intrauterine device insertion: a randomized controlled trial in adolescents and young women. Obstet Gynecol. 2017;130(4):795–802. https://doi.org/10.1097/AOG.0000000000002242.
4. American College of O, Gynecologists. ACOG commit tee opinion no. 557: management of acute abnormal uterine bleeding in nonpregnant reproductive-aged women. Obstet Gynecol. 2013;121(4):891–6. https://doi.org/10.1097/01.AOG.0000428646.67925.9a.
5. Bassuk SS, Manson JE. Oral contraceptives and menopausal hormone therapy: relative and attributable risks of cardiovascular disease, cancer, and other health outcomes. Ann Epidemiol. 2015;25(3):193–200. https://doi.org/10.1016/j.annepidem.2014.11.004.
6. Bednarek PH, Creinin MD, Reeves MF, Cwiak C, Espey E, Jensen JT, Post-Aspiration IUDRSTG. Prophylactic ibuprofen does not improve pain with IUD insertion: a randomized trial. Contraception. 2015;91(3):193–7. https://doi.org/10.1016/j.contraception.2014.11.012.
7. Black AFD, Rowe T, Collins J, Miller D, Brown T, David M, Dunn S, Fisher WA, Fleming N, Fortin CA, Guilbert E, Hanvey L, Lalonde A, Miller R, Morris M, O'Grady T, Pymar H, Smith T, Henneberg E, Society of Obstetrics and Gynaecology of Canada. Canadian contraception concensus. J Obstet Gynaecol Can. 2004;26(4):347–87.. 389–436
8. Bonny AE, Lange HL, Rogers LK, Gothard DM, Reed MD. A pilot study of depot medroxyprogesterone acetate pharmacokinetics and weight gain in adolescent females. Contraception. 2014;89(5):357–60. https://doi.org/10.1016/j.contraception.2014.01.017.
9. Bonny AE, Ziegler J, Harvey R, Debanne SM, Secic M, Cromer BA. Weight gain in obese and nonobese adolescent girls initiating depot medroxyprogesterone, oral contraceptive pills, or no hormonal contraceptive method. Arch Pediatr Adolesc Med. 2006;160(1):40–5. https://doi.org/10.1001/archpedi.160.1.40.
10. Brener N, Kann L, Shanklin S. Methodology of the youth risk behavior surveillance system – 2013. MMWR Recomm Rep (Morb Mortal Wkly Rep Recomm Rep/Centers Dis Control). 2013;62(RR01):1–20.
11. Committee on Adolescent Health C, Committee on Gynecologic P. Committee opinion no. 582: addressing health risks of noncoital sexual activity. Obstet Gynecol. 2013;122(6):1378–82. https://doi.org/10.1097/01.AOG.0000438963.23732.80.

12. Committee on Adolescent Health Care Long-Acting Reversible Contraception Working Group TACoO, Gynecologists. Committee opinion no. 539: adolescents and long-acting reversible contraception: implants and intrauterine devices. Obstet Gynecol. 2012;120(4):983–8. https://doi.org/10.1097/AOG.0b013e3182723b7d.
13. Committee on Health Care for Underserved W. Committee opinion no 707: access to emergency contraception. Obstet Gynecol. 2017;130(1):e48–52. https://doi.org/10.1097/AOG.0000000000002162.
14. Committee on Practice Bulletins-Gynecology L-ARCWG. Practice bulletin no. 186: long-acting reversible contraception: implants and intrauterine devices. Obstet Gynecol. 2017;130(5):e251–69. https://doi.org/10.1097/AOG.0000000000002400.
15. Committee Opinion No. 602. Depot medroxyprogesterone acetate and bone effects. Obstet Gynecol. 2014;123(6):1398–402. https://doi.org/10.1097/01.AOG.0000450758.95422.c8.
16. Committee opinion no. 606: Options for prevention and management of heavy menstrual bleeding in adolescent patients undergoing cancer treatment. Obstet Gynecol. 2014;124(2 Pt 1):397–402. https://doi.org/10.1097/01.AOG.0000452745.44206.c3
17. Committee opinion no. 607: Gynecologic concerns in children and adolescents with cancer. Obstet Gynecol. 2014;124(2 Pt 1):403–8. https://doi.org/10.1097/01.AOG.0000452746.44206.18
18. Curtis KM, Tepper NK, Jatlaoui TC, Berry-Bibee E, Horton LG, Zapata LB, Simmons KB, Pagano HP, Jamieson DJ, Whiteman MK. U.S. medical eligibility criteria for contraceptive use, 2016. MMWR Recomm Rep. 2016;65(3):1–103. https://doi.org/10.15585/mmwr.rr6503a1.
19. Darney P, Patel A, Rosen K, Shapiro LS, Kaunitz AM. Safety and efficacy of a single-rod etonogestrel implant (Implanon): results from 11 international clinical trials. Fertil Steril. 2009;91(5):1646–53. https://doi.org/10.1016/j.fertnstert.2008.02.140.
20. Deans EI, Grimes DA. Intrauterine devices for adolescents: a systematic review. Contraception. 2009;79(6):418–23. https://doi.org/10.1016/j.contraception.2008.12.009.
21. Denford S, Abraham C, Campbell R, Busse H. A comprehensive review of reviews of school-based interventions to improve sexual-health. Health Psychol Rev. 2017;11(1):33–52. https://doi.org/10.1080/17437199.2016.1240625.
22. Diedrich JT, Zhao Q, Madden T, Secura GM, Peipert JF. Three-year continuation of reversible contraception. Am J Obstet Gynecol. 2015;213(5):662 e661–8. https://doi.org/10.1016/j.ajog.2015.08.001.
23. Divasta AD, Laufer MR, Gordon CM. Bone density in adolescents treated with a GnRH agonist and add-back therapy for endometriosis. J Pediatr Adolesc Gynecol. 2007;20(5):293–7. https://doi.org/10.1016/j.jpag.2007.04.008.
24. Eisenberg D, McNicholas C, Peipert JF. Cost as a barrier to long-acting reversible contraceptive (LARC) use in adolescents. J Adolesc Health. 2013;52(4 Suppl):S59–63. https://doi.org/10.1016/j.jadohealth.2013.01.012.
25. Eisenberg DL, Schreiber CA, Turok DK, Teal SB, Westhoff CL, Creinin MD, Investigators AI. Three-year efficacy and safety of a new 52-mg levonorgestrel-releasing intrauterine system. Contraception. 2015;92(1):10–6. https://doi.org/10.1016/j.contraception.2015.04.006.
26. Green DM, Whitton JA, Stovall M, Mertens AC, Donaldson SS, Ruymann FB, Pendergrass TW, Robison LL. Pregnancy outcome of female survivors of childhood cancer: a report from the childhood cancer survivor study. Am J Obstet Gynecol. 2002;187(4):1070–80. https://doi.org/10.1067/mob.2002.126643.
27. Gronich N, Lavi I, Rennert G. Higher risk of venous thrombosis associated with drospirenone-containing oral contraceptives: a population-based cohort study. CMAJ. 2011;183(18):E1319–25. https://doi.org/10.1503/cmaj.110463.
28. Hatcher RATJ, Neson AL, Cates W, Kowal D, Policar MS. Contraceptive technology. New York: Ardent Media; 2013.
29. Heerman WJ, Hotop A, Omlung K, Armstrong S, Mathieu I, Sherwood NE, Barkin SL. A tool kit to enhance the informed consent process for community-engaged pediatric research. IRB: Ethics Hum Res. 2016;38(5):8–14.
30. Heinemann K, Reed S, Moehner S, Minh TD. Risk of uterine perforation with levonorgestrel-releasing and copper intrauterine devices in the European Active Surveillance Study on Intrauterine Devices. Contraception. 2015;91(4):274–9. https://doi.org/10.1016/j.contraception.2015.01.007.
31. Hickman LC, Llarena NC, Valentine LN, Liu X, Falcone T. Preservation of gonadal function in women undergoing chemotherapy: a systematic review and meta-analysis of the potential role for gonadotropin-releasing hormone agonists. J Assist Reprod Genet. 2018. https://doi.org/10.1007/s10815-018-1128-2
32. Hubacher D, Lopez L, Steiner MJ, Dorflinger L. Menstrual pattern changes from levonorgestrel subdermal implants and DMPA: systematic review and evidence-based comparisons. Contraception. 2009;80(2):113–8. https://doi.org/10.1016/j.contraception.2009.02.008.
33. Jacob MS, Kulie P, Benedict C, Ordoobadi AJ, Sikka N, Steinmetz E, McCarthy ML. Use of a midstream clean catch mobile application did not lower urine contamination rates in an emergency department. Am J Emerg Med. 2017. https://doi.org/10.1016/j.ajem.2017.07.016
34. Jatlaoui TC, Riley HE, Curtis KM. The safety of intrauterine devices among young women: a systematic review. Contraception. 2017;95(1):17–39. https://doi.org/10.1016/j.contraception.2016.10.006.
35. Kaunitz AM. Emergency contraception. 2018. http://www.uptodate.com/contents/emergency-contraception?source=search_result&search=Emergency+contraception&selectedTitle=1%7E137. Accessed 26 Feb 2018 2018.
36. Kohler PK, Manhart LE, Lafferty WE. Abstinence-only and comprehensive sex education and the initiation of sexual activity and teen pregnancy. J Adolesc Health. 2008;42(4):344–51. https://doi.org/10.1016/j.jadohealth.2007.08.026.

37. Lopez LM, Ramesh S, Chen M, Edelman A, Otterness C, Trussell J, Helmerhorst FM. Progestin-only contraceptives: effects on weight. Cochrane Database Syst Rev. 2016;8:CD008815. https://doi.org/10.1002/14651858.CD008815.pub4.
38. Loren AW, Mangu PB, Beck LN, Brennan L, Magdalinski AJ, Partridge AH, Quinn G, Wallace WH, Oktay K, American Society of Clinical O. Fertility preservation for patients with cancer: American Society of Clinical Oncology clinical practice guideline update. J Clin Oncol. 2013;31(19):2500–10. https://doi.org/10.1200/JCO.2013.49.2678.
39. McNicholas C, Maddipati R, Zhao Q, Swor E, Peipert JF. Use of the etonogestrel implant and levonorgestrel intrauterine device beyond the U.S. Food and Drug Administration-approved duration. Obstet Gynecol. 2015;125(3):599–604. https://doi.org/10.1097/AOG.0000000000000690.
40. McNicholas C, Peipert JF. Long-acting reversible contraception for adolescents. Curr Opin Obstet Gynecol. 2012;24(5):293–8. https://doi.org/10.1097/GCO.0b013e32835686d5.
41. Meirow D, Rabinovici J, Katz D, Or R, Shufaro Y, Ben-Yehuda D. Prevention of severe menorrhagia in oncology patients with treatment-induced thrombocytopenia by luteinizing hormone-releasing hormone agonist and depo-medroxyprogesterone acetate. Cancer. 2006;107(7):1634–41. https://doi.org/10.1002/cncr.22199.
42. Mestad R, Secura G, Allsworth JE, Madden T, Zhao Q, Peipert JF. Acceptance of long-acting reversible contraceptive methods by adolescent participants in the Contraceptive CHOICE Project. Contraception. 2011;84(5):493–8. https://doi.org/10.1016/j.contraception.2011.03.001.
43. Milbourne A. Heavy or irregular uterine bleeding during chemotherapy. 2018. https://www.uptodate.com/contents/heavy-or-irregular-uterine-bleeding-during-chemotherapy?search=chemoterapy%20menstrual%20bleeding&source=search_result&selectedTitle=8~150&usage_type=default&display_rank=8.
44. Miller L, Hughes JP. Continuous combination oral contraceptive pills to eliminate withdrawal bleeding: a randomized trial. Obstet Gynecol. 2003;101(4):653–61.
45. Morch LS, Skovlund CW, Hannaford PC, Iversen L, Fielding S, Lidegaard O. Contemporary hormonal contraception and the risk of breast cancer. N Engl J Med. 2017;377(23):2228–39. https://doi.org/10.1056/NEJMoa1700732.
46. Mueller TE, Gavin LE, Kulkarni A. The association between sex education and youth's engagement in sexual intercourse, age at first intercourse, and birth control use at first sex. J Adolesc Health. 2008;42(1):89–96. https://doi.org/10.1016/j.jadohealth.2007.08.002.
47. Ngo LL, Braaten KP, Eichen E, Fortin J, Maurer R, Goldberg AB. Naproxen sodium for pain control with intrauterine device insertion: a randomized controlled trial. Obstet Gynecol. 2016;128(6):1306–13. https://doi.org/10.1097/AOG.0000000000001746.
48. Ngo LL, Ward KK, Mody SK. Ketorolac for pain control with intrauterine device placement: a randomized controlled trial. Obstet Gynecol. 2015;126(1):29–36. https://doi.org/10.1097/AOG.0000000000000912.
49. Patel A, Schwarz EB, Society of Family P. Cancer and contraception. Release date May 2012. SFP guideline #20121. Contraception. 2012;86(3):191–8. https://doi.org/10.1016/j.contraception.2012.05.008.
50. Pierce SJ, Gazvani MR, Farquharson RG. Long-term use of gonadotropin-releasing hormone analogs and hormone replacement therapy in the management of endometriosis: a randomized trial with a 6-year follow-up. Fertil Steril. 2000;74(5):964–8. https://doi.org/10.1016/s0015-0282(00)01537-5.
51. Practice Bulletin No. 152: emergency contraception. Obstet Gynecol. 2015;126 (3):e1–11. https://doi.org/10.1097/AOG.0000000000001047
52. Quaas AM, Ginsburg ES. Prevention and treatment of uterine bleeding in hematologic malignancy. Eur J Obstet Gynecol Reprod Biol. 2007;134(1):3–8. https://doi.org/10.1016/j.ejogrb.2007.03.012.
53. Rosenstock JR, Peipert JF, Madden T, Zhao Q, Secura GM. Continuation of reversible contraception in teenagers and young women. Obstet Gynecol. 2012;120(6):1298–305. https://doi.org/10.1097/AOG.0b013e31827499bd.
54. Rowe P, Farley T, Peregoudov A, Piaggio G, Boccard S, Landoulsi S, Meirik O, Research IUDRGotUUW-WBSPo, Development, Research Training in Human R. Safety and efficacy in parous women of a 52-mg levonorgestrel-medicated intrauterine device: a 7-year randomized comparative study with the TCu380A. Contraception. 2016;93(6):498–506. https://doi.org/10.1016/j.contraception.2016.02.024.
55. Secura GM, Madden T, McNicholas C, Mullersman J, Buckel CM, Zhao Q, Peipert JF. Provision of no-cost, long-acting contraception and teenage pregnancy. N Engl J Med. 2014;371(14):1316–23. https://doi.org/10.1056/NEJMoa1400506.
56. Simmons KB, Edelman AB. Hormonal contraception and obesity. Fertil Steril. 2016;106(6):1282–8. https://doi.org/10.1016/j.fertnstert.2016.07.1094.
57. Society for Adolescent H, Medicine. Abstinence-only-until-marriage policies and programs: an updated position paper of the Society for Adolescent Health and Medicine. J Adolesc Health. 2017;61(3):400–3. https://doi.org/10.1016/j.jadohealth.2017.06.001.
58. Tepper NK, Dragoman MV, Gaffield ME, Curtis KM. Nonoral combined hormonal contraceptives and thromboembolism: a systematic review. Contraception. 2017;95(2):130–9. https://doi.org/10.1016/j.contraception.2016.10.005.
59. Waimey KE, Duncan FE, Su HI, Smith K, Wallach H, Jona K, Coutifaris C, Gracia CR, Shea LD, Brannigan RE, Chang RJ, Zelinski MB, Stouffer RL, Taylor RL, Woodruff TK. Future directions in oncofertility and fertility preservation: a report from the 2011 Oncofertility consortium conference. J Adolesc Young Adult Oncol. 2013;2(1):25–30. https://doi.org/10.1089/jayao.2012.0035.
60. WHO. Medical eligibility criteria for contraceptive use. 5th ed. Geneva: WHO; 2015.
61. Winther JF, Boice JD Jr, Svendsen AL, Frederiksen K, Olsen JH. Induced abortions in Danish cancer survivors: a population-based cohort study. J Natl Cancer Inst. 2009;101(9):687–9. https://doi.org/10.1093/jnci/djp064.

62. Xiao S, Coppeta JR, Rogers HB, Isenberg BC, Zhu J, Olalekan SA, McKinnon KE, Dokic D, Rashedi AS, Haisenleder DJ, Malpani SS, Arnold-Murray CA, Chen K, Jiang M, Bai L, Nguyen CT, Zhang J, Laronda MM, Hope TJ, Maniar KP, Pavone ME, Avram MJ, Sefton EC, Getsios S, Burdette JE, Kim JJ, Borenstein JT, Woodruff TK. A microfluidic culture model of the human reproductive tract and 28-day menstrual cycle. Nat Commun. 2017;8:14584. https://doi.org/10.1038/ncomms14584.
63. Zigler RE, McNicholas C. Unscheduled vaginal bleeding with progestin-only contraceptive use. Am J Obstet Gynecol. 2017;216(5):443–50. https://doi.org/10.1016/j.ajog.2016.12.008.

Female Sexual Function in Childhood, Adolescent, and Young Adult Cancer Survivors

Terri L. Woodard, Andrea Bradford, and Sukhkamal Campbell

T. K. Woodruff et al. (eds.), *Textbook of Oncofertility Research and Practice*,
https://doi.org/10.1007/978-3-030-02868-8_14

Key Points
- Female survivors of childhood, adolescent, and young adult cancers are at risk for impaired sexual functioning, which can negatively impact overall quality of life.
- Cancer treatment can profoundly affect sexual functioning through a variety of physiologic and psychosocial mechanisms.
- While nonmedical and medical interventions for sexual dysfunction exist, access to care is dependent on effective screening and assessment of sexual concerns. Multidisciplinary teams are particularly useful in providing comprehensive care that optimizes sexual functioning.
- Many sexual concerns can be addressed with brief interventions, if detected early; however, more complex cases should be referred to sexual health professionals.

14.1 Scope of the Problem

For most individuals, healthy sexual functioning represents an important component of overall health and quality of life. Previous studies have demonstrated a positive association between sexual function and overall health status [1, 2].

Cancer and its treatment affect multiple facets of life, including sexual well-being. Sexual functioning may be impacted through physiologic and/or psychosocial mechanisms. Unfortunately, it appears that survivors of cancer are at risk for persistent or worsening sexual problems [3]. As the number of survivors increases, the recognition of sexual well-being as an important quality of life issue continues to become more pressing [4, 5].

While there is growing literature on sexual function in adults diagnosed with cancer, research that addresses the sexual concerns of young adult and childhood cancer survivors is severely lacking [6], even though it is a priority concern in this population. In 2010, LIVE**STRONG** conducted a survey of more than 3000 cancer survivors, of which over 30% of respondents were adolescent and young adult (AYA) cancer survivors. Sexual functioning and satisfaction was one of the three top physical concerns reported, with 46% of people experiencing problems in this area. Unfortunately, the majority of these survivors (71%) reported that they did not receive care for sexual problems [7].

While many survivors of childhood cancer do not report problems with sexual functioning, there is evidence that there is a higher risk of impairment in this population. A survey of 599 young men and women aged 18–39 who were diagnosed with cancer at age 21 or younger revealed that 42.7% reported at least one problematic sexual symptom, with women having significantly higher symptom scores (21.6) than men (10.6) [8]. In a separate cohort study of adult female survivors of childhood cancer, women with a history of childhood cancer had poorer overall sexual functioning and significantly lower levels of sexual interest, desire, arousal, and satisfaction compared with their healthy siblings. Survivors with ovarian failure reported lower sexual functioning scores compared with those who had normal menses, though interestingly, sexual functioning scores did not improve with the addition of hormonal therapy (such as oral contraceptives or traditional hormone replacement therapy) [9].

In a recent 2-year longitudinal study, 123 young adult cancer patients (ages 18–39) completed the Medical Outcomes Study Sexual Functioning Scale within the first 4 months of diagnosis and again at 6 and 24 months after diagnosis. At both time points, more than half of the participants reported problems with sexual functioning. The probability of sexual problems increased over time ($P < 0.01$) and was greater for female cancer patients ($P < 0.001$), those treated with chemotherapy ($P < 0.05$), and those with lower social support ($P < 0.05$) [10].

Adolescent and young adult survivors may not only be at special risk of certain sexual complications, but they may also differ from middle aged and older survivors in their preferences for sexual health education and intervention. For instance, some evidence suggests that younger survivors have stronger preferences for web-based education versus conventional printed teaching materials and may also prefer face-to-face interactions to a greater extent than older survivors [11]. Younger survivors may also be especially responsive to peer-mediated interventions, which not only educate but can also be uniquely helpful sources of social support and effective role modeling [12].

As healthcare providers who strive to optimize the survivorship experience of patients, it is important to acknowledge how sexual functioning interfaces with other quality-of-life measures. Young adult survivors of childhood cancer with sexual dysfunction report decreased physical functioning, poorer general health, greater fatigue, and poorer mental health [13]. Sexual dysfunction is also correlated with lower life satisfaction and more distress [8].

14.2 Barriers to Care

There are a number of barriers that make addressing sexual concerns in this patient population challenging. Sex and sexuality are sensitive topics that are difficult for many people to discuss; they may be especially difficult for younger people who may feel embarrassed and/or lack the knowledge and vocabulary to speak freely about sexual problems. In addition, some providers experience discomfort talking with younger patients about sexual issues because they are not certain of what is "age appropriate" or, in the case of minors, they fear offending parents by bringing up the discussion [14]. Additionally, time constraints and a lack of knowledge of providers also influence whether providers address sexual concerns in their patients [15].

Many young people desire information about sexual health and sexual concerns, but most are not getting the counseling and care that they need, even though they represent an especially vulnerable group that may be more at risk for sexual problems. Patients who were diagnosed and treated at a very young age may have never grasped a complete understanding of how their treatment has impacted their reproductive health. Thus, it is important that providers are equipped with the confidence and skills that enable them to discuss sexual issues with patients in an age-appropriate manner [16].

14.3 Sexual Development

When considering sexual function and well-being in the adolescent and young adult population, it is important to do so in a developmental context. Normal sexual development is variable between individuals, and it is influenced not only by age but by culture and personal experiences. Sexual development begins at birth. It includes the physical changes that occur with growing older as well as the beliefs and behaviors that people exhibit about sex.

14.3.1 Infancy and Childhood

In infancy, children are curious about their genitals and may touch them in private and/or public. They are completely uninhibited. During early childhood, children remain openly curious about their own bodies and start to develop a curiosity about other's bodies. As they become a little older and have more interaction with peers, they begin to develop an awareness of the differences between boys and girls. It is generally at this time that they become aware of the concept of gender and adopt a stable sense of gender identity. They also begin to ask questions about sex.

Upon reaching school age, children begin to grasp a better understanding of societal norms with regard to sex and sexuality. They tend to become more modest and may desire more privacy, such as when changing their clothing. They remain curious about sex but are often more reluctant to talk about it with adults. It is not uncommon for them to develop a sexual attraction and interest in other people during this stage.

14.3.2 Preadolescence

Puberty begins during preadolescence. Preadolescents may become even more self-conscious as they experience physical changes in their bodies. Masturbation becomes more common. Although they generally do not have a lot of sexual experience, they are aware of different types of sexual activity as well as differences in sexual preferences and orientation. It is during this period when "group dating" often begins; some may even start to partner off as "boyfriend and girlfriend." Sexual exploration and experience varies but often involves "making out."

14.3.3 Adolescence

Adolescence is a complex time when the individual transitions from a child to an adult. Important developmental milestones include establishing autonomy, solidifying identity, and sexual emergence. While there is a wide range of diversity in development and life experiences during this developmental period, it is generally characterized by an increased interest in romantic and sexual relationships. Adolescents can and do form emotional attachments to romantic partners. There is also an increase in genital sex behaviors, such as sexual intercourse.

14.4 Sexual Development in Survivors of Childhood Cancer

Young adult survivors of childhood cancer may not reach sexual development milestones at the same rate as their peers as a result of medical and psychosocial challenges that are the result of their cancer experience. For example, cancer treatment can cause failed puberty, which is characterized by delayed or absent physical maturation. When a patient's disease isolates and alienates her from peers and the "normal" developmental experience, her psychosexual identity may not be well established and romantic relationships may not have the opportunity to form. As a result, the individual may not have ample opportunity to learn and adopt normal healthy sexual behaviors.

Childhood cancer survivors experience a delay in dating and initiation of social contacts compared with their peers [17]. Not only are they more likely to marry later [18–20], but they are also significantly more likely to be unmarried than their siblings [9]. They exhibit a later time of first sexual intercourse [17, 21, 22] and are less likely to be sexually active in general. They also report lower satisfaction with sexual experiences [17].

14.5 Risk Factors for Sexual Dysfunction

Since altered sexual development may influence sexual function in survivors of childhood cancer, multiple studies have attempted to identify specific risk factors for sexual dysfunction. Older age, being female, and having health problems are factors that have been associated with sexual dysfunction in this population [8]. In a separate study, older age at the time of sexual function assessment, having ovarian failure at a younger age, a history of treatment with cranial radiation, and having a cancer diagnosis during adolescence were identified as risk factors for poorer sexual functioning [9]. Psychosocial risk factors relevant to young cancer survivors include body image disturbances, depression and anxiety, and relationship difficulties with a partner [23, 24].

14.6 Long-Term and Late Effects of Cancer Treatment on Sexual Functioning

Cancer and its treatment can have profound effects on long-term sexual functioning. These effects can be the result of physiologic factors, psychosocial factors, or, most frequently, a combination of both [25].

14.6.1 Physiologic Effects

Cancer treatment modalities such as surgery, chemotherapy, irradiation, and hormonal therapy can cause hormonal, vascular, and/or neurologic changes that affect sexual function [25]. Primary hypogonadism (ovarian failure) can result from treatment with chemotherapy (particularly alkylating agents), surgery (bilateral oophorectomy), and abdominal/pelvic irradiation. Ovarian failure results in hypoestrogenism; if survivors were prepubertal at the time of failure, puberty will not occur. In such instances, hormone replacement therapy must be given to promote normal development of adult height and secondary sexual characteristics. If failure occurs post puberty, hypoestrogenism can result in menopausal symptoms such as hot flashes and vaginal dryness.

Central hypogonadism can occur when patients receive cranial radiation that affects the hypothalamic-pituitary-gonadal axis. As a result, the pituitary does not release the gonadotropins (FSH and LH) that direct ovarian function. In these cases, patients also may experience pubertal failure that can be treated with gonadotropin and/or hormone replacement. Conversely, cranial irradiation that includes the hypothalamus may lead to premature activation of the hypothalamic-pituitary-gonadal axis, resulting in precocious puberty.

Surgery that affects the vulva and vagina can cause dryness, sensory changes, and pain. Pelvic irradiation often leads to decreased blood flow that may lead to complications such as vaginal strictures and fistulas [26]. Survivors that receive these therapies may experience diminished sensation, pain, postcoital bleeding, and difficulties with vaginal penetration. Both pelvic surgery and radiation can cause nerve damage, resulting in weakening of the pelvic musculature that leads to discomfort during intercourse as well as urine and/or fecal incontinence. Patients who receive hematopoietic stem cell transplants are at risk for graft versus host disease of the vagina, which is associated with vaginal dryness, shortening, and pain [27].

Although the majority of studies of young female cancer survivors pertain to breast cancer, recent studies have also examined sexual adjustment in young women with gynecologic [28] and gastrointestinal tract cancers [29] and have found similar rates of sexual problems. As with breast cancer, less radical or invasive treatment (e.g., radical trachelectomy rather than radical hysterectomy for cervical cancer) appears to be associated with a greater likelihood of sexual functioning returning to baseline and lower rates of sexual dysfunction in the long term [28, 29].

14.6.2 Psychosocial Effects

Sexual functioning is also influenced by psychological and social factors. A diagnosis of cancer is life changing and often introduces challenges in peoples' lives beyond the obvious medical consequences. Distress, depression, or anxiety related to a cancer diagnosis may negatively affect a woman's sexual functioning. Treatment-related bodily disfigurements (e.g., as a result of a mastectomy [30], presence of a stoma [31], hair loss [32]) have been shown to be associated with emotional distress and poorer quality of life in cancer survivors in general but may be less of a problem in childhood cancer survivors [33]. However, these physical changes can negatively influence body image and self-esteem, decreasing one's confidence in engaging in sexual activity and/or sexual relationships. Survivors of human papillomavirus (HPV)-related cancers may harbor guilt and fears about transmission or recurrence of cancer, which may in turn lead to avoidance of sexual activity [34]. Cancer-related infertility is also intertwined with sexual health; a woman might be reluctant to pursue and/or maintain romantic relationships because she believes that a potential partner might reject her because of her inability to have a biological child.

14.6.3 Social Effects

Personal relationships are also affected by cancer and cancer therapy. For young people, feelings of alienation and isolation are common [35]. Concerns about attractiveness or competence as a romantic partner may lead survivors to avoid dating and going out. Friendships may wane if the patient is unable to "keep up" with the developmental and social milestones of her peers. Changes in existing romantic relationships may result if the partner takes on a new role as a caregiver, introducing a degree of intimacy that may be perceived as premature for the relationship or for the partner's life stage. Alternatively, partners who become more distant or "shielded" from the realities of the disease and its treatment may have difficulty empathizing with the survivor. Partners of young survivors may feel disappointed when, even after completion of successful cancer treatment, their relationships do not simply "return to normal." Studies of young breast cancer survivors have found that sexual difficulties are influenced by perceptions of supportiveness or how well their partners understand of their feelings [23]. Finally, the financial impact of cancer and cancer therapy can be an additional stressor that influences intimate relationships.

14.6.4 Cultural Effects

Cultural norms for gender roles and sexual activity influence the onset and course of sexual problems; indeed, some studies have noted significant geographical and cultural variation in sexual attitudes and satisfaction [36]. Culture further plays a large role in patient's perspectives and decisions regarding their cancer diagnoses and their treatment plans. Although in the USA research on cancer survivorship and sexual health is disproportionately based on data from White, college-educated survivors, emerging research has aimed to document the experiences of underrepresented groups. Unfortunately, little of this research has specifically focused on young survivors.

Cultural influences on sexual difficulties are often related in some ways to expectations tied to feminine roles and behaviors. For instance, in a review of sexual concerns in young breast cancer survivors, Hungr et al. noted that some Hispanic/Latina survivors, especially those who identify more closely with traditional cultures, may be more likely to have internalized ideals related to femininity and fertility, complicating their sexual adjustment after treatment [37]. Beliefs about one's obligations toward a partner, similarly, may influence the experiences of sexuality and intimacy. For instance, a qualitative study of Asian American breast cancer survivors described women's experiences of feeling obligated to their partners and, concurrently, wishing to not burden their partners or families [38]. Spiritual beliefs, likewise, can shape the ways in which women understand and cope with cancer, with potentially positive or negative influences on sexual adjustment. Understanding the cultural contexts that shape sexual attitudes and expectations can help clinicians understand the onset or maintenance of sexual problems.

Equally important to consider are ways in which culture influences help seeking and interactions with health care providers. Survivors from historically marginalized populations may employ a self-protective "healthy suspicion" in their interactions with clinicians. For example, in a survey of African American breast cancer survivors, higher levels of medical mistrust were associated with more severe sexual problems [39], suggesting that health disparities in sexual outcomes may be related to missed opportunities for culturally competent care. Cultural beliefs about sharing intimate details with strangers may also limit the extent to which some populations are willing to discuss sexual problems. Finally, survivors who are stigmatized in their culture for their sexual identities or practices face negative consequences for being "outed" and may feel reluctant to disclose their concerns. Interventions for sexual health in cancer survivors that are responsive to these systemic disparities are still early in their development and implementation [40, 41].

14.7 Female Sexual Dysfunction

Since women who are survivors of childhood and adolescent cancer are at risk for sexual problems, it is important that they are screened for female sexual dysfunction (FSD). Accurate diagnosis is vital so that proper care can be given.

A sexual complaint is diagnosed as a dysfunction when the criteria from the American Psychiatric Association's Diagnostic and Statistical Manual (DSM) [42] for sexual dysfunctions are met and the complaint results in significant distress. The newly published *Diagnostic and Statistical Manual of Mental Disorders*, 5th edition (DSM-5), created new diagnostic classifications including female sexual interest/arousal disorder (FSIAD), female orgasmic disorder, and genito-pelvic pain/penetration disorder (GPPPD) (see ▫ Table 14.1). Along with information obtained from a thorough clinical interview, physical examination, and indicated laboratory testing, DSM-5 criteria should be used to establish the diagnosis and etiology of sexual dysfunction in women.

14.7.1 Female Sexual Interest/Arousal Disorder (FSIAD)

The diagnosis of female sexual interest/arousal disorder is characterized by a lack of or significantly reduced sexual interest/arousal. It must be manifested by at least three of the following (in any combination): (1) absent/reduced interest in sexual activity, (2) absent/reduced sexual/erotic thoughts or fantasies, (3) no or reduced initiation of sexual activity and being unreceptive to a partner's attempts to initiate sex, (4) absent or reduced sexual excitement/pleasure during sex in all or almost all (approximately 75–100%) of sexual encounters, (5) absent or reduced sexual interest/arousal in response to any internal or external sexual/erotic cues (e.g., verbal, visual), and (6) absent or reduced genital or nongenital sensations during sexual activity during sex in almost all or all (approximately 75–100%) of sexual encounters. FSIAD is the most commonly reported sexual dysfunction in both cancer survivors and the general population.

14.7.2 Female Orgasmic Disorder

The diagnosis of female orgasmic disorder (FOD) requires the presence of (1) a marked delay in, marked infrequency of, or absence of orgasm and/or (2) a markedly reduced intensity of orgasmic sensations. Problems with orgasm should be

Table 14.1 DSM-5 classification of female sexual dysfunction

Disorder	Diagnostic criteria
Female orgasmic disorder (FOD)	(1) A marked delay in, marked infrequency of, or absence of orgasm and/or (2) a markedly reduced intensity of orgasmic sensations
Female sexual interest/arousal disorder (FSIAD)	Requires at least three of the following (in any combination): (1) absent/reduced interest in sexual activity, (2) absent/reduced sexual/erotic thoughts or fantasies, (3) no or reduced initiation of sexual activity and being unreceptive to a partner's attempts to initiate sex, (4) absent or reduced sexual excitement/pleasure during sex in all or almost all (approximately 75–100%) of sexual encounters, (5) absent or reduced sexual interest/arousal in response to any internal or external sexual/erotic cues (e.g., verbal, visual), and (6) absent or reduced genital or non-genital sensations during sexual activity during sex in almost all or all (approximately 75–100%) of sexual encounters
Genito-pelvic pain/penetration disorder (GPPPD)	Persistent or recurrent difficulties with one or more of (1) vaginal penetration during intercourse; (2) marked vulvovaginal or pelvic pain during intercourse or penetration attempts; (3) marked fear of anxiety about vulvovaginal or pelvic pain in anticipation of, during, or as a result of vaginal penetration; and (4) marked tensing or tightening of the pelvic floor muscles during attempted vaginal penetration

considered in the context of health status, partner factors, and other sexual problem (e.g., pain) that may interfere with sexual stimulation. Clinically, it is important to distinguish FOD that is generalized to all sexual stimulation versus problems that are more situation or context dependent. In general, the onset of FOD due to physiological etiology (such as neuropathy or effects of a medication) tends to be more global or generalized in presentation than situational FOD. Lifelong FOD, though not directly related to cancer, may be compounded by the effects of treatment.

14.7.3 Genito-Pelvic Pain/Penetration Disorder (GPPPD)

The diagnosis of genito-pelvic pain/penetration disorder (GPPPD) requires persistent or recurrent difficulties with one or more of (1) vaginal penetration during intercourse; (2) marked vulvovaginal or pelvic pain during intercourse or penetration attempts; (3) marked fear of anxiety about vulvovaginal or pelvic pain in anticipation of, during, or as a result of vaginal penetration; and (4) marked tensing or tightening of the pelvic floor muscles during attempted vaginal penetration. Pain with vaginal penetration is a common problem reported by cancer survivors who have undergone pelvic radiation, pelvic surgery, or treatment that disrupts the hormonal milieu.

The DSM-5 requires that a woman must have symptoms 75–100% of the time to make a diagnosis of sexual disorder, except when there is a substance or medication-induced disorder. The symptoms have to be present for at least 6 months and should not be better explained by a nonsexual mental disorder, a consequence of severe relationship distress (e.g., partner violence) or other significant stressors.

Each of the sexual dysfunction categories can be further described by using specifiers such as "lifelong versus acquired" and "generalized versus situational." The severity of the problem should also be documented—specifically, whether it is mild, moderate, or severe. Finally, associated features should be noted, including the presence of (1) partner factors (partner sexual problem and/or health status); (2) relationship factors (difficult communication, differences in desire for sexual activity); (3) individual vulnerability factors (poor body image, history of sexual or emotional abuse), psychiatric comorbidity (depression and/or anxiety), or stressors (job loss, bereavement); (4) cultural or religious factors (attitudes about sexuality); and (5) medical factors relevant to prognosis, course, or treatment.

14.8 Screening and Assessment

The Children's Oncology Group Long-Term Follow-Up Guidelines for Survivors of Childhood, Adolescent, and Young Adult Cancer (COG-LTFU Guidelines) provide evidence-based recommendations for screening and management of late effects of cancer treatment, including psychosexual dysfunction [43].

It has been recommended that sexual health status in women cancer survivors should be assessed at regular intervals and at least annually [44, 45] as well as anytime a woman voices a sexual concern. There are a number of screening instruments that can be used in an office setting that will allow quick identification, some of which have been developed and/or validated for use in cancer survivors [46–48]. Simply asking the patient about her sexual function and activity validates that it is an important part of overall health. However, routine assessment strategies in isolation are unlikely to enhance care for sexual problems [49]; ideally, screening is one component of a model implemented by well-trained staff who can deliver brief intervention and referrals at the point of care.

When introducing the topic of sexual functioning, it is important to communicate with the patient in a comfortable, nonjudgmental manner. It is helpful to broach the discussion by normalizing the presence of sexual concerns, which lets the patient know that she is not the only person experiencing her problem. Questions should start as open ended and become more directed. No assumptions should be made about her sexuality or sexual behaviors (i.e., assuming sexual orientation or practice of monogamy).

A complete history should be elicited with special emphasis on the gynecologic and sexual history. Medications should be thoroughly reviewed, as many can have negative effects on sexual function [50]. The physical examination should include a thorough pelvic examination [51]. Both external and internal genitalia should be evaluated for abnormalities, such as atrophy, scarring, and strictures. Laboratory evaluation (such as sex hormones and thyroid function tests) can be added as indicated.

Although the focus of this article is on sexual functioning of adolescent and young adult female cancer survivors, it is imperative that other aspects of sexual health are discussed. Discussions about pregnancy, sexual assault, and STI prevention are particularly important in this population, as they are vulnerable to reproductive health complications as it relates to immune compromise, incompatibility between desired contraception methods and treatment, and pregnancy complications [14].

14.9 Treatment

Some specialty cancer centers have recognized that women with a history of cancer have unique needs with regard to sexual functioning and have developed supportive services that can help patients anticipate and manage sexual issues before, during, and after cancer treatment. Often, these expert teams are multidisciplinary and may include gynecologists, psychologists, sex therapists, and pelvic floor physical therapists who can assess patients and provide a comprehensive treatment plan to optimize sexual functioning.

Treatment plans should be tailored to the individual patient and focus on the physical, psychological, and social factors that contribute to her sexual problem [44]. While there are few FDA-approved treatments for sexual dysfunction in women, there are still a considerable number of treatments that can be utilized to improve women's sexual satisfaction and well-being.

14.9.1 Education and Setting of Expectations

Healthcare providers can play a major role in helping women with sexual concerns or sexual dysfunction by providing accurate, unbiased sexual health education. Women who were diagnosed at a very young age might have some educational deficits in this area. It is not uncommon for some to have erroneous knowledge and beliefs about sex, including basic anatomy and physiology. Furthermore, socially influenced ideas of what "normal" sex and sexuality are can promote unrealistic expectations about how an individual woman's sex life should be. It is imperative to educate women that "normal" sexual functioning is variable between women and even throughout an individual woman's life. It should also be emphasized that the overall goal of healthy sexual functioning should be the achievement of sexual satisfaction and that she should be encouraged to define what that means for her as an individual and as part of a couple.

Lifestyle modification should be encouraged, as overall well-being influences sexual functioning. Women should be counseled to adopt healthy lifestyle behaviors, such as smoking cessation, limiting alcohol consumption, exercising most days of the week, getting adequate sleep, eating a healthy diet, and reducing stress as much as possible. The conditions surrounding sexual experiences should be optimized as well. Women should be informed of the importance of adequate sexual stimulation and arousal, which can be achieved with prolonged foreplay and the use of sexual aids. If patients experience difficulty with sexual intercourse, they should be encouraged to explore alternative means of expressing sexual intimacy and incorporate sexual activities that don't require intercourse. If intercourse is desired, the use of vaginal lubricants and moisturizers can make sexual activity easier and more comfortable.

14.9.2 Non-pharmacologic Therapies

Significant improvements in sexual function after intervention with traditional sex therapy and/or cognitive-behavioral therapy have been observed [52]. Traditional sex therapy is a behavioral treatment that aims to improve an individual/couple's erotic experiences while reducing anxiety and self-consciousness about sexual activity [53]. Education is an important component of sex therapy, as it is often therapeutic to normalize variations in sexual experiences and dispel sexual myths or unhelpful sexual beliefs. Other common sex therapy exercises include relaxation training and sensate focus, a graded series of mutually pleasurable touching exercises that emphasizes mutual enjoyment without demand for intercourse or other sexual "performance." Cognitive-behavioral sex therapy includes traditional behavioral sex therapy components but places a greater emphasis on modifying thought patterns or beliefs that interfere with intimacy and sexual pleasure [53]. Directed masturbation has been demonstrated to be efficacious in the treatment of orgasmic disorders [54–56]. Mindfulness-based cognitive-behavioral treatments have also shown excellent promise for sexual desire problems [57].

In light of pressures encouraging greater efficiency of health services, many recent studies have emphasized brevity and accessibility in the design of counseling interventions for sexual problems. For example, Brotto et al. demonstrated that a three-session mindfulness-based cognitive-behavioral intervention was successful in improving sexual desire and arousal problems in gynecologic cancer survivors [57]. A two-session counseling intervention that included education and support regarding cancer and reproductive issues was found to lessen anxiety about sexual and romantic relationships in adolescents and young adults with cancer [58]. Finally, a single half-day group behavioral therapy intervention delivered to 46 women with ovarian cancer appeared to result in enhanced sexual function through 2 and 6 months post-treatment [59].

Pelvic floor therapy is a type of physical therapy that can help strengthen the muscles of the pelvic floor and increase blood supply and innervation to the pelvic floor muscles. A pelvic floor exercise program has been shown to improve pelvic floor strength and sexual functioning in survivors of gynecologic cancers [60]. Dilator therapy is often recommended to selected patients for the prevention of vaginal stenosis in patients who received pelvic radiotherapy [61]; however, evidence that it prevents vaginal stenosis or improves quality of life is mixed [62]. Adherence to long-term use is often poor [63]. Data on the use of dilators for the treatment of sexual dysfunction in the adolescent population and younger is nonexistent.

14.9.3 Pharmacologic Therapies

For women who are prematurely postmenopausal as a result of their cancer treatment, hormonal replacement therapy can restore the normal hormonal milieu. However, only conjugated equine estrogen and ospemifene are FDA approved for the specific treatment of female sexual dysfunction. Vaginal estrogen can be prescribed in a variety of forms and is effective in the treatment of vulvovaginal atrophy (VVA), a common cause of painful intercourse. However, the use of estrogen in any form in patients with a history of hormone-sensitive cancer is controversial. Ospemifene is a selective estrogen receptor modulator that acts directly on the vulvovaginal tissues to reverse atrophy without exerting estrogenic effects on the uterus and breast; however, it has not been specifically studied in cancer survivors [64]. Finally, vaginal dehydroepiandrosterone has been used for the treatment of VVA; its use is associated with lower levels of systemic estrogen and testosterone, but its long-term safety profile is unknown [65].

The role of testosterone therapy for the treatment of female sexual dysfunction is even more controversial. Although it is not FDA approved for this indication, it is frequently prescribed off label. Testosterone has been shown to improve sexual satisfaction, general well-being, and mood [66]; however, safety concerns such as potential development of breast cancer and negative effects on cardiovascular health have limited its use [51].

Bupropion is a mild dopamine and norepinephrine reuptake inhibitor/nicotinic acetylcholine receptor antagonist that is used as an antidepressant and smoking cessation aid. Prior studies have shown that it is also useful treating low desire in women [67], including those with SSRI-induced low desire [68, 69], and women receiving adjuvant hormonal therapy for breast cancer [70]. Flibanserin is a 5-HT1A receptor agonist/5-HT2 receptor antagonist that was recently approved by the FDA for the treatment of premenopausal women with hypoactive sexual desire disorder (HSDD) [71, 72]. However, there are no data on its use in cancer survivors.

There are multiple sexual enhancement products that are available over the counter. While most have not been rigorously tested for efficacy and safety, many women with a history of cancer express interest in their use [73]. Most pharmacologic interventions for the treatment of sexual dysfunction have not been tested in cancer survivors [74], highlighting the importance of more research in this area.

A recent prospective study examined the effect of ospemifene, a selective estrogen receptor modulator, on quality of life and sexual function in women with cervical cancer [75]. The study included 52 women ages 18–60 with a previous diagnosis of stage I–IIa cervical cancer who also suffered from vulvovaginal atrophy. Patients had 6 months of therapy with ospemifene and performed a vaginal health index survey measuring sexual function/quality of life at baseline and after 6 months of therapy. Ospemifene improved vulvovaginal atrophy substantially for women with and without a uterus; on exam, improvements in vaginal dryness, redness, and mucosal friability were noted [75].

14.10 When to Refer

Most sexual problems, especially when detected early, can be addressed through relatively brief intervention. Complex cases warrant referral to professionals who have specialized training in sexual health and medicine. Organizations such as the International Society for the Study of Women's Sexual Health (▶ www.ISSWSH.org); the American Association of Sexuality Educators, Counselors and Therapists (▶ www.AASECT.org); and the Society for Sex Therapy and Research (▶ www.SSTARNET.org) have online tools that can assist with locating healthcare providers that specialize in sexual health issues.

14.11 Conclusion

Healthy sexual functioning is important for girls and women who have/had cancer. The ability to function sexually and experience sexual satisfaction significantly contributes to overall quality of life and can have implications for a woman's ability to develop and sustain intimate relationships [74]. Survivors of childhood, adolescent, and young adult cancers are at risk for sexual problems as a result of their cancer experience.

It is imperative that providers are proactive about addressing sexual concerns in this population. There are a range of treatments that can be used to optimize sexual health and function of survivors. Engaging girls and women in conversations about how cancer and cancer treatment might affect their sexual well-being at baseline can empower them to seek care for these problems if and when they develop.

Review Questions and Answers

Q1. What percentage of survivors of childhood cancer experience sexual problems?

A1. 42.7%

Q2. What are the three categories of female sexual dysfunction defined in the DSM-5?

A2. Female orgasmic disorder, female sexual interest/arousal disorder, and genito-pelvic pain/penetration disorder.

Q3. Name several non-pharmacologic therapies for the treatment of female sexual dysfunction.

A3. Sex therapy, cognitive-behavioral therapy, and pelvic floor physical therapy.

Q4. Name several risk factors for sexual dysfunction in female survivors of childhood cancer.

A4. Older age at cancer diagnosis, having other health problems, ovarian failure, and a history of cranial radiation.

References

1. Davison SL, Bell RJ, La China M, Holden SL, Davis SR. The relationship between self-reported sexual satisfaction and general well-being in women. J Sex Med. 2009;6(10):2690–7.
2. Field N, Mercer CH, Sonnenberg P, Tanton C, Clifton S, Mitchell KR, et al. Associations between health and sexual lifestyles in Britain: findings from the third National Survey of Sexual Attitudes and Lifestyles (Natsal-3). Lancet (London, England). 2013;382(9907):1830–44.
3. Kornblith AB, Ligibel J. Psychosocial and sexual functioning of survivors of breast cancer. Semin Oncol. 2003;30(6):799–813.
4. Robison LL, Hudson MM. Survivors of childhood and adolescent cancer: life-long risks and responsibilities. Nat Rev Cancer. 2014;14(1):61–70.
5. DeSimone M, Spriggs E, Gass JS, Carson SA, Krychman ML, Dizon DS. Sexual dysfunction in female cancer survivors. Am J Clin Oncol. 2014;37(1):101–6.
6. Cantrell MA, Conte T, Hudson M, Shad A, Ruble K, Herth K, et al. Recruitment and retention of older adolescent and young adult female survivors of childhood cancer in longitudinal research. Oncol Nurs Forum. 2012;39(5):483–90.
7. Rechis R, Boerner L, Nutt S, Shaw K, Berno D, Duchover Y. How cancer has affected post-treatment survivors: a LIVESTRONG report. 2010. https://www.livestrong.org/sites/default/files/what-we-do/reports/LSSurvivorSurveyReport.pdf.
8. Zebrack BJ, Foley S, Wittmann D, Leonard M. Sexual functioning in young adult survivors of childhood cancer. Psychooncology. 2010;19(8):814–22.
9. Ford JS, Kawashima T, Whitton J, Leisenring W, Laverdiere C, Stovall M, et al. Psychosexual functioning among adult female survivors of childhood cancer: a report from the childhood cancer survivor study. J Clin Oncol Off J Am Soc Clin Oncol. 2014;32(28): 3126–36.
10. Acquati C, et al. Sexual functioning among young adult cancer patients: a 2 year longitudinal study. Cancer. 2018;124(2):398–405.
11. Stabile C, et al. Sexual health needs and educational intervention preferences for women with cancer. Breast Cancer Res Treat. 2017;165(1):77–84.
12. D'Agostino NM, Penney A, Zebrack B. Providing developmentally appropriate psychosocial care to adolescent and young adult cancer survivors. Cancer. 2011;177(S10):2329–34.
13. Bober SL, Zhou ES, Chen B, Manley PE, Kenney LB, Recklitis CJ. Sexual function in childhood cancer survivors: a report from Project REACH. J Sex Med. 2013;10(8):2084–93.
14. Murphy D, Klosky JL, Termuhlen A, Sawczyn KK, Quinn GP. The need for reproductive and sexual health discussions with adolescent and young adult cancer patients. Contraception. 2013;88(2):215–20.
15. Wiggins DL, Wood R, Granai CO, Dizon DS. Sex, intimacy, and the gynecologic oncologists: survey results of the New England Association of Gynecologic Oncologists (NEAGO). J Psychosoc Oncol. 2007;25(4):61–70.
16. D'Agostino NM, Penney A, Zebrack B. Providing developmentally appropriate psychosocial care to adolescent and young adult cancer survivors. Cancer. 2011;117(10 Suppl):2329–34.
17. van Dijk EM, van Dulmen-den Broeder E, Kaspers GJ, van Dam EW, Braam KI, Huisman J. Psychosexual functioning of childhood cancer survivors. Psychooncology. 2008;17(5):506–11.
18. Langeveld NE, Stam H, Grootenhuis MA, Last BF. Quality of life in young adult survivors of childhood cancer. Support Care Cancer Off J Multinatl Assoc Support Care Cancer. 2002;10(8):579–600.
19. Pui CH, Cheng C, Leung W, Rai SN, Rivera GK, Sandlund JT, et al. Extended follow-up of long-term survivors of childhood acute lymphoblastic leukemia. N Engl J Med. 2003;349(7):640–9.
20. Rauck AM, Green DM, Yasui Y, Mertens A, Robison LL. Marriage in the survivors of childhood cancer: a preliminary description from the Childhood Cancer Survivor Study. Med Pediatr Oncol. 1999;33(1):60–3.
21. Kokkonen J, Vainionpaa L, Winqvist S, Lanning M. Physical and psychosocial outcome for young adults with treated malignancy. Pediatr Hematol Oncol. 1997;14(3):223–32.
22. Puukko LR, Hirvonen E, Aalberg V, Hovi L, Rautonen J, Siimes MA. Sexuality of young women surviving leukaemia. Arch Dis Child. 1997;76(3):197–202.
23. Fobair P, Stewart SL, Chang S, D'Onofrio C, Banks PJ, Bloom JR. Body image and sexual problems in young women with breast cancer. Psycho-Oncology. 2006;15:579–94.
24. Rosenberg SM, Tamimi RM, Gelber S, Ruddy KJ, Bober SL, Kereakoglow S, Borges VF, Come SE, Schapira L, Partridge AH. Treatment-related amenorrhea and sexual functioning in young breast cancer survivors. Cancer. 2014;120:2264–71.
25. Schover LR, van der Kaaij M, van Dorst E, Creutzberg C, Huyghe E, Kiserud CE. Sexual dysfunction and infertility as late effects of cancer treatment. EJC Suppl EJC Off J EORTC Eur Org Res Treat Cancer. 2014;12(1): 41–53.
26. Spunt SL, Sweeney TA, Hudson MM, Billups CA, Krasin MJ, Hester AL. Late effects of pelvic rhabdomyo-

14

sarcoma and its treatment in female survivors. J Clin Oncol Off J Am Soc Clin Oncol. 2005;23(28):7143–51.
27. Zantomio D, Grigg AP, MacGregor L, Panek-Hudson Y, Szer J, Ayton R. Female genital tract graft-versus-host disease: incidence, risk factors and recommendations for management. Bone Marrow Transplant. 2006;38(8):567–72.
28. Fleming ND, et al. Quality of life after radical trachelectomy for early stage cervical cancer: a 5 year prospective evaluation. Gynecol Oncol. 2016;143(3): 596–603.
29. Peri G, et al. Young patients and gastrointestinal (GI) tract malignancies – are we addressing the unmet needs? BMC Cancer. 2016;16:630.
30. Aerts L, Christiaens MR, Enzlin P, Neven P, Amant F. Sexual functioning in women after mastectomy versus breast conserving therapy for early-stage breast cancer: a prospective controlled study. Breast (Edinburgh, Scotland). 2014;23(5):629–36.
31. Sprangers MA, Taal BG, Aaronson NK, te Velde A. Quality of life in colorectal cancer. Stoma vs. nonstoma patients. Dis Colon Rectum. 1995;38(4):361–9.
32. Choi EK, Kim IR, Chang O, Kang D, Nam SJ, Lee JE, et al. Impact of chemotherapy-induced alopecia distress on body image, psychosocial well-being, and depression in breast cancer patients. Psychooncology. 2014;23(10):1103–10.
33. Lehmann V, Hagedoorn M, Gerhardt CA, Fults M, Olshefski RS, Sanderman R, et al. Body issues, sexual satisfaction, and relationship status satisfaction in long-term childhood cancer survivors and healthy controls. Psychooncology. 2015;25(2):210–6.
34. Taberna M, Inglehart RC, Pickard RK, Fakhry C, Agrawal A, Katz ML, Gillison ML. Significant changes in sexual behavior after a diagnosis of human papillomavirus-positive and human papillomavirus-negative oral cancer. Cancer. 2017;123:1156–65.
35. Warner EL, Kent EE, Trevino KM, Parsons HM, Zebrack BJ, Kirchhoff AC. Social well-being among adolescents and young adults with cancer: a systematic review. Cancer. 2016;122:1029–37.
36. Lauman EO, Paik A, Glasser DB, Kang J-H, Levinson B, Moreira ED Jr, Nicolosi A, Gingell C. A cross national study of subjective sexual well being among older women and men: findings from the Global Study of Sexual Attitudes and Behaviors. Arch Sex Behav. 2006;35(2):143–59.
37. Hungr C, et al. Self-image and sexuality issues among young women with breast cancer: practical recommendations. Rev Investig Clin. 2017;69(2): 114–22.
38. Ashing T, Padilla F, Tejero J, Kagawa-Singer M. Understanding the breast cance experience of Asian American women. Psycho-Oncology. 2003;12:38–58.
39. Barsevick AM, Leader A, Bradley PK, Avery T, Dean LT, DiCarlo M, Hegarty SE. Post-treatment problems of African American breast cancer survivors. Support Care Cancer. 2016;24(120):4979–86.
40. JohnsonTurbes A, Schlueter D, Moore AR, Buchanan ND, Fairley TL. Evaluation of a web-based program for African American young breast cancer survivors. Am J Prev Med. 2015;49(6):S543–9.
41. Schover LR, Rhodes MM, Baum G, Adams JH, Jenkins R, Lewis P, Jackson KE. Sisters peer counseling in reproductive issues after treatment (SPIRIT): a peer counseling program to improve reproductive health among African American breast cancer survivors. Cancer. 2011;117(21):4983–92.
42. American Psychiatric Association, American Psychiatric Association DSM-5 Task Force. Diagnostic and statistical manual of mental disorders: DSM-5. 5th ed. Washington, DC: American Psychiatric Association; 2013. p. xliv, 947.
43. Children's Oncology Group. Long-term follow-up guidelines for survivors of childhood, adolescent and young adult cancer 2013 [9/26/2015]. Version 4.0.
44. Metzger ML, Meacham LR, Patterson B, Casillas JS, Constine LS, Hijiya N, et al. Female reproductive health after childhood, adolescent, and young adult cancers: guidelines for the assessment and management of female reproductive complications. J Clin Oncol Off J Am Soc Clin Oncol. 2013;31(9):1239–47.
45. Network NCC. NCCN guidelines: survivorship 2015 [cited 2015 9/01/2015]. Version 2.2015.
46. Baser RE, Li Y, Carter J. Psychometric validation of the Female Sexual Function Index (FSFI) in cancer survivors. Cancer. 2012;118(18):4606–18.. Epub 2012/02/24
47. Flynn KE, Lin L, Cyranowski JM, Reeve BB, Reese JB, Jeffery DD, et al. Development of the NIH PROMIS (R) sexual function and satisfaction measures in patients with cancer. J Sex Med. 2013;10(Suppl 1):43–52. Pubmed Central PMCID: PMC3729213, Epub 2013/03/21.
48. Althof SE, Parish SJ. Clinical interviewing techniques and sexuality questionnaires for male and female cancer patients. J Sex Med. 2013;10(Suppl 1):35–42. Epub 2013/02/15.
49. Bradford A, Fellman B, Urbauer D, Bevers T. Effect of routine screening for sexual problems in a breast cancer survivorship clinic. Psycho-Oncology. 2016;25(11):1375.
50. Clayton A, Ramamurthy S. The impact of physical illness on sexual dysfunction. Adv Psychosom Med. 2008;29:70–88.
51. Dizon DS, Suzin D, McIlvenna S. Sexual health as a survivorship issue for female cancer survivors. Oncologist. 2014;19(2):202–10.
52. Gunzler C, Berner MM. Efficacy of psychosocial interventions in men and women with sexual dysfunctions – a systematic review of controlled clinical trials: part 2 – the efficacy of psychosocial interventions for female sexual dysfunction. J Sex Med. 2012;9(12):3108–25.
53. Kingsberg SA, Woodard T. Female sexual dysfunction: focus on low desire. Obstet Gynecol. 2015;125(2): 477–86.
54. Riley AJ, Riley EJ. A controlled study to evaluate directed masturbation in the management of primary orgasmic failure in women. Br J Psychiatry J Ment Sci. 1978;133:404–9.
55. Reisinger JJ. Effects of erotic stimulation and masturbatory training upon situational orgasmic dysfunction. J Sex Marital Ther. 1978;4(3):177–85.
56. Andersen BL. A comparison of systematic desensitization and directed masturbation in the treatment of

primary orgasmic dysfunction in females. J Consult Clin Psychol. 1981;49(4):568–70.
57. Brotto LA, Basson R, Luria M. A mindfulness-based group psychoeducational intervention targeting sexual arousal disorder in women. J Sex Med. 2008;5(7):1646–59.
58. Canada AL, Schover LR, Li Y. A pilot intervention to enhance psychosexual development in adolescents and young adults with cancer. Pediatr Blood Cancer. 2007;49(6):824–8.
59. Bober SL, et al. Improvement in sexual function after ovarian cancer: effects of sexual therapy and rehabilitation after treatment for ovarian cancer. Cancer. 2018;124(1):176–82.
60. Yang EJ, Lim JY, Rah UW, Kim YB. Effect of a pelvic floor muscle training program on gynecologic cancer survivors with pelvic floor dysfunction: a randomized controlled trial. Gynecol Oncol. 2012;125(3):705–11.
61. Bakker RM, ter Kuile MM, Vermeer WM, Nout RA, Mens JW, van Doorn LC, et al. Sexual rehabilitation after pelvic radiotherapy and vaginal dilator use: consensus using the Delphi method. Int J Fynecolog Cancer Off J Int Gynecol Cancer Soc. 2014;24(8):1499–506.
62. Miles T, Johnson N. Vaginal dilator therapy for women receiving pelvic radiotherapy. Cochrane Database Syst Rev. 2014;9:CD007291.
63. Law E, Kelvin JF, Thom B, Riedel E, Tom A, Carter J, et al. Prospective study of vaginal dilator use adherence and efficacy following radiotherapy. Radiother Oncol J Eur Soc Ther Radiol Oncol. 2015;116(1):149–55.
64. Portman DJ, Bachmann GA, Simon JA. Ospemifene, a novel selective estrogen receptor modulator for treating dyspareunia associated with postmenopausal vulvar and vaginal atrophy. Menopause (New York, NY). 2013;20(6):623–30.
65. Labrie F, Martel C, Berube R, Cote I, Labrie C, Cusan L, et al. Intravaginal prasterone (DHEA) provides local action without clinically significant changes in serum concentrations of estrogens or androgens. J Steroid Biochem Mol Biol. 2013;138:359–67.
66. Davis SR, Goldstat R, Papalia MA, Shah S, Kulkarni J, Donath S, et al. Effects of aromatase inhibition on sexual function and well-being in postmenopausal women treated with testosterone: a randomized, placebo-controlled trial. Menopause (New York, NY). 2006;13(1):37–45.
67. Segraves RT, Clayton A, Croft H, Wolf A, Warnock J. Bupropion sustained release for the treatment of hypoactive sexual desire disorder in premenopausal women. J Clin Psychopharmacol. 2004;24(3): 339–42.
68. Safarinejad MR. Reversal of SSRI-induced female sexual dysfunction by adjunctive bupropion in menstruating women: a double-blind, placebo-controlled and randomized study. J Psychopharmacol (Oxford, England). 2011;25(3):370–8.
69. Pereira VM, Arias-Carrion O, Machado S, Nardi AE, Silva AC. Bupropion in the depression-related sexual dysfunction: a systematic review. CNS Neurol Disord Drug Targets. 2014;13(6):1079–88.
70. Mathias C, Cardeal Mendes CM, Ponde de Sena E, Dias de Moraes E, Bastos C, Braghiroli MI, et al. An open-label, fixed-dose study of bupropion effect on sexual function scores in women treated for breast cancer. Ann Oncol Off J Eur Soc Med Oncol/ESMO. 2006;17(12):1792–6.
71. Katz M, DeRogatis LR, Ackerman R, Hedges P, Lesko L, Garcia M Jr, et al. Efficacy of flibanserin in women with hypoactive sexual desire disorder: results from the BEGONIA trial. J Sex Med. 2013;10(7):1807–15.
72. Dhanuka I, Simon JA. Flibanserin for the treatment of hypoactive sexual desire disorder in premenopausal women. Expert Opin Pharmacother. 2015;22:1–7.
73. Herbenick D, Reece M, Hollub A, Satinsky S, Dodge B. Young female breast cancer survivors: their sexual function and interest in sexual enhancement products and services. Cancer Nurs. 2008;31(6):417–25.
74. Lindau ST, Abramsohn EM, Matthews AC. A manifesto on the preservation of sexual function in women and girls with cancer. Am J Obstet Gynecol. 2015;213(2):166–74. Epub 2015/03/31. eng.
75. De Rosa N, Lavitola G, Giampaolino P, Morra I, Nappi C, Bifulco G. Impact of ospemifene on quality of life and sexual function in young survivors of cervical cancer: a prospective study. Biomed Res Int. 2017;2017: 7513610.

Pregnancy Considerations in Patients with Cancer and Cancer Survivors

Yuriko Iwahata, Hideyuki Iwahata, and Nao Suzuki

T. K. Woodruff et al. (eds.), *Textbook of Oncofertility Research and Practice*,
https://doi.org/10.1007/978-3-030-02868-8_15

Key Points

- Cancer care providers should prioritize cancer therapy rather than fertility.
- Cancer care providers should discuss treatment-related infertility risks and fertility preservation options to CAYA cancer patients prior to initiation of cancer therapy and refer to FP program or reproductive specialists as early as possible.
- Cancer care providers should know the detailed gonadotoxicity of cancer therapy and pregnancy/neonatal outcome after initiation of cancer therapy.
- Cancer treatments—Including chemotherapy, radiation therapy, and surgery—Are possible during pregnancy. Chemotherapy should be avoided during the first trimester. Radiation therapy is administered only in rare cases and the abdomen should be shielded.

15.1 Introduction

The face of both life-threatening cancer diagnosis and the desire to have a child in the future simultaneously present a struggle both for patients with cancer and for clinicians. Although improvement in multimodality treatment has enabled many cancer patients to survive a malignancy, these cancer treatments can result in gonadal dysfunction and infertility, especially for child, adolescents, and young adults (CAYA) and patients younger than 39 years old. The purpose of this chapter is to provide an overview of gonadotoxicity of cancer treatment, pregnancy outcome of women with a history of cancer, and the management of women diagnosed with cancer during pregnancy.

15.2 Becoming Pregnant After a Cancer Diagnosis

15.2.1 The Importance of Fertility-Related Discussion Before Cancer Therapy

It is important for oncologists to discuss about treatment-related infertility risks and fertility preservation (FP) options with CAYA cancer patients prior to initiation of potentially gonadotoxic therapies [21]. Although it is rational for most cancer patients to prioritize survival rather than fertility, having a child is an important life event after being treated for cancer [4, 5]. The American Society of Clinical Oncology (ASCO) guideline, American Society for Reproductive Medicine (ASRM), and National Comprehensive Cancer Network (NCCN) recommend the early provision of information on the risks to fertility associated with cancer treatment and on fertility preservation to all patients in reproductive age [10, 15, 23]. Despite these guidelines, many patients do not recall having fertility-related discussions with their physicians [27].The barriers to these conversations and referrals include a patient's poor prognosis, a disease requiring immediate treatment, marital or parenthood status, unclear referral paths for FP, and the cost of FP in insurance [27, 40]. To overcome unclear referral paths for FP, it has been reported that a formal oncofertility program with multidisciplinary team encouraging oncologists to address treatment-related infertility, discussing FP options, and referring to reproductive specialists prior to cancer treatment can increase discussions about FP and access to reproductive procedures [40]. Although it is sometimes difficult to deal with additional critical subjects after discussing the cancer treatment plan, the sooner the patient's fertility issues are addressed, the greater the chance that the patients can choose FP measures with minimum delay for cancer therapy [19].

Furthermore, explaining fertility issues to prepubertal child cancer patients is challenging. According to Anderson et al., while the negative effect of treatment on the ovarian function was discussed with 86% of the postpubertal girls and their parents, it was discussed with only 60% of the prepubertal girls [3]. Even adult patients who were not informed, did not undergo FP options, and later become infertile will later express regret associated with increased anxiety and depression during survivorship [40]. Although there are many reasons to not pursue FP procedures, just counseling a woman about reproductive health risks lowers long-term regret and increases satisfaction with life [29]. We believe it is important to continue to remind young patients of infertile potential and ovarian function assessment, in case these discussions either did not happen at cancer diagnosis, happened with parents, or have since been forgotten [20].

15.2.2 Gonadotoxicity of Cancer Therapies in CAYA Patients

Cancer treatments, including chemotherapy, radiation therapy, and surgery, can affect fertility by impacting the neuroendocrine axis, the primordial and growing follicles in the ovaries, and the reproductive organs such as uterus necessary for carrying a pregnancy to term. The human ovary contains a fixed number of primordial follicles at birth, estimated to be one million. These are progressively lost in a bi-exponential fashion as women age and approximately 400,000 follicles remain by the onset of puberty. During menopause, at an average age of 50–51 years, approximately less than 1000 oocytes remain [24, 41]. Both chemotherapy and radiation therapy will accelerate oocyte depletion, leading to a primary ovarian insufficiency (POI), which is defined as amenorrhea due to the premature depletion of functional ovarian follicles, in women <40 years [28, 41].

Radiation therapy can disrupt the functioning of the hypothalamic-pituitary axis, directly cause ovarian failure, or damage the uterus making it unable to accommodate the growth of a fetus to full term [43]. The impact of radiation on the body is largely dependent on the cumulative dose, location of the treatment, as well as the age of the patient [21]. Wallace et al have reported that the effective sterilizing dose (ESD), the dose of fractionated RT (Gy) at which premature ovarian failure occurs immediately following treatment in 97.5% of patients, decreases as age at treatment increases. ESD at birth is 20.3 Gy; at 10 years 18.4 Gy; at 20 years 16.5 Gy; and at 30 years 14.3 Gy [41]. Women who received abdominal or directed pelvic irradiation at high doses are at greater risk for subsequent infertility. Furthermore, a high dose of cranial irradiation may prevent secretion of gonadotrophin-releasing hormone (GnRH) and lead to lack of follicle-stimulating hormone (FSH) and luteinizing hormone (LH) resulting in affected release of estradiol and progesterone.

Certain chemotherapeutic agents can also negatively impact future fertility for young cancer survivors. Chemotherapeutic treatments can be gonadotoxic to primordial follicles as they cause DNA strand breaks, trigger apoptosis, and reduce stromal function within the ovary [31]. It has been reported that while reduction of the ovarian reserve may be caused from chemotherapy, there is also evidence that chemotherapy may impact the neuroendocrine axis. After receiving chemotherapy, many cancer survivors have growth hormone deficiency, hypothyroidism, or pubertal abnormalities [36]. Moreover, since it is known that gonadal damage in prepubertal children caused by chemotherapy and radiation may result in omission or delayed puberty, and abnormal development of secondary sex characteristics, it is important for providers to observe growth rates [36].

15.2.3 Pregnancy and Neonatal Outcomes After Cancer Therapy

It has been reported that female cancer survivors treated with pelvic radiotherapy had a twofold increased risk of low birth weight and preterm delivery among their infants [17]. It is associated with reduced adult uterine volume and reduced blood supply of the uterus [12, 22, 30, 35]. Also, pelvic irradiation significantly increased the risk of stillbirth and neonatal death at doses greater than 10 Gy [38]. Radiation to the brain also increases the chance of a miscarriage [16], possibly through dysfunction of the hypothalamic-pituitary-ovarian-axis function [7, 35]. However, no evidence has been reported [35].

While none of these studies found a statistically significant association between chemotherapy treatment during childhood and an increased risk for preterm birth or low birth weight [37], among chemotherapies, alkylating agents, including cyclophosphamides, procarbazine, and busulfan, are strongly associated with ovarian failure in a dose-dependent manner [24, 37]. Estimates of dosing thresholds vary among reports; the ASCO identifies a cyclophosphamide dose ≥ 7.5 g/m^2 in female younger than 20 years and a dose ≥ 5 g/m^2 in female older than 40 years as a high risk for amenorrhea after therapy [24, 26].

15.3 Cancer Diagnosis During Pregnancy

The approximate incidence of cancer diagnosed during pregnancy is 1 per 1000 pregnancies in the USA (Smith et al.). The most common types of cancer for women in the reproductive age group are breast cancer, hematological cancer, melanoma, cervical cancer, and thyroid in the USA (Smith et al.). After diagnosis of malignancy has been established during pregnancy, the patients should be referred to a multidisciplinary team containing, besides the oncology team, an obstetrician and a neonatologist [42]. If chemotherapy cannot be delayed until after delivery, and if termination is not desired, or if termination is prohibited by law, chemotherapy during pregnancy can be considered.

Chemotherapy should be administered only after the 12th–14th week of pregnancy until a gestational week of 35th–37th [2]. Exposure during the first trimester increases the risk of spontaneous abortion, fetal death, and major malformations, and direct effects of the tumor sometimes confound the risks of fetal loss [2, 9]. The estimated incidence for major malformations during the first trimester is 10–20% [1], while the administration of chemotherapy after the first trimester does not result in an increased rate of malformation [17]. During the second and third trimester, although the damage is suggested to be less extensive since it is after the organogenesis period [2, 37], the eyes and genitalia, the central nervous system (CNS), and the hematopoietic system remain vulnerable to exposure [2, 9, 37]. The risks of fetal growth restriction (FGR), preterm labor, and low birth weight are increased during the second and third trimesters [9, 44]. The placenta plays a role as barrier and may protect the fetus from cytotoxic agents in maternal blood [2]. This information may prevent termination of pregnancy permitting treatment of disease during a pregnancy [25].

According to the recommendation from NCCN, radiation therapy during pregnancy is contraindicated [11]. However, in very rare cases, when radiation therapy is needed, it should be delivered in low therapeutic doses with adequate uterine shielding to minimize fetal exposure [11]. The successful use of radiation therapy in pregnancy, particularly in breast cancer, Hodgkin lymphoma, brain cancer, and head and neck tumors, with appropriate shielding describes healthy pregnancy outcomes showing fetal exposure to be approximately 30–100 mGy from first and second trimester when tumor site dosing ranged from 30 to 80 Gy in the mother. However, fetal radiation doses >100 mGy are associated with fetal malformation and mental retardation [34, 37].

Surgery is possible at any time during pregnancy depending on the anatomic location of the tumor. In general, abdominal surgery is often deferred to the second trimester because the risk of miscarriage is decreased and the size of the uterus still allows a certain degree of access [13, 14]. Van Calsteren et al. have reported that surgery was performed in 65.7% of women with any cancer treatment during pregnancy [8].

Whether or not pregnancy negatively influences maternal prognosis has been a topic to be discussed. The mortality for pregnant patients with cancer is not different from nonpregnant patients when corrected for stage and age at diagnosis [39]. It has been reported that patients with cancer during pregnancy present with a more advanced stage of disease because of delay in diagnosis [39]. Since stage of diagnosis is strongly correlated to prognosis, a higher stage at time of diagnosis (due to patient and doctor's delay) may contribute to a worse maternal outcome, and this should be avoided where possible.

15

15.4 Contraceptive Use to Avoid Pregnancy

Many cancer units do not routinely bring up contraception necessity and many women during or following cancer treatment believe they are infertile. Even though chemotherapy and radiation reduce fertility and may cause ovarian failure, many patients still remain fertile [18, 32]. In the USA, due to this imprecise recognition among the patients, many women patients and cancer survivors aged 15–30 who got pregnant unintentionally were more likely to terminate a pregnancy than age-matched controls [16, 33]. For this reason, here we aim to emphasize that contraception counseling is important. Women should be counseled that irregular menses or amenorrhea does not always mean that they are infertile.

Contraception is a key to avoid unintended pregnancy; however, all contraception is not the same. The selection of contraception for cancer patients depends on the following factors: type of malignancy, disease status (active vs. remission), and other medical comorbidities. Combined hormone contraception should be avoided for hormone-dependent malignancy, such as breast cancer, because it may be able to effect prognosis or increase the possibility of recurrence. For patients who are contraindicated from utilizing estrogen therapy, other options include intrauterine devices (IUDs), barrier, or behavioral methods [17].

Furthermore the general recommendation of the optimal time point to attempt conception is 2–5 years after completion of chemotherapy because that is the timeframe when most relapses occur [17]. Some oncologists recommend 6 months after completion of chemotherapy because this timeframe can eliminate any eggs damaged by chemotherapy or radiation and it has been suggested that it takes approximately 6 months for a new cohort of follicles to be recruited for growth and maturation. However these recommendations are largely anecdotal, and there is no solid evidence to suggest that postponing conception will alter the outcome of cancer and pregnancy [6, 21].

15.5 Conclusion

There are many gaps in our knowledge, and we should keep continuing to develop the databases of obstetrical outcomes of cancer survivors and surviving offspring. Such a database would enhance the field-wide knowledge of the effects of cancer therapy and the risks on future offspring. Taken together, these understandings will improve the patients' long-term QOL and address one of the most difficult problems facing an emerging group of cancer patients.

Review Questions and Answers

Q1. Why is it important to discuss treatment-related fertility risks and FP options prior to cancer therapy?

A1. It may be possible to preserve fertility if cancer patients are provided the information of the risk of infertility and FP options prior to initiation of cancer treatment. And also, understanding the treatment's effect on fertility and patients' ability to make decision can improve the long-term QOL during cancer survivorship.

Q2. Are patients who experience oligomenorrhea or amenorrhea after chemotherapy always infertile?

A2. No. irregular menses or amenorrhea after cancer therapy does not always imply infertility. Reproductive-aged cancer patients should use contraceptives to avoid unintended pregnancy from the start of chemotherapy to at least 6 months after completion of chemotherapy.

Q3. Does the age of exposure to chemotherapy matter to infertility?

A3. Even though older women have a much higher reported incidence of acute POI, occurring during or immediately following treatment, chemotherapy may damage to follicles at all ages. The age-related difference may be because of older women having a smaller primordial follicle reserve at the start of treatment compared with young women, so that the loss from that already reduced follicle pool is more likely to induce POI.

Q4. What are the consequences of cancer treatment on pregnancy outcomes in cancer survivors?

A4. Female survivors exposed to abdominal irradiation had a significantly increased risk of low birth weight, preterm birth among their infant, and a small increased risk of miscarriage. The effects of chemotherapy in childhood cancer may vary among the reports, and it differs in each diagnosis and the kind of chemotherapeutic agents.

Q5. What are the effects of cancer treatment during pregnancy on fetal and child development?

A5. Chemotherapy in the first trimester is contraindicated because of an increased risk of congenital malformations and fetal death. The important risk of chemotherapy during second and the third trimester are preterm birth and low birth weight. Studies regarding radiation during pregnancy are insufficient.

References

1. Amant F, Han SN, Gziri MM, Dekrem J, Van Calsteren K. Chemotherapy during pregnancy. Curr Opin Oncol. 2012;24(5):580–6. https://doi.org/10.1097/CCO.0b013e328354e754.
2. Amant F, Han SN, Gziri MM, Vandenbroucke T, Verheecke M, Van Calsteren K. Management of cancer in pregnancy. Best Pract Res Clin Obstet Gynaecol. 2015;29(5):741–53. https://doi.org/10.1016/j.bpobgyn.2015.02.006.
3. Anderson RA, Weddell A, Spoudeas HA, Douglas C, Shalet SM, Levitt G, Wallace WH. Do doctors discuss fertility issues before they treat young patients with cancer? Hum Reprod. 2008;23(10):2246–51. https://doi.org/10.1093/humrep/den252.
4. Armuand GM, Wettergren L, Rodriguez-Wallberg KA, Lampic C. Desire for children, difficulties achieving a pregnancy, and infertility distress 3 to 7 years after cancer diagnosis. Support Care Cancer: Off J Multinatl Assoc Support Care Cancer. 2014;22(10):2805–12. https://doi.org/10.1007/s00520-014-2279-z.
5. Armuand GM, Wettergren L, Rodriguez-Wallberg KA, Lampic C. Women more vulnerable than men when facing risk for treatment-induced infertility: a qualitative study of young adults newly diagnosed with cancer. Acta Oncol (Stockholm, Sweden). 2015;54(2):243–52. https://doi.org/10.3109/0284186x.2014.948573.
6. Arnon J, Meirow D, Lewis-Roness H, Ornoy A. Genetic and teratogenic effects of cancer treatments on gametes and embryos. Hum Reprod Update. 2001;7(4):394–403.
7. Bath LE, Anderson RA, Critchley HO, Kelnar CJ, Wallace WH. Hypothalamic-pituitary-ovarian dysfunction after prepubertal chemotherapy and cranial irradiation for acute leukemia. Hum Reprod. 2001;16:1838–44.
8. Calsteren KV, Heyns L, Smet FD, Eycken LV, Gziri MM, Gemert WV, Halaska M, Vergote I, Ottevanger N, Amant F. Cancer during pregnancy: an analysis of 215 patients emphasizing the obstetrical and the neonatal outcomes. J Clin Oncol. 2010;28(4):683–9. https://doi.org/10.1200/jco.2009.23.2801.
9. Cardonick E, Iacobucci A. Use of chemotherapy during human pregnancy. Lancet Oncol. 2004;5(5):283–91. https://doi.org/10.1016/S1470-2045(04)01466-4.
10. Coccia PF, Altman J, Bhatia S, Borinstein SC, Flynn J, George S, Goldsby R, Hayashi R, Huang MS, Johnson RH, Beaupin LK, Link MP, Oeffinger KC, Orr KM, Pappo AS, Reed D, Spraker HL, Thomas DA, von Mehren M, Wechsler DS, Whelan KF, Zebrack BJ, Sundar H, Shead DA. Adolescent and young adult oncology. Clinical practice guidelines in oncology. J Natl Compr Cancer Netw: JNCCN. 2012;10(9):1112–50.
11. Coccia PF, Pappo AS, Beaupin L, Borges VF, Borinstein SC, Chugh R, Dinner S, Folbrecht J, Frazier AL, Goldsby R, Gubin A, Hayashi R, Huang MS, Link MP, Livingston JA, Matloub Y, Millard F, Oeffinger KC, Puccetti D, Reed D, Robinson S, Rosenberg AR, Sanft T, Spraker-Perlman HL, von Mehren M, Wechsler DS, Whelan KF, Yeager N, Gurski LA, Shead DA. Adolescent and young adult oncology, version 2.2018, NCCN clinical practice guidelines in oncology. J Natl Compr Cancer Netw: JNCCN. 2018;16(1):66–97. https://doi.org/10.6004/jnccn.2018.0001.
12. Critchley HO, Wallace WH, Shalet SM, Mamtora H, Higginson J, Anderson DC. Abdominal irradiation in childhood; the potential for pregnancy. Br J Obstet Gynaecol. 1992;99(5):392–4.
13. Doll DC, Ringenberg QS, Yarbro JW. Management of cancer during pregnancy. Arch Intern Med. 1988;148(9):2058–64.
14. Duncan PG, Pope WD, Cohen MM, Greer N. Fetal risk of anesthesia and surgery during pregnancy. Anesthesiology. 1986;64(6):790–4.
15. Fertility preservation and reproduction in patients facing gonadotoxic therapies: a committee opinion. Fertil Steril. 2013;100(5):1224–31. https://doi.org/10.1016/j.fertnstert.2013.08.041
16. Green DM, Whitton JA, Stovall M, Mertens AC, Donaldson SS, Ruymann FB, Pendergrass TW, Robison LL. Pregnancy outcome of female survivors of childhood cancer: a report from the Childhood Cancer Survivor Study. Am J Obstet Gynecol. 2002;187(4):1070–80.
17. Hideyuki IYI, Teresa KW. Pregnancy and cancer. Glob J Reprod Med. 2017;1:4.
18. Hodgson DC, Pintilie M, Gitterman L, Dewitt B, Buckley CA, Ahmed S, Smith K, Schwartz A, Tsang RW, Crump M, Wells W, Sun A, Gospodarowicz MK. Fertility among female hodgkin lymphoma survivors attempting pregnancy following ABVD chemotherapy. Hematol Oncol. 2007;25(1):11–5. https://doi.org/10.1002/hon.802.
19. Jeruss JS. Discussing fertility preservation with breast cancer patients. Cancer Treat Res. 2010;156:461–6. https://doi.org/10.1007/978-1-4419-6518-9_35.
20. Knight S, Lorenzo A, Maloney AM, Srikanthan A, Donen R, Greenblatt E, Gupta A. An approach to fertility preservation in prepubertal and postpubertal females: a critical review of current literature. Pediatr Blood Cancer. 2015;62(6):935–9. https://doi.org/10.1002/pbc.25440.
21. Kong BY, Skory RM, Woodruff TK. Creating a continuum of care: integrating obstetricians and gynecologists in the care of young cancer patients. Clin Obstet Gynecol. 2011;54(4):619–32. https://doi.org/10.1097/GRF.0b013e318236ea2c.
22. Larsen EC, Schmiegelow K, Rechnitzer C, Loft A, Muller J, Andersen AN. Radiotherapy at a young age reduces uterine volume of childhood cancer survivors. Acta Obstet Gynecol Scand. 2004;83(1):96–102.

23. Lee SJ, Schover LR, Partridge AH, Patrizio P, Wallace WH, Hagerty K, Beck LN, Brennan LV, Oktay K. American Society of Clinical Oncology recommendations on fertility preservation in cancer patients. J Clin Oncol. 2006;24(18):2917–31. https://doi.org/10.1200/jco.2006.06.5888.
24. Levine JM, Kelvin JF, Quinn GP, Gracia CR. Infertility in reproductive-age female cancer survivors. Cancer. 2015;121:1532–9.
25. Litton JK, Warneke CL, Hahn KM, Palla SL, Kuerer HM, Perkins GH, Mittendorf EA, Barnett C, Gonzalez-Angulo AM, Hortobagyi GN, Theriault RL. Case control study of women treated with chemotherapy for breast cancer during pregnancy as compared with nonpregnant patients with breast cancer. Oncologist. 2013;18(4):369–76. https://doi.org/10.1634/theoncologist.2012-0340.
26. Loren AW, Mangu PB, Beck LN, Brennan L, Magdalinski AJ, Partridge AH, Quinn G, Wallace WH, Oktay K, American Society of Clinical O. Fertility preservation for patients with cancer: American Society of Clinical Oncology clinical practice guideline update. J Clin Oncol. 2013;31(19):2500–10. https://doi.org/10.1200/JCO.2013.49.2678.
27. Micaux Obol C, Armuand GM, Rodriguez-Wallberg KA, Ahlgren J, Ljungman P, Wettergren L, Lampic C. Oncologists and hematologists' perceptions of fertility-related communication – a nationwide survey. Acta Oncol (Stockholm, Sweden). 2017;56(8):1103–10. https://doi.org/10.1080/0284186x.2017.1310394.
28. Morgan S, Anderson RA, Gourley C, Wallace WH, Spears N. How do chemotherapeutic agents damage the ovary? Hum Reprod Update. 2012;18(5):525–35.
29. Niemasik EE, Letourneau J, Dohan D, Katz A, Melisko M, Rugo H, Rosen M. Patient perceptions of reproductive health counseling at the time of cancer diagnosis: a qualitative study of female California cancer survivors. J Cancer Surviv. 2012;6(3):324–32. https://doi.org/10.1007/s11764-012-0227-9.
30. Nussbaum Blask AR, Nicholson HS, Markle BM, Wechsler-Jentzch K, O'Donnell R, Byrne J. Sonographic detection of uterine and ovarian abnormalities in female survivors of Wilms' tumor treated with radiotherapy. AJR Am J Roentgenol. 1999;172(3):759–63. https://doi.org/10.2214/ajr.172.3.10063876.
31. Oktem O, Oktay K. Quantitative assessment of the impact of chemotherapy on ovarian follicle reserve and stromal function. Cancer. 2007;110(10):2222–9. https://doi.org/10.1002/cncr.23071.
32. Partridge AH, Gelber S, Peppercorn J, Ginsburg E, Sampson E, Rosenberg R, Przypyszny M, Winer EP. Fertility and menopausal outcomes in young breast cancer survivors. Clin Breast Cancer. 2008;8(1):65–9. https://doi.org/10.3816/CBC.2008.n.004.
33. Patel A, Schwarz EB. Cancer and contraception. Release date May 2012. SFP guideline #20121. Contraception. 2012;86(3):191–8. https://doi.org/10.1016/j.contraception.2012.05.008.
34. Peccatori FA, Azim HA Jr, Orecchia R, Hoekstra HJ, Pavlidis N, Kesic V, Pentheroudakis G. Cancer, pregnancy and fertility: ESMO Clinical Practice Guidelines for diagnosis, treatment and follow-up. Ann Oncol. 2013;24(6):160–70.
35. Reulen RC, Zeegers MP, Wallace WH, Frobisher C, Taylor AJ, Lancashire ER, Winter DL, Hawkins MM. Pregnancy outcomes among adult survivors of childhood cancer in the British Childhood Cancer Survivor Study. Cancer Epidemiol Biomark Prev. 2009;18(8):2239–47. https://doi.org/10.1158/1055-9965.epi-09-0287.
36. Rose SR, Schreiber RE, Kearney NS, Lustig RH, Danish RK, Burghen GA, Hudson MM. Hypothalamic dysfunction after chemotherapy. J Pediatr Endocrinol Metab: JPEM. 2004;17(1):55–66.
37. Sabeti Rad Z. The effect of maternal malignancy on fertility, pregnancy, and neonatal outcomes. Lund: Lund university; 2017.
38. Signorello LB, Mulvihill JJ, Green DM, Munro HM, Stovall M, Weathers RE, Mertens AC, Whitton JA, Robison LL, Boice JD Jr. Stillbirth and neonatal death in relation to radiation exposure before conception: a retrospective cohort study. Lancet (London, England). 2010;376(9741):624–30. https://doi.org/10.1016/s0140-6736(10)60752-0.
39. Stensheim H, Moller B, van Dijk T, Fossa SD. Cause-specific survival for women diagnosed with cancer during pregnancy or lactation: a registry-based cohort study. J Clin Oncol. 2009;27(1):45–51. https://doi.org/10.1200/jco.2008.17.4110.
40. Vu JV, Llarena NC, Estevez SL, Moravek MB, Jeruss JS. Oncofertility program implementation increases access to fertility preservation options and assisted reproductive procedures for breast cancer patients. J Surg Oncol. 2017;115(2):116–21. https://doi.org/10.1002/jso.24418.
41. Wallace WH, Thomson AB, Kelsey TW. The radiosensitivity of the human oocyte. Hum Reprod. 2003;18(1):117–21.
42. Wang E. Pregnancy in cancer patients and survivors. In: Gracia C, Woodruff TK, editors. Oncofertility medical practice: clinical issues and implementation. New York: Springer New York; 2012. p. 129–48. https://doi.org/10.1007/978-1-4419-9425-7_10.
43. Wo JY, Viswanathan AN. The impact of radiotherapy on fertility, pregnancy, and neonatal outcomes of female cancer patients. Int J Radiat Oncol Biol Phys. 2009;73(5):1304–12. https://doi.org/10.1016/j.ijrobp.2008.12.016.
44. Zemlickis D, Lishner M, Degendorfer P, Panzarella T, Sutcliffe SB, Koren G. Fetal outcome after in utero exposure to cancer chemotherapy. Arch Intern Med. 1992;152(3):573–6.

Assessing Testicular Reserve in the Male Oncology Patient

James A. Kashanian and Robert E. Brannigan

T. K. Woodruff et al. (eds.), *Textbook of Oncofertility Research and Practice*,
https://doi.org/10.1007/978-3-030-02868-8_16

Key Points

- All patients should be counseled on the possibility of infertility arising as a consequence of oncology treatments.
- Normal testicular function is based on an intact hypothalamic-pituitary-gonadal (HPG) axis.
- Testicular function comprises reproductive and androgenic function, and males may have a congenital or acquired defect in reproductive function (spermatogenesis), androgenic function (testosterone), or both.
- A serum testosterone level, a serum FSH level, and a semen analysis are currently the most robust biomarkers for assessing testicular reserve in the male cancer survivor.

16.1 Overview

Over the past decade, numerous professional organizations have published fertility preservation recommendations that call for the seamless coordination of oncology care with concurrent fertility preservation care. For interested males, the cryopreservation of sperm prior to the initiation of cancer therapy has become an important aspect of comprehensive cancer care. Because fertility preservation is a major concern for many male patients diagnosed with malignancy, it is of utmost importance for healthcare providers to discuss fertility preservation with affected patients as soon as possible after a cancer diagnosis is made.

In its updated guidelines published in 2013, the American Society of Clinical Oncology (ASCO) recommended that all patients should be counseled on the possibility of infertility arising as a consequence of oncology treatments. Additionally, these guidelines call for clinicians to offer early referral to fertility preservation specialists to further discuss these issues and help deliver fertility preservation care if the patient is interested [1].

Despite these guidelines, it is estimated that less than half of male pubertal cancer patients are referred for fertility preservation consultation or sperm cryopreservation. Furthermore, less than half of pediatric oncology specialists are familiar with the ASCO recommendations on fertility preservation. This marked disparity exists despite the fact that published studies demonstrate that one of the biggest regrets male cancer survivors have is not discussing the deleterious reproductive effects of cancer therapy and options for fertility preservation [2].

While some men may permanently lose the ability to produce viable sperm as a result of their cancer therapies, others will, over time, have the return of sperm to the ejaculate. The proper determination of posttreatment fertility is an important aspect of ongoing care and can be a fluid situation changing over weeks, months, and even years. Clinicians must be familiar with the reproductive toxicities associated with various cancer treatment regimens, as these side effects can impact the endocrine system which drives male reproduction, the testes in which sperm production occurs, and the excurrent ductal system, which is responsible for sperm transport into the female reproductive tract. Finally, clinicians must be capable of accurately counseling patients as they consider their reproduction options.

Normal testicular function is based on an intact hypothalamic-pituitary-gonadal (HPG) axis. The HPG axis drives male sexual development and fertility. This process is initiated by gonadotropin-releasing hormone (GnRH) that is secreted by the hypothalamus in a pulsatile manner. The distinct frequency and amplitude of these pulses directly stimulates luteinizing hormone (LH) and follicle-stimulating hormone (FSH) secretion by the anterior pituitary gland. FSH and LH support testicular Sertoli cell and Leydig cell function, respectively.

Testicular function comprises reproductive and androgenic function, and males may have a congenital or acquired defect in reproductive function (spermatogenesis), androgenic function (testosterone), or both. In the assessment of male reproductive and androgenic testicular function, it is important to delineate between primary and secondary causes. Etiologies of primary testicular dysfunction are vast and can include cryptorchidism, disorders of sexual development (DSDs), trauma, infection, iatrogenic causes, and medication use. Cancer therapies, including surgery, chemotherapy, and radiation therapy, can also cause primary testicular failure and adversely affect fertility. Causes of secondary testicular failure can include genetic abnormalities affecting the HPG axis, brain tumors, trauma, and iatrogenic causes. Again, cancer therapies such as surgery, chemotherapy, and radiation therapy can also impact the HPG axis, leading to secondary testicular failure and adversely affecting fertility. The effects of cancer therapy, whether causing primary or secondary testicular failure side effects, occur in a dose-dependent and treatment-dependent manner [3–6]. Spermatogenesis, for example, is often impacted by chemotherapy in a dose-dependent fashion [3]. A history of chemotherapy is also often associated with an increase in posttreatment gonadotropin (LH and FSH) levels, a sign that the pituitary gland is actively compensating for impaired testicular production of testosterone and sperm, respectively [7]. Likewise, radiation therapy can affect testicular function by potentially damaging both germ cells and Leydig cells. Transient effects on spermatogenesis are common at very low doses (≤2 Gy) of radiation therapy. Cumulative doses >2 Gy can result in transient or even permanent azoospermia [8]. At doses in excess of 20 Gy, Leydig cell testosterone production is commonly affected, with some men developing lasting primary hypogonadism [8].

Biomarkers are, by definition, measurable indicators of a physiological state within an organism. Sensitivity, specificity, low cost, and attainability are hallmark features of an ideal biomarker, including biomarkers to monitor male androgenic and reproductive function [9]. As will be detailed below, numerous biomarkers have been investigated in order to quantify animal and human reproductive function [9]. When assessing testicular reserve in a male cancer survivor, clinicians should keep in mind that the minimum initial evaluation of the patient should include a full medical history, physical examination, and measurement of serum testosterone and FSH levels [10].

16.2 Evaluation

A full medical history, including a detailed accounting of all oncology treatments, is the first step in a comprehensive reproductive evaluation of male cancer survivors. Modes of therapy, dosage, and duration of treatment often impact the severity and duration of testicular dysfunction. A complete genitourinary exam is also an essential component of the evaluation of a male cancer survivor. Particular attention should be paid to the patient's overall appearance, with an assessment for clinical signs of low androgen levels. This can include changes such as a decrease in muscle mass and body hair. A breast exam should be conducted to assess for gynecomastia, which is a common sign of hyperestrogenemia. Additionally, a careful scrotal exam should be performed. This includes documentation of the size, consistency, and location of the testicles bilaterally. Assessment for the presence and condition of the epididymis and vas deferens is also important. The clinician should assess these structures meticulously in order to assess for changes that might suggest evidence of inflammation and/or obstruction that can sometimes result in response to the tumor or iatrogenically as an outcome of cancer therapies. While not a foolproof determinant of reproductive potential, testicular size can be a meaningful predictor of testicular function (hormone and sperm production) [11].

16.3 Hormones

Serum testosterone and FSH levels are useful in determining reproductive potential and facilitating the differentiation between subtypes of subfertility and infertility [10]. Endocrine abnormalities are highly prevalent in the setting of certain types of cancer. For example, among testicular cancer survivors, half will have at least one abnormality long term in testosterone, LH, or FSH following treatment [7].

FSH acts on testicular Sertoli cells to support spermatogonial proliferation and maturation through meiosis. FSH levels have been shown to be inversely correlated to testicular spermatogenic function and are commonly used as a barometer for spermatogenesis. Schoor et al. published data demonstrating that 8% of men with nonobstructive azoospermia will have a serum FSH level greater than 7.6 mIU/ml and a testicular long axis of <4.6 cm. These authors also showed that over 90% of men with normal sperm production will have an FSH in the normal range [12]. Several other groups have critically assessed the role of FSH as a biomarker for spermatogenesis and have reported similar findings. These authors have collectively recommended FSH reference ranges for adult men with the upper limit of normal for FSH being between 7.5 and 7.8 mIU/ml [13, 14]. Since there is minimal diurnal variation in FSH levels, a single level is sufficient to assess spermatogenesis [15].

Occasionally, an oncology patient will be found to have an abnormally low serum FSH level. This can result from tumor involvement with the hypothalamus and/or pituitary gland or cancer treatments (especially radiation therapy or surgical procedures) involving these same structures. For patients affected by abnormally low FSH levels, recombinant FSH (r-FSH) therapy typically results in normalization of FSH levels and restoration of fertility potential.

LH stimulates testicular Leydig cell testosterone production. Serum levels of LH help to delineate if the origin of androgenic testicular failure is secondary to a central cause (low LH) or to a primary testicular cause (normal or increased LH). Sometimes, an oncology patient will be found to have abnormally low serum LH levels. As is the case for low FSH, this can result from tumor involvement with the hypothalamus and/or pituitary gland or cancer treatments involving these same structures. For patients affected by abnormally low LH levels, hCG therapy typically results in normalization of testosterone levels and restoration of fertility potential.

Testosterone is the male sex hormone that stimulates male muscle mass production, hair growth, libido, erections, bone health, and RBC production. Testosterone is also paramount in supporting spermatogenesis [16–18]. LH stimulates testicular Leydig cells to produce testosterone, which has autocrine, paracrine, and endocrine effects. Low levels of testosterone, although not necessarily predictive of spermatogenic failure, can potentiate poor sperm production and low sperm concentrations in the semen. Testosterone levels peak early in the morning, and AM levels are preferred for evaluation purposes. In the setting of post-cancer treatment, the best predictors of low testosterone are increasing patient age and low residual testicular volume <12 cc [19].

Inhibin B is a dimer molecule comprised of alpha and beta subunits and is secreted by Sertoli cells in the testicle. Inhibin B exerts negative feedback on FSH secretion by the anterior pituitary gland, and there is thus an inverse relationship between serum inhibin B and serum FSH levels. Inhibin B levels are positively correlated with testicle volume and sperm concentration. In infertile patients, inhibin B levels are decreased and FSH levels are increased. In general, the more pronounced the degree of spermatogenic impairment and the earlier the state of spermatogenic disruption, the lower the inhibin B level.

In patients with a history of receiving chemotherapy or radiation therapy, inhibin B levels are often diminished [20]. Some investigators postulate that inhibin B and inhibin B/FSH ratios are more sensitive markers of male infertility than FSH levels alone [21]. Others have shown that levels of inhibin B can predict basal and reserve Sertoli cell activity [22]. Despite these findings, inhibin B has a limited role in serving as a marker of spermatogenesis, with conflicting results being reported in the literature. For example, inhibin B levels are not reliable predictors of the presence of some foci of spermatogenesis in men with azoospermia [23]. Because of the inconsistent results, most clinicians do not routinely use serum inhibin B as a marker for predicting spermatogenesis.

Anti-Müllerian hormone (*AMH*) is another hormone that has garnered attention as a possible reproductive biomarker in males. In females, AMH serves as a biomarker for ovarian reserve. In males, some authors have suggested that this protein may be helpful to determine gonadal function, including FSH activity upon the testicle and androgen action within the testicle [24]. Several studies have specifically investigated the role of AMH as a marker for spermatogenesis [25] and, more specifically, chemotherapy-induced testicular toxicity [26]. To date, AMH has not been found to be a reliable predictor of spermatogenesis in men with infertility, including men with a history of cancer treatments. AMH is thus not routinely used to determine testicular reserve, in contrast to its effective role in determining ovarian reserve.

Estrogen is formed in males by the peripheral aromatization of testosterone in the adipose, brain, skin, and bone tissue. Estrogen's role in spermatogenic maturation is still being delineated. In excess levels, it inhibits GnRH and LH release. At this time, estrogen is not routinely used in the evaluation of testicular reserve following cancer therapy, but it is a lab value often checked in the clinical evaluation of an infertile male. For cancer survivors with obesity, estradiol serum levels should be assessed to ensure that levels are not elevated, which can result in suppression of testosterone production.

16.4 Semen Testing

Cryopreservation of sperm prior to the commencement of gonadotoxic cancer treatment is the preferred approach for fertility preservation in males. Sperm banking should be considered for all patients diagnosed with any malignancy, especially males diagnosed with testicular cancer, leukemia, and lymphoma. The importance of sperm cryopreservation is evident in studies revealing that most cancer patients remain interested in future fertility and continue storage of banked sperm even after completion of cancer treatment [27, 28]. Men who cryopreserve sperm are more likely to be young and single compared to those who opt against sperm banking. Additionally, men who bank sperm are more likely to father a child after treatment, whether it be by natural means or IVF [29, 30]. While interest in fertility preservation is high, approximately 10–15% of oncology patients who desire to bank sperm are unable to do so for a variety of reasons, including psychosocial issues, anejaculation, necrospermia, or azoospermia [28, 31]. For these males, sperm can often be surgically extracted from the testicles for cryopreservation. Also, while high percentages of patients opt to bank sperm, there are those men who choose not to do so. Proper reproductive counseling is imperative for these men who decide against sperm cryopreservation before commencing oncologic therapy, as they may put themselves at risk of permanent infertility.

At baseline, before initiation of cancer therapy, patients with certain malignancies may have significantly lower sperm concentration and worse semen quality compared to fertile controls [28, 31, 32]. Six to 11.8% of all oncology patients will be azoospermic at the time of presentation [31, 33–35]. This is in stark contrast to the incidence of azoospermia in the general population, which is 1% [36]. Overall tumor burden and tumor stage are factors that can impact these parameters in some men [37, 38]. Chemotherapeutic regimens can also have an array of effects on spermatogenesis. This can range from no or minimal impact on semen parameters to temporary oligospermia or azoospermia with significant recovery to normospermia [4], to irreversible oligospermia, or to azoospermia [3]. The latter outcome is particularly associated with alkylating agent in chemotherapy. Similarly, radiation therapy can also affect quantitative semen characteristics in the short and long term, but semen parameters will often return to baseline by 24 months after treatment [32]. The ultimate effects on spermatogenesis, however, depend largely on the dose and location of radiation therapy being delivered. Bujan et al. demonstrated that 6% of men remained azoospermic at 12 months and 2% at 24 months following radiation therapy for testicular cancer [32].

Unlike in females, where ovarian reserve is established in utero and declines over time, spermatogenesis commences at puberty and continues throughout life. Because of this, the semen analysis is currently the gold standard for assessing fertility status in the male. This test is readily available at most tertiary care centers and can be performed at any age after puberty. The rapid increase in spermatogonial density and testicular volume associated with increasing gonadotropin levels starts at an average age of 11 years [39]. However, when assessing one's ability to produce a semen specimen, the focus should be on Tanner stage and not on chronological age [40]. In a study from Children's Hospital of Philadelphia assessing semen quality in AYA patients, 64.5%, 80.5%, and 90.3% of patients had sperm present on semen analysis in age groups 11–14, 14–17, and 17–30 years, respectively [40]. Average sperm concentration was 20.0, 33.8, and 40.0 million sperm/ml in age groups 11–14, 14–17, and 17–30 years, respectively [40].

Semen analysis testing is an easy, cost-effective, and noninvasive mode of determining fertility potential in the male. Important parameters that comprise a formal semen analysis include the semen volume, sperm concentration, sperm motility, and sperm morphology. In 2010, the World Health Organization (WHO) published the fifth edition of the *Laboratory Manual for the Examination and Processing of Human Semen*. Normal reference ranges were based on semen parameters of men whose partners became pregnant within 12 months of trying to conceive. Cutoffs above the fifth percentile were considered normal [41]. ◘ Table 9.1 represents normal reference ranges of bulk semen parameters for the WHO IV and WHO V editions.

Although these values are all taken into account when discussing male fertility, there is no algorithm available to reliably predict future fertility in men based on varying levels of sperm concentration, motility, and morphology. Calculations of the total sperm count, total motile

Table 9.1 Bulk semen parameters

	WHO fourth edition	WHO fifth edition
Volume	≥2.0 ml	≥1.5 ml
Sperm concentration	≥20 million sperm per ml	≥15 million sperm per ml
Sperm motility	≥50% total motility	≥40% total motility
Sperm morphology	≥14% normal forms	>4% normal forms
White blood cells	$\leq 1.0 \times 10^6$ per ml	$<1.0 \times 10^6$ per ml

sperm count, and morphology cutoffs have all been fraught with inaccuracy in predicting absolute fertility potential.

Furthermore, some men have an absence of sperm in ejaculated semen, or azoospermia. In a systemic review in 2016, 7% of AYA cancer patients were unable or failed to cryopreserve, the majority of these being secondary to azoospermia [42]. But even in the most challenging of cases, options for fertility are available. Live births are possible in azoospermic men via sperm retrieval with microdissection testicular sperm extraction and subsequent use with IVF [43].

16.5 Future Direction

16

In this evolving age of personalized medicine, increasing attention has been focused on the genetics of male fertility. As in other disease states, biomarkers are frequently used for diagnosis and stratification, treatment selection, monitoring of disease progression, and establishing patients' responses to therapy [44]. Although semen analysis testing is still recognized as a surrogate marker of male fertility, the exponential growth of biomarkers derived from proteomics, epigenomics, and genomics has contributed to a new direction of male fertility research. This shift in investigative focus could prove to be the next frontier in directed personalized medicine. However, although many studies have evaluated the genetic basis of male fertility, basic science and translational research have not resulted in a wealth of clinically useful diagnostic tests. Ideally, insights would be gained into genetic susceptibility to various cancer therapies, as well as propensity of an individual to regain reproductive function after completion of cancer treatment.

More than 3000 genes (about 4% of human genome) are expressed in the testicles alone, and hundreds of these genes influence reproductive function in humans [45]. Additionally, there are over 4000 proteins expressed in the seminal plasma. Because of this, significant attention has been focused on the proteomes of the testicles, sperm, seminal fluid, and epididymis [46]. It is thought that these proteins might represent a rich source of potential biomarkers for male fertility [47], and characterization of the reproductive proteome might ultimately lead to significant improvement in the evaluation of the male reproductive tract [48, 49].

This enhanced understanding of fertility markers at the level of the individual might facilitate the development of more comprehensive prognostic models for patients. The benefit of this approach would be potentially enhanced diagnostic capabilities, reduced cost, and personalized fertility treatments that anticipate reproductive success at baseline (before cancer treatment) and post-cancer therapy. This field is still quite young, and it is estimated that more than 1000 biomarkers would be needed to accurately evaluate male fertility potential [50]. Although much more clinical insight is needed, the implications of a more personalized approach to infertility risk stratification would be an enormously useful tool for clinicians and patients alike.

In conclusion, a serum testosterone level, a serum FSH level, and a semen analysis are currently the most robust biomarkers for assessing testicular reserve in the male cancer survivor. As the era of "personalized medicine" progresses, panels of biomarkers that stratify baseline fertility potential and posttreatment infertility risk will facilitate clinical decision-making for both healthcare providers and their patients.

Review Questions and Answers

Q1. A comprehensive urologic physical exam should include:

(a) Overall appearance, including muscle mass and body hair

(b) A breast exam to assess for gynecomastia

(c) Testicular exam documenting the size, consistency, and location of the testicles bilaterally
(d) Assessment of spermatic cord structures for the presence and condition of the epididymis and vas deferens
(e) All of the above.

A1. (e)

Q2. When assessing testicular function, the minimum hormone evaluation should include:
(a) FSH and LH
(b) LH and Testosterone
(c) FSH and Testosterone
(d) AMH and Testosterone
(e) Inhibin B and Testosterone

A2. (c)

Q3. FSH
(a) Is produced in the hypothalamus and acts on testicular Sertoli cells to support spermatogonial proliferation and maturation
(b) Is produced in the anterior pituitary and acts on testicular Sertoli cells to support spermatogonial proliferation and maturation
(c) Is produced in the hypothalamus and acts on testicular Leydig cells to stimulate testosterone production
(d) Is produced in the anterior pituitary and acts on testicular Leydig cells to stimulate testosterone production
(e) Is produced in the testicle and acts on Sertoli cells to support spermatogonial proliferation and maturation

A3. (b)

Q4. LH
(a) Is produced in the hypothalamus and acts on testicular Sertoli cells to support spermatogonial proliferation and maturation
(b) Is produced in the anterior pituitary and acts on testicular Sertoli cells to support spermatogonial proliferation and maturation
(c) Is produced in the hypothalamus and acts on testicular Leydig cells to stimulate testosterone production
(d) Is produced in the anterior pituitary and acts on testicular Leydig cells to stimulate testosterone production
(e) Is produced in the testicle and acts on Sertoli cells to support spermatogonial proliferation and maturation

A4. (d)

Q5. Testosterone is responsible for supporting
(a) Muscle mass
(b) Hair growth
(c) Libido and erections
(d) Bone health
(e) Red blood cell production
(f) All of the above

A5. (f)

References

1. Loren AW, Mangu PB, Beck LN, Brennan L, Magdalinski AJ, Partridge AH, et al. Fertility preservation for patients with cancer: American Society of Clinical Oncology clinical practice guideline update. J Clin Oncol Off J Am Soc Clin Oncol. 2013;31(19):2500–10.
2. Stein DM, Victorson DE, Choy JT, Waimey KE, Pearman TP, Smith K, et al. Fertility preservation preferences and perspectives among adult male survivors of pediatric cancer and their parents. J Adolesc Young Adult Oncol. 2014;3(2):75–82.
3. Green DM, Liu W, Kutteh WH, Ke RW, Shelton KC, Sklar CA, et al. Cumulative alkylating agent exposure and semen parameters in adult survivors of childhood cancer: a report from the St Jude Lifetime Cohort Study. Lancet Oncol. 2014;15(11):1215–23.
4. Howell SJ, Shalet SM. Testicular function following chemotherapy. Hum Reprod Update. 2001;7(4):363–9.
5. De Mas P, Daudin M, Vincent MC, Bourrouillou G, Calvas P, Mieusset R, et al. Increased aneuploidy in spermatozoa from testicular tumour patients after chemotherapy with cisplatin, etoposide and bleomycin. Hum Reprod (Oxford, Engl). 2001;16(6):1204–8.
6. Stahl O, Eberhard J, Cavallin-Stahl E, Jepson K, Friberg B, Tingsmark C, et al. Sperm DNA integrity in cancer patients: the effect of disease and treatment. Int J Androl. 2009;32(6):695–703.
7. Sprauten M, Brydoy M, Haugnes HS, Cvancarova M, Bjoro T, Bjerner J, et al. Longitudinal serum testosterone, luteinizing hormone, and follicle-stimulating hormone levels in a population-based sample of

long-term testicular cancer survivors. J Clin Oncol Off J Am Soc Clin Oncol. 2014;32(6):571–8.
8. Shalet SM. Effect of irradiation treatment on gonadal function in men treated for germ cell cancer. Eur Urol. 1993;23(1):148–51. discussion 52.
9. Dere E, Anderson LM, Hwang K, Boekelheide K. Biomarkers of chemotherapy-induced testicular damage. Fertil Steril. 2013;100(5):1192–202.
10. The optimal evaluation of the infertile male: best practice statement. American Urological Association. Reviewed and validity confirmed 2011.
11. Bahk JY, Jung JH, Jin LM, Min SK. Cut-off value of testes volume in young adults and correlation among testes volume, body mass index, hormonal level, and seminal profiles. Urology. 2010;75(6):1318–23.
12. Schoor RA, Elhanbly S, Niederberger CS, Ross LS. The role of testicular biopsy in the modern management of male infertility. J Urol. 2002;167(1):197–200.
13. Barbotin AL, Ballot C, Sigala J, Ramdane N, Duhamel A, Marcelli F, et al. The serum inhibin B concentration and reference ranges in normozoospermia. Eur J Endocrinol/Eur Fed Endocr Soc. 2015;172(6):669–76.
14. Gordetsky J, van Wijngaarden E, O'Brien J. Redefining abnormal follicle-stimulating hormone in the male infertility population. BJU Int. 2012;110(4):568–72.
15. Spratt DI, O'Dea LS, Schoenfeld D, Butler J, Rao PN, Crowley WF Jr. Neuroendocrine-gonadal axis in men: frequent sampling of LH, FSH, and testosterone. Am J Phys. 1988;254(5 Pt 1):E658–66.
16. Huang HF, Boccabella AV. Dissociation of qualitative and quantitative effects of the suppression of testicular testosterone upon spermatogenesis. Acta Endocrinol. 1988;118(2):209–17.
17. Jarow JP, Zirkin BR. The androgen microenvironment of the human testis and hormonal control of spermatogenesis. Ann N Y Acad Sci. 2005;1061:208–20.
18. Tsai MY, Yeh SD, Wang RS, Yeh S, Zhang C, Lin HY, et al. Differential effects of spermatogenesis and fertility in mice lacking androgen receptor in individual testis cells. Proc Natl Acad Sci U S A. 2006;103(50):18975–80.
19. Puhse G, Secker A, Kemper S, Hertle L, Kliesch S. Testosterone deficiency in testicular germ-cell cancer patients is not influenced by oncological treatment. Int J Androl. 2011;34(5 Pt 2):e351–7.
20. Marchetti C, Hamdane M, Mitchell V, Mayo K, Devisme L, Rigot JM, et al. Immunolocalization of inhibin and activin alpha and betaB subunits and expression of corresponding messenger RNAs in the human adult testis. Biol Reprod. 2003;68(1):230–5.
21. Grunewald S, Glander HJ, Paasch U, Kratzsch J. Age-dependent inhibin B concentration in relation to FSH and semen sample qualities: a study in 2448 men. Reproduction (Cambridge, England). 2013;145(3):237–44.
22. Adamopoulos D, Kapolla N, Nicopoulou S, Pappa A, Koukkou E, Gregoriou A. Assessment of Sertoli cell functional reserve and its relationship to sperm parameters. Int J Androl. 2003;26(4):215–25.
23. Tunc L, Kirac M, Gurocak S, Yucel A, Kupeli B, Alkibay T, et al. Can serum Inhibin B and FSH levels, testicular histology and volume predict the outcome of testicular sperm extraction in patients with non-obstructive azoospermia? Int Urol Nephrol. 2006;38(3–4):629–35.
24. Grinspon RP, Rey RA. New perspectives in the diagnosis of pediatric male hypogonadism: the importance of AMH as a sertoli cell marker. Arq Bras Endocrinol Metabologia. 2011;55(8):512–9.
25. Tuttelmann F, Dykstra N, Themmen AP, Visser JA, Nieschlag E, Simoni M. Anti-Mullerian hormone in men with normal and reduced sperm concentration and men with maldescended testes. Fertil Steril. 2009;91(5):1812–9.
26. Levi M, Hasky N, Stemmer SM, Shalgi R, Ben-Aharon I. Anti-Mullerian hormone is a marker for chemotherapy-induced testicular toxicity. Endocrinology. 2015;156:3818–27. en20151310.
27. Johnson MD, Cooper AR, Jungheim ES, Lanzendorf SE, Odem RR, Ratts VS. Sperm banking for fertility preservation: a 20-year experience. Eur J Obstet Gynecol Reprod Biol. 2013;170(1):177–82.
28. Bizet P, Saias-Magnan J, Jouve E, Grillo JM, Karsenty G, Metzler-Guillemain C, et al. Sperm cryopreservation before cancer treatment: a 15-year monocentric experience. Reprod Biomed Online. 2012;24(3):321–30.
29. Girasole CR, Cookson MS, Smith JA Jr, Ivey BS, Roth BJ, Chang SS. Sperm banking: use and outcomes in patients treated for testicular cancer. BJU Int. 2007;99(1):33–6.
30. Pacey A, Merrick H, Arden-Close E, Morris K, Rowe R, Stark D, et al. Implications of sperm banking for health-related quality of life up to 1 year after cancer diagnosis. Br J Cancer. 2013;108(5):1004–11.
31. van Casteren NJ, Boellaard WP, Romijn JC, Dohle GR. Gonadal dysfunction in male cancer patients before cytotoxic treatment. Int J Androl. 2010;33(1):73–9.
32. Bujan L, Walschaerts M, Moinard N, Hennebicq S, Saias J, Brugnon F, et al. Impact of chemotherapy and radiotherapy for testicular germ cell tumors on spermatogenesis and sperm DNA: a multicenter prospective study from the CECOS network. Fertil Steril. 2013;100(3):673–80.
33. Crha I, Ventruba P, Zakova J, Huser M, Kubesova B, Hudecek R, et al. Survival and infertility treatment in male cancer patients after sperm banking. Fertil Steril. 2009;91(6):2344–8.
34. Molnar Z, Benyo M, Bazsane Kassai Z, Levai I, Varga A, Jakab A. Influence of malignant tumors occurring in the reproductive age on spermiogenesis: studies on patients with testicular tumor and lymphoma. Orv Hetil. 2014;155(33):1306–11.
35. Zakova J, Lousova E, Ventruba P, Crha I, Pochopova H, Vinklarkova J, et al. Sperm cryopreservation before testicular cancer treatment and its subsequent utilization for the treatment of infertility. Sci World J. 2014;2014:575978.
36. Gangel EK. American Urological Association Inc, American Society for Reproductive Medicine. AUA and ASRM produce recommendations for male infertility. American Urological Association, Inc and American Society for Reproductive Medicine. Am Fam Physician. 2002;65(12):2589–90.
37. Smit M, van Casteren NJ, Wildhagen MF, Romijn JC, Dohle GR. Sperm DNA integrity in cancer patients before and after cytotoxic treatment. Hum Reprod (Oxford, Engl). 2010;25(8):1877–83.

38. Gandini L, Lombardo F, Salacone P, Paoli D, Anselmo AP, Culasso F, et al. Testicular cancer and Hodgkin's disease: evaluation of semen quality. Hum Reprod (Oxford, Engl). 2003;18(4):796–801.
39. Masliukaite I, Hagen JM, Jahnukainen K, et al. Establishing reference values for age-related spermatogonial quantity in prepubertal human testes: a systematic review and meta-analysis. Fertil Steril. 2016;106(7):1652–1657 e1652.
40. DiNofia AM, Wang X, Yannekis G, et al. Analysis of semen parameters in a young cohort of cancer patients. Pediatr Blood Cancer. 2017;64(2):381–6.
41. World Health Organization. WHO laboratory manual for the examination and processing of human semen. 5th ed. Geneva: World Health Organization; 2010. xiv, 271 p.
42. Ferrari S, Paffoni A, Filippi F, Busnelli A, Vegetti W, Somigliana E. Sperm cryopreservation and reproductive outcome in male cancer patients: a systematic review. Reprod Biomed Online. 2016;33(1):29–38.
43. Choi BB, Goldstein M, Moomjy M, Palermo G, Rosenwaks Z, Schlegel PN. Births using sperm retrieved via immediate microdissection of a solitary testis with cancer. Fertil Steril. 2005;84(5):1508.
44. Plebani M. Proteomics: the next revolution in laboratory medicine? Clin Chim Acta Int J Clin Chem. 2005;357(2):113–22.
45. Zorrilla M, Yatsenko AN. The genetics of infertility: current status of the field. Curr Genet Med Rep. 2013;1(4):1–22.
46. Upadhyay RD, Balasinor NH, Kumar AV, Sachdeva G, Parte P, Dumasia K. Proteomics in reproductive biology: beacon for unraveling the molecular complexities. Biochim Biophys Acta. 2013;1834(1):8–15.
47. Gilany K, Minai-Tehrani A, Savadi-Shiraz E, Rezadoost H, Lakpour N. Exploring the human seminal plasma proteome: an unexplored gold mine of biomarker for male infertility and male reproduction disorder. J Reprod Infertility. 2015;16(2):61–71.
48. Kolialexi A, Mavrou A, Spyrou G, Tsangaris GT. Mass spectrometry-based proteomics in reproductive medicine. Mass Spectrom Rev. 2008;27(6):624–34.
49. Fernandez Encinas A, Garcia-Peiro A, Ribas-Maynou J, Abad C, Amengual MJ, Navarro J, et al. Characterization of nuclease activity in human seminal plasma and its relationship with semen parameters, sperm DNA fragmentation and male infertility. J Urol. 2016;195(1):213–9.
50. Zhu WB, Long XY, Fan LQ. Male fecundity prognosis and infertility diagnosis in the era of personalised medicine. Asian J Androl. 2010;12(4):463–7.

Male Fertility Preservation: Current Options and Advances in Research

Kathrin Gassei, Hanna Valli-Pulaski, Allison G. Close, Erika D. Friehling, Rajeev Chaudhry, Patrick J. Fox, Glenn M. Cannon, Thomas M. Jaffe, Lillian R. Meacham, and Kyle E. Orwig

T. K. Woodruff et al. (eds.), *Textbook of Oncofertility Research and Practice*,
https://doi.org/10.1007/978-3-030-02868-8_17

Key Points
- Fertility preservation options for pubertal boys and adult men include sperm banking and testicular sperm extraction (TESE).
- For prepubertal boys, there are no standard of care options. The only option for prepubertal boys is testicular tissue cryopreservation, which is still considered experimental.
- Experimental techniques currently in the pipeline for restoring fertility with cryopreserved testicular tissues include spermatogonial stem cell transplantation, de novo testicular morphogenesis, testicular tissue grafting and xenografting, and testicular tissue organ culture.
- Many centers around the world are actively cryopreserving testicular tissues for prepubertal boys who are at risk for infertility in anticipation that those samples can be use in the future for reproductive purposes.

17.1 Introduction

Improvements in cancer therapies have resulted in improved 5-year survival rates [68] and an increasing focus on quality of life after cure. Cancer survivors report that parenthood is important to them, and distress over infertility has long-term psychological and relationship implications [152]. Therefore, the American Society for Clinical Oncology [96, 100] and the American Society for Reproductive Medicine [37, 38] recommend that patients be educated about the reproductive risks associated with their therapy as well as options for preserving fertility.

Whole-body radiation, radiation to the hypothalamus, pituitary, or testes, and alkylating and heavy metal chemotherapies are particularly toxic to male fertility [54, 67, 80, 94, 97, 105, 171]. This is an important public health concern because nearly 25,000 males under the age of 44 will be diagnosed with cancer each year in the United States. Epidemiological data [54, 68, 106] indicate that most of these patients will survive their cancer, but many will receive treatments that put them at significant risk for infertility. The Childhood Cancer Survivor Study (CCSS) has shown that male survivors of childhood cancer are half as likely to achieve a pregnancy with their partner compared to their male siblings [54]. When rates of infertility were studied in the CCSS, 46% of cancer survivors compared to 18% of siblings reported experiencing infertility [172].

Patients and families with children facing a cancer diagnosis and planning for treatment may be ill-prepared to discuss, think about, or take action to preserve their future fertility before initiating treatment. Unfortunately, while healthcare professionals acknowledge the need to discuss fertility preservation with their patients, fertility counseling is not consistently implemented [154, 155]. Consequently, many families are inadequately informed of the risk of infertility [154] and the options they have to preserve their child's fertility [140]. Insufficient training for medical staff to counsel patients on this sensitive topic has been identified as an important factor, along with patient factors such as degree of disease, age, and cultural/religious concerns [48]. Both parents and adolescent cancer patients identify fertility as an important life goal after cancer [87].

Spermatogonial stem cells (SSCs) are at the foundation of spermatogenesis and maintain continuous sperm production throughout the postpubertal life of men [27, 123, 161, 165]. Spermatogenesis is an extraordinarily productive process that generates more than 100 million sperm each day from the testes of adult men [156]. Because spermatogenesis is such a productive system, it can sometimes become an unintended target of cancer therapies that are toxic to rapidly dividing cells. Therapies that deplete the stem cell pool and/or damage the somatic niche can cause temporary or permanent infertility. Infertility in male cancer survivors is due to impaired spermatogenesis, which can be characterized as oligospermia (<15 million sperm/ml of semen) or azoospermia (no sperm in the semen). High-dose alkylating agents (e.g., cyclophosphamide, busulfan, melphalan, chlorambucil), bleomycin, testicular radiation >400 cGy, or genitourinary surgery are associated with the highest risk of developing azoospermia [20, 97, 105, 107, 171, 172]. In contrast to spermatogenesis, the steroidogenic function of the testes appears to be less affected by cancer therapy and the testosterone-producing Leydig cells appear to be fairly resistant to damage by chemotherapy [22].

17.2 Sperm Banking: The Gold Standard Procedure for Male Fertility Preservation

Boys who have reached Tanner III of pubertal development and adult men have the option to cryopreserve a semen sample containing sperm before initiating treatment, which can be thawed at a later date to achieve pregnancy by intrauterine insemination [3], in vitro fertilization (IVF, [159]), or IVF with intracytoplasmic sperm injection (ICSI, [118]). Unfortunately, only about 24% of adult men freeze a semen sample before initiating their therapy [153]. Some males as young as 12 or 13 years of age are capable of producing a semen sample. Semen is produced via masturbation, but other methods such as vibratory stimulation [151] or electroejaculation [2, 45] have been used. Ideally, patients should provide two to three specimens obtained at 2–3 day intervals. Standard semen analysis would be performed by the andrology laboratory, and results will be available within 1 day to confirm whether the semen specimens contain sperm. Some patients have asked if it is safe to preserve sperm if they have just started chemotherapy. There is insufficient data and no consensus about best practices in this scenario. Please see the following references for discussion [15, 21, 104].

17.3 Testicular Sperm Extraction (TESE)

For patients who did not preserve a semen sample and have persistent azoospermia after cancer therapy, there is the option to retrieve rare sperm directly from the testis during a surgical procedure called testicular sperm extraction (TESE). This is possible because a few SSCs may survive the gonadotoxic therapy and produce focal areas of spermatogenesis in the seminiferous tubules. Hsiao and colleagues recently described their experience with 73 patients with postchemotherapy azoospermia [70]. They reported that sperm were successfully retrieved from 37% of patients on initial attempt, with an overall success rate of 42.9%. Fertilization rate with the retrieved sperm was 57%; the pregnancy rate was 50%; and the live birth rate was 42%. Success in retrieving sperm was treatment dependent in that study, with the lowest sperm recovery success rates (21%) in patients receiving alkylating chemotherapy [70]. Picton and colleagues surveyed results from a total of five centers (including the Hsiao et al. study) and reported an overall sperm recovery rate of 44% in azoospermic patients undergoing TESE after chemotherapy [124].

There are currently no standard options to treat the infertility of adult patients who did not cryopreserve a semen sample and were not successful with the TESE/ICSI procedure. Adoption and third-party reproduction are family-building options for these patients, but most cancer survivors prefer to have their own biological children [96]. Therefore, sperm banking should be discussed with all pubertal, adolescent, and adult males who are able to produce a semen sample.

17.4 TESE for Men and Adolescent Boys with Klinefelter Syndrome

TESE is also used effectively for Klinefelter Syndrome (KS) patients who typically have a 46, XXY karyotype and azoospermia, often characterized as a Sertoli cell only phenotype. However, germ cells are sometimes present in the testes of KS patients, which produce focal areas of spermatogenesis in the testes. Success rates for retrieving sperm by TESE from the testes of KS patients are consistently above 50% (50–72%) [14, 88, 114, 130, 147, 183] and are similar to the success rates reported for TESE in azoospermic patients without Klinefelter syndrome. Most importantly, pregnancy rates and live birth rates after ICSI are similar in couples with or without KS, and children fathered by KS patients have a normal karyotype [14, 147, 183]. The infertility phenotype of KS patients is considered progressive, with rapid declines in spermatogenesis during the teenage years [5, 103, 174]. Previous studies in adult KS patients reported that sperm recovery rates were significantly lower after the age of 35 [14, 114, 130]. Therefore, early intervention may be important to preserve the fertility of Klinefelter patients. In fact, some centers have protocols to retrieve sperm by TESE from adolescent boys with KS based on the understanding that the likelihood of retrieving sperm in later years will be reduced [103, 112]. Other groups, however, did not find that performing TESE at a younger age increased the chances of successful sperm retrieval [126, 174], and there is considerable debate about the benefit of early fertility intervention for KS patients [112, 134].

Typically, pubertal development is determined by Tanner staging of pubic hair and genitalia development, testicular size, and hormone levels. In most boys, the median age of onset of spermatogenesis is 13–14 years, correlating to a genital Tanner stage III. However, in patients with KS, the early stages of pubertal development that consist of increase in size of the testes are not reliable since testicular size is often diminished. It is currently unknown when spermatogenesis starts in boys with KS. While it seems to be commonly accepted that there is a progressive depletion of germ cells in the testes of KS patients after the onset of puberty, the evidence to support this notion is equivocal with small patient populations, lack of controls, and no longitudinal data. In addition, the standard therapy for boys with KS is testosterone replacement therapy in order to trigger entry and progression of puberty, secondary sexual characteristics, bone development, and longitudinal growth. However, testosterone supplementation also suppresses spermatogenesis (if present) even further through negative feedback on the hypothalamus-pituitary-gonadal axis. Some argue that any intervention to preserve fertility for KS patients should ideally precede hormone replacement therapy [169], although recent studies have shown that testosterone replacement therapy might not negatively affect spermatogenesis in KS patients [42, 103]. The risks of invasive surgical procedures like TESE for boys should be carefully weighed against the possible benefits for this unique patient population. Systematic, longitudinal studies are needed to characterize spermatogenic decline in KS patients.

17.5 Gonadal Shielding

Gonadal shielding can be used to protect the testes from scatter radiation using lead shielding. The proper shielding technique should be carefully evaluated on a case-by-case basis depending on total radiation dose, fractionation, and the specific mode of delivery of the external beam therapy [39, 142, 180]. However, when the testicular tissue requires radiation therapy as a part of cancer treatment, shielding cannot be used. At other times, the proximity of the testes to the target of radiation results in scatter radiation to the testes, which can also result in impaired spermatogenesis.

17.6 Testicular Tissue Banking: An Experimental Procedure for Fertility Preservation

There are currently no standard of care options to preserve the future fertility of prepubertal boys who are not yet producing sperm. This is an important human health concern because, with improved therapies, the event-free survival rate of children with cancer is 85% [69], and these survivors can look forward to a full and productive life after cure. We estimate that each year in the United States, more than 2000 boys will receive gonadotoxic treatments for cancer or other conditions (e.g., myeloablative conditioning prior to bone marrow transplantation) that put them at high risk for infertility [166]. Prepubertal boys are not producing sperm, but they do have spermatogonial stem cells (SSCs) in their testes that are poised to initiate sperm production at the time of puberty [119]. There are several methods in the research pipeline, including SSC transplantation, testicular tissue grafting or xenografting, testicular tissue organ culture, and de novo testicular morphogenesis that might be used to restore spermatogenesis or fertility from cryopreserved SSCs and/or testicular tissue. Induced pluripotent stem cell (iPSC) technologies may also be a fertility option for cancer survivors in the future. These methods are reviewed in this chapter.

Anticipating that new therapies will be available in the future, many centers in the United States and abroad have determined that it is reasonable to preserve testicular tissue for young patients who are at risk for infertility and have no other options to preserve their fertility [50, 53, 81, 116, 124, 139, 141, 178]. Testicular tissue-based fertility preservation methods for children are considered experimental and should be performed with institutional review board (IRB) oversight and approval. Although no pregnancies from cryopreserved testicular tissues have been reported in humans to date, two centers reported that the majority of parents consented to fertility preservation procedures on behalf of their children [49, 176, 178].

17.7 Considerations for Testicular Tissue Collection, Processing, and Freezing

Testicular tissue for cryopreservation is obtained via needle biopsy, wedge biopsy, or orchiectomy, ideally before the initiation of gonadotoxic treatment (surgery, chemotherapy, radiation). There is insufficient experience or evidence to recommend a particular surgical approach or orchiectomy, and each center will make those decisions based on individual and/or institutional biases about what is in the best interest of the patient in the short term and long term. Needle biopsy may be the least invasive but has an increased risk of unmitigated bleeding and recovers the least amount of tissue for downstream fertility applications. Wedge resection is more invasive than needle biopsy but may allow recovery of more testicular tissue (depending on surgeon preference), and bleeding can be controlled during surgery. Orchiectomy (removal of an entire testis) is the most invasive procedure but allows for the greatest recovery of testicular tissue for downstream fertility applications, and bleeding can be controlled during surgery. Collection of more tissue at the time of surgery should correlate with increased recovery of SSCs and greater flexibility for future fertility applications. However, limited tissue should not be a deterrent to enrollment in a testicular tissue cryopreservation protocol. There are several experimental cell-based and tissue-based options under development with different requirements for the amount of cells/tissue that will be needed.

There are no established "best practices" for processing and freezing testicular tissue or cells. Two labs examined the postthaw recovery of spermatogonia from cryopreserved human testis cell suspensions versus intact pieces of testicular tissue. Yango and colleagues reported that recovery of SSEA4$^+$ (undifferentiated spermatogonia marker) spermatogonia from cryopreserved fetal testicular tissue was similar to cryopreserved testicular cells, but recovery of SSEA4$^+$ cells from cryopreserved adult testicular cells was greater than cryopreserved testicular tissue [182]. Pacchiarotti and coworkers reported that cryopreservation of testicular tissue was comparable in most aspects to cryopreservation of a cell suspension. However, while the viability of total cells from the cryopreserved tissue was higher than the cryopreserved cell suspension, the recovery of SSEA4$^+$ and VASA$^+$ (pan germ cell marker) germ cells from cryopreserved tissue pieces tended to be greater than cryopreserved cell suspensions. These differences were not significant [117].

For fertility preservation, most centers are freezing intact pieces of testicular tissue for patients because this preserves the option for both tissue-based and cell-based therapies in the future [11, 50, 53, 81, 115, 124, 164, 178]. Biopsied testicular tissues are typically cut into small pieces (1–9 mm^3), suspended in a DMSO-based freezing medium, and frozen at a controlled slow rate using a programmable freezing machine (◘ Fig. 17.1) [50, 81, 82, 116, 124, 164, 177, 178]. Some centers have reported using an ethylene glycol-based freezing medium instead of DMSO [19, 93, 163], and some centers have reported that the viability of vitrified testicular tissue is similar to tissue frozen at a controlled slow rate [13, 26, 127, 138]. This may improve access to testicular tissue freezing technology in centers that do not have programmable freezing machines. The experimental endpoints that have been used to evaluate freezing protocols have been varied and include cell viability, immunocytochemistry for spermatogonial markers, ultrastructural, histological and/or immunohistochemical examination of cultured or grafted tissue, and hormone production. Systematic studies on prepubertal human testicular tissues with evaluation of both cell-based and tissue-based endpoints are needed. It is possible that the optimal freezing condition depends on the intended use of the tissue or cells.

17.8 Testicular Cell-Based Methods to Preserve and Restore Male Fertility

Spermatogonial Stem Cell Transplantation Spermatogonial stem cell transplantation was first described by Ralph Brinster and colleagues in 1994, who demonstrated that SSCs could be isolated and transplanted to regenerate spermatogenesis in infertile recipient mice [17, 18]. SSC transplantation has now been reported in mice, rats, pigs, goats, bulls, sheep, dogs, and monkeys, and donor-derived progeny have been produced by

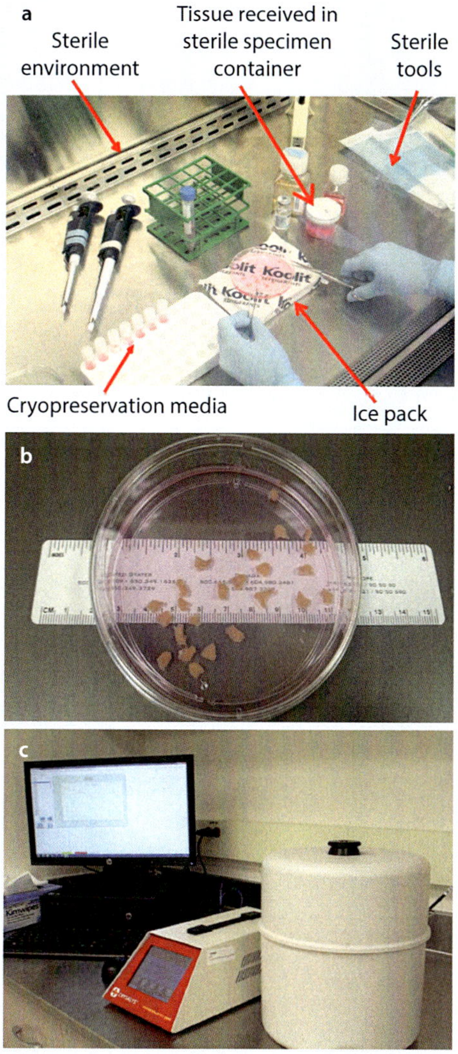

Fig. 17.1 Testicular tissue cryopreservation. Testicular tissues are transported on ice from the operating room to the andrology lab in a sterile specimen container containing medium. (**a**) The tissue is kept cool and processed in a sterile environment with sterile tools. (**b**) Most centers cut the testicular tissue into small pieces (1–9 mm^3) and deposit these pieces in cryovials with DMSO-based freezing medium. (**c**) Controlled slow rate freezing using a freezing machine

natural breeding in mice, rats, goats, and sheep [16, 60–62, 72, 73, 84, 108, 110, 113, 148, 157]. SSCs from donors of all ages, newborn to adult, are competent to regenerate spermatogenesis [137, 157], and SSCs can be cryopreserved and retain spermatogenic function upon thawing and transplantation [28, 29, 60]. Thus, it appears feasible that a testicular tissue biopsy (containing SSCs) could be obtained from a prepubertal boy prior to gonadotoxic therapy, frozen, thawed at a later date, and transplanted back into his testes to regenerate spermatogenesis. If spermatogenesis from transplanted cells is robust, this approach may restore natural fertility, allowing survivors to achieve pregnancy with their partner by natural intercourse and have biological children.

Radford and colleagues already reported cryopreserving testicular cells for 11 adult non-Hodgkin's lymphoma patients in 1999 and subsequently reported transplanting autologous frozen and thawed testis cells back into the testes of seven survivors [128, 129]. The fertility outcomes for patients in that study have not been reported, and even if the men fathered children, it would not be possible to ascertain whether the sperm arose from transplanted stem cells or surviving endogenous stem cells. This uncertainty will always plague the interpretation of human SSC transplant studies where it is not ethically possible to genetically mark the transplanted cells because the genetic modification would be transmitted to the progeny. Therefore, large epidemiological datasets generated over decades will be required to prove the fertility benefit of SSC transplantation. Nonetheless, this study demonstrates that patients are willing to pursue experimental stem cell-based options even when there is no guarantee of a fertile outcome. There are no published reports of SSC transplantation in humans since Radford's follow-up report of his non-Hodgkin's lymphoma patients in 2003 [128].

17.9 Translating Spermatogonial Stem Cell Transplantation into the Clinic: Challenges and Opportunities

Considering the progress in several animal models and the fact that testicular tissues have already been cryopreserved for hundreds of human patients worldwide [50, 53, 81, 116, 128, 129, 139, 141, 178], it seems reasonable to expect that SSC transplantation and/or other stem cell technologies will impact the fertility clinic in the next decade. However, there are several safety and feasibility issues that must be considered.

Spermatogonial Stem Cell Culture Based on our experiences at the Fertility Preservation Program in Pittsburgh [116] and published reports [50, 81], it is reasonable to expect that 50–1000 mg of testicular tissue can be obtained by wedge biopsy or needle biopsy from a single testis of a prepubertal boy. This is a small amount of tissue relative to the size of adult human testes that can range from 11 to 26 g in size [167]. It is widely believed that the number of stem cells in biopsies from prepubertal boys will be small and that SSCs will have to be expanded in culture prior to transplant. Conditions for maintaining and expanding rodent SSCs in culture are well established, and SSCs maintained in long-term culture (e.g., several months to 1 year) remain competent to regenerate spermatogenesis and restore fertility [56, 76, 77, 92, 133, 136].

If cultured human SSCs function like cultured rodent SSCs, it should be feasible to expand a few stem cells obtained from the testis biopsy of a prepubertal boy to a number sufficient to produce robust spermatogenesis upon transplantation back into his testes when he is an adult. Several studies have reported culturing human SSCs [1, 4, 9, 23, 24, 44, 51, 55, 58, 89, 98, 99, 102, 109, 111, 125, 139, 141, 158, 175, 184], including two studies in which cultures were established from the testes of prepubertal patients [139, 175]. Human SSC cultures have been evaluated by quantitative PCR or immunocytochemistry for spermatogonial markers or xenotransplantation into mouse testes. Strategies to isolate and culture human spermatogonia have been unique to each study, and to date, no approach has been independently replicated in another laboratory. Also, the field is frustrated by the lack of a functional assay to test the full spermatogenic potential of cultured human cells.

17

Malignant Contamination A testicular biopsy obtained from a cancer patient could harbor malignant cells, especially for patients with leukemia. Kim and colleagues [83] reported that 20% of boys with acute lymphocytic anemia had malignant cells in their testicular tissue prior to the initiation of oncologic treatment. Jahnukainen and colleagues [74] reported the transmission of leukemia after transplantation of testis cells from terminally ill leukemic rats into the testes of nonleukemic recipients. The same group further demonstrated that transplantation of as few as 20 leukemic cells was sufficient for disease transmission, leading to terminal leukemia within 3 weeks.

Because infertility is not life threatening and fertility treatments are elective, it is essential that the risk of cancer recurrence after transplant be reduced to zero. Fluorescence-activated cell sorting (FACS) and magnetic-activated cell sorting (MACS) strategies to isolate and enrich therapeutic spermatogonia from testis cell suspension while removing malignant contamination have been explored with mixed results. Fujita and coworkers isolated germ cells from the testes of leukemic mice in the forward scatter high and side scatter low fraction (positive selection), which was then further divided into fractions that were CD45/MHC class I antigens (H-2K^b/H-2D^b) double-positive and CD45/MHC class I double-negative cells. All recipient males injected with the CD45$^+$/MHC class I$^+$ cells developed terminal leukemia within 40 days. All mice injected with CD45$^-$/MHC class I$^-$ cells survived for 300 days without the onset of leukemia and produced donor-derived offspring [40]. In a subsequent study, the same group reported that seven out of eight human leukemic cell lines expressed the cell surface antigens CD45 and MHC class I [41]. In a rat model of Roser's T-cell leukemia, Hou and colleagues concluded that single parameter selection using either leukemic (CD4 and MHC Class I) or SSC (Ep-CAM) markers was not sufficient to eliminate malignant contamination [66], but malignant contamination was successfully removed using a combination of leukemia and SSC markers (plus/minus selection) [32, 59]. Using similar positive/negative selection strategies, Hermann and colleagues isolated VASA+ germ cells in the THY-1$^+$/CD45$^-$ fraction of leukemia-contaminated prepubertal nonhuman primate testis cells [59], and this fraction did not produce tumors in mice. Dovey and colleagues contaminated human testis cells with MOLT-4 acute lymphoblastic leukemia cells and demonstrated by xenotransplantation that the Ep-CAM^{lo}/HLA-ABC$^-$/CD49e$^-$ fraction was enriched 12-fold for transplantable human SSCs and was devoid of malignant contamination [32]. Collectively, these results are encouraging, but caution is still warranted as Geens and colleagues concluded, using EL-4 lymphoma contaminated mouse and human testis cells, that FACS- and MACS-based methods were insufficient to remove malignant contamination [47].

It will not be possible to perform comprehensive in vivo testing on patient samples because this would limit the amount of sample available for fertility therapy. More sensitive PCR-based methods have been described for detection of minimal residual disease (MRD), and this approach has identified malignant contamination in many ovarian tissue samples that were preserved for leukemia patients, even after negative histology and immunocytochemistry examination [30, 135]. However, in one of those studies, Dolmans and colleagues obtained disparate results from histology, qRT-PCR, and xenografting of ovarian tissues from leukemia patients. Quantitative RT-PCR to detect MRD revealed the possibility of malignant contamination in 9 of the 16 samples that was not detected by histological examination. However, when those ovarian tissues were grafted into recipient mice, only five of the nine samples with positive MRD had evidence of leukemic cells 3 months after transplantation [30]. Were the MRD results in the other four cases nefarious or were they accurate and the leukemic cells simply failed to survive freezing, thawing, and grafting? In the absence of a definitive and practical test of malignant contamination, alternatives to autologous transplantation are needed for patients with hematogenous cancers, testis cancers, or cancers that metastasize to the testes.

De Novo Testicular Morphogenesis Testicular cells (including germ cells, Sertoli cells, peritubular myoid cells, and Leydig cells) have the remarkable ability to reorganize to form normal looking seminiferous tubules when grafted under the skin of recipient mice [8, 33, 43, 64, 86]. Ina Dobrinski and colleagues disaggregated neonatal pig and sheep testis cells, pelleted them by centrifugation, and grafted under the skin of immune-deficient mice. When grafts were recovered between 16 and 41 weeks after transplant, cells had reorganized to form seminiferous tubules with complete spermatogenesis [8, 64]. In a remarkable extension of this approach, Kita and colleagues [86] mixed fetal or neonatal testis cells from mice or rats with GFP^+-cultured mouse germline stem cells and growth factor-reduced matrigel (extracellular matrix) and grafted under the skin of immune-deficient mice. Seven to 10 weeks after grafting, seminiferous tubules with complete spermatogenesis originating from both intrinsic germ cells and cultured (GFP^+) germ cells were observed. Tubules were dissected and GFP^+ round spermatids were recovered and injected into mouse oocytes. The resulting embryos were transferred to recipient females, which gave birth to ten mouse pups, including four with the GFP transgene. In vitro organoid systems have also been developed. In mice and rats, the most promising results have been achieved using 3D scaffolds [6, 95, 160], where postmeiotic cells and spermatozoa developed. In vitro organoid cultures have been less successful with human cells. Maintenance of early and late spermatogonia was reported by several studies [10, 122, 170]; however, only two of the studies observed the presence of postmeiotic markers [122, 170]. These reports used pubertal or adult human tissues that already contain postmeiotic cells, which can make it difficult to determine the origin of the cells expressing the postmeiotic markers. To date, no human sperm has been produced using this model. One day it may be possible to "build a testis," in vitro or in vivo, on the scaffold of a decellularized human testis [12].

17.10 Testicular Tissue-Based Methods to Preserve and Restore Male Fertility

Testicular Tissue Grafting and Xenografting Testicular tissue grafting may provide an alternative approach for generating fertilization competent sperm from small testicular biopsies. In contrast to the SSC transplantation method in which SSCs are removed from their cognate niches and transplanted into recipient seminiferous tubules, grafting involves transplantation of the intact SSC/niche unit in pieces of testicular tissue. Honaramooz and colleagues reported that grafted testicular tissue from newborn mice, rats, pigs, and goats, in which spermatogenesis was not yet established, could mature and produce complete spermatogenesis when xenografted into nude mice [65]. The same group later reported the production of live offspring from sperm obtained from mouse testicular tissue grafts [149]. Fertilization-competent sperm was also produced from xenografts of prepubertal nonhuman primate testicular tissue transplanted into mice [63]. These results suggest that it may be possible to obtain fertilization-competent sperm by xenografting small pieces of testicular tissue from a prepubertal cancer patient under the skin of mice or other animal recipients such as pigs that are already an established source for human food consumption, replacement heart valves [7, 75], and potentially other organs [25]. Xenografting would also circumvent the issue of malignant contamination. However, the xenografting approach raises concerns about xenobiotics because viruses from mice, pigs, and other species can be transmitted to human cells [85, 173]. There is no evidence to date that xenografted human testicular tissue can produce spermatogenesis or sperm in mice [46, 52, 146, 150, 168, 179]. However, there is reason for optimism because Sato and colleagues observed primary spermatocytes 1 year after xenografting testicular tissue from a 3-month-old boy who clearly did not have spermatocytes at the time of transplantation [146]. Xenografting of human testicular tissue to species other than mice has not been tested to our knowledge.

If malignant contamination of the testicular tissue is not a concern, autologous testicular tissue grafting can be considered. Luetjens and colleagues demonstrated that fresh autologous testicular tissue grafts from prepubertal marmosets could produce complete spermatogenesis when transplanted into the scrotum, but not under the skin [101]. Frozen and thawed grafts did not produce complete spermatogenesis in that study, but those grafts were only transplanted under the skin. Therefore, additional experimentation is merited. Testicular tissue grafting will not restore natural fertility, but could generate haploid sperm that can be used to fertilize oocytes by ICSI.

Testicular Tissue Organ Culture Sato and colleagues reported that intact testicular tissues from newborn mice (2.5–3.5 days old) could be maintained in organ culture and mature to produce spermatogenesis, including the production of fertilization-competent haploid germ cells [144, 145]. Testicular tissues from neonatal mice were minced into pieces (1–3 mm^3) and placed in culture at the gas–liquid interface on a slab of agarose that was soaked in medium. Haploid round spermatids and sperm were recovered from the tissue after 3–6 weeks in culture and used to fertilize mouse eggs by ICSI. The resulting embryos were transferred to pseudopregnant females and gave rise to healthy offspring that matured to adulthood and were fertile. If testicular tissue organ culture can be translated to humans, it will provide an alternative to autologous SSC transplantation, autologous grafting, and xenografting in cases where there is concern about malignant contamination of the testicular tissue. The same authors were also successful to produce haploid germ cells in an organ culture of frozen and thawed testicular tissues, which is particularly relevant to the cancer survivor paradigm. However, the fertilization potential of those sperm was not tested [144]. In the initial studies, the testicular tissue deteriorated with time. However, when tissues were maintained in a microfluidics device with continuous media flow to deliver nutrients and remove waste, testicular tissues could be maintained for up to 6 months with continuous production of testosterone and fertilization-competent sperm [91]. To make the microfluidics system more accessible, Komeya and colleagues [90] developed a pumpless microfluidics device that could maintain spermatogenesis in cultured seminiferous tubules for up to 3 months. Testicular tissue organ culture is a promising technology that now needs to be replicated in other laboratories and extended nonhuman primate and human tissues to set the stage for clinical translation.

17.11 Induced Pluripotent Stem Cell-Based Methods to Preserve and Restore Male Fertility

Several groups have now reported that it is possible to produce germ cells from pluripotent embryonic stem cells (ESCs) or induced pluripotent stem cells (iPSCs) [31, 34, 35, 57, 71, 78, 79, 120, 121, 131, 132, 143, 162, 181]. Hayashi and coworkers reported that it is possible to differentiate ESCs or iPSCs into epiblast-like cells (EpiLCs) that then give rise to primordial germ cell-like cells (PGCLCs) when cultured in the presence of BMP4 [57]. The resulting germ cells were transplanted into the seminiferous tubules of infertile recipient mice where they regenerated spermatogenesis and produced haploid gametes that were used to fertilize mouse oocytes by ICSI. The embryos were transferred to recipient females and gave rise to live offspring. However, some of the offspring developed tumors in the neck area and died prematurely, suggesting that further optimization of the culture and differentiation protocols will be required [57]. Two groups recently reported the differentiation of human pluripotent stem cells into putative hPGCLCs exhibiting gene expression patterns similar to bona fide human PGCs [71, 143]. Of course, functional validation by generation of progeny is not possible in studies with human cells.

An important implication of the iPSC to germ cell differentiation technology, if responsibly developed, is that it will no longer be necessary to preserve fertility before the initiation of gonadotoxic treatments. An adult survivor of a childhood cancer who desires to start his family and discovers that he is infertile can theoretically produce sperm and biological offspring from his own skin, blood, or other somatic cell type. This scenario applies not only to childhood cancer survivors, but all survivors who did not preserve semen or testicular tissue prior to gonadotoxic therapy. Nonhuman primate and human pluripotent stem cells have also been differentiated to the germ lineage, producing putative transplantable germ cells and even rare cells that appear to be haploid [31, 34–36, 78, 79, 120, 121, 132, 162, 181]. The challenge with the human studies is that it is not possible to test the spermatogenic potential or fertilization potential of putative germ cells, which are the gold standards in animal studies. Thus, the burden of proof required of human studies is much lower than animal studies. Spermatogenic lineage development and testicular anatomy in nonhuman primates is similar to humans [165], and this may serve as a platform for safety and feasibility studies in which putative germ cells can be tested by transplantation and the resulting gametes can be tested by fertilization [60], embryo transfer and production of live offspring. Perhaps one day, it will be possible to build a human testis in vitro or in vivo on a decellularized human testis scaffold, and this will provide the ultimate platform to test the spermatogenic potential of experimentally derived human germ cells.

17.12 Conclusions

Many centers worldwide are actively preserving testicular tissue or testicular cells for cancer patients in anticipation that those samples can be used in the future for reproductive purposes. Therefore, it is incumbent on the medical and research communities to responsibly develop the technologies that will allow patients to use their samples to achieve their family-building goals. This is important because cancer survivors report that fertility has a significant impact on their quality of life after cure. It seems reasonable to assume that similar quality of life issues are relevant to men who are infertile due to genetic (e.g., Klinefelter), surgical, age-related, accidental, or other causes. The first, best, and proven approach for fertility preservation in males is to freeze sperm that can be obtained in a semen sample or extracted from the testis. With IVF and IVF with ICSI, only a relatively small number of sperm are required to achieve fertilization and pregnancy. Unfortunately, sperm banking is not an option for all patients, including prepubertal boys who are not yet producing sperm.

There are several testicular cell- and tissue-based technologies in the research pipeline that may have application for patients who cannot preserve sperm. All of the technologies described in this chapter are dependent on stem cells (SSCs or iPSCs) with the potential to generate or regenerate autologous spermatogenesis. Spermatogonial stem cell transplantation, de novo testicular morphogenesis, testicular tissue organ culture, testicular tissue grafting/xenografting, and iPSC-derived germ cells have all produced spermatogenesis with sperm that are competent to fertilize oocytes and give rise to viable offspring in mice. Several of these methods have also been translated to larger animal models, including nonhuman primates, indicating a potential for application in the human fertility clinic.

The greatest challenge in the development of stem cell technologies for treatment of human male infertility is the lack of experimental tools for testing the spermatogenic and fertile potential of human cells. This means that human studies cannot be held to the same standard for burden of proof that is required of animal studies. While it is not realistic or possible to demonstrate the fertilization potential of human stem cell-derived gametes, it may be possible to develop systems to test the spermatogenic potential of human cells, such as de novo testicular morphogenesis or engraftment of a decellularized testis. Progress along these lines will provide powerful tools to ensure responsible development and validation of stem cell technologies before they are translated to the male fertility clinic.

Acknowledgments The authors would like to thank the Scaife Foundation, the Richard King Mellon Foundation, the Magee-Womens Research Institute and Foundation, the Children's Hospital of Pittsburgh Foundation, and the University of Pittsburgh Departments of Obstetrics, Gynecology and Reproductive Sciences and Urology, which have generously provided funds to support the Fertility Preservation Program in Pittsburgh (▶ https://fertilitypreservationpittsburgh.org/). It is in this context that we have had the opportunity to meet the infertile patients that fuel our passion for fertility research. The Orwig lab is supported by the Magee-Women's Research Institute and Foundation, the *Eunice Kennedy Shriver* National Institute of Child Health and Human Development grants HD075795 and HD076412, the US-Israel Binational Science Foundation, and gift funds from Montana State University, Sylvia Bernassoli, and Julie and Michael McMullen.

Review Questions and Answers

Q1. What are the standard of care fertility preservation options for pubertal boys and adult males?

A1. Sperm banking is the gold standard for male fertility preservation. If no sperm is present in the ejaculate, testicular sperm extraction (TESE) could be considered.

Q2. Which fertility preservation options are available for prepubertal boys?

A2. Currently, there are no standard of care options available. The only option for prepubertal boys is testicular tissue freezing, which is still considered experimental.

Q3. How is testicular tissue obtained from prepubertal patients?

17

A3. Either through needle biopsy, wedge biopsy, or orchiectomy

Q4. What are the possible future options for using stored testicular tissue?

A4. Methods to restore fertility using cryopreserved testicular tissue in the future include spermatogonial stem cell transplantation, de novo testicular morphogenesis, testicular tissue grafting and xenografting, and testicular tissue organ culture.

References

1. Abdul Wahab AY, Md Isa ML, Ramli R. Spermatogonial stem cells protein identification in in vitro culture from non-obstructive azoospermia patient. Malay J Med Sci. 2016;23(3):40–8.
2. Adank MC, van Dorp W, Smit M, van Casteren NJ, Laven JSE, Pieters R, van den Heuvel-Eibrink MM. Electroejaculation as a method of fertility preservation in boys diagnosed with cancer: a single-center experience and review of the literature. Fertil Steril. 2014;102(1):199–205.e191. https://doi.org/10.1016/j.fertnstert.2014.03.038.
3. Agarwal A, Allamaneni SR. Artificial insemination. In: Falcone T, Hurd W, editors. Clinical reproductive medicine and surgery. Philadelphia: Elsevier; 2007. p. 539–48.
4. Akhondi MM, Mohazzab A, Jeddi-Tehrani M, Sadeghi MR, Eidi A, Khodadadi A, Piravar Z. Propagation of human germ stem cells in long-term culture. Iran J Reprod Med. 2013;11(7):551–8.
5. Aksglaede L, Wikstrom AM, Rajpert-De Meyts E, Dunkel L, Skakkebaek NE, Juul A. Natural history of seminiferous tubule degeneration in Klinefelter syndrome. Hum Reprod Update. 2006;12(1):39–48. https://doi.org/10.1093/humupd/dmi039.
6. Alves-Lopes JP, Söder O, Stukenborg J-B. Use of a three-layer gradient system of cells for rat testicular organoid generation. Nat Protoc. 2018;13:248. https://doi.org/10.1038/nprot.2017.140.
7. Andreas M, Wallner S, Ruetzler K, Wiedemann D, Ehrlich M, Heinze G, Binder T, Moritz A, Hiesmayr MJ, Kocher A, Laufer G. Comparable long-term results for porcine and pericardial prostheses after isolated aortic valve replacement. Eur J Cardiothorac Surg. 2014; https://doi.org/10.1093/ejcts/ezu466.
8. Arregui L, Rathi R, Megee SO, Honaramooz A, Gomendio M, Roldan ER, Dobrinski I. Xenografting of sheep testis tissue and isolated cells as a model for preservation of genetic material from endangered ungulates. Reproduction. 2008;136(1):85–93. https://doi.org/10.1530/REP-07-0433.
9. Baert Y, Braye A, Struijk RB, van Pelt AM, Goossens E. Cryopreservation of testicular tissue before long-term testicular cell culture does not alter in vitro cell dynamics. Fertil Steril. 2015a;104(5):1252.e1241–4. https://doi.org/10.1016/j.fertnstert.2015.07.1134.
10. Baert Y, De Kock J, Alves-Lopes JP, Söder O, Stukenborg J-B, Goossens E. Primary human testicular cells self-organize into organoids with testicular properties. Stem Cell Rep. 2017;8(1):30–8. https://doi.org/10.1016/j.stemcr.2016.11.012.
11. Baert Y, Onofre J, Van Saen D, Goossens E. Cryopreservation of human testicular tissue by isopropyl-controlled slow freezing. In: Alves MG, Oliveira PF, editors. Sertoli cells: methods and protocols. New York: Springer; 2018. p. 287–94. https://doi.org/10.1007/978-1-4939-7698-0_20.
12. Baert Y, Stukenborg JB, Landreh M, De Kock J, Jornvall H, Soder O, Goossens E. Derivation and characterization of a cytocompatible scaffold from human testis. Human Reprod (Oxford, England). 2015b;30(2):256–67. https://doi.org/10.1093/humrep/deu330.

13. Baert Y, Van Saen D, Haentjens P, In't Veld P, Tournaye H, Goossens E. What is the best cryopreservation protocol for human testicular tissue banking? Hum Reprod. 2013; https://doi.org/10.1093/humrep/det100.
14. Bakircioglu ME, Ulug U, Erden HF, Tosun S, Bayram A, Ciray N, Bahceci M. Klinefelter syndrome: does it confer a bad prognosis in treatment of nonobstructive azoospermia? Fertil Steril. 2011;95(5):1696–9. https://doi.org/10.1016/j.fertnstert.2011.01.005.
15. Brannigan RE, Sandlow JI. Cryopreservation of sperm after chemotherapy. J Androl. 2008;29(3):e1–2. https://doi.org/10.2164/jandrol.107.004713.
16. Brinster CJ, Ryu BY, Avarbock MR, Karagenc L, Brinster RL, Orwig KE. Restoration of fertility by germ cell transplantation requires effective recipient preparation. Biol Reprod. 2003;69(2):412–20. https://doi.org/10.1095/biolreprod.103.016519.
17. Brinster RL, Avarbock MR. Germline transmission of donor haplotype following spermatogonial transplantation. Proc Natl Acad Sci U S A. 1994;91(24):11303–7.
18. Brinster RL, Zimmermann JW. Spermatogenesis following male germ-cell transplantation. Proc Natl Acad Sci U S A. 1994;91(24):11298–302.
19. Brook PF, Radford JA, Shalet SM, Joyce AD, Gosden RG. Isolation of germ cells from human testicular tissue for low temperature storage and autotransplantation. Fertil Steril. 2001;75(2):269–74.
20. Bucci LR, Meistrich ML. Effects of busulfan on murine spermatogenesis: cytotoxicity, sterility, sperm abnormalities, and dominant lethal mutations. Mutat Res. 1987;176(2):259–68.
21. Carson SA, Gentry WL, Smith AL, Buster JE. Feasibility of semen collection and cryopreservation during chemotherapy. Human Reprod (Oxford, England). 1991;6(7):992–4.
22. Chemaitilly W, Sklar CA. Endocrine complications in long-term survivors of childhood cancers. Endocr Relat Cancer. 2010;17(3):R141–59. https://doi.org/10.1677/ERC-10-0002.
23. Chen B, Wang YB, Zhang ZL, Xia WL, Wang HX, Xiang ZQ, Hu K, Han YF, Wang YX, Huang YR, Wang Z. Xeno-free culture of human spermatogonial stem cells supported by human embryonic stem cell-derived fibroblast-like cells. Asian J Androl. 2009;11(5):557–65. https://doi.org/10.1038/aja.2009.21.
24. Chikhovskaya JV, van Daalen SKM, Korver CM, Repping S, van Pelt AMM. Mesenchymal origin of multipotent human testis-derived stem cells in human testicular cell cultures. MHR: Basic Sci Reprod Med. 2014; 20(2):155–67. https://doi.org/10.1093/molehr/gat076.
25. Cozzi E, White DJ. The generation of transgenic pigs as potential organ donors for humans. Nat Med. 1995;1(9):964–6.
26. Curaba M, Poels J, van Langendonckt A, Donnez J, Wyns C. Can prepubertal human testicular tissue be cryopreserved by vitrification? Fertil Steril. 2011;95(6):2123.e2129–12. https://doi.org/10.1016/j.fertnstert.2011.01.014.
27. de Rooij DG, Grootegoed JA. Spermatogonial stem cells. Curr Opin Cell Biol. 1998;10(6):694–701.
28. Dobrinski I, Avarbock MR, Brinster RL. Transplantation of germ cells from rabbits and dogs into mouse testes. Biol Reprod. 1999;61(5):1331–9.
29. Dobrinski I, Avarbock MR, Brinster RL. Germ cell transplantation from large domestic animals into mouse testes. Mol Reprod Dev. 2000;57(3):270–9. https://doi.org/10.1002/1098-2795(200011)57:3<270::AID-MRD9>3.0.CO;2-Z.
30. Dolmans MM, Marinescu C, Saussoy P, Van Langendonckt A, Amorim C, Donnez J. Reimplantation of cryopreserved ovarian tissue from patients with acute lymphoblastic leukemia is potentially unsafe. Blood. 2010;116(16):2908–14. https://doi.org/10.1182/blood-2010-01-265751.
31. Dominguez AA, Chiang HR, Sukhwani M, Orwig KE, Reijo Pera RA. Human germ cell formation in xenotransplants of induced pluripotent stem cells carrying X chromosome aneuploidies. Sci Rep. 2014;4:6432. https://doi.org/10.1038/srep06432.
32. Dovey SL, Valli H, Hermann BP, Sukhwani M, Donohue J, Castro CA, Chu T, Sanfilippo JS, Orwig KE. Eliminating malignant contamination from therapeutic human spermatogonial stem cells. J Clin Invest. 2013; 123(4):1833–43. https://doi.org/10.1172/JCI65822.
33. Dufour JM, Rajotte RV, Korbutt GS. Development of an in vivo model to study testicular morphogenesis. J Androl. 2002;23(5):635–44.
34. Durruthy Durruthy J, Ramathal C, Sukhwani M, Fang F, Cui J, Orwig KE, Reijo Pera RA. Fate of induced pluripotent stem cells following transplantation to murine seminiferous tubules. Hum Mol Genet. 2014;23(12):3071–84. https://doi.org/10.1093/hmg/ddu012.
35. Easley CA, Phillips BT, McGuire MM, Barringer JM, Valli H, Hermann BP, Simerly CR, Rajkovic A, Miki T, Orwig KE, Schatten GP. Direct differentiation of human pluripotent stem cells into haploid spermatogenic cells. Cell Rep. 2012;2(3):440–6. https://doi.org/10.1016/j.celrep.2012.07.015.
36. Easley CA, Simerly CR, Schatten G. Stem cell therapeutic possibilities: future therapeutic options for male-factor and female-factor infertility? Reprod BioMed Online. 2013;27(1):75–80. https://doi.org/10.1016/j.rbmo.2013.03.003.
37. Ethics Committee of the American Society for Reproductive Medicine. Fertility preservation and reproduction in cancer patients. Fertil Steril. 2005;83(6):1622–8.
38. Practice Committee of American Society for Reproductive Medicine. Fertility preservation in patients undergoing gonadotoxic therapy or gonadectomy: a committee opinion. Fertil Steril. 2013;100(5):1214–23. https://doi.org/10.1016/j.fertnstert.2013.08.012.
39. Fraass BA, Kinsella TJ, Harrington FS, Glatstein E. Peripheral dose to the testes: the design and clinical use of a practical and effective gonadal shield. Int J Radiat Oncol Biol Phys. 1985;11(3):609–15.
40. Fujita K, Ohta H, Tsujimura A, Takao T, Miyagawa Y, Takada S, Matsumiya K, Wakayama T, Okuyama A. Transplantation of spermatogonial stem cells isolated from leukemic mice restores fertility without inducing leukemia. J Clin Investig. 2005;115(7):1855–61. https://doi.org/10.1172/Jci124189.
41. Fujita K, Tsujimura A, Miyagawa Y, Kiuchi H, Matsuoka Y, Takao T, Takada S, Nonomura N, Okuyama A. Isolation of germ cells from leukemia and lymphoma cells in a human in vitro model: potential clinical applica-

tion for restoring human fertility after anticancer therapy. Cancer Res. 2006;66(23):11166–71. https://doi.org/10.1158/0008-5472.CAN-06-2326.
42. Garolla A, Selice R, Menegazzo M, Valente U, Zattoni F, Iafrate M, Prayer-Galetti T, Gardiman MP, Ferlin A, Di Nisio A, Foresta C. Novel insights on testicular volume and testosterone replacement therapy in Klinefelter patients undergoing testicular sperm extraction. A retrospective clinical study. Clin Endocrinol. 2018;88:711–8. https://doi.org/10.1111/cen.13572.
43. Gassei K, Schlatt S, Ehmcke J. De novo morphogenesis of seminiferous tubules from dissociated immature rat testicular cells in xenografts. J Androl. 2006;27(4):611–8. https://doi.org/10.2164/jandrol.05207.
44. Gat I, Maghen L, Filice M, Wyse B, Zohni K, Jarvi K, Lo KC, Gauthier Fisher A, Librach C. Optimal culture conditions are critical for efficient expansion of human testicular somatic and germ cells in vitro. Fertil Steril. 2017;107(3):595–605.e597. https://doi.org/10.1016/j.fertnstert.2016.12.028.
45. Gat I, Toren A, Hourvitz A, Raviv G, Band G, Baum M, Lerner-Geva L, Inbar R, Madgar I. Sperm preservation by electroejaculation in adolescent cancer patients. Pediatr Blood Cancer. 2014;61(2):286–90. https://doi.org/10.1002/pbc.24752.
46. Geens M, De Block G, Goossens E, Frederickx V, Van Steirteghem A, Tournaye H. Spermatogonial survival after grafting human testicular tissue to immunodeficient mice. Hum Reprod. 2006;21(2):390–6. https://doi.org/10.1093/humrep/dei412.
47. Geens M, Van de Velde H, De Block G, Goossens E, Van Steirteghem A, Tournaye H. The efficiency of magnetic-activated cell sorting and fluorescence-activated cell sorting in the decontamination of testicular cell suspensions in cancer patients. Hum Reprod. 2007;22(3):733–42.
48. Gilbert E, Adams A, Mehanna H, Harrison B, Hartshorne GM. Who should be offered sperm banking for fertility preservation? A survey of UK oncologists and haematologists. Ann Oncol. 2011;22(5):1209–14. https://doi.org/10.1093/annonc/mdq579.
49. Ginsberg JP. New advances in fertility preservation for pediatric cancer patients. Curr Opin Pediatr. 2011;23(1):9–13. https://doi.org/10.1097/MOP.0b013e3283420fb6.
50. Ginsberg JP, Carlson CA, Lin K, Hobbie WL, Wigo E, Wu X, Brinster RL, Kolon TF. An experimental protocol for fertility preservation in prepubertal boys recently diagnosed with cancer: a report of acceptability and safety. Human Reprod (Oxford, England). 2010;25(1):37–41. https://doi.org/10.1093/humrep/dep371.
51. Goharbakhsh L, Mohazzab A, Salehkhou S, Heidari M, Zarnani AH, Parivar K, Akhondi MM. Isolation and culture of human spermatogonial stem cells derived from testis biopsy. Avicenna J Med Biotechnol. 2013;5(1):54–61.
52. Goossens E, Geens M, De Block G, Tournaye H. Spermatogonial survival in long-term human prepubertal xenografts. Fertil Steril. 2008;90(5):2019–22. https://doi.org/10.1016/j.fertnstert.2007.09.044.
53. Goossens E, Van Saen D, Tournaye H. Spermatogonial stem cell preservation and transplantation: from research to clinic. Hum Reprod. 2013;28(4):897–907. https://doi.org/10.1093/humrep/det039.
54. Green DM, Kawashima T, Stovall M, Leisenring W, Sklar CA, Mertens AC, Donaldson SS, Byrne J, Robison LL. Fertility of male survivors of childhood cancer: a report from the Childhood Cancer Survivor Study. J Clin Oncol. 2010;28(2):332–9. https://doi.org/10.1200/JCO.2009.24.9037.
55. Guo Y, Liu L, Sun M, Hai Y, Li Z, He Z. Expansion and long-term culture of human spermatogonial stem cells via the activation of SMAD3 and AKT pathways. Exp Biol Med (Maywood). 2015;240(8):1112–22. https://doi.org/10.1177/1535370215590822.
56. Hamra FK, Chapman KM, Nguyen DM, Williams-Stephens AA, Hammer RE, Garbers DL. Self renewal, expansion, and transfection of rat spermatogonial stem cells in culture. Proc Natl Acad Sci U S A. 2005;102(48):17430–5. https://doi.org/10.1073/pnas.0508780102.
57. Hayashi K, Ohta H, Kurimoto K, Aramaki S, Saitou M. Reconstitution of the mouse germ cell specification pathway in culture by pluripotent stem cells. Cell. 2011;146(4):519–32. https://doi.org/10.1016/j.cell.2011.06.052.
58. He Z, Kokkinaki M, Jiang J, Dobrinski I, Dym M. Isolation, characterization, and culture of human spermatogonia. Biol Reprod. 2010;82(2):363–72. https://doi.org/10.1095/biolreprod.109.078550.
59. Hermann BP, Sukhwani M, Salati J, Sheng Y, Chu T, Orwig KE. Separating spermatogonia from cancer cells in contaminated prepubertal primate testis cell suspensions. Hum Reprod. 2011;26(12):3222–31. https://doi.org/10.1093/humrep/der343.
60. Hermann BP, Sukhwani M, Winkler F, Pascarella JN, Peters KA, Sheng Y, Valli H, Rodriguez M, Ezzelarab M, Dargo G, Peterson K, Masterson K, Ramsey C, Ward T, Lienesch M, Volk A, Cooper DK, Thomson AW, Kiss JE, Penedo MC, Schatten GP, Mitalipov S, Orwig KE. Spermatogonial stem cell transplantation into rhesus testes regenerates spermatogenesis producing functional sperm. Cell Stem Cell. 2012;11(5):715–26. https://doi.org/10.1016/j.stem.2012.07.017.
61. Herrid M, Olejnik J, Jackson M, Suchowerska N, Stockwell S, Davey R, Hutton K, Hope S, Hill JR. Irradiation enhances the efficiency of testicular germ cell transplantation in sheep. Biol Reprod. 2009;81(5):898–905. https://doi.org/10.1095/biolreprod.109.078279.
62. Honaramooz A, Behboodi E, Megee SO, Overton SA, Galantino-Homer H, Echelard Y, Dobrinski I. Fertility and germline transmission of donor haplotype following germ cell transplantation in immunocompetent goats. Biol Reprod. 2003;69(4):1260–4. https://doi.org/10.1095/biolreprod.103.018788.
63. Honaramooz A, Li MW, Penedo MCT, Meyers S, Dobrinski I. Accelerated maturation of primate testis by xenografting into mice. Biol Reprod. 2004;70(5):1500–3. https://doi.org/10.1095/biolreprod.103.025536.
64. Honaramooz A, Megee SO, Rathi R, Dobrinski I. Building a testis: formation of functional testis tissue after transplantation of isolated porcine (Sus scrofa) testis cells. Biol Reprod. 2007;76(1):43–7. https://doi.org/10.1095/biolreprod.106.054999.
65. Honaramooz A, Snedaker A, Boiani M, Scholer H, Dobrinski I, Schlatt S. Sperm from neonatal mammalian testes grafted in mice. Nature. 2002;418(6899):778–81. https://doi.org/10.1038/nature00918.

66. Hou M, Andersson M, Zheng C, Sundblad A, Soder O, Jahnukainen K. Decontamination of leukemic cells and enrichment of germ cells from testicular samples from rats with Roser's T-cell leukemia by flow cytometric sorting. Reproduction. 2007;134(6):767–79. https://doi.org/10.1530/REP-07-0240.
67. Howell SJ, Shalet SM. Spermatogenesis after cancer treatment: damage and recovery. JNCI Monogr. 2005;2005(34):12–7. https://doi.org/10.1093/jncimonographs/lgi003.
68. Howlader N, Noone AM, Krapcho M, Miller D, Bishop K, Kosary CL, Yu M, Ruhl J, Tatalovich Z, Mariotto A, Lewis DR, Chen HS, Feuer EJ, Cronin KA. SEER cancer statistics review, 1975–2014. Bethesda, MD: National Cancer Institute; 2017.. https://seer.cancer.gov/csr/1975_2014/. Accessed 2/19/2018.
69. Howlader N, Noone AM, Krapcho M, Neyman N, Aminou R, Waldron W, Altekruse SF, Kosary CL, Ruhl J, Tatalovich Z, Cho H, Mariotto A, Eisner MP, Lewis DR, Chen HS, Feuer EJ, Cronin KA, Edwards BK. SEER cancer statistic review 1975–2008. Bethesda, MD: National Cancer Institute; 2010.. http://seer.cancer.gov/csr/1975_2008/.
70. Hsiao W, Stahl PJ, Osterberg EC, Nejat E, Palermo GD, Rosenwaks Z, Schlegel PN. Successful treatment of postchemotherapy azoospermia with microsurgical testicular sperm extraction: the weill cornell experience. J Clin Oncol. 2011;29(12):1607–11. https://doi.org/10.1200/jco.2010.33.7808.
71. Irie N, Weinberger L, Tang WW, Kobayashi T, Viukov S, Manor YS, Dietmann S, Hanna JH, Surani MA. SOX17 is a critical specifier of human primordial germ cell fate. Cell. 2015;160(1–2):253–68. https://doi.org/10.1016/j.cell.2014.12.013.
72. Izadyar F, Den Ouden K, Stout TA, Stout J, Coret J, Lankveld DP, Spoormakers TJ, Colenbrander B, Oldenbroek JK, Van der Ploeg KD, Woelders H, Kal HB, De Rooij DG. Autologous and homologous transplantation of bovine spermatogonial stem cells. Reproduction. 2003;126(6):765–74.
73. Jahnukainen K, Ehmcke J, Quader MA, Saiful Huq M, Epperly MW, Hergenrother S, Nurmio M, Schlatt S. Testicular recovery after irradiation differs in prepubertal and pubertal non-human primates, and can be enhanced by autologous germ cell transplantation. Human Reprod (Oxford, England). 2011;26(8):1945–54. https://doi.org/10.1093/humrep/der160.
74. Jahnukainen K, Hou M, Petersen C, Setchell B, Soder O. Intratesticular transplantation of testicular cells from leukemic rats causes transmission of leukemia. Cancer Res. 2001;61(2):706–10.
75. Jamieson SW, Madani MM. The choice of valve protheses*. J Am Coll Cardiol. 2004;44(2):389–90. https://doi.org/10.1016/j.jacc.2004.04.021.
76. Kanatsu-Shinohara M, Muneto T, Lee J, Takenaka M, Chuma S, Nakatsuji N, Horiuchi T, Shinohara T. Long-term culture of male germline stem cells from hamster testes. Biol Reprod. 2008;78(4):611–7. https://doi.org/10.1095/biolreprod.107.065615.
77. Kanatsu-Shinohara M, Ogonuki N, Inoue K, Miki H, Ogura A, Toyokuni S, Shinohara T. Long-term proliferation in culture and germline transmission of mouse male germline stem cells. Biol Reprod. 2003;69(2):612–6. https://doi.org/10.1095/biolreprod.103.017012.
78. Kee K, Angeles VT, Flores M, Nguyen HN, Reijo Pera RA. Human DAZL, DAZ and BOULE genes modulate primordial germ-cell and haploid gamete formation. Nature. 2009;462(7270):222–5. https://doi.org/10.1038/nature08562.
79. Kee K, Gonsalves JM, Clark AT, Pera RA. Bone morphogenetic proteins induce germ cell differentiation from human embryonic stem cells. Stem Cells Dev. 2006;15(6):831–7. https://doi.org/10.1089/scd.2006.15.831.
80. Kenney LB, Cohen LE, Shnorhavorian M, Metzger ML, Lockart B, Hijiya N, Duffey-Lind E, Constine L, Green D, Meacham L. Male reproductive health after childhood, adolescent, and young adult cancers: a report from the Children's Oncology Group. J Clin Oncol. 2012;30(27):3408–16. https://doi.org/10.1200/jco.2011.38.6938.
81. Keros V, Hultenby K, Borgstrom B, Fridstrom M, Jahnukainen K, Hovatta O. Methods of cryopreservation of testicular tissue with viable spermatogonia in pre-pubertal boys undergoing gonadotoxic cancer treatment. Human Reprod (Oxford, England). 2007;22(5):1384–95. https://doi.org/10.1093/humrep/del508.
82. Keros V, Rosenlund B, Hultenby K, Aghajanova L, Levkov L, Hovatta O. Optimizing cryopreservation of human testicular tissue: comparison of protocols with glycerol, propanediol and dimethylsulphoxide as cryoprotectants. Hum Reprod. 2005;20(6):1676–87. https://doi.org/10.1093/humrep/deh797.
83. Kim TH, Hargreaves HK, Brynes RK, Hawkins HK, Lui VK, Woodard J, Ragab AH. Pretreatment testicular biopsy in childhood acute lymphocytic leukaemia. Lancet. 1981;2(8248):657–8.
84. Kim Y, Turner D, Nelson J, Dobrinski I, McEntee M, Travis AJ. Production of donor-derived sperm after spermatogonial stem cell transplantation in the dog. Reproduction. 2008;136(6):823–31. https://doi.org/10.1530/REP-08-0226.
85. Kimsa MC, Strzalka-Mrozik B, Kimsa MW, Gola J, Nicholson P, Lopata K, Mazurek U. Porcine endogenous retroviruses in xenotransplantation – molecular aspects. Viruses. 2014;6(5):2062–83. https://doi.org/10.3390/v6052062.
86. Kita K, Watanabe T, Ohsaka K, Hayashi H, Kubota Y, Nagashima Y, Aoki I, Taniguchi H, Noce T, Inoue K, Miki H, Ogonuki N, Tanaka H, Ogura A, Ogawa T. Production of functional spermatids from mouse germline stem cells in ectopically reconstituted seminiferous tubules. Biol Reprod. 2007;76(2):211–7. https://doi.org/10.1095/biolreprod.106.056895.
87. Klosky JL, Simmons JL, Russell KM, Foster RH, Sabbatini GM, Canavera KE, Hodges JR, Schover LR, McDermott MJ. Fertility as a priority among at-risk adolescent males newly diagnosed with cancer and their parents. Support Care Cancer. 2015;23(2):333–41. https://doi.org/10.1007/s00520-014-2366-1.
88. Koga M, Tsujimura A, Takeyama M, Kiuchi H, Takao T, Miyagawa Y, Takada S, Matsumiya K, Fujioka H, Okamoto Y, Nonomura N, Okuyama A. Clinical comparison of successful and failed microdissection testicular sperm extraction in patients with nonmosaic Klinefelter syndrome. Urology. 2007;70(2):341–5. https://doi.org/10.1016/j.urology.2007.03.056.

89. Kokkinaki M, Djourabtchi A, Golestaneh N. Long-term culture of human SSEA-4 positive spermatogonial stem cells (SSCs). J Stem Cell Res Ther. 2011;S2:003. https://doi.org/10.4172/2157-7633.S2-003.
90. Komeya M, Hayashi K, Nakamura H, Yamanaka H, Sanjo H, Kojima K, Sato T, Yao M, Kimura H, Fujii T, Ogawa T. Pumpless microfluidic system driven by hydrostatic pressure induces and maintains mouse spermatogenesis in vitro. Sci Rep. 2017;7(1):15459. https://doi.org/10.1038/s41598-017-15799-3.
91. Komeya M, Kimura H, Nakamura H, Yokonishi T, Sato T, Kojima K, Hayashi K, Katagiri K, Yamanaka H, Sanjo H, Yao M, Kamimura S, Inoue K, Ogonuki N, Ogura A, Fujii T, Ogawa T. Long-term ex vivo maintenance of testis tissues producing fertile sperm in a microfluidic device. Sci Rep. 2016;6:21472. https://doi.org/10.1038/srep21472.. http://www.nature.com/articles/srep21472 - supplementary-information.
92. Kubota H, Avarbock MR, Brinster RL. Growth factors essential for self-renewal and expansion of mouse spermatogonial stem cells. Proc Natl Acad Sci U S A. 2004;101(47):16489–94. https://doi.org/10.1073/pnas.0407063101.
93. Kvist K, Thorup J, Byskov AG, Hoyer PE, Mollgard K, Yding Andersen C. Cryopreservation of intact testicular tissue from boys with cryptorchidism. Human Reprod (Oxford, England). 2006;21(2):484–91. https://doi.org/10.1093/humrep/dei331.
94. Lambertini M, Del Mastro L, Pescio MC, Andersen CY, Azim HA, Peccatori FA, Costa M, Revelli A, Salvagno F, Gennari A, Ubaldi FM, La Sala GB, De Stefano C, Wallace WH, Partridge AH, Anserini P. Cancer and fertility preservation: international recommendations from an expert meeting. BMC Med. 2016;14(1):1. https://doi.org/10.1186/s12916-015-0545-7.
95. Lee JH, Kim HJ, Kim H, Lee SJ, Gye MC. In vitro spermatogenesis by three-dimensional culture of rat testicular cells in collagen gel matrix. Biomaterials. 2006a;27(14):2845–53. https://doi.org/10.1016/j.biomaterials.2005.12.028.
96. Lee SJ, Schover LR, Partridge AH, Patrizio P, Wallace WH, Hagerty K, Beck LN, Brennan LV, Oktay K. American Society of Clinical Oncology recommendations on fertility preservation in cancer patients. J Clin Oncol. 2006b;24(18):2917–31. https://doi.org/10.1200/JCO.2006.06.5888.
97. Levine J, Canada A, Stern CJ. Fertility preservation in adolescents and young adults with cancer. J Clin Oncol. 2010;28(32):4831–41. https://doi.org/10.1200/JCO.2009.22.8312.
98. Lim JJ, Sung SY, Kim HJ, Song SH, Hong JY, Yoon TK, Kim JK, Kim KS, Lee DR. Long-term proliferation and characterization of human spermatogonial stem cells obtained from obstructive and non-obstructive azoospermia under exogenous feeder-free culture conditions. Cell Prolif. 2010;43(4):405–17. https://doi.org/10.1111/j.1365-2184.2010.00691.x.
99. Liu S, Tang Z, Xiong T, Tang W. Isolation and characterization of human spermatogonial stem cells. Reprod Biol Endocrinol: RB&E. 2011;9:141. https://doi.org/10.1186/1477-7827-9-141.
100. Loren AW, Mangu PB, Beck LN, Brennan L, Magdalinski AJ, Partridge AH, Quinn G, Wallace WH, Oktay K, American Society of Clinical Oncology. Fertility preservation for patients with cancer: American Society of Clinical Oncology clinical practice guideline update. J Clin Oncol. 2013;31(19):2500–10. https://doi.org/10.1200/JCO.2013.49.2678.
101. Luetjens CM, Stukenborg J-B, Nieschlag E, Simoni M, Wistuba J. Complete spermatogenesis in orthotopic but not in ectopic transplants of autologously grafted marmoset testicular tissue. Endocrinology. 2008;149(4):1736–47. https://doi.org/10.1210/en.2007-1325.
102. Medrano JV, Rombaut C, Simon C, Pellicer A, Goossens E. Human spermatogonial stem cells display limited proliferation in vitro under mouse spermatogonial stem cell culture conditions. Fertil Steril. 2016; https://doi.org/10.1016/j.fertnstert.2016.07.1065.
103. Mehta A, Paduch DA, Schlegel PN. Successful testicular sperm retrieval in adolescents with Klinefelter syndrome treated with at least 1 year of topical testosterone and aromatase inhibitor. Fertil Steril. 2013;100(4):e27. https://doi.org/10.1016/j.fertnstert.2013.08.001.
104. Meistrich ML. Potential genetic risks of using semen collected during chemotherapy. Human Reprod (Oxford, England). 1993;8(1):8–10.
105. Meistrich ML. Male gonadal toxicity. Pediatr Blood Cancer. 2009;53(2):261–6. https://doi.org/10.1002/pbc.22004.
106. Meistrich ML, Vassilopoulou-Sellin R, Lipshultz LI. Adverse effects of treatment: gonadal dysfunction. In: DeVita VT, Hellman S, Rosenberg SA, editors. Principles and practice of oncology. 7th ed. Philadelphia: Lippincott Williams & Wilkins; 2004. p. 2560–74.
107. Meistrich ML, Wilson G, Brown BW, da Cunha MF, Lipshultz LI. Impact of cyclophosphamide on long-term reduction in sperm count in men treated with combination chemotherapy for Ewing and soft tissue sarcomas. Cancer. 1992;70(11):2703–12.
108. Mikkola M, Sironen A, Kopp C, Taponen J, Sukura A, Vilkki J, Katila T, Andersson M. Transplantation of normal boar testicular cells resulted in complete focal spermatogenesis in a boar affected by the immotile short-tail sperm defect. Reprod Domest Anim. 2006;41(2):124–8. https://doi.org/10.1111/j.1439-0531.2006.00651.x.
109. Mirzapour T, Movahedin M, Tengku Ibrahim TA, Koruji M, Haron AW, Nowroozi MR, Rafieian SH. Effects of basic fibroblast growth factor and leukaemia inhibitory factor on proliferation and short-term culture of human spermatogonial stem cells. Andrologia. 2012;44:41–55. https://doi.org/10.1111/j.1439-0272.2010.01135.x.
110. Nagano M, Brinster CJ, Orwig KE, Ryu BY, Avarbock MR, Brinster RL. Transgenic mice produced by retroviral transduction of male germ-line stem cells. Proc Natl Acad Sci U S A. 2001;98(23):13090–5. https://doi.org/10.1073/pnas.231473498.
111. Nowroozi MR, Ahmadi H, Rafiian S, Mirzapour T, Movahedin M. In vitro colonization of human spermatogonia stem cells: effect of patient's clinical characteristics and testicular histologic findings. Urology. 2011;78(5):1075–81. https://doi.org/10.1016/j.urology.2011.06.035.

112. Oates RD. Sperm retrieval in adolescents with Klinefelter syndrome. Fertil Steril. 2013;100(4):943–4. https://doi.org/10.1016/j.fertnstert.2013.07.003.
113. Ogawa T, Dobrinski I, Avarbock MR, Brinster RL. Transplantation of male germ line stem cells restores fertility in infertile mice. Nat Med. 2000;6(1):29–34. https://doi.org/10.1038/71496.
114. Okada H, Goda K, Yamamoto Y, Sofikitis N, Miyagawa I, Mio Y, Koshida M, Horie S. Age as a limiting factor for successful sperm retrieval in patients with nonmosaic Klinefelter's syndrome. Fertil Steril. 2005;84(6):1662–4. https://doi.org/10.1016/j.fertnstert.2005.05.053.
115. Onofre J, Baert Y, Faes K, Goossens E. Cryopreservation of testicular tissue or testicular cell suspensions: a pivotal step in fertility preservation. Hum Reprod Update. 2016;22(6):744–61. https://doi.org/10.1093/humupd/dmw029.
116. Orwig KE, Shaw PH, Sanfilippo JS, Kauma SW, Nayak S, Cannon GM. (http://www.mwrif.org/220) Fertility preservation program of Magee-Womens Hospital in Pittsburgh. http://www.mwrif.org/220
117. Pacchiarotti J, Ramos T, Howerton K, Greilach S, Zaragoza K, Olmstead M, Izadyar F. Developing a clinical-grade cryopreservation protocol for human testicular tissue and cells. Biomed Res Int. 2013;2013:10. https://doi.org/10.1155/2013/930962.
118. Palermo G, Joris H, Devroey P, Van Steirteghem AC. Pregnancies after intracytoplasmic injection of single spermatozoon into an oocyte. Lancet. 1992;340(8810):17–8.
119. Paniagua R, Nistal M. Morphological and histometric study of human spermatogonia from birth to the onset of puberty. J Anat. 1984;139(Pt 3):535–52.
120. Panula S, Medrano JV, Kee K, Bergstrom R, Nguyen HN, Byers B, Wilson KD, Wu JC, Simon C, Hovatta O, Reijo Pera RA. Human germ cell differentiation from fetal- and adult-derived induced pluripotent stem cells. Hum Mol Genet. 2011;20(4):752–62. https://doi.org/10.1093/hmg/ddq520.
121. Park TS, Galic Z, Conway AE, Lindgren A, van Handel BJ, Magnusson M, Richter L, Teitell MA, Mikkola HK, Lowry WE, Plath K, Clark AT. Derivation of primordial germ cells from human embryonic and induced pluripotent stem cells is significantly improved by coculture with human fetal gonadal cells. Stem Cells. 2009;27(4):783–95. https://doi.org/10.1002/stem.13.
122. Pendergraft SS, Sadri-Ardekani H, Atala A, Bishop CE. Three-dimensional testicular organoid: a novel tool for the study of human spermatogenesis and gonadotoxicity in vitro†. Biol Reprod. 2017;96(3):720–32. https://doi.org/10.1095/biolreprod.116.143446.
123. Phillips BT, Gassei K, Orwig KE. Spermatogonial stem cell regulation and spermatogenesis. Philos Trans R Soc Lond Ser B Biol Sci. 2010;365(1546):1663–78. https://doi.org/10.1098/rstb.2010.0026.
124. Picton HM, Wyns C, Anderson RA, Goossens E, Jahnukainen K, Kliesch S, Mitchell RT, Pennings G, Rives N, Tournaye H, van Pelt AM, Eichenlaub-Ritter U, Schlatt S. A European perspective on testicular tissue cryopreservation for fertility preservation in prepubertal and adolescent boysdagger. Human Reprod (Oxford, England). 2015;30(11):2463–75. https://doi.org/10.1093/humrep/dev190.
125. Piravar Z, Jeddi-Tehrani M, Sadeghi MR, Mohazzab A, Eidi A, Akhondi MM. In vitro culture of human testicular stem cells on feeder-free condition. J Reprod Infertility. 2013;14(1):17–22.
126. Plotton I, Giscard d'Estaing S, Cuzin B, Brosse A, Benchaib M, Lornage J, Ecochard R, Dijoud F, Lejeune H. Preliminary results of a prospective study of testicular sperm extraction in young versus adult patients with nonmosaic 47,XXY Klinefelter syndrome. J Clin Endocrinol Metab. 2015;100(3):961–7. https://doi.org/10.1210/jc.2014-3083.
127. Poels J, Van Langendonckt A, Many MC, Wese FX, Wyns C. Vitrification preserves proliferation capacity in human spermatogonia. Human Reprod (Oxford, England). 2013;28(3):578–89. https://doi.org/10.1093/humrep/des455.
128. Radford J. Restoration of fertility after treatment for cancer. Horm Res. 2003;59(Suppl 1):21–3. https://doi.org/10.1159/000067840.
129. Radford JA, Shalet SM, Lieberman BA. Fertility after treatment for cancer. BMJ. 1999;319(7215):935–6.
130. Ramasamy R, Ricci JA, Palermo GD, Gosden LV, Rosenwaks Z, Schlegel PN. Successful fertility treatment for Klinefelter's syndrome. J Urol. 2009;182(3):1108–13. https://doi.org/10.1016/j.juro.2009.05.019.
131. Ramathal C, Angulo B, Sukhwani M, Cui J, Durruthy-Durruthy J, Fang F, Schanes P, Turek PJ, Orwig KE, Reijo Pera R. DDX3Y gene rescue of a Y chromosome AZFa deletion restores germ cell formation and transcriptional programs. Sci Rep. 2015;5:15041. https://doi.org/10.1038/srep15041.
132. Ramathal C, Durruthy-Durruthy J, Sukhwani M, Arakaki JE, Turek PJ, Orwig KE, Reijo Pera RA. Fate of iPSCs derived from azoospermic and fertile men following xenotransplantation to murine seminiferous tubules. Cell Rep. 2014;7(4):1284–97. https://doi.org/10.1016/j.celrep.2014.03.067.
133. Richardson TE, Chapman KM, Tenenhaus Dann C, Hammer RE, Hamra FK. Sterile testis complementation with spermatogonial lines restores fertility to DAZL-deficient rats and maximizes donor germline transmission. PloS One. 2009;4(7):e6308. https://doi.org/10.1371/journal.pone.0006308.
134. Rives N, Milazzo JP, Perdrix A, Castanet M, Joly-Helas G, Sibert L, Bironneau A, Way A, Mace B. The feasibility of fertility preservation in adolescents with Klinefelter syndrome. Human Reprod (Oxford, England). 2013;28(6):1468–79. https://doi.org/10.1093/humrep/det084.
135. Rosendahl M, Andersen MT, Ralfkiaer E, Kjeldsen L, Andersen MK, Andersen CY. Evidence of residual disease in cryopreserved ovarian cortex from female patients with leukemia. Fertil Steril. 2010;94(6):2186–90. https://doi.org/10.1016/j.fertnstert.2009.11.032.
136. Ryu BY, Kubota H, Avarbock MR, Brinster RL. Conservation of spermatogonial stem cell self-renewal signaling between mouse and rat. Proc Natl Acad Sci U S A. 2005;102(40):14302–7. https://doi.org/10.1073/pnas.0506970102.
137. Ryu BY, Orwig KE, Avarbock MR, Brinster RL. Stem cell and niche development in the postnatal rat testis. Dev Biol. 2003;263(2):253–63.

138. Sa R, Cremades N, Malheiro I, Sousa M. Cryopreservation of human testicular diploid germ cell suspensions. Andrologia. 2012;44(6):366–72. https://doi.org/10.1111/j.1439-0272.2012.01290.x.
139. Sadri-Ardekani H, Akhondi MA, van der Veen F, Repping S, van Pelt AM. In vitro propagation of human prepubertal spermatogonial stem cells. JAMA J Am Med Assoc. 2011;305(23):2416–8. https://doi.org/10.1001/jama.2011.791.
140. Sadri-Ardekani H, Akhondi MM, Vossough P, Maleki H, Sedighnejad S, Kamali K, Ghorbani B, van Wely M, van der Veen F, Repping S. Parental attitudes toward fertility preservation in boys with cancer: context of different risk levels of infertility and success rates of fertility restoration. Fertil Steril. 2013;99(3):796–802. https://doi.org/10.1016/j.fertnstert.2012.11.030.
141. Sadri-Ardekani H, Mizrak SC, van Daalen SK, Korver CM, Roepers-Gajadien HL, Koruji M, Hovingh S, de Reijke TM, de la Rosette JJ, van der Veen F, de Rooij DG, Repping S, van Pelt AM. Propagation of human spermatogonial stem cells in vitro. JAMA. 2009;302(19):2127–34. https://doi.org/10.1001/jama.2009.1689.
142. Sanghvi PR, Kaurin DG, McDonald TL, Holland JM. Testicular shielding in low-dose total body irradiation. Bone Marrow Transplant. 2007;39(4):247–8. https://doi.org/10.1038/sj.bmt.1705574.
143. Sasaki K, Yokobayashi S, Nakamura T, Okamoto I, Yabuta Y, Kurimoto K, Ohta H, Moritoki Y, Iwatani C, Tsuchiya H, Nakamura S, Sekiguchi K, Sakuma T, Yamamoto T, Mori T, Woltjen K, Nakagawa M, Yamamoto T, Takahashi K, Yamanaka S, Saitou M. Robust in vitro induction of human germ cell fate from pluripotent stem cells. Cell Stem Cell. 2015;17(2):178–94. https://doi.org/10.1016/j.stem.2015.06.014.
144. Sato T, Katagiri K, Gohbara A, Inoue K, Ogonuki N, Ogura A, Kubota Y, Ogawa T. In vitro production of functional sperm in cultured neonatal mouse testes. Nature. 2011;471(7339):504–7. https://doi.org/10.1038/nature09850.
145. Sato T, Katagiri K, Kubota Y, Ogawa T. In vitro sperm production from mouse spermatogonial stem cell lines using an organ culture method. Nat Protoc. 2013;8(11):2098–104. https://doi.org/10.1038/nprot.2013.138.. http://www.nature.com/nprot/journal/v8/n11/abs/nprot.2013.138.html - supplementary-information.
146. Sato Y, Nozawa S, Yoshiike M, Arai M, Sasaki C, Iwamoto T. Xenografting of testicular tissue from an infant human donor results in accelerated testicular maturation. Hum Reprod. 2010;25(5):1113–22. https://doi.org/10.1093/humrep/deq001.
147. Schiff JD, Palermo GD, Veeck LL, Goldstein M, Rosenwaks Z, Schlegel PN. Success of testicular sperm extraction [corrected] and intracytoplasmic sperm injection in men with Klinefelter syndrome. J Clin Endocrinol Metab. 2005;90(11):6263–7. https://doi.org/10.1210/jc.2004-2322.
148. Schlatt S, Foppiani L, Rolf C, Weinbauer GF, Nieschlag E. Germ cell transplantation into X-irradiated monkey testes. Human Reprod (Oxford, England). 2002; 17(1):55–62.
149. Schlatt S, Honaramooz A, Boiani M, Scholer HR, Dobrinski I. Progeny from sperm obtained after ectopic grafting of neonatal mouse testes. Biol Reprod. 2003;68(6):2331–5. https://doi.org/10.1095/biolreprod.102.014894.
150. Schlatt S, Honaramooz A, Ehmcke J, Goebell PJ, Rubben H, Dhir R, Dobrinski I, Patrizio P. Limited survival of adult human testicular tissue as ectopic xenograft. Hum Reprod. 2006;21(2):384–9. https://doi.org/10.1093/humrep/dei352.
151. Schmiegelow ML, Sommer P, Carlsen E, Sønksen JOR, Schmiegelow K, Muller JR. Penile vibratory stimulation and electroejaculation before anticancer therapy in two pubertal boys. J Pediatr Hematol Oncol. 1998;20(5):429–30.
152. Schover LR. Patient attitudes toward fertility preservation. Pediatr Blood Cancer. 2009;53(2):281–4. https://doi.org/10.1002/pbc.22001.
153. Schover LR, Brey K, Lichtin A, Lipshultz LI, Jeha S. Knowledge and experience regarding cancer, infertility, and sperm banking in younger male survivors. J Clin Oncol. 2002a;20(7):1880–9. https://doi.org/10.1200/Jco.2002.07.175.
154. Schover LR, Brey K, Lichtin A, Lipshultz LI, Jeha S. Knowledge and experience regarding cancer, infertility, and sperm banking in younger male survivors. J Clin Oncol. 2002b;20(7):1880–9.
155. Schover LR, Brey K, Lichtin A, Lipshultz LI, Jeha S. Oncologists' attitudes and practices regarding banking sperm before cancer treatment. J Clin Oncol. 2002c;20(7):1890–7.
156. Sharpe RM. Regulation of spermatogenesis. In: Knobil E, Neill JD, editors. The physiology of reproduction. New York: Raven Press, Ltd.; 1994. p. 1363–434.
157. Shinohara T, Orwig KE, Avarbock MR, Brinster RL. Remodeling of the postnatal mouse testis is accompanied by dramatic changes in stem cell number and niche accessibility. Proc Natl Acad Sci U S A. 2001;98(11):6186–91.
158. Smith JF, Yango P, Altman E, Choudhry S, Poelzl A, Zamah AM, Rosen M, Klatsky PC, Tran ND. Testicular niche required for human spermatogonial stem cell expansion. Stem Cells Transl Med. 2014;3(9):1043–54. https://doi.org/10.5966/sctm.2014-0045.
159. Steptoe PC, Edwards RG. Birth after the reimplantation of a human embryo. Lancet. 1978;2(8085):366.
160. Stukenborg JB, Schlatt S, Simoni M, Yeung CH, Elhija MA, Luetjens CM, Huleihel M, Wistuba J. New horizons for in vitro spermatogenesis? An update on novel three-dimensional culture systems as tools for meiotic and post-meiotic differentiation of testicular germ cells. Mol Hum Reprod. 2009;15(9):521–9. https://doi.org/10.1093/molehr/gap052.
161. Tegelenbosch RA, de Rooij DG. A quantitative study of spermatogonial multiplication and stem cell renewal in the C3H/101 F1 hybrid mouse. Mutat Res. 1993;290(2):193–200.
162. Teramura T, Takehara T, Kawata N, Fujinami N, Mitani T, Takenoshita M, Matsumoto K, Saeki K, Iritani A, Sagawa N, Hosoi Y. Primate embryonic stem cells proceed to early gametogenesis in vitro. Cloning Stem Cells. 2007;9(2):144–56. https://doi.org/10.1089/clo.2006.0070.

163. Unni S, Kasiviswanathan S, D'Souza S, Khavale S, Mukherjee S, Patwardhan S, Bhartiya D. Efficient cryopreservation of testicular tissue: effect of age, sample state, and concentration of cryoprotectant. Fertil Steril. 2012;97(1):200–208 e201. https://doi.org/10.1016/j.fertnstert.2011.10.018.
164. Valli H, Gassei K, Orwig KE. Stem cell therapies for male infertility: where are we now and where are we going? In: Carrell DT, Schlegel PN, Racowsky C, Gianaroli L, editors. Biennial review of infertility, vol. 4. Cham: Springer International Publishing; 2015a. p. 17–39. https://doi.org/10.1007/978-3-319-17849-3_3.
165. Valli H, Phillips BT, Gassei K, Nagano MC, Orwig KE. Spermatogonial stem cells and spermatogenesis. In: Plant TM, Zeleznik AJ, editors. Knobil and Neill's physiology of reproduction, vol. 1. 4th ed. San Diego: Elsevier; 2015b. p. 595–635.
166. Valli H, Phillips BT, Shetty G, Byrne JA, Clark AT, Meistrich ML, Orwig KE. Germline stem cells: toward the regeneration of spermatogenesis. Fertil Steril. 2014a;101(1):3–13. https://doi.org/10.1016/j.fertnstert.2013.10.052.
167. Valli H, Sukhwani M, Dovey SL, Peters KA, Donohue J, Castro CA, Chu T, Marshall GR, Orwig KE. Fluorescence- and magnetic-activated cell sorting strategies to isolate and enrich human spermatogonial stem cells. Fertil Steril. 2014b;102(2):566–80. https://doi.org/10.1016/j.fertnstert.2014.04.036.
168. Van Saen D, Goossens E, Bourgain C, Ferster A, Tournaye H. Meiotic activity in orthotopic xenografts derived from human postpubertal testicular tissue. Hum Reprod. 2011;26(2):282–93. https://doi.org/10.1093/humrep/deq321.
169. Verit FF, Verit A. Klinefelter syndrome: an argument for early aggressive hormonal and fertility management. Fertil Steril. 2012;98(5):e25; author reply e26. https://doi.org/10.1016/j.fertnstert.2012.08.031.
170. von Kopylow K, Schulze W, Salzbrunn A, Schaks M, Schäfer E, Roth B, Schlatt S, Spiess A-N. Dynamics, ultrastructure and gene expression of human in vitro organized testis cells from testicular sperm extraction biopsies. MHR: Basic Sci Reprod Med. 2018;24(3):123–34. https://doi.org/10.1093/molehr/gax070.
171. Wallace WH, Anderson RA, Irvine DS. Fertility preservation for young patients with cancer: who is at risk and what can be offered? Lancet Oncol. 2005;6(4):209–18. https://doi.org/10.1016/S1470-2045(05)70092-9.
172. Wasilewski-Masker K, Seidel KD, Leisenring W, Mertens AC, Shnorhavorian M, Ritenour CW, Stovall M, Green DM, Sklar CA, Armstrong GT, Robison LL, Meacham LR. Male infertility in long-term survivors of pediatric cancer: a report from the childhood cancer survivor study. J Cancer Surviv. 2014;8(3):437–47. https://doi.org/10.1007/s11764-014-0354-6.
173. Weiss RA. The discovery of endogenous retroviruses. Retrovirology. 2006;3:67. https://doi.org/10.1186/1742-4690-3-67.
174. Wikstrom AM, Raivio T, Hadziselimovic F, Wikstrom S, Tuuri T, Dunkel L. Klinefelter syndrome in adolescence: onset of puberty is associated with accelerated germ cell depletion. J Clin Endocrinol Metab. 2004;89(5):2263–70. https://doi.org/10.1210/jc.2003-031725.
175. Wu X, Schmidt JA, Avarbock MR, Tobias JW, Carlson CA, Kolon TF, Ginsberg JP, Brinster RL. Prepubertal human speratogonia and mouse gonocytes share conserved gene expression of germline stem cell regulatory molecules. Proc Natl Acad Sci U S A. 2009;106(51):21672–7. https://doi.org/10.1073/pnas.0912432106.
176. Wyns C, Collienne C, Shenfield F, Robert A, Laurent P, Roegiers L, Brichard B. Fertility preservation in the male pediatric population: factors influencing the decision of parents and children. Hum Reprod. 2015; https://doi.org/10.1093/humrep/dev161.
177. Wyns C, Curaba M, Martinez-Madrid B, Van Langendonckt A, Francois-Xavier W, Donnez J. Spermatogonial survival after cryopreservation and short-term orthotopic immature human cryptorchid testicular tissue grafting to immunodeficient mice. Hum Reprod. 2007;22(6):1603–11. https://doi.org/10.1093/humrep/dem062.
178. Wyns C, Curaba M, Petit S, Vanabelle B, Laurent P, Wese JF, Donnez J. Management of fertility preservation in prepubertal patients: 5 years' experience at the Catholic University of Louvain. Human Reprod (Oxford, England). 2011;26(4):737–47. https://doi.org/10.1093/humrep/deq387.
179. Wyns C, Van Langendonckt A, Wese FX, Donnez J, Curaba M. Long-term spermatogonial survival in cryopreserved and xenografted immature human testicular tissue. Hum Reprod. 2008;23(11):2402–14. https://doi.org/10.1093/humrep/den272.
180. Yadav P, Kozak K, Tolakanahalli R, Ramasubramanian V, Paliwal BR, Welsh JS, Rong Y. Adaptive planning using megavoltage fan-beam CT for radiation therapy with testicular shielding. Med Dosim. 2012;37(2):157–62. https://doi.org/10.1016/j.meddos.2011.06.005.
181. Yamauchi K, Hasegawa K, Chuma S, Nakatsuji N, Suemori H. In vitro germ cell differentiation from cynomolgus monkey embryonic stem cells. PloS one. 2009;4(4):e5338. https://doi.org/10.1371/journal.pone.0005338.
182. Yango P, Altman E, Smith JF, Klatsky PC, Tran ND. Optimizing cryopreservation of human spermatogonial stem cells: comparing the effectiveness of testicular tissue and single cell suspension cryopreservation. Fertil Steril. 2014;102(5):1491–1498 e1491. https://doi.org/10.1016/j.fertnstert.2014.07.1250.
183. Yarali H, Polat M, Bozdag G, Gunel M, Alpas I, Esinler I, Dogan U, Tiras B. TESE-ICSI in patients with non-mosaic Klinefelter syndrome: a comparative study. Reprod BioMed Online. 2009;18(6):756–60.
184. Zheng Y, Thomas A, Schmidt CM, Dann CT. Quantitative detection of human spermatogonia for optimization of spermatogonial stem cell culture. Human Reprod (Oxford, England). 2014;29(11):2497–511. https://doi.org/10.1093/humrep/deu232.

Male Sexuality

Anne Katz, Brooke Cherven, Linda Ballard, Chad Ritenour, and Lillian R. Meacham

T. K. Woodruff et al. (eds.), *Textbook of Oncofertility Research and Practice*,
https://doi.org/10.1007/978-3-030-02868-8_18

Key Points
- Male sexuality and sexual functioning may be impacted by all treatment modalities
- Attainment of developmental milestones may be delayed by cancer treatment
- Sexual functioning of young adult men is often not addressed by cancer care providers
- Both pharmacologic and psycho-educational and/or sexual interventions may help the young adult cancer survivor

18.1 Normal Sexual Development and Function

A review of the anatomy of the male reproductive system as well as endocrinology and physiology is important in the consideration of sexual function in male survivors of pediatric and adolescent cancer. Sexual differentiation occurs in the fetus at 6–12 weeks gestation. In the presence of hormonally functioning testes, the phallus and scrotum form and the Wolffian ducts emerge while the Mullerian ducts regress. In mid-gestation, the hypothalamic-pituitary-testicular axis matures. Gonadotropin-releasing hormone (GnRH) produced in the medial basal hypothalamus is released into the hypophyseal portal circulation and regulates the secretion of luteinizing hormone (LH) and follicle-stimulating hormone (FSH). LH regulates testosterone production from the Leydig cells in the testes, while FSH is important for spermatogenesis. The hypothalamic-pituitary axis is quiescent after a brief burst of activity in early infancy until puberty which begins at age 11.5–12 years in males. As the physical transition from child to adult occurs with the acquisition of secondary sexual characteristics, sexual behaviors also emerge. Although the average age of ejacularche is 13 years, the onset of masturbation and sexual activities with others is modified by social mores, family beliefs, and the individual's health and beliefs.

To understand the pathophysiologic causes of sexual dysfunction, it is important to know the male genitourinary anatomy and normal physiologic functions related to sexual activity [4]. The penis is composed of a single corpus spongiosum surrounding the urethra and paired corpora cavernosa which fill with blood during an erection. The innervation to the penis is through somatic, parasympathetic, and sympathetic nerves. The somatic nerves have both sensory and motor functions. The parasympathetic nerves arise from the sacral cord at S2 and S4 and traverse the retroperitoneal space as the nervi erigentes signal vasodilation of the corpora, and this initiates an erection. The counterbalancing sympathetic nervous system regulates contraction of the vasa deferentia, seminal vesicles, prostate, and bladder neck during sexual activity which results in emission. In addition, the sympathetic nervous system mediates detumescence.

18.2 Erectile Dysfunction (ED)

Erectile dysfunction has been defined by the NIH as the "persistent inability to attain and maintain an erection sufficient to permit satisfactory sexual performance" [5]. Erectile function is the result of a complex interplay between vascular, neurologic, hormonal, and psychological factors and may significantly impact quality of life. Epidemiological data have shown a high prevalence and incidence of ED worldwide. The first large, community-based study of ED was the Massachusetts Male Aging Study (MMAS) [1]. The study reported an overall prevalence of 52% ED in noninstitutionalized men aged 40–70 years in the Boston area; Furlow reported a rate of 12% in males above age 18 [6], while other surveys reported ranges of 25–30% in men aged 60–70 [7, 8].

18.2.1 Etiology

The pathophysiology of ED may be vascular, neurogenic, anatomical, hormonal, drug induced, and/or psychogenic. ED may also be a result of a mix of etiologies (see Table 18.1). Systemic diseases such as chronic liver, kidney disease, diabetes, or cancer have been associated with ED [4]. Cardiovascular diseases are strongly associated with ED, which may be the complaint that leads to discovery of an underlying diagnosis of hypertension or coronary artery disease. Anatomical disorders include Peyronie's disease, congenital malformations, and genitourinary trauma. Hormonal disorders include hypogonadism and hyperprolactinemia. Medications associated with ED include primarily

18

Table 18.1 Male sexual dysfunction

Dysfunction by the activities of the sexual cycles	Causes of sexual dysfunction
Libido/desire:	Psychogenic
Hypoactive sexual desire	Androgen deficiency
15% adult men	Major psychological disorders
	Chronic medical conditions
	Drugs (antihypertensives, psychotropics, dopamine blockers)
	Substance abuse (alcohol, narcotics)
Erection/erectile dysfunction:	Psychogenic
12% in >18 years old	Androgen deficiency
25–50% in 60–70 years old	Major psychological disorders
52% in mass male aging study	Chronic medical conditions (diabetes, vascular, cardiac, hepatic, renal, pulmonary cancer)
	Penile disease (Peyronie's disease, congenital malformations)
	Drugs (antihypertensives, anticholinergics, psychotropics)
	Substance abuse (cigarette smoking, alcohol, narcotics)
Ejaculation:	Psychogenic
Premature ejaculation	Poor health status
Prevalence 20–30%	Sympathetic denervation (diabetes, surgery, or radiation)
Problems of emission or retrograde ejaculation	Drugs (sympatholytic, antihypertensive, MAO inhibitors, CNS depressants, antipsychotics)
	Androgen deficiency
Orgasm:	Psychogenic
Orgasmic dysfunction	Drugs (SSRI, TCA, MAO inhibitors)
Relatively rare – prevalence 3–10%	Substance abuse
	CNS disease (multiple sclerosis, Parkinson's disease, Huntington's chorea, lumbar sympathectomy)
Detumescence:	Structural abnormalities (Peyronie's disease, phimosis)
Failure of detumescence (priapism)	Primary priapism (idiopathic)
	Secondary priapism due to disease (sickle cell, amyloidosis, inflammatory, solid tumors, trauma) or due to drugs (phenothiazine, trazodone, cocaine)

antihypertensive agents and psychogenic drugs. In addition, the normal aging process has been shown to result in a decrease in sexual responsiveness and is reflected in the increased incidence of complaints of ED in older age groups [1].

18.2.2 Diagnosis

The first step in screening for ED is a detailed sexual and medical history of the patient. Partners, when available, should be included.

18.2.2.1 Sexual History

The sexual history should include information about previous and current sexual relationships, onset, severity and duration of the erectile problem, and previous consultations and treatments. A detailed description should be made of the rigidity and duration of both sexually stimulated and morning erections and of problems with arousal, ejaculation, and orgasm [9]. Assessment of other areas of sexual dysfunction such as ejaculation, libido, and orgasm should be included in the history. Several patient questionnaires have been developed for assessment of ED, including the Sexual Health Inventory for Men (SHIM) and the International Index of Erectile Function (IIEF) [9]. Either of these questionnaires may be used as an adjunct to diagnosis of ED; however, they focus on heterosexual intercourse and are thus not of use in men who have sex with men.

18.2.2.2 Medical History

Men with ED should be screened for symptoms of possible hypogonadism, including decreased energy, libido, and fatigue, as well as for symptomatic lower urinary tract infections. Any history of heart disease, hypertension, diabetes mellitus, neurologic disorders, and renal disease should be reviewed. Lifestyle factors that include smoking, obesity, high-fat diet, use of recreational drugs and alcohol, and lack of exercise may be contributing factors. Mental health history and current psychological status are important considerations as depression is a common comorbidity in ED. Medications, including antihypertensive, cardiac, psychotropic, and hypoglycemic agents, are often associated with ED. It may be difficult, however, to separate the medication from the underlying disease as the causative agent of the ED. History of cancer of the pelvic organs, testes, prostate, central nervous system, and spinal tumors and associated treatments including surgery and radiation may contribute to ED.

18.2.2.3 Physical Examination

The physical examination should be focused on the genitourinary, endocrine, vascular, and neurological systems. The exam may reveal unsuspected diagnoses, such as Peyronie's disease (an acquired, localized fibrotic disorder of the tunica albuginea resulting in penile deformity, mass, and/or pain), or hypogonadism. Signs of hypogonadism include decreased volume and/or turgor of the testes, alterations in secondary sexual characteristics, and gynecomastia. Blood pressure and femoral and peripheral pulses can reflect vascular health. A thorough neurological exam, including visual fields, should be assessed for symptoms of pituitary tumors.

18.2.2.4 Laboratory Testing

Laboratory testing should be tailored to the patient's complaints and risk factors. Testing may include fasting glucose or HbA1c, urinalysis, blood chemistry panel, and lipid profile. ED may be an early manifestation of coronary artery disease [10]. Concern for associated cardiovascular disease may warrant further investigation and/or referral to a cardiologist. Hormonal tests include a morning sample for a total testosterone. However, the threshold of testosterone to maintain erectile function is low, and ED is usually a symptom of more severe cases of hypogonadism. Additional hormonal tests, such as prolactin and luteinizing hormone, are performed when low testosterone levels are detected. If any abnormality is observed, referral to an endocrinologist may be indicated.

18.2.2.5 Specialized Diagnostic Tests

While most patients with ED can be diagnosed with a thorough history and physical exam, some patients may need referral to a urologist for specific diagnostic tests. These may include nocturnal penile tumescence and rigidity test, intracavernosal injection test, duplex ultrasound of the penis, arteriography, and dynamic infusion cavernosometry or cavernosography.

18.2.3 Treatment Options

The primary goal in the management strategy of a patient with ED is to determine and treat its underlying etiology when possible. The American Urological Association (AUA) has issued evidence-based guidelines for the diagnosis and treatment of erectile dysfunction [11]. Originally written in 1996, the guidelines have been reviewed and revised in 2005 and 2011 and provide detailed descriptions of recommended strategies for ED management.

ED may be associated with modifiable or reversible risk factors, including lifestyle and/or medications. These factors may be modified either before or in conjunction with specific therapies. Screening for cardiovascular disease must be done prior to treatment, due to the potential risks associated with sexual activity in patients with heart disease [12]. Guidelines developed by the Princeton Consensus Panel [11] describe three levels (high, intermediate, low) of cardiovascular risk factors. Patients in the high and intermediate categories should be evaluated by a cardiologist prior to initiating therapies for ED.

The currently available therapies that should be considered for the treatment of erectile dysfunction include the following: pharmacologic (oral phosphodiesterase type 5 [PDE-5] inhibitors), intraurethral alprostadil, intracavernous vasoactive drug injection, vacuum constriction devices, and penile prosthesis implantation. These appropriate treatment options should be applied in a stepwise fashion with increasing invasiveness and risk balanced against the likelihood of efficacy [11], and referral for management by urology may be appropriate. PDE-5 inhibitors are contraindicated in men taking nitrates and should be used cautiously in men taking alpha-adrenergic blocker medications. The choice of a specific PDE-5 inhibitor (short or long acting) depends on the frequency of intercourse and the patient's personal experience.

Surgical correction may be needed for patients with ED due to penile abnormalities, e.g., hypospadias, congenital curvature, or Peyronie's disease, with preserved rigidity. Endocrine therapy for hypogonadism or hyperprolactinemia is an appropriate intervention for patients with a definite endocrinopathy. Combination therapy of a PDE-5 inhibitor and testosterone may be useful for hypogonadal men who do not respond to PDE-5 therapy alone. Testosterone therapy should be supervised by an endocrinologist and requires close monitoring for side effects (liver, prostate). Testosterone should be used cautiously in patients with unstable cardiac disease or concern for prostate disease [13].

Psychosexual therapy may be useful in combination with both medical and surgical treatment for men with ED. For some patients, brief education, support, and reassurance may be sufficient to restore sexual function, and for others, referral for more specialized and intensive counseling may be necessary.

18.3 Ejaculatory Dysfunction

18.3.1 Premature (or Rapid) Ejaculation

Premature ejaculation (PE) is a common male sexual dysfunction. Prevalence rates are quite variable ranging from 20% to 30% in multiple studies of adult males [9, 14], while European studies indicate an approximate prevalence of 5% [10]. PE can be difficult to define, and few men present for treatment. It is defined in the DSM-VI as persistent or rapid ejaculation with minimal sexual stimulation that occurs before or shortly after penetration and, importantly, before the person wishes it.

18.3.1.1 Etiology

The etiology and pathophysiology of PE are unknown. A significant proportion of men with ED also experience PE, and it can be difficult to distinguish between them. The fear of losing an erection may cause rapid ejaculation before the man or his partner is satisfied. Other potential risk factors for PE include a genetic predisposition, poor overall health status and obesity, prostate inflammation, thyroid hormone disorders, emotional problems and stress, and traumatic sexual experiences [10].

18.3.1.2 Diagnosis

The diagnosis of PE is based on the patient's medical and sexual history. Important criteria include whether PE is situational, such as with a specific partner or certain circumstances, and lifelong or acquired and impact on sexual activity and quality of life for both the patient and partner. Physical exam may assist in identifying associated underlying conditions, such as endocrinopathies and urological disorders.

There are several patient questionnaires for use in diagnosing PE. The most commonly used is the Premature Ejaculation Diagnostic Tool (PEDT) [15].

18.3.1.3 Treatment

Treatment approaches may include behavioral modification therapies and/or psychotherapy, decrease in sensory input, or controlled use of medications that have delayed ejaculation as part of their side effect profile. Although not approved by the FDA for this indication, oral antidepressants (SSRIs) and topical anesthetic agents have been shown to delay ejaculation in men with PE and have minimal side effects when used for the treatment of PE. Treatment with oral antidepressants should be started at the lowest possible dose that is compatible with a reasonable chance of success, and some men may be advised to take the SSRI before planned sexual activity rather than daily. In patients with concomitant PE and ED, the ED should be treated first [14]. Regular follow-up is important to evaluate efficacy and side effects. Support and education of the patient and, when possible, the partner are an integral part of PE therapy [14].

18.3.2 Inhibited Ejaculation

The prevalence of inhibited ejaculation is estimated at 1.5 in 1000 of the general male population [9]. Rates of inhibited ejaculation increase with age, with an overall incidence of 3% in men aged 50–54 years [16]. This disorder may be lifelong or acquired and situational or partner specific and is described as delayed or absent ejaculation.

18.3.2.1 Etiology

The majority of patients who report inhibited ejaculation have no clear etiology. There is an association with reports of personal or relationship distress and general health issues [9]. Any medical disease, drug, or surgical procedure that interferes with either central (including spinal or supraspinal) control of ejaculation or the autonomic innervation to the seminal tract, including the sympathetic innervation to the seminal vesicles, the prostatic urethra, and the bladder neck, or sensory innervation to the anatomical structures involved in the ejaculation process can result in delayed ejaculation, anejaculation, and anorgasmia [17]. Specific causes of delayed or absent ejaculation include medications, sympathetic denervation, hormone deficiency, lower urinary tract infections, and spinal cord injury.

18

18.3.2.2 Treatment

Treatments include psychosexual counseling, medication therapy or discontinuation of interfering medication, hormone replacement, and vibratory stimulation.

18.3.3 Retrograde Ejaculation (RE)

18.3.3.1 Etiology

Retrograde ejaculation results from damage to the sympathetic innervation of the ejaculatory system and bladder neck. RE may be caused by anatomic abnormalities such as urethral strictures, bladder neck resection, or fibrosis. Neurologic causes include multiple sclerosis, spinal cord injury, retroperitoneal lymphadenectomy, prostate or colorectal surgery, or diabetic neuropathy. Pharmacologic agents can also result in RE, primarily antihypertensive drugs, alpha-adrenergic blocking drugs, antipsychotics, and antidepressants [9].

18.3.3.2 Diagnosis

Patients with absent or low-volume ejaculate should be tested using semen analysis and urinalysis. Diagnosis is confirmed by the presence of sperm in a post-ejaculation urine sample. Diagnosis may result following evaluation for infertility due to azoospermia.

18.3.3.3 Treatment

In cases of pharmacologic etiology, discontinuation of the medication may resolve the problem. Pharmacotherapy is most often used for neurologic causes, particularly if partial nerve damage exists. Current drugs include alpha-adrenergic agents such as ephedrine or tricyclic antidepressants with anticholinergic effects. Successful response is most likely found in patients with partial nerve damage.

18.3.4 Painful Ejaculation or Dysorgasmia

Ejaculatory pain, although rare, may result from epididymal congestion after vasectomy, duct infection or obstruction, testicular torsion, mass lesion, lower urinary tract infection, or prostatitis. It is also quite common after radical prostatectomy. Psychogenic causes should also be considered.

18.4 Psychosexual Problems

Sexual dysfunction often has psychosocial components as an underlying cause and/or a consequence. Relationship status, strain with partner, life changes, and stress can all impact sexual function. Any patients with sexual dysfunction problems should be evaluated for psychological issues. Even if a problem is found to have a known physical cause, there may still be underlying psychological causes or implications.

Erectile dysfunction and ejaculatory problems can often be associated with psychological problems, particularly depression and anxiety. In the Massachusetts Male Aging Study, researchers found that ED was associated with depressive symptoms (OR 1.82, 95% CI, 1.21–2.73) [1].

Hypoactive sexual desire (HSD), or decreased libido, is a subjective report of the absence or decrease in frequency of sexual desire. It is often associated with other sexual dysfunctions, such as ED, and is influenced by social and cultural norms [9]. Depression and relationship conflict can influence sexual desire, and patients reporting HSD may benefit from referral to a psychologist.

18.5 Sexuality in Survivors of Childhood Cancer

18.5.1 Risk for Sexual Dysfunction in Survivors of Childhood Cancer

Survivors of childhood cancer should receive lifelong, specialized follow-up for late effects of cancer treatment. Survivorship care is individualized based on diagnosis and treatment exposures and is best directed by a Survivorship Healthcare Plan (SHP) which includes a detailed medical summary of cancer treatment, individualized late-effect risk profile, and surveillance plan for early detection of late effects. An SHP is created using the Children's Oncology Group Long-Term Follow-Up Guidelines for Survivors of Childhood, Adolescent, and Young Adult Cancer [18]. These guidelines are evidence-based screening recommendations created by multidisciplinary teams of expert clinicians in the field of childhood cancer survivorship. In addition to screening recommendations for a variety of health problems, the guidelines detail specific treatments which are associated with potential sexual dysfunction, such as radiation and surgery (Table 18.3) [19].

The impact of cancer treatment on sexuality has not been studied extensively in survivors of childhood cancer. Relander [20] found that among male survivors, 60% reported normal sexual function, with higher rates of sexual dysfunction reported in patients treated for tumors of the hypothalamic-pituitary region and patients who received testicular radiation or high doses of alkylating agents. The self-report of sexual function, however, in general is not specific to types of problems. The limited evidence of association of childhood cancer treatment with erectile dysfunction, ejaculatory problems, and psychosexual problems as well as psychosocial implications of sexual dysfunction in survivors will be discussed below.

18.5.2 Erectile Dysfunction

18.5.2.1 Etiology in Survivors

Specific treatment-related risk factors in survivors include cranial, pelvic, or spinal surgery, radiation, and hormonal deficiency, as well as those risk factors found in the general population such as increasing age and emotional distress [21]. Untreated hypoandrogenism may impact erectile function. In a report from the Childhood Cancer Survivor Study, radiation therapy to the testes was associated with ED as was pelvic radiation, thought to be caused by effects on the corpora cavernosa or penile bulb [22]. The study found that exposures as low as 10 Gy were associated with ED, suggesting that males treated at a young age may be vulnerable to permanent changes of the penile structure [22]. Treatment-related comorbidities such as obesity, diabetes mellitus, hyperlipidemia, renal disease, cardiac dysfunction, and/or depression and anxiety may cause or worsen ED, and many survivors are at a higher risk than their peers for these conditions [23, 24]. See Table 18.2 for a list of health conditions associated with sexual dysfunction with bolded items indicating those that can be seen in survivors depending on their treatment exposure history. Specific childhood cancer treatments which may increase risk for sexual dysfunction are found in Table 18.3.

18.5.2.2 Incidence in Survivors

The specific incidence of ED in childhood cancer survivors has not been well studied. Some studies report an incidence to be around 20% in survivors

Table 18.2 Health condition associated with sexual dysfunction

Vascular disease	*Cardiovascular disease (hypertension, atherosclerosis, hyperlipidemia)*
	Diabetes mellitus
Neurogenic	*Central causes*
	Degenerative disorders (multiple sclerosis, Parkinson's disease, etc.)
	Stroke
	Central nervous system tumors
	Peripheral causes
	Spinal cord trauma or diseases
	Polyneuropathy
	Types 1 and 2 diabetes mellitus
	Chronic renal failure
Anatomic or structural	Hypospadias/epispadias
	Micropenis
	Congenital curvature of the penis
	Peyronie's disease
Hormonal	*Hypogonadism*
	Hyperprolactinemia
Medication side effect	Antihypertensives (diuretics are the most common medication causing ED)
	Antidepressants (selective serotonin reuptake inhibitors, tricyclics)
	Antipsychotics (including neuroleptics)
	Antiandrogens
	GnRH analogues and antagonists
	Recreational drugs (alcohol, heroin, cocaine, marijuana, methadone)
Psychogenic	*Generalized*
	Lack of arousability and disorders of sexual intimacy
	Situational
	Partner-related, performance-related issues due to distress
Trauma	Penile fracture
	Peyronie's disease

Italics indicates conditions for which many survivors are at risk because of their treatment history
See the Children's Oncology Group Long-term Follow-up Guidelines for treatment exposures associated with risk for various health conditions. ► www.survivorshipguidelines.org

18

[2, 22, 25]. In a study of 1622 adult survivors of childhood cancer, Ritenour et al., using the International Index of Erectile Function, found that 12% met the criteria for erectile dysfunction, compared with only 4% of their healthy siblings (relative risk 2.66, 95% CI, 1.41–5.01). Survivors were also twice as likely than their siblings to report treatment for ED [22]. Similar to the

Table 18.3 Cancer treatment exposures associated with increased risk for sexual dysfunction

Chemotherapy	Radiation sites	Surgery
None	Pelvis	Spinal cord surgery
	Spine	Pelvic surgery
	Testicular	Cystectomy
		Retroperitoneal tumor or node dissection

According to the Children's Oncology Group Long-term Follow-up Guidelines

general population, sexual dysfunction was more common in older survivors, regardless of the previous treatment [25].

18.5.3 Ejaculatory Problems

18.5.3.1 Etiology in Survivors

Surgical procedures and/or pelvic radiation involving the bladder or other pelvic organs may also impact nerve and blood vessel function. Retroperitoneal lymph node dissection techniques have been known to cause retrograde ejaculation, and while procedures have been improved, they continue to carry a risk. Patients with impaired spinal cord function may have difficulty with ejaculation [9].

Patients with comorbid conditions related to their cancer diagnosis and treatments may experience ejaculatory dysfunction due to medication therapy such as antihypertensives and antidepressants.

18.5.3.2 Incidence in Survivors

Sundberg compared young adult male survivors with healthy peers and found that survivors more frequently reported sexual dysfunction compared with peers; this includes premature ejaculation in 9% of survivors compared to 7% of peers and orgasmic difficulty during intercourse among 10% of survivors compared with 3% of peers [3]. Jonker-Pool et al. conducted a meta-analysis of research focused on survivors of testicular cancer, a common diagnosis in the young adult population, which revealed that ejaculatory dysfunction was reported in 44% of survivors and was related to surgery in the retroperitoneal area [26].

18.5.4 Psychosexual Issues in Survivors

Much of what is known about sexual dysfunction in survivors of childhood cancer has been assessed through the lens of sexuality, satisfaction with sexuality, impact on quality of life, and life satisfaction. A recent study examined body image and sexual satisfaction in a group of 87 survivors and age-/gender-matched controls [27]. While results from this study indicate comparable satisfaction and psychosexual development, other studies have found that survivors report problems in categories of the NHSLS such as decreased desire and arousal as well as a negative impact from health problems on sexual satisfaction.

Zebrack surveyed 599 survivors of childhood cancer aged 18–39 and found that 20% of males reported lack of sexual interest and being unable to relax and enjoy sex and 16% reported at least some difficulty in becoming sexually aroused [2]. Van Dijk et al. surveyed 60 survivors (31 males) between the ages of 16 and 40 who were diagnosed under the age of 21 to assess the relationship of psychosexual function and quality of life and found that many survivors experienced problems [28]. Sexual problems included just over 40% of respondents who seldom or were never able to feel themselves sexually attractive and 44% felt almost no sexual attraction and seldom satisfied with their sexual lives. Forty-four percent were seldom/never able to see themselves as sexually attractive toward others [28].

Those who reported sexual dysfunction also had poorer health-related quality of life, and the association between the two was stronger among males than females [2]. When comparing survivors by gender, females were more likely to report sexual function problems, but having a sexual function problem had a larger impact on quality of life in males. This finding is echoed by van Dijk's study where 18% of male survivors surveyed felt a limitation in their sexual life due to their illness, mainly associated with uncertainty about their own body, difficulty with emotions, scars, and possible fertility problems [28]. Interestingly, a study of survivors of cancer to the lower bone extremity found that those who had an amputation or Van Nes rotationplasty reported better sexual functioning than those who had a limb salvage procedure [29].

Young adult patients experience significant interruptions to the developmental milestones that should be achieved in the years between ages 19 and 35. These include identity formation, self-focus, development of intimate and sexual relationships, and career and employment decisions [30]. Cancer delays or arrests the attainment of these milestones and increased dependence on parents both instrumentally and economically. It also isolates young adults from their peers and complicates existing relationships [31]. Alterations to body image and potential fertility are both concerns for young adults and may prevent them from establishing committed relationships [32].

18.5.5 Cancer's Impact on Normal Sexual Development and Activity

Cancer diagnosis can often impact the trajectory of typical childhood development, especially for those patients whose treatment may interrupt normal adolescence. Research has found that survivors have fewer sexual partners and often reach sexual milestones later than healthy peers. Survivors are often older at the time of the first relationship and at the time of the first sexual intercourse [33]. Van Dijk found this to be true especially for survivors who had received cancer treatment during adolescence [28]. These findings are echoed through a qualitative study of adolescent survivors who describe the challenges of forming romantic relationships while undergoing treatment and the need to prioritize getting through treatment over dating [34].

The diagnosis of testicular cancer provides a clear example of how normal sexual development can negatively impact on the lives of young adults [35]. From the embarrassment of finding a lump in the testicle that may lead to a delay in diagnosis to the feeling of being "damaged goods" and different from peers to fear of rejection and feeling less masculine than others, the experience of living with this cancer has far-reaching effects on global aspects of life. Concerns about disclosing a history of cancer coupled with uncertainty related to future fertility create additional stress and anxiety for these young men, and some may choose to delay or even avoid sexual relationships. Young adult men with testicular cancer have reported low libido, erectile dysfunction, and ejaculatory disorders [35, 36].

Young adult men diagnosed with Hodgkin or non-Hodgkin lymphoma also report significant sexual problems including lack of libido and erectile dysfunction. In one study [37], 39% of young adult survivors reported persistent sexual problems that did not resolve. Another study conducted in this population reported 20–54% of men experiencing sexual problems that were emotionally distressing [38].

Young men with colorectal cancer also experience sexual problems that are both functional and psychosocial with negative impacts on body image from scarring and especially if a permanent stoma is required [39].

18.5.6 Relationships and Intimacy

Cancer diagnosis and treatment can have effects on future relationships. Over one-third of adolescent and young adult cancer survivors report cancer having a negative impact on dating, and 40–60% report a negative impact on their sexual function/intimate relations, with a larger perceived impact seen in older childhood cancer survivors (30–39 years of age) compared with adolescents aged 15–20 years [40]. In a qualitative study of adolescent survivors, Stinson et al. found that the adolescents expected cancer to have little impact on future sexual relationships, but parents in the same study worried that their child's history of cancer could impact future relations [34]. Survivors often struggle with the disclosure of their cancer history with a new romantic partner, and this can be particularly stressful if they are concerned about their future fertility and its potential impact on forming a relationship [41].

Young adult survivors experience significant distress when a relationship ends and tend to stay in poor relationships longer in part due to the fear that they may not be able to find another partner [42]. Much of the research in relationships of young adult survivors is in women with breast cancer and their experience cannot be assumed to be the same for young men. This is an area where additional studies are needed.

There is also an overwhelming gap in the literature about the experiences of young men who have sex with men or identify themselves as gay or bisexual. Websites dedicated to gay cancer survivors are silent on the issue of young adults, and websites targeted at young adult cancer survivors ignore those who are gay. This is another area that is ripe for research that may have a significant impact on the lives of young adult cancer survivors.

18.5.7 How to Approach Cancer Survivors

It is crucial that providers who are caring for survivors of childhood cancer obtain a thorough history to assess for any sexual functioning problems. Bolte et al. suggest using the Permission, Limited Information, Specific Suggestions, Intensive Therapy (PLISSIT) model when communicating with adolescent and young adult survivors about sexuality after cancer treatment [43, 44] (Table 18.4). Talking about sexuality and sexual functioning can be uncomfortable for providers, but they may find general open-ended questions helpful in initiating the conversation. Using language such as "tell me what your friends are talking about with sex…what are you wondering about…" can help providers quickly gauge where patients are developmentally and identify their concerns (see Table 18.4 for more suggestions).

When referring to a urologist, providers should ensure the urologist is familiar with the context of the patient's health in terms of previous treatment by providing a thorough health history and risk for late effects, such as that provided in a Survivorship Healthcare Plan. Survivors may also benefit from a referral to psychology.

18.5.8 Challenges and Future Directions

Assessing the true incidence of sexual dysfunction is difficult. Many survivors transition to adult care which makes it difficult to ascertain the prevalence of late effects and the impact of late effects on the quality of life. Since these are not problems often seen in the pediatric realm, many survivors are not aware that they might be at increased risk of developing sexual health problems. Ensuring that survivors, especially as they transition to adult care, are aware of their risk and confident in talking with a healthcare provider about sexual function will be important to empower them to receive the care they need. Educating adult providers about the risks for sexual dysfunction associated with cancer treatment in childhood and its long-lasting impact on health is always important. It is also important to advocate for and conduct studies that examine the unique needs of these survivors so that effective interventions can be planned and tested.

Table 18.4 Using the PLISSIT model for communicating with male cancer survivors

PLISSIT model	Example question
Permission: offering permission for sexual challenges to exist and permission to initiate discussion and legitimize concerns	Some survivors experience sexual problems after cancer treatment. What questions do you have about this?
Limited information: address myths, reeducate patients about sexual health, provide resources	You received radiation to your pelvis which can sometimes cause erectile dysfunction. How have your erections been affected if at all?
Specific suggestions: individualize recommendations, avoid medical jargon	Many people benefit from treatment with medication or other interventions. Let's talk briefly about what can be done to help you
Intensive therapy: provide opportunities for patients to express feelings of fear and frustration around changes in sexuality after cancer treatment or refer for specialist care depending on the issue	Having erectile dysfunction can often be stressful and impact relationships. I can refer you to a sexuality counselor who can provide you with more information. How does that sound?

Review Questions and Answers

Q1. What treatments place a young adult male at a greater risk for erectile dysfunction?
   (a) All chemotherapy
   (b) Pelvic radiation
   (c) Antidepressants particularly SSRIs

A1. (b)

Q2. True or False? Ejaculatory disorders are associated with retroperitoneal lymph node dissection

A2. True

Q3. True or False? Young adult cancer survivors are more likely to end relationships because they are mature and have experienced personal growth

A3. False

Q4. Young adult cancer survivors with Hodgkin lymphoma are at risk for which of the following sexual problems
   (a) Anejaculation
   (b) Erectile dysfunction
   (c) Dysorgasmia
   (d) None of the above

A4. (b)

References

1. Feldman HA, et al. Impotence and its medical and psychosocial correlates: results of the Massachusetts Male Aging Study. J Urol. 1994;151(1):54–61.
2. Zebrack BJ, et al. Sexual functioning in young adult survivors of childhood cancer. Psychooncology. 2010;19(8):814–22.
3. Sundberg KK, et al. Sexual function and experience among long-term survivors of childhood cancer. Eur J Cancer. 2011;47(3):397–403.
4. Kandeel FR, Koussa VK, Swerdloff RS. Male sexual function and its disorders: physiology, pathophysiology, clinical investigation, and treatment. Endocr Rev. 2001;22(3):342–88.
5. Online NCS. Impotence. 1992;10(4):1–31.
6. Furlow WL. Prevalence of impotence in the United States. Med Asp Hum Sex. 1985;19:13–6.
7. Schiavi RC, et al. Healthy aging and male sexual function. Am J Psychiatry. 1990;147(6):766–71.
8. Diokno AC, Brown MB, Herzog AR. Sexual function in the elderly. Arch Intern Med. 1990;150(1):197–200.
9. Porst H, Buvat J. Standard practice in sexual medicine. Maiden: Blackwell Publishing; 2006.
10. Wespes E, et al. EAU guidelines on erectile dysfunction: an update. Eur Urol. 2006;49(5):806–15.
11. Montague DK, et al. Clinical guidelines panel on erectile dysfunction: summary report on the treatment of organic erectile dysfunction. The American Urological Association. J Urol. 1996;156(6):2007–11.
12. Nehra A, et al. The Princeton III consensus recommendations for the management of erectile dysfunction and cardiovascular disease. Mayo Clin Proc. 2012;87(8):766–78.
13. Bhasin S, et al. Testosterone therapy in adult men with androgen deficiency syndromes: an endocrine society clinical practice guideline. J Clin Endocrinol Metab. 2006;91(6):1995–2010.
14. Montague DK, et al. AUA guideline on the pharmacologic management of premature ejaculation. J Urol. 2004;172(1):290–4.
15. Symonds T, et al. Development and validation of a premature ejaculation diagnostic tool. Eur Urol. 2007;52(2):565–73.
16. Blanker MH, et al. Erectile and ejaculatory dysfunction in a community-based sample of men 50 to 78 years old: prevalence, concern, and relation to sexual activity. Urology. 2001;57(4):763–8.
17. Coolen LM, et al. Central regulation of ejaculation. Physiol Behav. 2004;83(2):203–15.
18. Children's Oncology Group. Long-term follow-up guidelines for survivors of childhood, adolescent and young adult cancers, version 5.0. Monrovia: Children's Oncology Group; 2013. Retrieved from http://www.survivorshipguidelines.org/pdf/2018/COG_LTFU_Guidelines_v5.pdf.
19. Landier W, et al. Development of risk-based guidelines for pediatric cancer survivors: the Children's Oncology Group long-term follow-up guidelines from the Children's Oncology Group late effects committee and nursing discipline. J Clin Oncol. 2004;22(24):4979–90.
20. Relander T, et al. Gonadal and sexual function in men treated for childhood cancer. Med Pediatr Oncol. 2000;35(1):52–63.
21. Kenney LB, et al. Male reproductive health after childhood, adolescent, and young adult cancers: a report from the Children's Oncology Group. J Clin Oncol. 2012;30(27):3408–16.
22. Ritenour CW, et al. Sexual health in male childhood cancer survivors: a report from the childhood cancer survivor study (CCSS). 13th international conference on long-term complications of treatment of children and adolescents for cancer poster presentation. Memphis, 2014.
23. Oeffinger KC, et al. Chronic health conditions in adult survivors of childhood cancer. N Engl J Med. 2006;355(15):1572–82.

24. Hudson MM, et al. Clinical ascertainment of health outcomes among adults treated for childhood cancer. JAMA. 2013;309(22):2371–81.
25. Bober SL, et al. Sexual function in childhood cancer survivors: a report from Project REACH. J Sex Med. 2013;10(8):2084–93.
26. Jonker-Pool G, et al. Sexual functioning after treatment for testicular cancer – review and meta-analysis of 36 empirical studies between 1975–2000. Arch Sex Behav. 2001;30(1):55–74.
27. Lehmann V, et al. Body issues, sexual satisfaction, and relationship status satisfaction in long-term childhood cancer survivors and healthy controls. Psychooncology. 2015;25(2):210–6.
28. van Dijk EM, et al. Psychosexual functioning of childhood cancer survivors. Psychooncology. 2008;17(5):506–11.
29. Barrera M, et al. Sexual function in adolescent and young adult survivors of lower extremity bone tumors. Pediatr Blood Cancer. 2010;55(7):1370–6.
30. Arnett J. Emerging adulthood(s). In: Lene A, Jensen, editors. Bridging cultural and developmental approaches to psychology. New syntheses in theory, research, and policy. New York: Oxford University Press; 2011.
31. Lewis P, Jordens CF, Mooney-Somers J, Smith K, Kerridge I. Growing up with cancer: accommodating the effects of cancer into young people's social lives. J Pediatric Oncol Nurs. 2013;30(6):311–9.
32. Zebrack BJ. Psychological, social, and behavioral issues for young adults with cancer. Cancer. 2011;117(10 Suppl):2289–94.
33. Stam H, Grootenhuis MA, Last BF. The course of life of survivors of childhood cancer. Psychooncology. 2005;14(3):227–38.
34. Stinson J, et al. A qualitative study of the impact of cancer on romantic relationships, sexual relationships, and fertility: perspectives of Canadian adolescents and parents during and after treatment. J Adolesc Young Adult Oncol. 2015;4(2):84–90.
35. Carpentier MY, Fortenberry JD, Ott MA, Brames MJ, Einhorn LH. Perceptions of masculinity and self-image in adolescent and young adult testicular cancer survivors: implications for romantic and sexual relationships. Psychooncology. 2011;20(7):738–45.
36. Kim C, McGlynn KA, McCorkle R, Li Y, Erickson RL, Ma S, et al. Sexual functioning among testicular cancer survivors: a case-control study in the U.S. J Psychosom Res. 2012;73(1):68–73.
37. Eeltink CM, Incrocci L, Witte BI, Meurs S, Visser O, Huijgens P, et al. Fertility and sexual function in female Hodgkin lymphoma survivors of reproductive age. J Clin Nurs. 2013;22:3513–21.
38. Arden-Close E, Eiser C, Pacey A. Sexual functioning in male survivors of lymphoma: a systematic review. J Sex Med. 2011;8:1833–40.
39. Donovan K, Thompson L, Hoffe S. Sexual function in colorectal cancer survivors. Cancer Control. 2010;17(1):44–51.
40. Bellizzi KM, et al. Positive and negative psychosocial impact of being diagnosed with cancer as an adolescent or young adult. Cancer. 2012;118(20):5155–62.
41. Thompson AL, Long KA, Marsland AL. Impact of childhood cancer on emerging adult survivors' romantic relationships: a qualitative account. J Sex Med. 2013;10(Suppl 1):65–73.
42. Thompson A, Marsland A, Marshal M, Tersak J. Romantic relationships of emerging adult survivors of childhood cancers. Psychooncology. 2008;18:767–74.
43. Bolte S, Zebrack B. Sexual issues in special populations: adolescents and young adults. Semin Oncol Nurs. 2008;24(2):115–9.
44. Annon J. The PLISSIT model: a proposed conceptual scheme for the behavioral treatment of sexual problems. J Sex Educ Ther. 1976;2:1–15.

Suggested Reading

Laumann EO, Paik A, Rosen RC. Sexual dysfunction in the United States: prevalence and predictors. JAMA. 1999;281(6):537–44.

Kolodyn RC, Masters WH, Johnson VE. Textbook of sexual medicine. Boston: Little Brown and Company; 1979. p. 1–28.

Govier FE, et al. Timing of penile color flow duplex ultrasonography using a triple drug mixture. J Urol. 1995;153(5):1472–5.

Lue TF, Tanagho E. Contemporary management of impotence and infertility. Baltimore: Williams & Wilkins; 1988.

Walsh PC, Wilson J. Harrison's principles of internal medicine. 11th ed. New York: McGraw-Hill Book Co.; 1987.

Ayta IA, McKinlay JB, Krane RJ. The likely worldwide increase in erectile dysfunction between 1995 and 2025 and some possible policy consequences. BJU Int. 1999;84(1):50–6.

Oncofertility in Clinical Practice

Contents

Setting Up an Oncofertility Program

Chelsea Webb Fox and H. Irene Su

T. K. Woodruff et al. (eds.), *Textbook of Oncofertility Research and Practice*,
https://doi.org/10.1007/978-3-030-02868-8_19

Key Points
- A clinical oncofertility program comprises a multidisciplinary team within an enabling framework.
- Developing standardized clinical pathways for oncofertility care will enable more universal access to care.
- Outreach efforts to inform the community about fertility preservation and the oncofertility program are integral to program success.

19.1 Introduction

In the United States, more than 160,000 women, men, and children who are younger than age 45 are diagnosed with cancer each year, with nearly one million cancer survivors of reproductive age [1, 13]. Moreover, young people with certain benign conditions may also face similar fertility-threatening treatments. The overarching goal of a clinical oncofertility program is to help these young patients and their physicians consider the impact of treatment on future fertility and facilitate fertility preservation efforts in what is often a limited time period before treatment begins. This chapter will discuss one approach to building an oncofertility program.

A comprehensive oncofertility program has multiple missions:
- Provide timely and comprehensive fertility risk and preservation consultations for patients facing fertility-threatening treatments
- Offer or refer patients to a range of appropriate fertility preservation treatments
- Coordinate care for and safely navigate medically complicated patients through fertility preservation treatments
- Serve as a resource for patients and healthcare providers who are seeking up-to-date fertility preservation information
- Offer or refer patients to reproductive health services, including contraceptive, sexual health, and menopause management

19

To fulfill these missions, a successful fertility preservation program requires an interdisciplinary team, a clear patient flow plan including the use of referral pathways to facilitate universal access to oncofertility services; access to equipment, supplies, and expertise for banking gametes, embryos, and gonadal tissue which often must occur on a short notice; and communication and marketing support. These represent the integral building blocks for any oncofertility program and are discussed in detail below.

19.2 The Oncofertility Team

19.2.1 Team Development

Care of oncofertility patients requires an interdisciplinary team (Table 19.1). Most often, the team is initially composed of a reproductive endocrinologist or an oncologist, who serves as a champion for program development. This individual seeks out potential team members, meets with them to discuss the oncofertility program, attains their input and commitment to collaborate on program execution, and generates a communication mechanism among team members for patient care. Early identification of key contacts facilitates the navigation of patients across specialties and within the tight timelines necessary for fertility preservation.

The oncofertility team does not need to be limited to a single institution. With few exceptions, the number of medically complex fertility preservation cases is limited at any one center. Therefore, having a forum to discuss oncofertility cases with like-minded colleagues is often invaluable. One source for peer-to-peer clinical care communication has been the Oncofertility Consortium FERTLINE, a national fertility preservation hotline.

19.2.2 Medical Team

The process begins with medical professionals addressing the possibility of infertility with patients who face exposure to fertility-threatening therapies before or during their reproductive years [2, 8]. The role of the treating oncologists, hematologists, rheumatologists, and their clinical staff is not to perform full oncofertility consultations but rather to address the issue of in fertility and refer patients who would like a more in-depth discussion to fertility specialists.

Table 19.1 The oncofertility team

Patient navigator	Responds to oncofertility requests
	Collects key clinical information on patients seeking care
	Provides basic information and resources regarding fertility risk and preservation options
	Triages patients
	Refers patients and providers to appropriate oncofertility medical providers
	Facilitates oncofertility appointments
Reproductive endocrinologist	Provides oncofertility consultations
	Directs fertility preservation treatments with input from oncology or rheumatology, anesthesia, pathology, and other medical specialties
	Provides or refers patients to reproductive health services, including contraceptive, sexual health, and menopause management
Reproductive urologist	Provides oncofertility consultations in males
	Performs testicular tissue biopsies or orchiectomies for banking
	Provides or refers patients to reproductive health services, including contraceptive, sexual health, and testicular failure management
Oncology, hematology, and rheumatology care teams	Address the possibility of infertility with patients treated before or during their reproductive years
	Refer patients who are interested in future fertility for fertility preservation consultations
Anesthesiologist	Provides anesthesia plan for fertility preservation surgeries
Pathology	Aids in shaping protocols for handling tissue for fertility preservation
Surgeon	Performs fertility preservation surgeries. This may be a reproductive endocrinologist, oncologist, urologist, or pediatric surgeon
Genetic counselor	Provides genetic counseling on inherited disease risk
Psychology and social work	Provide counseling and support services
Cell and tissue banking personnel	Performs clinical tissue banking
Financial counselor	Discusses out-of-pocket expenses for oncofertility counseling and fertility preservation with patients
	Checks insurance benefits, file insurance appeals
	Facilitates application to aid programs such as Sharing Hope
Marketing personnel	Publicizes the oncofertility program

For any oncofertility program, it can be very helpful to have a designated oncofertility patient navigator to whom medical providers direct inquiries and refer patients to reproductive endocrinologists for consultation. Patient navigators are frequently nurses or other allied healthcare professionals who can respond to oncofertility requests, obtain key clinical data on patients, provide basic information and resources to both patients and providers regarding fertility risk and fertility preservation options, and facilitate fertility appointments. A challenge is financial support for patient navigators. Some solutions to this challenge include a dedicated oncofertility navigator supported by cancer and/or infertility programs, training oncology or infertility patient navigators for oncofertility navigation, and automating referral processes (see Clinical Pathway below).

The reproductive endocrinologist and urologist provide oncofertility consultations and perform fertility preservation procedures. At the initial consultation, they will review individualized fertility risk and both standard of care and experimental options for fertility preservation. These physicians need to take into account diagnosis, proposed treatment, and other medical and social circumstances to *individualize* fertility risk and options for fertility preservation. For patients who contemplate undergoing fertility preservation treatments, the reproductive endocrinologist or urologist then communicates with the oncology team, anesthesia, and other relevant medical personnel to discuss safety, timing, and coordination of fertility preservation procedures and cancer treatment. Importantly, the reproductive health needs of young patients extend beyond fertility preservation, and thus, oncofertility consultation presents an important opportunity to discuss (or refer to care) contraception, pregnancy, sexual health, and gonadal failure risks and management.

An experienced anesthesia team plays a central role in evaluating patients for surgical fertility preservation procedures. While egg retrieval, the mainstay of female fertility preservation, is a common surgical procedure, oncofertility patients may pose complex medical scenarios that require advanced planning. Many egg retrievals and testicular biopsies are performed in ambulatory surgery centers, which benefit from adjacent embryology laboratories, surgical and embryology equipment, and surgical team expertise. While these surgicenters may facilitate gamete retrieval, they often have limited advanced cardiopulmonary monitoring and support. For challenging fertility preservation patients—for example, lymphoma patients with mediastinal or neck masses—the choice to undergo egg retrieval in the in vitro fertilization (IVF) surgicenter, with specialized equipment such as retrieval equipment and gamete incubators, is weighed against moving the surgery to the hospital operating room, where more intensive monitoring and resuscitation are available. Therefore, it is key to have an experienced anesthesiologist as part of the oncofertility team to formulate a sound plan for surgical retrievals in these complex cases.

The pathologist is a crucial contact for discussing disposition of ovarian and testicular tissue obtained for banking. Removal of ovarian or testicular tissue for fertility preservation requires maintaining sterility, keeping the tissue at 0–5 °C during transport, and minimizing time from removal to processing for freezing. Pathology examination protocols vary by site. Ideally, the minimum amount of tissue required for pathology exam (if any) should be prespecified and removed after the tissue in its entirety has been transported to the lab for preservation procedures. The protocol for handling tissue for banking needs to be worked out in advance, with the input of a pathologist.

The surgeon is the part of the team that harvests ovarian or testicular tissue. This person may be a reproductive endocrinologist, oncologist, urologist, or, in the case of infants and children, a pediatric surgeon. It is imperative that the surgeon understand the guidelines that determine the suitability and handling of tissue to be removed for fertility preservation.

Genetic counselors can help determine if there are heritable conditions that patients may transmit to their offspring. In embryo banking cases, the possibility of preimplantation genetic testing may be considered.

Psychologists and social workers can help young patients and their families with counseling needs during these often emotional and stressful circumstances.

19.2.3 Laboratory Team

Freezing of cells and tissues must be performed by laboratory personnel who are highly experienced in clinical tissue banking. In most centers, this will be embryologists, andrology lab personnel, or bone marrow lab personnel. These personnel are familiar with:

- Sterile technique and good tissue banking procedures.
- Tissue dissection and preparation.
- Addition of cryoprotectant solutions.
- Loading of tissues into vials.
- Labeling and documentation.
- Programming and use of slow cooling freezing equipment.
- Manual seeding.
- Storage in liquid nitrogen.

- Preparation of cryopreserved tissue for shipping.
- In some practices, isolation of oocytes, in vitro maturation (IVM), and oocyte and embryo cryopreservation; if these services are not available locally, the practice will need to be able to refer patients out to other facilities, using resources such as FERTLINE.

19.2.4 Financial Counseling, Marketing, and Public Relations Team

The financial counselor can help check insurance benefits, prepare letters of medical necessity, file insurance appeals, act as advocate for patients, and facilitate application to financial assistance programs such as Fertile Hope's Sharing Hope program. The counselor also clearly conveys the out-of-pocket costs for fertility preservation treatments to each patient.

Marketing and public relations personnel can help educate oncology, rheumatology, and primary care practices about oncofertility as well as the local community about fertility preservation programs for cancer patients. This team helps to build websites, create informational materials, and leverage social media approaches to publicize the program.

19.3 Clinical Pathway for Oncofertility Care and Patient Flow

Despite long-standing clinical guidelines supporting fertility risk counseling [2, 8] and evidence that oncofertility care preserves fertility options and improves quality of life for patients, a significant gap in care exists. Aggregate data from the Quality of Oncology Practice Initiative shows a stagnant 40% rate of fertility risk discussion and <30% rate of discussing fertility preservation options from 2013 to 2016. Lack of access to specialized care, fragmented multispecialty care, and inadequate infrastructure to support timely counseling and referrals contribute to this care gap [3, 5, 7, 11, 14]. This care gap can be minimized through the design and implementation of an oncofertility clinical pathway (◘ Fig. 19.1), which includes detailed protocols to deliver high-quality oncofertility care. While tailoring to individual programs is needed, considerations for an oncofertility clinical pathway and incorporation of electronic health record (EHR) technology include:

1. *Assessment and documentation of fertility risk*: Fertility risk discussions prior to cancer treatment have become a quality measure for cancer program accreditation [4]. Healthcare providers who administer fertility-threatening treatments need to inform patients of risks, document risk discussion, and refer patients accordingly. Materials for both healthcare provider and patient education (oral, printed materials, and web-based resources) will support this goal (◘ Table 19.2). EHR supports both back end algorithms that generate prompts for at-risk patients and dissemination of standardized risk counseling language embedded in EHR for documentation; EHR tools have been used in established programs and can be shared [6, 9, 10, 12].
2. *Referral to fertility risk and preservation counseling* must occur in a timely fashion to allow consideration of the full range of

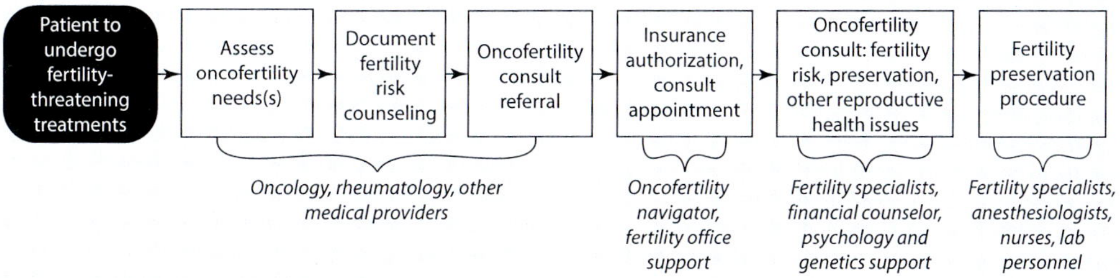

◘ **Fig. 19.1** Clinical pathway for oncofertility care

Table 19.2 Educational and financial resources for providers and patients

Site and type of information	What organization provides this resource?	Geared toward
FERTLINE: 866-708-FERT (3378) National hotline to connect providers and patients with fertility preservation programs	Oncofertility Consortium	Patients and providers
► www.savemyfertility.org Online fertility preservation toolkit and mobile application for patients and providers	Oncofertility Consortium	Patients and providers
► http://www.sart.org/ Locate US fertility specialists and view individual clinic IVF success rates	Society of Assisted Reproductive Technology	Patients and providers
► https://www.livestrong.org/we-can-help/fertility-services/ Navigation for cancer survivors on finding reproductive specialists and potential discounts on fertility services and medications	LIVESTRONG Fertility	Patients
► www.allianceforfertilitypreservation.org Fertility scout tool provides navigation for patients to find fertility specialists	Alliance for Fertility Preservation	Patients and providers
► http://www.cancercare.org/connect_workshops/359-young_adult_survivorship_fertility_sexuality_intimacy_2013-06-28 Audio recording discussing fertility, sexuality, and intimacy for young adult cancer survivors	Cancer*Care*	Patients
► https://www.livestrong.org/we-can-help/health-care-professionals Online training to help healthcare providers offer better fertility care to cancer patients	LIVESTRONG Fertility	Providers
► http://store.asrm.org Principles of fertility preservation for reproductive health providers certificate course, eLearning CME activity	American Society for Reproductive Medicine	Providers
► www.rhoinstitute.org ECHO web-based communication skill-building training program for oncology health professionals to communicate with patients on reproductive health	H. Lee Moffitt Cancer Center and Research Institute	Providers

fertility preservation options. For most programs, consultations occur within 24–72 h of referral. To execute referrals, patients can be prompted to contact the fertility specialist (risk of loss to follow-up), patient navigators can be notified of these referrals and contact patients (financial cost of navigation), or automated EHR processes may be set in place. As an example, our institution has generated a dedicated order for fertility preservation counseling that places referrals into respective work queues for male and female fertility specialists' administrative staff. There is a dedicated staff member who checks for these referrals daily, obtains insurance authorizations, and contacts the patient to schedule the appointment promptly. This EHR build prevented loss of referrals at the patient, oncology authorization staff, general gynecology, and urology staff levels.

Key treatment information including proposed cancer treatment and dosing is needed to estimate fertility risk in advance of the fertility preservation consultation to help the oncofertility team prepare for the visit. Figure 19.2 is an example of a referral form that is currently in use at our institution and incorporated into the EHR referral order.

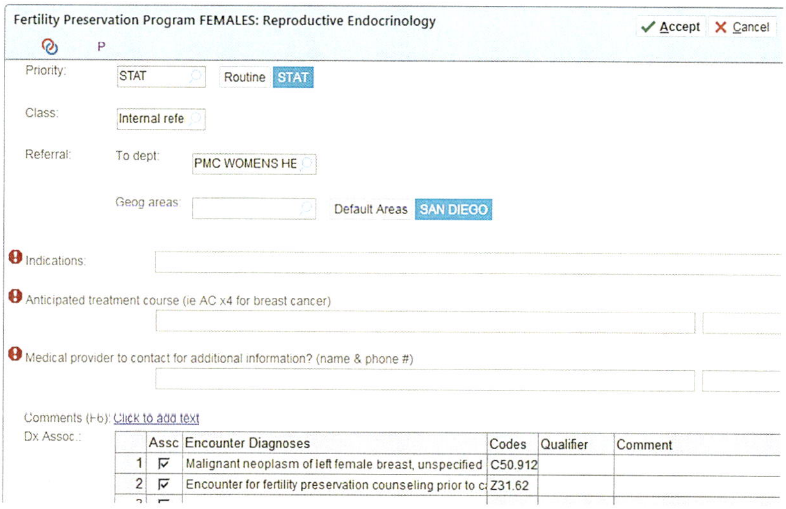
Fertility Preservation Program FEMALES: Reproductive Endocrinology
✓ Accept ✗ Cancel
P
Priority: STAT Routine STAT
Class: Internal refe
Referral: To dept: PMC WOMENS HE
Geog areas: Default Areas SAN DIEGO
Indications:
Anticipated treatment course (ie AC x4 for breast cancer)
Medical provider to contact for additional information? (name & phone #)
Comments (F6): Click to add text
Dx Assoc.:

	Assc	Encounter Diagnoses	Codes	Qualifier	Comment
1	☑	Malignant neoplasm of left female breast, unspecified	C50.912		
2	☑	Encounter for fertility preservation counseling prior to c	Z31.62		

Fig. 19.2 Oncofertility consultation referral order in electronic health record. As part of the order, patients receive instructions that they will be contacted within 3 days by the oncofertility program staff, as well as the phone number of the oncofertility program

3. *Fertility risk and preservation consultation* entails a discussion of the risks posed by the proposed cancer treatment on future fertility, an evaluation of the patient's medical fitness to undergo fertility preservation treatments, a discussion of the specific options for fertility preservation, referring patients to resources on fertility preservation, and a review of the costs associated with fertility preservation procedures. Applications for financial assistance programs are initiated. Because the reproductive health needs of young patients are broader than fertility preservation, this consultation also provides the opportunity to discuss contraception, sexual health, pregnancy, and management of gonadal failure. Telemedicine consultations are underway for a variety of medicine disciplines, and active program development to enable telemedicine consultations and insurance billing for these consultations has been initiated to reach geographically diverse young patients.

   Most decisions on whether to pursue treatment are made over the ensuing days and involve communication among the patient, their support system, the reproductive endocrinologist or urologist, and the treating oncologist or rheumatologist. Referrals to psychology and social work are generated as needed, and a bioethicist should be available for consultation when ethically challenging situations arise. For programs with research protocols, the research staff is contacted.
4. *Fertility preservation procedures*: For patients who elect to undergo ovarian stimulation for egg or embryo banking, a protocol is selected to minimize treatment time, tentative egg retrieval dates are established, and fertility-threatening treatment start dates are planned. Women who elect to use anonymous donor sperm are directed to sperm banks. Anesthesia consultations are initiated. During the time of ovarian stimulation, close communication between the fertility preservation team and the medical oncology or rheumatology team provides a continuous update on patient status. In addition, appropriate infectious disease testing of the patient or couple is undertaken. Of note, in the United States, infectious disease testing should be performed at FDA-approved labs if the gametes or embryos are to be used in third-party reproduction in the future. Surgical dates are set for patients who decide to preserve ovarian and testicular tissue or undergo other fertility preservation surgeries such as ovarian transposition. Pathology is contacted regarding disposition of the tissue to maximize future fertility potential.

   After fertility preservation treatment is completed, a summary of the procedure is communicated to the patient and their oncology, hematology, or rheumatology team. Annual follow-up of the patient regarding banked tissues is encouraged.
5. *Improvement of the clinical pathway*: Clinical pathways can be improved periodically, engaging the oncofertility team at regular intervals to review performance data, troubleshoot, and design adaptations.

19.4 Laboratory and Storage Considerations

Handling reproductive tissues requires appropriate laboratory expertise, equipment, and FDA registration. For storage facilities, there are also state-specific licensure requirements. Once licensed, there are regular monitoring updates and reporting schedules. As most tissues for fertility preservation are stored long term, banking at off-site storage facilities may be a consideration for the program and the patient.

19.5 Communication and Marketing

One barrier to fertility preservation referrals is the lack of awareness of fertility preservation programs. It is crucial to inform both the medical and general communities of the presence of an oncofertility program. Good marketing staff help to facilitate these outreach efforts. For individual programs, experiences include:

- A dedicated telephone number (Oncofertility FERTLINE) to reach the fertility preservation program. This is publicized clearly in all of the outreach efforts on behalf of the program.
- Grand rounds to primary care physicians, hematologists, oncologists, rheumatologists, and other medical professionals who care for this population.
- Attendance at tumor boards.
- Distribution of fertility preservation educational materials and resources to medical practices.
- Creation of the oncofertility program website. Presence on or links to local cancer program websites are important.
- Work with local advocacy groups such as Young Survivalors Coalition (targeting individuals with breast cancer) and Stupid Cancer (targeting young adult cancer survivors).
- Holding continuing medical education programs on oncofertility.

19

19.6 Financial Considerations

Most fertility preservation treatments are not covered by insurance. In the United States, there are few state and no national laws that mandate health insurance coverage of fertility preservation services for iatrogenic infertility at the time of this writing. Many oncofertility centers have a negotiated package price for patients undergoing fertility preservation treatments. Some programs have lowered global rates for all fertility preservation patients. Other centers participate in financial assistance programs such as the Sharing Hope program. Finally, some oncofertility programs have undertaken fundraising to help patients defray the significant costs of fertility preservation services.

19.7 Summary

Establishing a clinical oncofertility program provides an invaluable resource to the local community. Diverse expertise is required to discuss and undertake fertility preservation options in young cancer patients facing fertility-threatening therapy. Outreach efforts to inform the community about fertility preservation and the oncofertility program are integral to the success of any program.

Acknowledgments This work was supported by a grant (HD080952-04).

Review Questions and Answers

Q1. What is the role of a clinical pathway in an oncofertility program?

A1. Introduce standardized processes for each step of patient flow to decrease variability and increase access.

Q2. A successful oncofertility program requires the collaboration of an interdisciplinary team (True/False).

A2. True. Effective collaboration and communication of an interdisciplinary team including the medical team and their staff, embryologists, and administrative staff are paramount in fertility preservation.

References

1. American Cancer Society. Cancer treatment & survivorship facts & figures 2016–2017, vol. 2016. Atlanta: American Cancer Society; 2016.

2. ASRM. Fertility preservation in patients undergoing gonadotoxic therapy or gonadectomy: a committee opinion. Fertil Steril. 2013;100(5):1224–31.
3. Clayman ML, Harper MM, Quinn GP, Reinecke J, Shah S. Oncofertility resources at NCI-designated comprehensive cancer centers. J Natl Compr Cancer Netw. 2013;11(12):1504–9.
4. The Commission on Cancer's (CoC). Cancer program standards: ensuring patient-centered care. In Ensuring patient-centered care, vol Standard 4.5, 2016 edn. Commission on Cancer, p 67.
5. Corney RH, Swinglehurst AJ. Young childless women with breast cancer in the UK: a qualitative study of their fertility-related experiences, options, and the information given by health professionals. Psychooncology. 2014;23(1):20–6. https://doi.org/10.1002/pon.3365.
6. Johnson RH, Kroon L. Optimizing fertility preservation practices for adolescent and young adult cancer patients. J Natl Compr Cancer Netw. 2013;11(1):71–7.
7. King JW, Davies MC, Roche N, Abraham JM, Jones AL. Fertility preservation in women undergoing treatment for breast cancer in the UK: a questionnaire study. Oncologist. 2012;17(7):910–6. https://doi.org/10.1634/theoncologist.2012-0064.
8. Loren AW, Mangu PB, Beck LN, Brennan L, Magdalinski AJ, Partridge AH, Quinn G, Wallace WH, Oktay K. Fertility preservation for patients with cancer: American Society of clinical oncology clinical practice guideline update. J Clin Oncol. 2013; https://doi.org/10.1200/JCO.2013.49.2678.
9. Nagel K, Cassano J, Wizowski L, Neal MS. Collaborative multidisciplinary team approach to fertility issues among adolescent and young adult cancer patients. Int J Nurs Pract. 2009;15(4):311–7.
10. Ogle SK, Hobbie WL, Carlson CA, Meadows AT, Reilly MM, Ginsberg JP. Sperm banking for adolescents with cancer. J Pediatr Oncol Nurs. 2008;25(2):97–101.
11. Quinn GP, Vadaparampil ST, Lee JH, Jacobsen PB, Bepler G, Lancaster J, Keefe DL, Albrecht TL. Physician referral for fertility preservation in oncology patients: a national study of practice behaviors. J Clin Oncol. 2009;27(35):5952–7. https://doi.org/10.1200/JCO.2009.23.0250.
12. Shnorhavorian M, Kroon L, Jeffries H, Johnson R. Creating a standardized process to offer the standard of care: continuous process improvement methodology is associated with increased rates of sperm cryopreservation among adolescent and young adult males with cancer. J Pediatr Hematol Oncol. 2012;34(8):e315–9.
13. Surveillance Epidemiology, and End Results (SEER). Program SEER*Stat database: incidence – SEER 18 regs research data + hurricane Katrina impacted Louisiana cases, Nov 2016 Sub (1973–2014 varying) – linked to county attributes – total U.S., 1969–2015 counties, National Cancer Institute, DCCPS, Surveillance Research Program, released April 2017, based on the November 2016 submission. http://www.seer.cancer.gov/seerstat.
14. Yee S, Fuller-Thomson E, Lau A, Greenblatt EM. Fertility preservation practices among Ontario oncologists. J Cancer Educ. 2012;27(2):362–8. https://doi.org/10.1007/s13187-011-0301-4.

Building a Pediatric Oncofertility Practice

Karen Burns and Lesley Breech

T. K. Woodruff et al. (eds.), *Textbook of Oncofertility Research and Practice*,
https://doi.org/10.1007/978-3-030-02868-8_20

Key Points
- A successful pediatric oncofertility practice takes a multidisciplinary approach.
- Team visibility and communication are key to obtaining consults.
- Visual aids will help in decision-making for patients/families.
- Make it easy to consult the fertility preservation team via multiple modalities – Phone, pager, email, EMR, etc.

20.1 Introduction

The rate of cure for childhood cancer is now nearly 90% due to tremendous therapeutic advances in the past 50 years. Childhood cancer survivors now comprise approximately 1 of every 530 young adults aged 20–39 living in the United States (▶ www.childrensoncologygroup.org). Today childhood cancer survivors are living well into adulthood. The goals of pediatric oncology treatment include achieving cure, but also doing so in a way that minimizes a lifetime of late effects. Once such late effect of therapy is the impact on fertility.

Pediatric patients present unique challenges not often encountered in the adult cancer arena. Patients under the age of 18 are not able to consent to treatment. Parents must consent with their child's best interest in mind. Many parents and patients have not yet considered future childbearing at the time of diagnosis. They may be prematurely forced to discuss the topic for the first time and under stressful conditions. Pediatric malignancies grow very rapidly, leaving a very short window between diagnosis and the initiation of possible gonadotoxic therapy. This results in a narrow time frame for a discussion of potential fertility preservation options. Finally, many pediatric malignancies occur prior to puberty. This limits the number of established fertility preservation options available to this population.

This chapter represents the experience of Cincinnati Children's Hospital Medical Center (CCHMC) in building an oncofertility program for pediatric, adolescent, and young adult patients. Our team comprises physicians and medical staff from the Cancer and Blood Diseases Institute (CBDI); Pediatric and Adolescent Gynecology, Pediatric Urology, Pathology, and Ethics team; and the University of Cincinnati Reproductive Endocrinology and Infertility (REI). CCHMC is a tertiary care center with >350 new patients in oncology and >100 bone marrow transplant patients per year. We are able to offer ovarian tissue cryopreservation for females as young as 1 month of age under an open IRB-approved study protocol. In collaboration with our REI team members, we also offer oocyte/embryo cryopreservation for postpubertal patients. For males, testicular cryopreservation is available for patients at all ages under an open IRB-approved study protocol, and sperm cryopreservation is available for postpubertal patients.

20.2 The Oncofertility Team

A successful pediatric oncofertility program involves a collaborative effort that crosses several disciplines. Our process flow is defined in a later section of this chapter. For now, we will begin by defining the key individuals on our team. Successful program development and implementation requires recognition of the valuable input of all stakeholders. Team members work closely together with the assistance and coordination of the fertility navigator throughout.

20.2.1 Primary Team Members

At our institution the fertility navigator's role is performed by a registered nurse with experience in both pediatric oncology and pediatric and adolescent gynecology. She receives the initial consult and orchestrates communication between the multiple specialties, keeping timeliness and patient/family experience as the highest priorities. She is the core team member. She facilitates the actual consultation, ensures appropriate laboratory testing is performed, assists in the consultation, and arranges the indicated follow-up dependent upon the patient/family decision for intervention. At our institution, she also helps to navigate the research process and financial considerations. She is critical in assisting the patient/family through the oncofertility process as seamlessly as possible.

The pediatric oncologist on the oncofertility team is responsible for assessing the risk of infertility from the proposed treatment plan. He or she discusses the patient's treatment plan and timeline with their primary oncology/bone marrow transplant team. They will frequently involve the radiation oncologist if patients are to receive radiation therapy that will affect gonadal tissue either directly or through scatter fields. The pediatric oncologist has knowledge of the cancer diagnosis as well as access to detailed treatment protocols. This allows an accurate and individualized risk assessment of the effect of treatment on future fertility for the patient.

Our pediatric and adolescent gynecologist plays a critical role in the consultation for female patients. He or she is able to meet with the patient and family to discuss the risk assessment and appropriate fertility preservation options. They are then able to perform select procedures at our freestanding pediatric hospital (in the case of ovarian tissue cryopreservation) or refer to the reproductive endocrinologist for rapid consultation (embryo and oocyte cryopreservation). The gynecology team also manages medical therapies, including hormone therapy for menstrual suppression during treatment and hormone replacement therapy for females experiencing premature ovarian insufficiency post-therapy.

Our pediatric urologist is likewise essential in the consultation process for male patients. He or she is able to meet with the patient and family to discuss the risk assessment and appropriate fertility preservation options. They are then able to perform testicular tissue cryopreservation procedures in appropriate candidates or initiate a rapid sperm banking referral.

Many pediatric centers do not perform oocyte harvesting or oocyte/embryo cryopreservation; thus it is necessary to have a relationship with a reproductive endocrinologist familiar with oncofertility. They should be equipped to schedule urgent office visits to discuss the process of hormonal stimulation and oocyte harvest. Good communication is critical to maintaining the timeline agreed upon with the primary oncology team.

A research coordinator is also a valuable member of the team. Ovarian and testicular tissue cryopreservation are the only fertility preservation options available to prepubertal patients. Both methods of preservation are only performed under IRB-approved research protocols. The research coordinator ensures all proper research protocols are followed and informed consent has been obtained. He or she ensures appropriate documentation, record keeping, and follow-up are performed.

The team is not limited to the members detailed above. Other potential members might include a social worker to help identify community resources for financial aid, a member of the hospital Ethics team to aid in complicated decisions, Global Health to ease cultural differences, and Pastoral Care to help patients and families work through religious concerns. A team psychologist can help families work through their thoughts about fertility preservation and the available options. Programs that plan to process their own specimens (testicular and ovarian tissue, oocyte, and embryo preservation) will also need to include team members from the laboratory who specialize in processing this tissue (Table 20.1).

20.3 Oncofertility Consultation Process

The oncofertility process begins when a patient initially presents to the oncology or bone marrow transplant (BMT) program for diagnosis and treatment of their underlying disease. The primary oncology/BMT team contacts the fertility navigator to initiate the fertility consult and risk assessment. Initial contact can occur by phone, communication via the electronic medical record, or by email. We have a new patient order set in our EMR system to help ensure the primary team addresses fertility consults up front. By also creating a separate specific email address, the primary team has an additional streamlined way to reach our team (▶ Box 20.1).

Box 20.1 Exclusion Criteria

- Exclusion criteria at time of diagnosis
  - Presented for phase I/palliative therapy only
  - Diagnosed with malignancy but undergoing surgery or observation only
- Consultation deferred at time of diagnosis
  - Acutely ill
  - Urgent need to start cancer therapy

Table 20.1 Medical care team

Primary medical team	Addresses diagnosis and treatment plan with patient and family
	Introduces the concept of impaired fertility from necessary treatment
Pediatric oncology	Specific oncologist(s) with interest in oncofertility. Works with oncofertility team and primary medical team to determine the risk of impaired fertility with the proposed treatment plan, works with primary medical team to form timeline
Pediatric and adolescent gynecology	Addresses risk of impaired fertility with patient and family, discusses available fertility preservation options, performs surgery for ovarian tissue cryopreservation
Pediatric urology	Addresses risk of impaired fertility with patient and family, discusses available fertility preservation options, performs surgery for testicular tissue cryopreservation
Oncofertility navigator	Orchestrates communication between multiple disciplines involved in consultation process, maintains timeline for fertility preservation procedures/treatment start date, participates in consultations with patient/family, helps navigate research process when applicable
Research coordinator	Ensures proper research protocols are followed and informed consent obtained for all research-based fertility preservation options
Reproductive endocrinology	Provides services for oocyte harvesting and oocyte/embryo cryopreservation, provides laboratory for semen collection/storage for sperm cryopreservation

The goal of our oncofertility program is to see ALL patients new to the oncology and BMT division. However, we recognize that not every patient will be an appropriate candidate for a discussion on fertility preservation. A patient may be deemed ineligible for the following reasons:

- Diagnosed with malignancy but planned therapy consists of surgery/observation only.
- Presents for phase I therapy or palliative therapy only.

If a new patient meets one or more of these criteria, we will meet with the primary medical team to discuss whether or not it is appropriate to approach the family about fertility preservation options. Certainly some families who seem ineligible by criteria alone have many questions regarding future fertility. Patients who are acutely ill at the time of presentation and require immediate oncologic treatment will have the fertility consult delayed until the patient's medical condition is stable and timing is appropriate. This decision is always made in conjunction with the treating medical team. Patients who have previously had a fertility consult (relapse, transfer of care) may have an abbreviated consult to ensure all fertility preservation needs have been met.

20

Once a patient is classified as eligible, the fertility navigator contacts the oncofertility pediatric oncologist to perform the risk assessment. This physician will discuss the proposed treatment plan (surgery, radiation, chemotherapy) and timeline with the primary medical team. He or she calculates a patient-specific infertility risk assessment (low, intermediate, high). This is done using a cyclophosphamide equivalent dosing (CED) calculation and radiation/surgical risk assessment with published dose guidelines [1]. A literature review is also performed and is especially critical with regimens using newer agents.

The risk assessment is then communicated back to the fertility navigator and documented in the electronic medical record. She advises the gynecology/urology team of the consultation. The fertility navigator facilitates timing of evaluation and testing for the patient to ensure all parameters are met in accordance with the fertility preservation and cancer treatment plan. In addition to the consultation with the provider and fertility navigator, the patient and family receive written information on the fertility preservation options available to them. Many families would like time to think about their decision prior to making a final choice. Thus, the fertility navigator reconnects with the family after 24–48 h and then begins to coordinate any necessary procedures or referrals. The consult is completed and documented in the electronic medical record using a

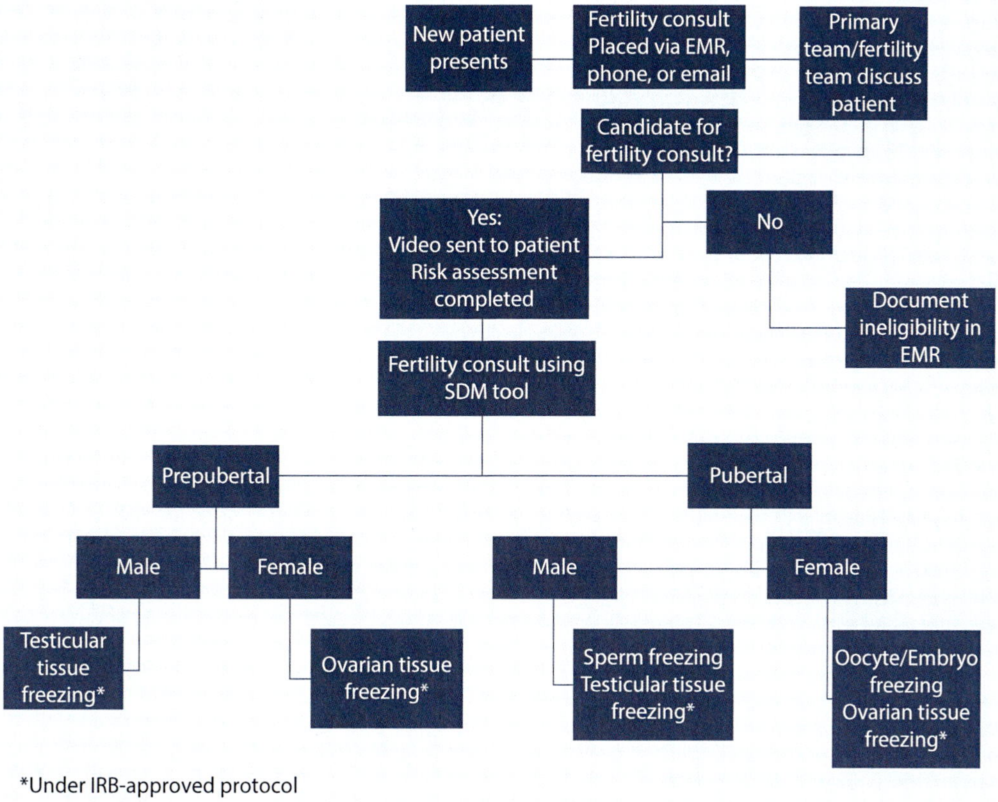

Fig. 20.1 Program workflow

standardized format. The primary medical team is updated regularly throughout the process to maintain good communication and best care for the patient (Fig. 20.1).

20.3.1 Laboratory Management

Assessment of fertilityat the time of evaluation informs patients/parents and the team about current fertility potential and allows informed decision-making regarding possible next steps. Our oncofertility team requests baseline laboratory studies on all patients who receive a consult. We request that these be drawn prior to starting chemotherapy. It allows a frame of reference for post-therapy values, as there can be some interpersonal variability in normal levels. For females, this includes baseline AMH, FSH, and LH. For males, we request baseline testosterone. Anyone who elects to have a cryopreservation technique is required to have infectious disease testing for HIV, hepatitis B, and hepatitis C drawn before the sample is frozen. It is important to use an FDA-approved lab (Table 20.2).

Table 20.2 Laboratory testing

Females	AMH
	LH
	FSH
	Estradiol
Males	Testosterone

We do not have a laboratory for long-term storage of cryopreserved specimens at our institution. At this time, cryopreserved ovarian tissue at CCHMC is placed in shipping media and shipped off-site for storage. Patients who opt for oocyte and/or embryo cryopreservation receive those services (evaluation, hormonal management, and tissue processing) through an adult-based Reproductive Endocrinology and Infertility (REI) facility. We maintain a strong collaborative relationship with the adult team to allow timely referrals as well as research and quality improvement work. Transportation for sperm banking services is sometimes difficult for patients due to timing and/or medical conditions prohibiting travel. A private, onsite room for semen collection (not the patient's hospital room) will help decrease anxiety and increase success rates.

We do perform tissue processing and short-term storage in-house. We partnered with our pathology laboratory colleagues to identify appropriately trained staff, space, equipment, and surveillance of the transiently stored tissue and storage tanks. Our entire team was trained in good tissue practices to ensure proper management and handling of human ovarian tissue.

Minimizing transfer costs for cryopreserved tissue can be helpful. There is a transfer fee associated with shipping specimens to the long-term cryopreservation facility. It is a flat fee independent of the number of specimens that is passed along to the patient. Batching specimens helps to defray the cost to the patient by dividing it among multiple samples.

20.3.2 Financial Concerns

Unfortunately, since many insurance providers do not provide full coverage for fertility preservation services, it is important to include financial counseling as part of the initial consultation. Fees may vary by institution. In some cases, discounts may be available for some or all of the services. It may be advantageous to attempt to process claims through the insurance carrier, before collecting any potential payment on the part of the patient. However, in order to store cryopreserved tissue for future use, payment is often due at the time of service. It is important to know the facilities and policies in your community to properly counsel families as they make their decision regarding fertility preservation.

Many assisted reproduction facilities offer discounted services for oncofertility patients. We have also found that combining fertility preservation procedure with other OR-related events (central line placement, etc.) when medically appropriate can help to bundle expenses and help to defray cost (Table 20.3).

Table 20.3 Potential costs to patient

Consultations	
Initial fertility consultation	Office visit cost and/or insurance co-pay
REI/urology consultation	Office visit cost and/or insurance co-pay
Fertility preservation intervention	
Sperm cryopreservation	Collection fee
	Shipment to storage facility
	Yearly storage fee
Testicular tissue preservation	Transportation fee if procedure not performed at local institution
	OR/surgery/anesthesia costs if not covered under another procedure
	Shipment to storage facility
	Yearly storage fee
Oocyte/embryo cryopreservation	Medication cost
	Procedural costs for retrieving oocytes
	Shipment to storage facility
	Yearly storage fee
Ovarian tissue cryopreservation	Transportation fee if procedure not performed at local institution
	OR/surgery/anesthesia cost if not covered under another procedure
	Shipment to storage facility
	Yearly storage fee
Future use of reproductive tissues	
Tissue reimplantation	Shipment of reproductive tissue to clinic/hospital of patient's choice
	OR/surgery/anesthesia costs if not covered under another procedure
In vitro fertilization	Shipment of reproductive tissue to clinic/hospital of patient's choice
	Medication costs
	Procedural costs for implanting an embryo

20.4 Consultation Aids

Most patients with a pediatric malignancy begin therapy very soon after diagnosis. The families receive a great deal of information in a very short and stressful time period. In addition to information about the diagnosis and therapy plan, they must also process the information related to fertility risk and preservation. We have aligned with two additional resources to aid in this process. Our first partnership is with the LiveWell Collaboration at the University of Cincinnati. Through this effort we were able to develop an animated video introducing the concept of oncofertility and fertility preservation. The video is available on our hospital network as well as a public Internet site (YouTube) for repeated viewings. New patients/families watch this prior to meeting with our team. Next, we worked with the James M. Anderson Center for Health Systems Excellence at CCHMC to develop a Shared Decision-Making (SDM) tool. Employing written materials with the consultation may allow patients and families a resource for reviewing information in their decision-making process. This gives the patient and family written information on risk and options in an easy-to-read format. It is easily reproducible so that each family can keep their copy for future reference. The SDM tool is used to walk the family through the process of understanding the individualized risk to their child as well as the options available specifically to them. The tool also allows stratification of factors that will be important for patients and families to consider in making their decision. For example, factors such as timing, additional surgical risk, cultural importance of fertility, religious considerations, and cost are outlined in the tool.

20.5 Documentation

Patients who receive a fertility consult have the encounter formally documented in our electronic medical record (EMR). It becomes part of their official medical chart. We have created a separate category specific to our team (labeled fertility consult) so that it is searchable in the EMR. It is important to document the diagnosis, date of diagnosis, treatment plan, and expected risk of infertility from therapy. The note should also capture the patient age and pubertal status as this will significantly impact potential therapeutic options. The note should detail the discussion with the patient and family: fertility preservation options available to the patient and risk/benefit of each. Finally, the note must communicate the next steps in the fertility preservation plan. If a family is uncertain as to how they would like to proceed, the note will state a timeline for follow-up. In this circumstance a follow-up note will be needed to document the decision and next steps in the oncofertility process.

Finally, a clinical database of consults is helpful. This can be maintained by the fertility navigator. This allows the team to track patients for follow-up during and after their cancer-directed therapy. Many times new questions arise and/or new options become available throughout the course of therapy. For example, a patient with acute lymphoblastic leukemia may be classified as having low risk of infertility due to therapy at diagnosis but then experiences a relapse and requires a bone marrow transplant. He or she is now at high risk of infertility from the planned therapy and may opt to choose a fertility preservation method. In another example, females at risk of premature ovarian insufficiency who did not have time to undergo oocyte or embryo cryopreservation prior to beginning therapy may elect to do so after completing therapy.

20.6 Communication and Institutional Awareness

Pediatric oncofertility is becoming more common but is still relatively rare in practice. Two of the greatest barriers are (1) not requesting the consult at all and (2) not initiating the consult in a timely manner. There are several ways one might address this issue:

- Initiating the consultation. An individual on the oncology team is designated as the person to initiate the consult on new patients. We have chosen to use our patient care manager (oncology navigator) for this role and added it to the checklist of our new diagnosis order set. This aligns the consult with our other new diagnosis consults and disease evaluation protocols. By relieving the primary oncologist from this obligation, it allows them to focus on their area of expertise – Developing the best treatment plan for the malignancy.

- Medical provider education. Healthcare professional education is key. Frequent in-service meetings for staff and physicians will increase awareness and knowledge. This in turn increases the volume of consultations. Our institution also has disease-specific team meetings. Having a presence at these meetings has helped to increase education and awareness.
- Ease of access. Consults are requested through the new patient order set in the EMR. We also have a designated email: fertilityconsult@cchmc.org. Our patient care managers communicate new consult requests via this email. It is checked several times per day by members of the fertility consult team. There is a member of the fertility consult team on call at all times. The call number is listed along with the hematology/oncology/BMT call schedule.
- Visibility. With the increasing use of technology among today's healthcare consumers, online access is critical. We have a designated fertility preservation landing page within the hospital website (▶ www.cincinnatichildrens.org). The page is also embedded within the oncology pages. It is easily accessible through the hospital search function as well as independent search functions under the title "Comprehensive Fertility Care and Preservation Program."
- Peer-to-peer information. Nothing emphasizes the credibility of information like someone who has already navigated the same stressful or overwhelming experience. Web-based video testimonials from current and former patients are available on our website for patients, families, and providers to review.

20.7 Cultural Considerations

Our hospital has become an international referral center for many conditions. It is important for team members to appreciate the beliefs of the different cultures and religions surrounding fertility, children, and afterlife. We work closely with our Global Health Division to understand regional customs prior to performing consultations. In addition, we make every attempt to provide written information in the family's native language and use an interpreter for all interactions. We have found that the importance of having one's own biological child varies greatly by culture. By addressing this issue, we are able to properly acknowledge the future fertility concerns of our international families. This in turn educates our team, and we gain a better understanding of fertility in each culture we encounter.

20

Review Questions and Answers

Q1. True or false: Fertility preservation procedures are usually covered by insurance.

A1. False. Most insurance policies do not cover fertility preservation. However, there may be financial assistance programs available, both on a national and local level. It is important to know what is available in your area.

Q2. Which of the following describe aspects of care that are unique to pediatric patients/families considering fertility preservation?
(a) Parents must consent for patients under the age of 18.
(b) There is often not much time between diagnosis and start of therapy with pediatric malignancies.
(c) All of the above.
(d) None of the above.

A2. (c)

Q3. True or false: Visual aids may help a family process information during the fertility preservation consultation.

A3. True. Our team uses both an animated video and written material during the consultation process.

Q4. Name several modalities a consulting team might use to reach the fertility team (and thus make obtaining a consult easy).

A4. Our team uses the following methods: specific pager, EMR order set and consult order, specific fertility email, specific fertility phone number, and on-call fertility team member listed on hospital call list. There are certainly other ways of reaching the fertility team, and institutions should use the methods that work best in their system.

Reference

1. Green DM, Nolan VG, Goodman PJ, Whitton JA, Srivastava D, Leisenring WM, Neglia JP, Sklar CA, Kaste SC, Hudson MM, Diller LR, Stovall M, Donaldson SS, Robison LL. The cyclophosphamide equivalent dose as an approach for quantifying alkylating agent exposure: a report from the Childhood Cancer Survivor Study. Pediatr Blood Cancer. 2014;61(1):53–67. https://doi.org/10.1002/pbc.24679.

The Fertility Preservation (FP) Consult

Barbara A. Lockart

T. K. Woodruff et al. (eds.), *Textbook of Oncofertility Research and Practice*,
https://doi.org/10.1007/978-3-030-02868-8_21

Key Points

- Information regarding impact treatment will have on future fertility and fertility preservation options should be provided to pediatric and adolescent patients and families prior to initiation of cancer treatment.
- Counseling patients and families includes consideration of the child's age and maturity level, family's health literacy, socioeconomic class, and cultural or religious background.
- Social workers, child life therapists, and psychologists can be utilized to provide reproductive information to children and adolescents in developmentally appropriate terms.
- Counseling childhood and AYA cancer patients should be ongoing throughout treatment and into survivorship.

The pace of pediatric oncology moves quickly, especially at the time of a cancer diagnosis. Families are overwhelmed by the diagnosis of a life-threatening illness in a previously healthy child, and they are inundated with information. Counseling a family on FP may not be an initial priority at the time of diagnosis, and, fortunately, the majority of childhood cancer survivors are not at risk for infertility [4, 21]. For those patients receiving treatment which may harm future fertility, counseling regarding the impact of treatment on fertility and preservation options prior to initiation of cancer therapy is important. For patients at risk for compromised fertility, the evidence supports a discussion regarding the risk of infertility and FP options prior to treatment initiation is extremely important [17, 20].

Educating families regarding side effects of treatment is the responsibility of both nurses and physicians. Fertility preservation as a patient right is supported by the American Society of Clinical Oncologists (ASCO), the American Society for Reproductive Medicine (ASRM), the American Academy of Pediatrics (AAP), and the Association of Pediatric Hematology and Oncology Nurses (APHON). These professional organizations support patient access to FP prior to treatment, as well as the need for ongoing emotional and physical support once treatment is completed [1, 5, 9, 14]. Current recommendations from ASCO, ASRM, AAP, and the nursing committee of the Children's Oncology Group (COG) endorse offering sperm banking to all adolescent and young adult males receiving cancer treatment. Oocyte harvesting is no longer considered experimental and should be discussed prior to treatment initiation with adolescent and young adult female patients at high risk for infertility [1, 9, 10, 14]. Nonexperimental methods of FP may not be available to a patient because of age, urgency to start treatment, or disease process. In such cases, the healthcare team is obligated to explain to families that experimental methods such as ovarian or testicular tissue cryopreservation may be an option for their child. Referral to an institution offering FP should be made as the family wishes.

The FP consult not only includes counseling with the patient and family but also with the oncology team, who are often unfamiliar with reproductive medicine technology. Conversely, reproductive medicine teams do not routinely encounter a critically ill pediatric or adolescent patient. The reproductive medicine team may require assistance in providing developmentally appropriate care to the patient, as well as caring for the entire family at a time of great stress. Utilization of a nurse or patient navigator to facilitate the coordination of patient care between the primary oncology team and reproductive medicine specialists is key to successfully caring for patients and families throughout treatment and into survivorship.

21.1 The Primary Treatment Team

The FP referral is often initiated by the patient's primary oncology team, either as a standard component of the new diagnosis workup or at the request of the family. Despite professional guidelines from ASCO and the AAP, research shows that many patients, especially female patients, are not satisfied with FP discussions prior to treatment [6, 8, 22]. Barriers to FP include healthcare provider discomfort with patient sexuality, cultural and religious influences, lack of knowledge regarding FP options, and concerns regarding the cost of FP [18]. A fertility preservation consultant is able to provide the family with FP information and allows the oncology team to focus on supporting the family through the new diagnosis discussion.

The fertility preservation consultant must meet with the primary team prior to counseling the patient and family. Information regarding diagnosis, medical and surgical history, Tanner stage, relapse information, planned cancer treatment, as well as previous cancer treatment is vital to assess the patient's risk of infertility. Another key component to counseling families is information regarding religious or cultural influences, family literacy level, preferred language, and any discussions the treatment team had with families regarding FP. A consult order in the electronic medical record formalizes the referral process and allows the FP team to track the number of patients referred to the service.

21.2 Assessing Risk of Infertility

A comprehensive medical history and physical exam, including Tanner staging, should be performed. Review of the treatment plan to assess the risk of infertility is vital. If the patient is eligible to enroll in a research study, the determination of patient eligibility is based upon planned treatment is required and should be verified prior to discussing FP options with families. The risk of infertility must be weighed with the cost, potential delay in treatment, cultural and ethical concerns regarding assisted reproduction, and health of the patient. The cyclophosphamide equivalent dose [13] has increasingly been used to estimate the potential risk of infertility due to alkylating agent exposure. When estimating the likelihood of infertility, previous chemotherapy, radiation, and surgeries must be included in the risk assessment.

Fertility preservation medical history

- Family medical history
- Genetic disorders
- Cancer syndromes
- Reproductive/sexual health
  - Biological children
  - Sexual transmitted infections
  - Sexual activity
    - Partners – male, female, both
    - Age at intercourse
    - Number of partners
    - Type of sex – oral, vaginal, anal
- Puberty history – Females
  - Tanner stage
  - Libido
  - Menstrual history
    - Age at which menstruation began
    - LMP
    - Frequency and duration of cycles
  - Pregnancies
    - Number
    - Terminations
- Puberty history – males
  - Tanner stage
  - Nocturnal emissions – age
  - Erectile dysfunction
  - Libido

21.3 Counseling Children and Adolescents

Information families provide to their children on the topics of sexuality and reproductive biology varies widely [15]. Healthcare providers counseling families on the topic of fertility preservation cannot assume either the parents or the patient possesses an understanding of basic reproductive biology. Therefore, any discussion on fertility preservation must include an explanation of puberty, reproductive health, pregnancy, menopause, and hormone regulation. Information provided to the patient should be developmentally appropriate and determined by the patient's age, cognitive ability to grasp the topic, and maturity level. Initiation of fertility preservation or reproductive health following cancer treatment is more successful if a healthcare provider begins the discussion [22]. Open-ended questions such as "have you thought about being a mom or dad in the future?" provide the patient the opportunity to express a vision of their future in a developmentally appropriate manner. Many pediatric hospitals employ child life therapists who are able to assist both the parents and the healthcare team to use developmentally appropriate language to explain reproduction and any FP procedures the patient might undergo.

There is never a "good time" to discuss the risk of infertility with a cancer patient, but waiting until after the initiation of treatment is not optimal and may mean FP is no longer feasible. The concepts of patient autonomy and informed decision-making require the patient and family to be provided with the information needed to determine if fertility preservation is a viable option as early as possible. Armuand et al. [3] report adult female cancer patients not provided information on FP options described a loss of control and report a greater sense of loss than male cancer patients. The researchers also state healthcare providers' assumptions about a patient's desire for FP rob the patient of autonomy.

During the course of the diagnosis and treatment discussions, the healthcare team reviews all potential side effects of treatment. A fertility preservation counselor or patient navigator is often the best professional to provide the patient and family information on FP options as well as reproductive health information during and following treatment. The impact of treatment on reproductive health and sexuality should also be included in the discussion. For example, a male patient at risk for retrograde ejaculation due to a reproperitoneal lymph node dissection should be informed of these side effects prior to surgery. Even patients whose treatment plan confers a low risk of infertility should be informed that treatment is unlikely to impact future reproductive health.

Parents of young children may prefer to discuss FP without their child present and may seek guidance from the healthcare team on how and when to begin the discussion with their child. Asking the parents if they wish to discuss FP with their child or if a discussion led by the healthcare team is desired provides the opportunity for families to choose the manner in which the information is delivered. Children can feel untethered if the adults around them are not providing information in an attempt to protect the child; therefore, it is important for the adults to structure the discussion, allow the patient to express concerns and fears, and have the parents and healthcare team respond to those concerns and fears. How adults respond to the child is more important than what is said [2]. A pediatric social worker or child life specialist may be helpful in providing the patient developmentally appropriate information.

It is best to begin with a basic explanation of reproduction, given in the patient and family's native language. Reassuring the patient that puberty and reproduction are a normal part of the human experience is vital. Quizzing the child is counterproductive and may inhibit any discussion on FP. Allowing the patient and family to ask questions is important, as well as giving them time to process the information provided. Patients may not be familiar with medical terms such as masturbation, oocyte, or testicles, requiring the healthcare provider to use slang terms to provide context to the discussion. Medications, stress, cognitive delays, language, fatigue, and cultural barriers may impact comprehension of the topic. The complex nature of the topic, as well as the seriousness of the cancer diagnosis, may necessitate several meetings with the family to adequately cover the topic. Do not assume that a child who is silent during the discussion is not paying attention or is not curious about the topic – embarrassment, fear, or anxiety may prevent him or her from engaging in a dialogue. Conversely, do not allow a parent to dominate the conversation or speak for the child (▶ Box 21.1).

Box 21.1 Guidelines for Counseling Families

1. Set the environment to allow for a private discussion
2. Lead the discussion
3. Do not assume the patient or family has knowledge of reproductive biology
4. Allow time to process information and formulate questions
5. Do not allow the parent to speak for the child
6. Do not assume a patient's silence means a lack of interest in the topic

Adolescence is often divided into three distinct phases of development. Therefore, counseling adolescents on reproductive health and FP is quite different than younger children. Early adolescence is from 11 to 13 years, middle adolescence is 14–16 years, and then late adolescence is 17–21 years of age [19]. Cognitive, emotional, and developmental needs of each stage of adolescent development influence how sensitive information such as FP is communicated with the patient.

Physical development does not correspond to the emotional and cognitive changes occurring during this time. A physically mature 14-year-old may be a concrete thinker, not quite able to grasp the significance of the decision to proceed with FP. If desired, the adolescent should be given the opportunity to discuss reproductive health and FP without parents present. To avoid any conflict between the adolescent and parents, the healthcare provider asks the adolescent if he or she wishes to have a parent or both parents present during the FP consult visit. This establishes that the adolescent is the patient and not the parent(s) [16].

21.4 Discussing Cost, Consent, and Disposal of Tissue in Event of Death

In addition to counseling families on the risk of infertility and FP options, families need to be informed of the cost of FP, the consent process, and tissue disposal. These topics may be even more sensitive for families than FP. Children may worry about the cost of FP and decline due to concerns of cost or financial burden to the family. The decision on what happens to tissue or sperm in the event of the patient's death may be influenced by religion or culture. These are sensitive topics and for most families should not be discussed in the presence of a minor child. The healthcare provider must not allow assumptions regarding a family's socioeconomic level, culture, or religion to influence what information a family is given. A 2014 study examining adult male survivors of childhood cancer and their parents identified many themes regarding FP decisions at the time of diagnosis. Cost of FP was not identified by any parent as a factor influencing their decision-making at the time of diagnosis [20].

Consent for medical procedures and research is guided by both legal and ethical principles. In the United States, the age of consent is typically 18 years of age. An adolescent may be asked to provide assent for medical procedures. Participation in experimental and standard of care fertility preservation requires both parental consent and adolescent assent. Maintaining the adolescent's "independence and enabling supportive collaboration with parents" is vital [12]. When enrollment in a research study is sought, the adolescent patient's refusal to assent to the study should supersede the parent's consent to study enrollment [11]. Consent and assent documents must include what will be done with the tissue or sperm in the event of death. When a minor child reaches the age of 18, the tissue or sperm bank must consent the patient.

21.5 Fertility Preservation and Sexual Health Counseling after Treatment Is Completed

Optimal care of childhood cancer patients includes educating and informing them of sexual and reproductive health issues throughout their developmental stages and lifespan. Patients treated for cancer prior to the start of puberty should be monitored for precocious or delayed puberty. Anticipatory guidance includes discussing how treatment may or may not impact sexual development and fertility throughout all phases of treatment, including survivorship. For example, parents of a child diagnosed with cancer at the age of 4 may not be concerned about pubertal development until their child is approaching puberty. As the patient matures, information is provided in a developmentally appropriate manner. Patients should be given the opportunity to discuss sexual health and reproductive issues, including contraception, without parents present, regardless of the patient's age.

Ongoing monitoring of hormone levels such as testosterone or estradiol may be indicated for patients who received gonadotoxic treatment. The Children's Oncology Group Survivorship Guidelines provide recommendations for monitoring the reproductive health of childhood cancer survivors post treatment. These guidelines may be incorporated into counseling patients [7]. Fertility preservation following cancer treatment may be appropriate after completion of cancer treatment for females who are at risk for premature menopause. Healthcare providers should review FP options following treatment with patients. Additionally, examining options such as adoption, use of donor oocytes or sperm, or gestational carrier should be discussed with adult survivors of childhood cancers who are infertile due to treatment.

21.6 Conclusion

Counseling patients and families on the topic of FP starts at the time of diagnosis and continues throughout the care trajectory. Discussions include not only FP options available but also reproductive health and parenting options. Healthcare providers should not wait for families to initiate a conversation on the topic of FP. Reassurance that this is a normal part of the human experience and important to the care of any cancer patient is vital. For families struggling emotionally with concerns about their child's future fertility, utilizing other services such as social work, chaplain services, or child life therapists will provide both information and emotional support to families during a very difficult time.

Review Questions and Answers

Q1. True or false? Barriers to fertility preservation include provider concerns about family's ability to pay for procedures, cultural and religious influences, discomfort with the topic, and lack of awareness of available options.

A1. True

Q2. True or false? A 16-year-old male who is staring at the floor when meeting with the provider to discuss sperm banking is not interested in his fertility.

A2. False

Q3. Sexual identity begins to emerge in:
(a) Early adolescence
(b) Middle adolescence
(c) Late adolescence

A3. (a)

Q4. True or False? Patients younger than 18 should be offered the opportunity to discuss fertility preservation without parents present.

A4. True

References

1. American Society for Reproductive Medicine and Society for Assisted Reproductive Technology: Ethics Committees. Fertility preservation and reproduction in cancer patients. Fertil Steril. 2005;86(6):1622–8.
2. Anderson S, Barton D, Bell B, Beniquez L, Bodiford C, Butler E, Thibodeau J. Hey, what do I say? A parent to parent guide on how to talk to children about sexuality. Planned Parenthood of New York City. 2009. www.ppnyc.org.
3. Armuand GM, Wettergren L, Rodriguez-Wallberg KA, Lampic C. Women more vulnerable than men when facing risk for treatment-induced infertility: a qualitative study of young adults newly diagnosed with cancer. Acta Oncol. 2015;54:243–52.
4. Barton SE, Najita JS, Ginsburg ES, Leisenring WM, Stovall M, Weathers RE, Sklar CA, Robison LL, Diller L. Infertility, infertility treatment, and achievement of pregnancy in female survivors of childhood cancer: a report from the Childhood Cancer Survivor Study cohort. Lancet Oncol. 2013;14(9):873–81.
5. Bashore L, Carr B, Lockart B, Schmidt D. Fertility preservation for pediatric, adolescent and young adult patients. 2012. Retrieved from www.aphon.org/files/public/onco-fertilitypaper.
6. Burns KC, Boudreau C, Panepinto JA. Attitudes regarding fertility preservation in female adolescent cancer patients. J Pediatr Hematol Oncol. 2006;28(6):350–4.
7. Children's Oncology Group. Long-term follow-up guidelines for survivors of childhood, adolescent, and young adult cancers and related health links Version 4. 2013.
8. Edge B, Holmes D, Makin G. Sperm banking in adolescent cancer patients. Arch Dis Child. 2006;91:149–52.
9. Fallat ME, Hutter J. Preservation of fertility in pediatric and adolescent patients with cancer. Pediatrics. 2008;121(5):1461–9. https://doi.org/10.1542/peds.2008-0593.
10. Fernbach A, Lockart B, Armus CL, Bashore LM, Levine J, Kroon L, Sylvain G, Rodgers C. Evidence-based recommendations for fertility preservation options for inclusion in treatment protocols for pediatric and adolescent patients diagnosed with cancer. J Pediatr Oncol Nurs. 2014;31(4):211–22. https://doi.org/10.1177/1043454214532025.
11. Giesbertz NAA, Bredenoord AL, van Delden JJM. Consent procedures in pediatric biobank. Eur J Hum Genet. 2014;23:1–6.
12. Grady C, Wiener L, Abdoler E, Trauernicht E, Zadeh S, Diekema DS, Wilfond BS, Wendler D. Assent in research: the voices of the adolescents. J Adolesc Health. 2014;54(5):515–20.
13. Green DM, Nolan VG, Goodman PJ, Whitton JA, Srivastava D, Leisenring WM, Neglia JP, Sklar CA, Kaste SC, Hudson MM, Diller LR, Stovall M, Donaldson SS, Robison LL. The cyclophosphamide equivalent dose as an approach for quantifying alkylating agent exposure. A report from the Childhood Cancer Survivor Study. Pediatr Blood Cancer. 2014;61(1):53–67.
14. Loren AW, Mangu PB, Nohr Beck L, Brennan L, Magdalinski AJ, Partridge AH, Quinn G, Wallace WH, Oktay K. Fertility preservation for patients with cancer: American Society of Clinical Oncology clinical practice guideline update. J Clin Oncol. 2013; Advance online publication. Retrieved from https://doi.org/10.1200/JCO.2013.49.2678.

15. Martino SC, Elliott MN, Corona R, Kanouse DE, Schuster MA. Beyond the "Big Talk": the roles of breadth and repetition in parent-adolescent communication about sexual topics. Pediatrics. 2008;121:e612.
16. National Sexual Violence Resource Center. An overview of adolescent sexual development. 2014. Retrieved from www.nsvrc.org/saam.
17. Nieman CL, Kinahan KE, Young SE, Rosenbloom SK, Yost KJ, Volpe T, Zoloth L, Woodruff TK. Fertility preservation and adolescent cancer patients: lessons from adult survivors of childhood cancer and their patients. Cancer Treat Res. 2007;138:201–17.
18. Quinn GP, Vadaparampil ST. Fertility preservation and adolescent young/adult cancer patients: physician communication challenges. J Adolesc Health. 2009;44:394–400.
19. Shafii T, Burstein GR. The adolescent sexual health visit. Obstet Gynecol Clin N Am. 2009;36:99–117.
20. Stein DM, Victorson DE, Choy JT, Waimey KE, Pearman TP, Smith K, Dreyfuss J, Kinahan KE, Sadhwani D, Woodruff TK, Brannigan RE. Fertility preservation preferences and perspectives among adult male survivors of pediatric cancer and their parents. J Adolesc Young Adult Oncol. 2014;3(2):75–85.
21. Wasilewski-Masker K, Seidel KD, Leisenring W, Mertens AC, Shnorhavorian M, Ritenour CW, Stovall M, Green DM, Sklar CA, Armstrong GT, Robison LL, Meacham LR. Male infertility in long-term survivors of pediatric cancer: a report from the Childhood Cancer Survivor Study. J Cancer Surviv. 2014;8(3):437–47.
22. Yeomanson DJ, Morgan S, Pacey AA. Discussing fertility preservation at the time of cancer diagnosis: dissatisfaction of young females. Pediatr Blood Cancer. 2013;60:1996–2000.

Genetic Counselors: Bridging the Oncofertility Information Gap

Allison L. Goetsch

T. K. Woodruff et al. (eds.), *Textbook of Oncofertility Research and Practice*,
https://doi.org/10.1007/978-3-030-02868-8_22

Key Points
- Genetic counselors believe fertility preservation discussions are an important part of their role as healthcare providers.
- Genetic counselors may use a nondirective approach to discuss fertility preservation with patients prior to cancer treatment or prophylactic surgery, effectively bridging the oncofertility information gap.

22.1 Introduction

As of January 1, 2016, it is estimated that there are more than 15 million cancer survivors in the United States, 8 million of whom are women [1]. By 2026, the American Cancer Society [1] estimates there will be more than 10 million female cancer survivors. Approximately 10% of individuals diagnosed with cancer are younger than 45 years of age and thus still within their reproductive years [1, 13]. Additionally, the 5-year relative survival rate for all cancers diagnosed between 2008 and 2014 is 67.5%, up from 49% between 1975 and 1977 [18]. The increase in survival rate can be attributed to progress in earlier diagnosis and improvements in treatment. With an increase in cancer survival, we can expect that more young women diagnosed with cancer will be seeking information about fertility preservation prior to cancer treatment. In fact, approximately 75% of young adult cancer survivors who have not previously had children express a desire for children in the future [13].

The goal of oncofertility is to balance life-preserving cancer treatments with fertility preserving options. Three main gaps have created an unmet need for preserving fertility in patients with cancer: an information gap, a data gap, and an option gap. The information gap, in particular, involves a lack of cancer patient understanding regarding the effects of cancer treatment on fertility and the option of fertility preservation. Many cancer patients do not recall discussing the impact of cancer treatment on fertility with their physician; because of this, multidisciplinary care that includes fertility treatment is especially valuable for bridging the information gap. In particular, genetic counselors—healthcare professionals specifically trained to deliver options and facilitate decision-making while focusing on psychosocial issues—are an untapped resource for educating cancer patients about fertility impairment and fertility preservation options. Genetic counselors possess the necessary skills to bridge the oncofertility information gap.

22.2 The Oncofertility Information Gap

Advances in cancer diagnostics and treatments have redefined the previous treatment-based approach to a broader perspective including survivorship and quality of life [12]. This new longer-term perspective on cancer care has revealed gaps in clinician-patient education, communication, and decision support with regard to fertility preservation that need to be addressed.

22.2.1 Lack of Oncofertility Patient Education and Communication

As part of their care, oncology healthcare providers should not only focus on the short-term goal of treatment and survival but also help cancer patients to preserve the best possible quality of life, including the possibility of having children [27]. If women are not informed of the risk that cancer treatment poses to their fertility, they may lose the opportunity to preserve their fertility prior to cancer treatment [16]. Even women who choose not to become parents value the opportunity to preserve their fertility [14]. Fertility preservation is especially important in adolescent and young adult patients with cancer, and unfortunately it is one of the most under-prescribed and least implemented services in their cancer care [5]. The National Comprehensive Cancer Network (NCCN) guidelines for young adults with cancer state that fertility preservation should be an essential part of cancer management, and the risk of infertility associated with cancer therapy should be discussed at the time of diagnosis [5]. Yet, while 75% of young women express interest in the opportunity to have children after a cancer diagnosis, as few as 34% of reproductive-age women treated for cancer recall having a discussion about the effects of cancer treatment on fertility [16]. The lack of patient education about fertility preservation is associated with the desire of the healthcare provider to start cancer treatment immediately, a lack of adequate knowledge regarding fertility preservation by the cancer care team, and insufficient provider-patient communication skills.

Studies show that few women with a new diagnosis of cancer are afforded the opportunity to discuss the benefits and limitations of fertility preservation options available to them. Many oncologists report little time to discuss future fertility or options for fertility preservation with their patients because the immediate focus is on cancer treatment. Providers also report they do not discuss fertility preservation with patients because fertility preservation techniques were not effective or useful or that fertility would not be affected by first-line chemotherapy [6, 8, 19].

In addition to their focus on the immediate need to start treatment, healthcare providers may not have adequate knowledge or sufficient communication skills to counsel concerned patients in a timely and supportive manner [21]. Hayat Roshanai et al. [11] found that physicians rarely ask about patients' concerns and questions in the oncology setting. However, some oncologists cite that lack of discussion is due to the perception that if a patient did not raise the issue themselves, then they were not interested [16].

Patient communication involves not only the transfer of information but also the provision of psychological and emotional support. Emotional support for young women with cancer is especially important because they experience greater distress and less emotional well-being than older women [12]. Counseling requires the ability to take into account a patient's individual background, provide information and support in a timely and accurate manner, and address the patient's emotional needs [21]. Kirkman et al. [14] found that the psychosocial needs of young women with cancer were not met and staff numbers in psychology and counseling were inadequate. In another study, women cancer survivors reported that fertility was a vital concern because they wanted to preserve not only quality of life after cancer but also protect their mental and emotional health [27]. Healthcare providers with proper training in counseling may be better equipped to provide emotional support to cancer patients and therefore facilitate discussions of fertility preservation and post-cancer quality of life.

To address psychosocial and behavioral issues, the NCCN provides a detailed list of support healthcare workers who can provide counseling to young adults with cancer. These patients need healthcare providers who are able to assess cognitive function, emotional issues, and evaluate other psychiatric symptoms, depression, and anxiety. Additionally, healthcare providers offering psychosocial support to young adult cancer patients need to be able to take into consideration patient existential/spiritual issues, personal relationships, decision-making preferences, and communication preferences that may affect cancer treatment and fertility preservation decisions [5].

22.2.2 Lack of Oncofertility Patient Decision Support

A lack of support for patient decision-making also contributes to the oncofertility information gap. Patients value fertility preservation and those healthcare providers who recognize that childbearing is a future option [14]. Patients want healthcare providers to offer options—including a discussion of the off-target effects of cancer treatment—and to support the decision to try for pregnancy after cancer treatment [14]. Patients can be particularly troubled when their fertility concerns are not well managed. In the Kirkman et al. [14] study, some women reported feeling excluded from discussions and decision-making about their own fertility. They were given minimal information and regret not being treated with consideration, especially when unwarranted assumptions were made about their fertility plans.

Healthcare providers should not assume they understand patient fears, priorities, or preferences related to their cancer treatment and fertility preservation. Doing so may influence the quality of the information a provider gives to a patient [19]. Alternatively, healthcare providers should be supportive of patient decisions and implement the use of the shared decision-making model [4].

22.2.3 Multidisciplinary Care

In 2013, The American Society of Clinical Oncology (ASCO) updated the clinical practice guidelines for Fertility Preservation, extending the responsibility for discussion and referral of fertility preservation beyond the oncologist to include other physician specialties and allied health professionals [17]. This recommendation supports a multidisciplinary approach in the cancer care setting including fertility preservation. Kirkman et al. [14] identified the multidisciplinary team approach to cancer care as especially valuable in a qualitative study of the significance of fertility and motherhood after a cancer diagnosis. Multidisciplinary care mitigates the need for the integration of the sensitive topic of fertility into an already overwhelming oncology consultation. Research suggests that the multidisciplinary approach and inclusion of healthcare workers who have special training to address fertility issues in the confusing period of time just after a cancer diagnosis would be well received by patients [15].

22.3 The Role of the Genetic Counselor

Genetic counselors are medical professionals who have undergone extensive graduate-level human genetics and psychosocial coursework. They possess the necessary skill set to deliver options and facilitate decision-making while also focusing on psychosocial concerns.

Genetic counselors facilitate informed medical decision-making by patients in many arenas, including genetic testing, family planning, medical screening, and treatment [7]. They are able to provide relevant information, reduce anxiety, and empower patients to make decisions through nondirective counseling. Nondirectiveness is an active counseling strategy which allows genetic counselors to support client autonomy and facilitate informed patient decision-making [2, 22, 25]. The goal of this approach is to increase patient self-esteem and enable patients to make independent, informed decisions free from coercion [23]. Nondirective counseling techniques employed by genetic counselors leave patients with greater sense of control over their lives and decisions [22].

Genetic counselors utilize their training and skills to reduce patient anxiety, enhance the patient's sense of control and mastery over life circumstances, increase patient understanding of the genetic disease and options for testing and disease management, and provide the individual and family with the tools required to adjust to potential outcomes [2]. The unique skill set of genetic counselors can be used to discuss the effects of cancer treatment on fertility and, through nondirective counseling, facilitate fertility preservation decision-making with patients during the sensitive window of time prior to cancer treatment or prophylactic surgery for women with a personal or family history suggestive of a hereditary or familial cancer.

22.4 Genetic Counselors and Fertility Preservation

It is recommended by the NCCN that individuals with a personal or family history suggestive of a hereditary or familial cancer be referred to a genetics expert, such as a genetic counselor, for further counseling and risk assessment. In addition to risk assessment, an appointment with a genetic counselor typically includes discussion of genetic testing, cancer risk-reducing options like prophylactic surgery, cancer treatment, risk to family members, and family planning considerations. The genetic counseling appointment is an opportune time to discuss the effect of cancer treatment on fertility and fertility preservation options.

While genetic counselors are a widely accepted addition to oncology and reproductive patient care, only one study to date has assessed genetic counselors' attitudes, knowledge, and discussion of fertility preservation in cancer patients. Several themes emerged from a survey of 218 oncology genetic counselors regarding care of breast and ovarian cancer patients by Volk et al. [24], including the general belief that fertility preservation discussions are important and part of the role of the genetic counselor. The study also identified barriers that prevent genetic counselors from discussing fertility preservation with their breast and ovarian cancer patients; the primary obstacle was the timing of cancer treatment.

22.4.1 Genetic Counselor Attitudes Toward Fertility Preservation

Almost all (98.7%) of the participating genetic counselors in the Volk et al. [24] study agreed or strongly agreed that breast and ovarian cancer patients should be told of the risk to fertility associated with cancer treatments. Approximately 70.2% of genetic counselors believed that discussing fertility preservation with their breast and ovarian cancer patients is part of their role as genetic counselors. A majority (61% and 65.4%, respectively) also stated that cancer patients and patients with an identified *BRCA1/2* pathogenic variant have asked about the potential threats to their fertility caused by treatment. In fact, most genetic counselors stated that fertility options were a major concern for all of their cancer patients (51.7%) as well as patients with a *BRCA1/2* pathogenic variant (63.8%).

The majority of genetic counselors in the Volk et al. [24] study stated that cancer patients have asked about fertility problems associated with both surgical and nonsurgical treatment options, patients with a *BRCA1/2* pathogenic variant have asked about problems associated with prophylactic bilateral salpingo-oophorectomy (BSO), and, in general, fertility is a major concern for both breast and ovarian cancer patients as well as patients with a *BRCA1/2* pathogenic variant.

22.4.2 Barriers to Discussions of Fertility Preservation by Genetic Counselors

The major barrier that prevents discussion of fertility preservation in genetic counseling sessions is the fact that breast and ovarian cancer patients are often seeing genetic counselors after cancer treatment (reported by 79.7% in the Volk et al. study). Only 29.5% of genetic counselors reported seeing breast and ovarian cancer patients prior to cancer treatment [24]. Ideally, discussion of fertility preservation should occur before cancer treatment. When genetic counseling sessions are held prior to cancer treatment or prophylactic surgery, genetic counselors can integrate fertility preservation into the medical management options discussion and facilitation of patient decision-making.

22.4.3 Hereditary Cancer Syndromes and Fertility Preservation

Hereditary breast and ovarian cancer (HBOC), caused by pathogenic variants in *BRCA1* and *BRCA2*, and Lynch syndrome, caused by pathogenic variants in *MSH2*, *MLH1*, *MSH6*, *PMS2*, and *EPCAM*, are responsible for the majority of hereditary gynecologic cancers. In fact, HBOC and Lynch syndrome underlie at least 20% of all ovarian cancer diagnoses [3, 10, 26]. Women with hereditary cancer syndromes undergoing cancer treatment or prophylactic cancer-risk-reducing surgery that impacts fertility should receive information regarding recurrence risk and family planning options, in addition to fertility preservation information. HBOC and Lynch syndrome are autosomal dominant genetic disorders with a 50% recurrence risk with each pregnancy. To reduce this risk, patients may pursue preimplantation genetic diagnosis (PGD) and embryo selection, which has been used in conjunction with in vitro fertilization (IVF) to screen embryos for an inherited genetic disorder.

The option to consider PGD should be included during any fertility preservation discussion with women diagnosed with a hereditary cancer syndrome associated with increased risk for gynecologic cancer. The majority of reproductive endocrinologists consult with a genetic counselor regarding PGD for hereditary cancer syndromes (92%) and recommend genetic counseling to cancer patients considering fertility preservation (82%) [9]. Women with hereditary cancer syndromes undergoing cancer treatment or prophylactic cancer-risk-reducing surgery that impacts fertility should receive genetic counseling [20]. Genetic counselors can address the associated effects on fertility, fertility preservation, and option to pursue PGD to reduce the risk to pass on the inherited cancer susceptibility to their future children.

22.5 Conclusion: Genetic Counselors Can Bridge the Oncofertility Information Gap

The goal of oncofertility is to balance life-preserving cancer treatments with fertility preservation options. Gaps in information, data, and options have led to an unmet need for preserving fertility in patients with cancer. The information gap, in particular, involves a lack of cancer patient education about fertility impairment associated with cancer treatment and fertility preservation options. As few as 34% of reproductive-age women treated for cancer recall discussing the effect of cancer treatment on fertility [16], yet NCCN guidelines for young adults with cancer state that fertility preservation should be an essential part of cancer management and the effects of treatment on fertility should be discussed at the time of diagnosis [5]. The oncofertility information gap can be attributed to the healthcare provider's desire to start treatment immediately, lack of adequate knowledge regarding fertility preservation, and insufficient communication and counseling skills.

The oncofertility information gap can be addressed with the implementation of a multidisciplinary approach to fertility preservation. Many patients have emphasized the importance of having access to not only fertility specialists and oncologists but also psychological support and counseling [14]. Meeting this need has led to recommendations for a healthcare worker with special training to address the sensitive topic of fertility preservation separate from the often overwhelming initial oncology consultation [15]. Genetic counselors possess the skill set to discuss the effects of cancer treatment on fertility and facilitate fertility preservation decision-making.

According to Volk et al. [24], genetic counselors believe that fertility preservation discussions are important and that they are a part of genetic counselors' role in cancer care. Genetic counselors possess the necessary skills to bridge the oncofertility information gap with their patients—those who have a personal or family history suggestive of familial or hereditary cancer. Unlike the traditional treatment-based discussions with patients, genetic counselors use a nondirective, patient-centered counseling approach to facilitate shared decision-making.

The NCCN guidelines for young adult cancer recommend a genetic and familial risk assessment within the first 2 months after the start of treatment [5]. However, because timing of cancer treatment is identified as the number one barrier to genetic counselors' ability to discuss potential threats to fertility and fertility preservation options, healthcare providers should refer young women diagnosed with cancer to a genetic counselor prior to cancer treatment. Genetic counselors have a unique skill set that allows them to discuss options, facilitate decision-making, and make valuable psychosocial assessments that may underlie cancer treatment and subsequent fertility preservation. Genetic counselors can effectively bridge the oncofertility information gap for patients with a personal or family history suggestive of a hereditary or familial cancer.

Acknowledgments This work was supported by the Oncofertility Consortium NIH 5UL1DE019587 and the Specialized Cooperative Centers Program in Reproduction and Infertility Research NIH P50HD076188.

Review Questions and Answers

Q1. For what indications should a patient be referred to a genetic counselor?

A1. Personal or family history suggestive of a hereditary or familial cancer or an individual with a hereditary cancer syndrome considering healthcare intervention which may impact fertility and/or family planning, such as prophylactic bilateral salpingo-oophorectomy, fertility preservation, or preimplantation genetic diagnosis.

Q2. How can a genetic counselor work with the oncology care team to increase oncofertility discussions and shared decision-making?

A2. A genetic counselor is part of the multidisciplinary cancer care team. They are allied health professionals with training in human genetics, psychosocial counseling, and facilitating of medical decision-making. The genetic counselor can integrate fertility preservation into their discussions with patients regarding cancer treatment, risk reduction, and recurrence risk/family planning.

References

1. American Cancer Society. Cancer treatment & survivorship facts & figures 2016–2017. Atlanta: American Cancer Society; 2016.
2. Bennett RL, Hampel HL, Mandell JB, Marks JH. Genetic counselors: translating genomic science into clinical practice. J Clin Invest. 2003;112(9):1274–9.
3. Berliner JL, Fay AM. Risk assessment and genetic counseling for hereditary breast and ovarian cancer: recommendations of the National Society of Genetic Counselors. J Genet Couns. 2007;16(3):241–60.
4. Clayman ML, Galvin KM, Arntson P. Shared decision making: fertility and pediatric cancers. In: Woodruff TK, Snyder KA, editors. Oncofertility. New York: Springer; 2007. p. 149–60.
5. Coccia PF, Altman J, Bhatia S, Borinstein SC, Flynn J, George S, Goldsby R, et al. Adolescent and young adult oncology. Clinical practice guidelines in oncology. J Natl Compr Cancer Netw. 2012;10(9):1112–50. Retrieved from http://www.ncbi.nlm.nih.gov/pubmed/22956810.
6. Duffy C, Allen SM, Dube C, Dickersin K. Oncologists' confidence in knowledge of fertility issues for young women with cancer. J Cancer Educ. 2012;27:369–76.
7. Elwyn G, Gray J, Clarke A. Shared decision making and non-directiveness in genetic counselling. J Med Genet. 2000;37:135–8.
8. Forman EJ, Anders CK, Behara MA. A nationwide survey of oncologist regarding treatment-related infertility and fertility preservation in female cancer patients. Fertil Steril. 2010;94:1652–6.
9. Goetsch AL, Wicklund C, Clayman ML, Woodruff TK. Reproductive endocrinologists' utilization of genetic counselors for oncofertility and preimplantation genetic diagnosis (PGD) treatment of BRCA1/2 mutation carriers. J Genet Couns. 2016;25(3):561–71. https://doi.org/10.1007/s10897-015-9908-7.
10. Hall MJ, Obeid EI, Schwartz SC, Mantia-Smaldone G, Forman AD, Daly MB. Genetic testing for hereditary cancer predisposition: BRCA1/2, Lynch syndrome, and beyond. Gynecol Oncol. 2016;140(3):566–74.
11. Hayat Roshanai A, Lampic C, Ingvoldstad C, Askmalm MS, Bjorvatn C, Rosenquist R, Nordin K. What information do cancer genetic counselees prioritize? J Genet Couns. 2012;21(4):510–26. https://doi.org/10.1007/s10897-011-9409-2.
12. Hershberger PE, Finnegan L, Pierce PF, Scoccia B. The decision-making process of young adult women with cancer who considered fertility cryopreservation. J Obstet Gynecol Neonatal Nurs. 2013;42(1):59–69. https://doi.org/10.1111/j.1552-6909.2012.01426.x.
13. Jeruss J, Woodruff T. Preservation of fertility for cancer patients. N Engl J Med. 2009;360(9):902–11. https://doi.org/10.1056/NEJMra0801454.
14. Kirkman M, Stern C, Neil S, Winship I, Mann GB, Shanahan K, Missen D, et al. Fertility management after breast cancer diagnosis : a qualitative investigation of women's experiences of and recommendations for professional care. Health Care Women Int. 2013;34(1):50–67.
15. Lee MC, Gray J, Han HS, Plosker S. Fertility and reproductive considerations in premenopausal patients with breast cancer. Cancer Control. 2010;17(3):162–72.
16. Letourneau JM, Ebbel EE, Katz PP, Katz A, Ai WZ, Chien AJ, Melisko ME, et al. Pretreatment fertility counseling and fertility preservation improve quality of life in reproductive age women with cancer. Cancer. 2012;118(6):1710–7. https://doi.org/10.1002/cncr.26459.
17. Loren AW, et al. Fertility preservation for patients with cancer: American Society of Clinical Oncology clinical practice guideline update. J Clin Onco. 2013;31(19):2500–10.
18. Noone AM, Howlader N, Krapcho M, Miller D, Brest A, Yu M, Ruhl J, Tatalovich Z, Mariotto A, Lewis DR, Chen HS, Feuer EJ, Cronin KA, editors. SEER cancer statistics review, 1975–2015. Bethesda: National Cancer Institute, https://seer.cancer.gov/csr/1975_2015/, based on November 2017 SEER data submission, posted to the SEER web site, April 2018.
19. Peddie VL, Porter M a, Barbour R, Culligan D, MacDonald G, King D, Horn J, et al. Factors affecting decision making about fertility preservation after cancer diagnosis: a qualitative study. BJOG. 2012;119(9):1049–57. https://doi.org/10.1111/j.1471-0528.2012.03368.x.
20. Shulman LP, Dungan JS. Cancer genetics: risks and mechanisms of cancer in women with inherited susceptibility to epithelial ovarian cancer. In: Woodruff TK, Zoloth L, Camp-Engelstein L, Rodriguez S, editors. Oncofertility ethical, legal, social, and medical perspectives. Boston: Springer; 2010. p. 69–85.
21. Tschudin S, Bitzer J. Psychological aspects of fertility preservation in men and women affected by cancer and other life-threatening diseases. Hum Reprod Update. 2010;15(5):587–97. https://doi.org/10.1093/humupd/dmp015.
22. Uhlmann WR, Schuette JL, Yashar BM. A guide to genetic counseling. Hoboken: Wiley; 2009.
23. Veach PM, LeRoy BS, Bartels DM. Facilitating the genetic counseling process: a practice manual. New York: Springer-Verlag; 2003.
24. Volk A, Aufox S, Fallen T, Beaumont J, Woodruff T. Genetic counselor attitudes, knowledge and discussions of fertility preservation in the hereditary breast and ovarian cancer clinic. Chicago. 2012. unpublished.
25. Weil J. Psychosocial genetic counseling. New York: Oxford University Press; 2000.
26. Wevers MR, Hahn DEE, Verhoef S, Bolhaar MDK, Ausems MGEM, Aaronson NK, Bleiker EM a. Breast cancer genetic counseling after diagnosis but before treatment: a pilot study on treatment consequences and psychological impact. Patient Educ Couns. 2012;89(1):89–95. https://doi.org/10.1016/j.pec.2012.03.019.
27. Yee S, Abrol K, McDonald M, Tonelli M, Liu KE. Addressing oncofertility needs: views of female cancer patients in fertility preservation. J Psychosoc Oncol. 2012;30(3):331–46. https://doi.org/10.1080/07347332.2012.664257.

Psychosocial Impact of Cancer-Related Infertility

Mollie Rose Canzona, Bansari G. Patel, and John M. Salsman

T. K. Woodruff et al. (eds.), *Textbook of Oncofertility Research and Practice*,
https://doi.org/10.1007/978-3-030-02868-8_23

Key Points

- While distress secondary to cancer-related infertility is prevalent across genders, women, in particular, face more difficult decisions with respect to options for fertility preservation. Options for women are expensive, time-consuming, invasive, and oftentimes experimental.
- Financial burden in the form of direct costs, such as medical bills and transportation expenses, and indirect costs like loss of salary and reduction in work results in significant psychosocial distress for patients.
- In addition to biologic infertility, concerns for personal health, longevity, pregnancy outcomes, and the well-being of offspring oftentimes dictate decisions surrounding future fertility after a cancer diagnosis.
- Oncologic providers should be prepared to deliver the latest information regarding the deleterious impact of cancer therapy on fertility, offer referrals to clinicians with appropriate expertise, and coordinate therapeutic counseling and peer support for reproductive-aged patients afflicted with cancer.

23.1 Introduction

According to the American Cancer Society, there will be an estimated 1,735,350 new cancer cases diagnosed in 2018. Adolescents and young adults (ages 15–39) represent approximately 70,000 of these cases [1]. All cancers directly or indirectly affect patients' ability to have children [2]. Cancer and cancer treatments can disrupt female and male fertility by damaging reproductive organs, suppressing reproductive function, destabilizing sexual health, or delaying reproduction [3, 4]. The ability to become a parent is one of the strongest predictors of well-being for cancer survivors [5]. For many patients, fertility remains a critical issue in the short and long term [6]. Cancer-related infertility is associated with psychosocial distress regardless of whether or not patients choose to engage in assisted reproductive technology. Over the past three decades, the 5-year relative survival rate for all cancers has significantly increased. Given the rise in survival rates, infertility concerns are becoming more prevalent. Cancer-related infertility is associated with long- and short-term psychological and social distress related to relationships, financial burden, complexity of fertility preservation procedures, alternate paths to parenthood, as well as concerns about patient health and the health of future or current offspring.

23.2 Prevalence of Distress Due to Cancer-Related Infertility

Threats to fertility can have a severe and enduring impact on cancer patients. For many, the struggle with infertility can be felt as intensely as the cancer diagnosis itself [7]. Hammond and colleagues found that 54% of male and female cancer survivors younger than age 40 expressed elevated reproductive concerns [8]. Reproductive concerns have been linked to lower physical and mental quality of life scores and heightened cancer-specific distress [9]. One study of gynecologic cancer patients revealed that 40% of participants met the clinical criteria for depression and over 50% of women experienced difficulty coming to terms with infertility, longed to give birth, or struggled with anger due to fertility concerns [3]. Another study found that women used a variety of potentially harmful strategies to cope with the risk of infertility, including denial of negative thoughts and avoidance [10]. Men also struggle with decisions around fertility and often experience regret for not taking steps to preserve their ability to become a parent [11].

23.3 Correlates of Distress Due to Cancer-Related Infertility

Individuals struggling with infertility suffer from depression and psychological distress at twice the rate of the normal population [12]. Cancer-related infertility can be even more devastating as it can deepen the sense of loss and fear experienced with cancer diagnosis [12]. Concerns about fertility come at a time when cancer patients may be confronting their own mortality, coping with uncertainty regarding prognosis, and navigating threats to their sense of self [13]. For some women and men, fertility is linked to their ideas of femininity and masculinity [14].

23.3.1 Relationship Concerns

Infertility concerns are not experienced in a bubble. Patients can be apprehensive about the implications of infertility for their current or future relational lives [15]. Patients may worry that fertility concerns will cause potential partners to reject them. They also believe their inability to have children will make it impossible to establish a long-term relationship [16]. Patients report that infertility is a sensitive topic that can cause relationships to end [12, 17]. Patients report uncertainty about when and how much to disclose to future or current partners and fear partners' reactions after disclosures are made [18]. Previously experienced rejection can deepen these concerns, postpone disclosure, and reinforce isolation [19]. Patients currently in romantic relationships express guilt about depriving their partner of the opportunity to have biological children and report disagreements with their partner regarding preferences for adoptive versus biological parenthood [20]. The fear surrounding communication and the desire to appear "normal" can perpetuate silence, which can heighten distress and lead to relational breakdowns [12, 16]. Despite these complications, research demonstrates that the cancer experience can strengthen the importance of parenthood in patients' lives [14].

23.3.2 Financial Burden

Many patients who want to become parents face another barrier that can exacerbate existing distress surrounding cancer and infertility: financial burden. Cancer patients often suffer from the adverse impact of disease and treatment-related costs, including direct costs such as medical bills, transportation expenses, and indirect costs like loss of salary and reduction in work. These hardships have mental and emotional consequences, which can be magnified when one is faced with the challenges of pursuing parenthood [21]. Fertility preservation treatments are expensive and often not covered by insurance plans [16]. Adoption has also become increasingly expensive. Costs of domestic adoptions range from $5000 to $40,000 with international adoptions ranging from $15,000 to $30,000 [22]. It is important for clinicians to be aware of and communicate with patients about the availability of reduced prices, payment plans, and other forms of financial assistance. Local and national resources are available through the Alliance for Fertility Preservation, National Adoption Foundation, and the Livestrong Foundation. However, patients may not qualify for assistance, or remaining costs may still be prohibitive [21]. Given these considerable constraints, many patients feel the goal of having biological children may be out of reach.

23.3.3 Sociodemographic Factors

It is important to note that sociodemographic factors also create disparities that can leave certain patients more vulnerable to psychosocial distress. Disparities associated with characteristics such as age, race/ethnicity, income, and education have been previously documented in oncology and fertility care [23, 24]. Letourneau and colleagues found that female cancer patients without a bachelor's degree or who were 35 years or older were less likely to be counseled about fertility preservation options [25]. Patients who do not understand how cancer and cancer treatments can impact fertility or are not given the opportunity to make the decision to protect their ability to become a parent may experience shock, anger, and hopelessness when they learn they no longer have a path to biological children [16].

23.3.4 Complexity of Fertility Preservation Options

Pursuing the goal of parenthood while simultaneously making difficult treatment decisions can be extraordinarily challenging – especially for women. For men, sperm cryopreservation (sperm banking) is the primary established nonexperimental fertility preservation method. Women, however, must process complex information about a variety of fertility preservation options, ranging from assisted reproductive techniques such as oocyte and embryo freezing to ovarian tissue cryopreservation or hormonal suppression [26]. They must also weigh their desire for biological children against the possibility of treatment delays with resultant prognosis implications as well as the risks and undetermined outcomes of fertility preservation procedures [26]. Being forced to make these decisions in the midst of this uncertainty provokes anxiety and can amplify the devastation associated with cancer diagnosis and treatment [27]. Due to physiologic differences in gamete production between genders, the emotional impact may be somewhat lessened for male cancer patients compared to females. For men, there is the hope that function may return. Many men will recover the ability to produce sperm within 1–3 years post treatment [21]. For women, recovery of reproductive potential is less likely [28]. This is especially problematic as up to 75% of female survivors report a desire for children [14]. So, while infertility causes distress for both sexes, it may be more prevalent in women due to the complicated decisions they must make, limited potential for return of fertility, and women's emotional investment in parenthood.

For cancer patients who wish to pursue paths to parenthood such as assisted reproductive technology or adoption, psychosocial distress is often intertwined with concerns about fertility perseveration procedures and their impact on patients' personal health and the health of potential offspring.

23.4 Distress About Fertility Preservation Procedures and Other Pathways to Parenthood

Several options exist for cancer patients who want to preserve their fertility. Embryo cryopreservation is a well-established procedure, resulting in cumulative pregnancy rates of up to 50% depending on maternal age at the time of cryopreservation [29]. Oocyte vitrification is also an established option for women who are not currently in stable heterosexual partnered relationships or do not want to utilize sperm donation [30]. Women can experience stress and confusion stemming from the invasiveness of these procedures, the attendant requirement to delay treatment, and uncertainty regarding the success of these efforts [12]. It is a complicated decision-making progress for those who are candidates for assisted reproductive technologies. This is troubling since decisional conflict is associated with greater emotional distress and regret [31]. While those women who have estrogen-sensitive tumors have historically been counseled against such procedures due to resultant elevation in estrogen levels, recent data indicate that these women can also safely undergo these procedures without a deleterious impact on prognosis [32]. Patients with a low egg reserve or certain hematologic malignancies, however, may not be candidates for assisted reproduction and may not be offered these well-established options. This can be devastating news for women and couples who have a strong preference for biological parenthood.

An additional concern for patients who wish to use assisted reproductive technology is the social stigma still associated with fertility impairment and perceptions of nontraditional family building [33]. Patients may feel uncomfortable talking openly about their fertility preservation efforts with friends and family. They also report the fear that others may view their desire to use technology to have a biological child as selfish when so many children are in need of a nurturing, supportive family [34]. Despite these challenges, some patients feel biological parenthood is their only option. Certain religious traditions bar the use of donor gametes. This creates a conundrum for distraught patients who feel they cannot honor their religious beliefs and their desire for children [14]. The path to parenthood for patients open to adoption is not without its own challenges. Patients may be concerned about discrimination from adoption agencies due to their cancer history. Some adoption agencies may require a letter from a physician confirming favorable prognosis before considering their application [22]. The cancer community's growing emphasis on treating long-term sequelae of cancer may inadvertently be driving discriminatory adoption practices. This may perpetuate and magnify suffering for patients who are already struggling with the life-altering consequences of cancer-related infertility. Public education and advocacy campaigns are needed to correct prejudicial adoption practices based on patient health history [22].

23.4.1 Concerns About Implications for Personal Health

Cancer survivors who retain their fertility are less likely than their peers to become parents. The exact reasons for this are unknown, but the research demonstrates survivors' concerns about parenthood extend beyond biological fertility [35–37]. Cancer-related threats to fertility are directly and indirectly associated with serious consequences for patients' personal health and well-being. For women cancer patients, fears regarding premature menopause or pregnancy complications can interfere with sexual functioning and sexual health-related quality of life [38]. Women with cancer are often told to postpone attempts to become pregnant for 2 years post treatment since this is the time period in which most cancer recurrences occur. Women may, however, interpret this as a sign that pregnancy and recurrence are linked [14]. A common myth among women is that the hormone fluctuation associated with pregnancy can trigger a cancer recurrence [20, 37]. Patients worry about the implications of having cancer for their general health and longevity. Many fear they will not live long enough to see potential children grow up or may be hesitant to become a parent due to perceived long-term physical and psychological consequences of having had cancer [16]. Financial burden can be intertwined with these concerns as patients may feel their health status will not allow them to provide adequately for future offspring [39].

23.4.2 Concerns About Future (or Current) Children's Health

Even when patients believe it is possible to carry a baby to term, they can have concerns about the impact their cancer history or cancer treatments may have on future children's health. Patients report the fear that past chemotherapy or radiation may cause birth defects [37]. One of the strongest predictors of distress for patients with familial cancer is the fear that future offspring would be more susceptible to developing childhood or adult cancer. In these instances, patients experience guilt, believing it is selfish or immoral to have children at risk for cancer [18]. Patients' perception of risk, their coping style, and their overall level of psychological distress influence the degree to which gene carrier status shapes childbearing decisions [14]. Women also report distress stemming from concerns about the well-being of future or current offspring. They may worry about the perceived emotional burden on the child of having a mother who is seriously ill. For women who already have children, they may be concerned that engaging in stressful and financially draining attempts to have additional children may negatively impact their existing children's lives [37]. There is evidence to suggest women are more concerned than men about the risk to potential offspring; however, there is not enough evidence to definitively state how men's concerns differ from women's sources of distress [40].

23.5 The Need for Enhanced Patient-Provider Communication and Psychosocial Counseling

Patients report a desire for health care professionals to be proactive about fertility discussions [28]. Patients want information about the risks of infertility and fertility preservation options [41]. However, all too often, cancer patients do not receive this information despite firm recommendations regarding dispersion of this information from the American Society of Clinical Oncology. In one study, only 50% of patients were told about fertility risks and options by their cancer providers [12]. This may be partially due to a difference in perception. While patients view fertility as important, providers have ranked the importance of fertility concerns as low for their patients [42]. Previous research found that providers do not broach the topic of infertility issues unless the patient raises it [43]. This is an important discrepancy to correct. Providers must appreciate that fertility issues are important to cancer patients and that "socially and emotionally, fertility can be about more than reproduction" [28]. For many, having biological children is a rite of passage that is central to identity and expectations for the future [44]. Failure to discuss the full biopsychosocial implications of infertility can have negative long-term impact on patients' quality of life. Unmet informational and support needs can lead to increases in decisional conflict, regret, and emotional distress [27]. Instead of assuming fertility is not a concern for particular patients, the most ethical approach is to bring up the topic of fertility with every patient [12].

Several misperceptions are particularly important to address in these conversations. There is a great deal of misunderstanding about the risks of fertility preservation options. Helping patients arrive at an accurate understanding of the risks and potential outcomes of pursuing parenthood after cancer is an important first step in preventing avoidable suffering. Fears about the implications of fertility preservation procedures for the health of the patient and his/her potential offspring need to be addressed [32]. Discussing issues surrounding romantic relationships and disclosure will provide an important source of support for patients who are struggling [18].

Providers who care for cancer patients should be prepared to deliver the latest information, offer referrals to clinicians with appropriate expertise, or coordinate therapeutic counseling and peer support [28]. Providers require support to effectively deliver care to patients who are at risk for infertility. Educational interventions should be aimed at improving the knowledge of risks, fertility preservation options, and other resources available to patients [12]. One study showed that the presence of a psychologist during discussions about preservation procedures improved communication between providers and patients [45]. Oncology nurses could fulfill a vital role in identifying patients at risk and facilitating the delivery of information and support [46]. One study suggests that patients prefer nurses to initiate these kinds of conversations [47]. Comprehensive reproductive health counseling that addresses a variety of paths to parenthood is needed to assist patients in this uncertain time. Pretreatment fertility counseling is associated with less regret and better quality of life after treatment [48]. However, fertility counseling alone may not be enough to support patients [49]. Additional methods of decision support are warranted. It is critical to create resources for patients to support informed decisions and to address psychosocial distress [18].

23.6 Summary

Women and men who are faced with cancer-related infertility experience significant distress related to romantic relationships, financial burden, and complexity of fertility preservation options. Patients who belong to certain sociodemographic groups may suffer these concerns disproportionately. Patients who wish to pursue parenthood report distress stemming from fertility preservation procedures and other paths to having a child. They may also experience concerns about the implications of fertility preservation for their personal health and the health of their future or current children. There is a need to enhance timely patient-provider communication and psychosocial counseling for cancer patients.

Review Questions and Answers

Q1. Individuals struggling with infertility suffer from depression and psychological distress at twice the rate of the normal population.

(a) True
(b) False

A1. (a)

Q2. Women deciding to use assisted reproductive technologies can experience stress and confusion stemming from:

(a) The invasiveness of fertility preservation procedures
(b) The potential requirement to delay treatment
(c) Uncertainty regarding the success of fertility preservation procedures
(d) a and b
(e) All of the above

A2. (e)

Q3. Cancer patients experience the following relationship concerns:

(a) Fear their inability to have children will make it impossible to establish a long-term relationship
(b) Uncertainty about when and how much to disclose to future or current partners.
(c) Guilt about depriving their partner of the opportunity to have biological children
(d) Disagreements with their partner regarding preferences for adoptive versus biological parenthood
(e) All of the above

A3. (e)

Q4. One of the strongest predictors of distress for patients with familial cancer is:

(a) The fear that pregnancy will cause cancer recurrence
(b) The fear that efforts to preserve fertility will be unsuccessful
(c) The fear that future offspring would be more susceptible to developing childhood or adult cancer
(d) The fear that they will be stigmatized for their efforts to become pregnant after cancer treatment
(e) All of the above

A4. (c)

Q5. Unmet informational and support needs can lead to increases in patient:

(a) Decisional conflict, regret, and memory loss
(b) Regret, concerns about friendships, and memory loss
(c) Concerns about friendships, distress, and decisional conflict
(d) Emotional distress, regret, and decisional conflict
(e) Memory loss, concerns about friendships, and emotional distress

A5. (d)

References

1. American Cancer Society. Cancer facts & figures 2018. https://www.cancer.org/research/cancer-facts-statistics/all-cancer-facts-figures/cancer-facts-figures-2018.html.
2. Schover L. Sexuality and fertility after cancer. New York: Wiley; 1997.
3. Carter J, Rowland K, Chi D, et al. Gynecologic cancer treatment and the impact of cancer-related infertility. Gynecol Oncol. 2005;97:90–5.
4. Dellapasqua S, Colleoni M, Gelber RD, Goldhirsch A. Adjuvant endocrine therapy for premenopausal women with early breast cancer. J Clin Oncol. 2005;23:1736–50. https://doi.org/10.1200/JCO.2005.11.050.
5. Grinyer A. Life after cancer in adolescence and young adulthood: the experience of survivorship, vol. 10. 1st ed. Florence: Routledge; 2009.
6. Zebrack BJ, Mills J, Weitzman TS. Health and supportive care needs of young adult cancer patients and survivors. J Cancer Surviv. 2007;1:137–45.
7. Surbone A, Petrek JA. Childbearing issues in breast carcinoma survivors. Cancer. 1997;79:1271–8.
8. Hammond C, Abrams JR, Syrjala KL. Fertility and risk factors for elevated infertility concern in 10-year hematopoietic cell transplant survivors and case-matched controls. J Clin Oncol. 2007;25:3511–7.
9. Wenzel L, Dogan-Ates A, Habbal R, et al. Defining and measuring reproductive concerns of female cancer survivors. J Natl Cancer Inst Monogr. 2005;34:94–8.
10. Quinn GP, Murphy D, Knapp CA, et al. Coping styles of female adolescent cancer patients with potential fertility loss. J Adolesc Young Adult Oncol. 2013;2:66–71.
11. Cella D, Najavits L. Letter to the editor: denial of infertility in patients with Hodgkin's disease. Psychosomatics. 1986;27:71.
12. Crawshaw MA, Sloper P. 'Swimming against the tide'—the influence of fertility matters on the transition to adulthood or survivorship following adolescent cancer. Eur J Cancer Care. 2010;19:610–20.
13. Tschudin S, Bitzer J. Psychological aspects of fertility preservation in men and women affected by cancer and other life-threatening diseases. Hum Reprod Updat. 2009;15(5):587–97.
14. Schover LR, Rybicki LA, Martin BA, Bringelsen KA. Having children after cancer. A pilot survey of survivors' attitudes and experiences. Cancer. 1999;86(4):697–709.
15. Lukse MP, Vacc NA. Grief, depression, and coping in women undergoing infertility treatment. Obstet Gynecol. 1999;93:245–51.
16. Nilsson J, Jervaeus A, Lampic C, et al. 'Will I be able to have a baby?' Results from online focus group discussions with childhood cancer survivors in Sweden. Hum Reprod (Oxford, England). 2014;29(12):2704–11.
17. Gorman JR, Bailey S, Pierce JP, Su HI. How do you feel about fertility and parenthood? The voices of young female cancer survivors. J Cancer Surviv. 2012;6:200–9.
18. Benedict C, Thom B, Friedman N, et al. Young adult female cancer survivors' unmet information needs and reproductive concerns contribute to decisional conflict regarding posttreatment fertility preservation. Cancer. 2016;122(13):2101–9.
19. Zebrack BJ, Casillas J, Nohr L, Adams H, Zeltzer LK. Fertility issues for young adult survivors of childhood cancer. Psychooncology. 2004;13:689–99.
20. Gorman JR, Su HI, Pierce JP, Roberts SC, Dominick SA, Malcarne VL. A multidimensional scale to measure the reproductive concerns of young adult female cancer survivors. J Cancer Surviv. 2014;8(2):218–28.
21. Kelvin JF. Fertility preservation before cancer treatment: options, strategies, and resources. Clin J Oncol Nurs. 2016;20:44–51.
22. Quinn GP, Zebrack BJ, Sehovic I, Bowman ML, Vadaparampil ST. Adoption and cancer survivors: findings from a learning activity for oncology nurses: adoption and cancer survivors. Cancer. 2015;121:2993–3000.

23. Burris J, Andrykowski M. Disparities in mental health between rural and nonrural cancer survivors: a preliminary study. Psychooncology. 2010;19:637–45.
24. Ashing-Giwa K, Gonzalez P, Lim JW, et al. Diagnostic and therapeutic delays among a multiethnic sample of breast and cervical cancer survivors. Cancer. 2010;116:3195–204.
25. Letourneau JM, Smith JF, Ebbel EE, et al. Racial, socioeconomic, and demographic disparities in access to fertility preservation in young women diagnosed with cancer. Cancer. 2012;118:4579–88.
26. Loren AW, Mangu PB, Beck LN, et al. Fertility preservation for patients with cancer: American Society of Clinical Oncology clinical practice guideline update. J Clin Oncol. 2013;31(19):2500–10.
27. Hershberger PE, Finnegan L, Pierce PF, Scoccia B. The decision-making process of young adult women with cancer who considered fertility cryopreservation. J Obstet Gynecol Neonatal Nurs. 2013;42:59–69.
28. Crawshaw M. Psychosocial oncofertility issues faced by adolescents and young adults over their lifetime: a review of the research. Hum Fertil (Cambridge, England). 2013;16(1):59–63.
29. Wang JX, Yap YY, Matthews CD. Frozen-thawed embryo transfer: influence of clinical factors on implantation rate and risk of multiple conception. Hum Reprod. 2001;16:2316–9.
30. Son WY, Yoon SH, Yoon HJ, et al. Pregnancy outcome following transfer of human blastocysts vitrified on electron microscopy grids after induced collapse of the blastocoele. Hum Reprod. 2003;18:137–9.
31. O'Connor AM, Jacobsen MJ, Stacey D. An evidence-based approach to managing women's decisional conflict. J Obstet Gynecol Neonatal Nurs. 2002;31:570–81.
32. Oktay K, Hourvitz A, Sahin G, et al. Letrozole reduces estrogen and gonadotropin exposure in women with breast cancer undergoing ovarian stimulation before chemotherapy. J Clin Endocrinol Metab. 2006;91:3885–90.
33. Slade P, O'Neill C, Simpson AJ, Lashen H. The relationship between perceived stigma, disclosure patterns, support and distress in new attendees at an infertility clinic. Hum Reprod (Oxford, England). 2007;22(8):2309–17.
34. Cahill LS. Moral concerns about institutionalized gamete donation. In: Cohen CB, editor. New ways of making babies. Bloomington: Indiana University Press; 1996. p. 70–87.
35. Syse A, Kravdal O, Tretli S. Parenthood after cancer – a population-based study. Psychooncology. 2007;16(10):920–7.
36. Magelssen H, Melve KK, Skjaerven R, Fossa SD. Parenthood probability and pregnancy outcome in patients with a cancer diagnosis during adolescence and young adulthood. Hum Reprod (Oxford, England). 2008;23(1):178–86.
37. Goncalves V, Sehovic I, Quinn G. Childbearing attitudes and decisions of young breast cancer survivors: a systematic review. Hum Reprod Updat. 2014;20(2):279–92.
38. Absolom K, Eiser C, Turner L, et al. Ovarian failure following cancer treatment: current management and quality of life. Hum Reprod (Oxford, England). 2008;23(11):2506–12.
39. Amir Z, Wilson K, Hennings J, Young A. The meaning of cancer: implications for family finances and consequent impact on lifestyle, activities, roles and relationships. Psychooncology. 2012;21(11):1167–74.
40. Zeltzer LK. Cancer in adolescents and young adults: psychosocial aspects in long-term survivors. Cancer. 1993;71(Suppl 10):3463–8.
41. Thewes B, Meiser B, Rickard J, et al. The fertility- and menopause-related information needs of younger women with a diagnosis of breast cancer: a qualitative study. Psychooncology. 2003;12:500–11.
42. Vadaparampil S, Quinn G, King L, et al. Barriers to fertility preservation among pediatric oncologists. Patient Educ Couns. 2008;72:402–10.
43. King L, Quinn GP, Vadaparampil ST, et al. Oncology nurses' perceptions of barriers to discussion of fertility preservation with patients with cancer. Clin J Oncol Nurs. 2008;12:467–76.
44. Gerrity DA. A biopsychosocial theory of infertility. Fam J. 2001;9:151–8.
45. Razzano A, Revelli A, Delle Piane L, et al. Fertility preservation program before ovarotoxic oncostatic treatments: role of the psychological support in managing emotional aspects. Gynecol Endocrinol. 2014;30(11):822–4.
46. Penrose R, Beatty L, Mattiske J, Koczwara B. The psychosocial impact of cancer-related infertility on women: a review and comparison. Clin J Oncol Nurs. 2013;17(2):188–93.
47. Koutsopoulou S, Papathanassoglou ED, Katapodi MC, Patiraki EI. A critical review of the evidence for nurses as information providers to cancer patients. J Clin Nurs. 2010;19(5–6):749–65.
48. Letourneau JM, Katz PP, Smith JF, et al. The impact of fertility counseling and fertility preservation on long-term psychosocial outcomes in young female cancer survivors. Fertil Steril. 2010;94:S65.
49. Balthazar U, Deal AM, Fritz MA, Kondapalli LA, Kim JY, Mersereau JE. The current fertility preservation consultation model: are we adequately informing cancer patients of their options? Hum Reprod. 2012;27:2413–9.

Oncofertility Consults in the REI Setting

Jason Elliott, Rhonda Zwingerman, Jinglan Han, Tamas Gotz, and Eileen McMahon

T. K. Woodruff et al. (eds.), *Textbook of Oncofertility Research and Practice*,
https://doi.org/10.1007/978-3-030-02868-8_24

24

Key Points
- An organized approach to oncofertility consultations is essential.
- Much of oncofertility treatment is similar to more common infertility therapies.
- Recognize that psychosocial aspects play a huge role in oncofertility care.
- Providing excellent oncofertility care is achievable by anyone willing to spend time learning the process.

24.1 Introduction

Developing familiarity in fertility preservation (FP) can be difficult for the new Reproductive Endocrinology and Infertility (REI) practitioner, as exposure to FP care varies considerably among REI training programs. Accordingly, for some REI fellows or new graduates, managing women being referred for FP can seem complicated, overwhelming, and stressful. The FP process at our institution is very robust, with a large proportion of women referred for consideration of FP being directly managed by the REI fellows and an experienced nurse practitioner, with supervision by attending REI staff. As a result, our REI fellows have the opportunity to manage complex FP patients throughout their training and have accumulated real-world experience in this area.

The goal of this chapter is to provide ten "Pearls of Practice" to assist new practitioners in acquiring comfort and competence in FP. After each pearl are clinical cases and a short description to further illustrate key points. We hope these tips help alleviate some of the anxiety about providing quality FP care to women in need.

But first, a few disclaimers. Much of the focus below is on more complex FP approaches such as oocyte or embryo cryopreservation procedures, but many of the pearls apply equally well to less complex FP modalities. We do not discuss FP for men, nor FP for non-oncology reasons (i.e., gender transitioning, oophorectomy for non-oncologic indications, or premature ovarian insufficiency (POI)). We also do not specifically address the unique concerns of pre-pubertal girls with cancer, although many components of these consultations may be similar.

Pearl #1: - **FP patients require close and ongoing communication between REI and oncology team members.**

Case 1a: - Gwen is referred by her breast surgeon after lumpectomy for an invasive ductal carcinoma. She is waiting to see a medical oncologist to discuss whether chemotherapy is warranted. The medical oncologist has learned that Gwen has been seen by REI and desires FP; however, the medical oncologist is opposed to FP as she wants Gwen to start chemotherapy immediately.

Case 1b: - Sadia has a large pelvic mass and is referred for consideration of FP by her gynecologic oncologist. An oocyte retrieval is planned but shortly before this occurs, the gynecologic oncologist expresses concern that only oocytes from the unaffected ovary should be retrieved to avoid disrupting the mass.

Case 1c: - Ying has locally advanced breast cancer. She has been seen and referred by the medical oncologist. The plan is for neoadjuvant chemotherapy to begin in 7 days. It is not clear from the referral whether the chemotherapy start date is fixed or flexible in the event that she wants to pursue FP.

Ongoing communication may seem like an obvious point, but one we believe needs emphasizing. If there are problems in communication between treatment teams, it makes organizing and proceeding with FP much more difficult than necessary. Asking the referring team, prior to seeing the woman initially, for the most complete information regarding diagnosis, probable treatment plan, and flexibility in timing of treatments allows the most efficient and effective FP consultation. On the other hand, waiting for the final oncologic treatment plan can lead to delays in proceeding with FP. It is important to recognize that treatment plans will sometimes change and the REI team needs to respond with agility and flexibility in terms of the options and timing of FP. It is important to provide updates back to the referring team so that everyone is "in the loop." A common misconception is the length of time required to perform some FP procedures, and some oncologic care providers are concerned that undergoing FP will delay the start of cancer treatment for an unacceptably long period, which is usually not the case. Furthermore, with good communication, both oncologic and REI team members develop more familiarity with each other's processes, and future referrals naturally become more streamlined over time.

Pearl #2: - **FP patients have multiple care providers, and frequently tests, procedures, and appointments outside of the fertility clinic compete for their time.**

Case 2a: - Rowena has breast cancer. She is still in the early days of completing investigations and planning cancer treatment. She is sure she wants to proceed with FP but is concerned that her numerous tests (PET scan, bone scan, CT scan, etc.) and specialist appointments (medical oncology, etc.) may interfere with the visits required for her FP cycle, including her oocyte retrieval.

Case 2b: - Gurpreet wants to undergo an IVF cycle for FP prior to starting her chemotherapy. She has also moved up her wedding date to before her chemotherapy begins. With good communication, both the FP and oncology teams can work to schedule all the needed tests and procedures and work around the very important personal schedule that Gurpreet has with her wedding.

As discussed in Pearl #1, it is important to remember that women considering FP have both medical and non-medical commitments. Asking about these and then coordinating with the woman and her other care providers can facilitate the best care. Women should not be forced to choose between FP and cancer investigations – and this can almost always be avoided with good communication between treatment teams.

Pearl #3: - **FP patients often have complex timelines that need to be considered when planning management.**

Case 3a: - Raihana has been diagnosed with breast cancer. She is being seen for FP before she has been scheduled for surgery. She asks whether it is best to have an oocyte retrieval prior to her breast surgery or between her surgery and the start of her chemotherapy.

Case 3b: - Maria is 36 years old and was recently diagnosed with an estrogen receptor-positive breast cancer. She knows she will be prescribed hormonal suppression for many years after completing her chemotherapy. She worries this will compromise her future fertility.

It is important to consider the timelines of various cancer treatments when discussing risks to fertility and how FP might ameliorate those risks. Decisions about when to do an FP cycle should be made jointly with the patient and oncology team to minimize disruptions and maximize patient convenience. As well, hormonally responsive cancers will often be treated for an extended period of time with hormonal suppression using selective estrogen receptor modulators (SERMs) or aromatasc inhibitors [1, 2]. These extended duration therapies have negative consequences on fertility due to age-related fertility decline and the inability to carry a pregnancy while using these agents. This may necessitate the use of a gestational carrier or a "holiday" from hormonal suppression with the support of the oncologist. The results of an international study assessing the safety of this approach are forthcoming [3].

Pearl #4: - **FP patients need to consider their short- and long-term reproductive goals.**

Case 4a: - Daphne is a 22-year-old woman diagnosed with non-Hodgkin lymphoma. She has been with her current boyfriend for only 2 months. Daphne has not previously considered whether or not she wanted children nor is she sure that she wants to have children with her current partner.

Case 4b: - Siobhan is a married 39-year-old woman who previously had not wanted children. Now with a new cancer diagnosis, she is facing the definitive loss of fertility and this is challenging her prior decision to not have children.

A cancer diagnosis can often lead to a re-prioritization of life goals, and having children can suddenly become more important, even if this wasn't a priority in the past. Similarly, if a woman is young or newly partnered, she may never have considered having children, nor be comfortable with the idea of doing so with her current partner. It is important to discuss short- and long-term fertility goals with women to try to understand their priorities and motivations. It is helpful to provide options and alternatives to fertility preservation (see Pearl #7), and recognize that some women may choose to cryopreserve a combination of oocytes and embryos to provide additional options in the future. This may involve using either their current partner's sperm (if applicable) or donor sperm. It can be an uncomfortable discussion to describe scenarios where the woman may no longer be in her current relationship in the future, but these possibilities are important to explore given the finality of creating embryos with another person prior to potentially sterilizing treatment. Although current statistics suggest that vitrified oocytes yield fewer blastocysts than fresh oocytes, and therefore cryopreserving embryos may be associated with superior longer-term success rates, ongoing improvements in oocyte cryopreservation may make this approach unnecessary in the future. In many cases, women considering the use of donor sperm can benefit from referral to a fertility counsellor for additional decisional support regarding third-party reproduction, assuming this can be arranged in a timely fashion.

Pearl #5: - FP patients may have medical comorbidities that prohibit FP treatment.

Case 5a: - Vidhi is a 25-year-old woman with acute lymphocytic leukemia (ALL). She is currently admitted to the hospital with SVC syndrome and shortness of breath. Her oncologists have asked for an FP consultation but indicate on the referral that Vidhi needs to start chemotherapy immediately.

Case 5b: - Sophie is a 36-year-old nulligravida referred for consideration of FP for right-sided invasive breast cancer. She has had a bilateral mastectomy and is awaiting adjuvant chemotherapy. At Sophie's FP consultation she tells you that she has lung metastases which make her severely short of breath when supine. She is being seen in a center that performs their oocyte retrievals under procedural sedation in an out-of-hospital setting where they cannot perform procedures on women who are at elevated risk of airway obstruction or respiratory compromise.

Case 5c: - Inez is 35 years old and was recently diagnosed with endometrial cancer. She was referred for FP. The FP team assesses Inez and although she is otherwise healthy, her BMI is 51. She is being seen in a center that performs their oocyte retrievals under procedural sedation in an out-of-hospital setting where they cannot perform procedures on women above a certain BMI due to respiratory depression risk.

It is imperative that FP clinicians understand the limitations and risks of the treatments they are proposing. Generally, if a woman is acutely unwell, her ability to tolerate a delay in oncologic treatment while waiting for 2 weeks to complete an ovarian stimulation cycle and oocyte retrieval will be poor. In such situations, the FP clinician will need to ensure the oncologist has explained to the woman that delaying her cancer treatments to undergo fertility preservation may be extremely risky. The logistics and technical aspects of performing oocyte retrieval and the related risks are also essential to consider. As with any other infertility patient, some women with cancer have medical co-morbidities that make ovarian stimulation or oocyte retrieval potentially dangerous. Although some women who are determined to proceed with fertility preservation are willing to undergo significant risk to achieve this, it must be balanced by clinicians' good judgement to ensure that patients are not placed at undue risk. Sometimes a frank, but honest, statement such as, "We cannot put your health at risk to preserve oocytes/embryos. In the event that you are not able to conceive with your own eggs in the future, alternative options are available such as donor oocytes". This may help to clarify the larger picture regarding the risk of undergoing FP and why this may not be an option for them.

Pearl #6: - FP patients may have a difficult time making decisions about FP treatment given uncertainty around cancer treatment, prognosis and likelihood of sterilization.

Case 6a: - Anjali is 33 years old and has a large pelvic mass. The diagnosis is not yet known, but a malignancy is strongly suspected. She has consented to surgery with many possible procedures planned, dependent upon what is found at the time of the surgery. She could have no reproductive organs removed, or could lose one or both ovaries and/or her uterus. At this point, no one can provide her with a definitive answer.

Case 6b: - Momoe has recently been diagnosed with Hodgkin's lymphoma. Her oncologist has planned a chemotherapy regimen of ABVD. Momoe is uncertain whether she should proceed with FP.

The uncertainty around the effects of cancer and its treatment on a woman's fertility can lead to difficult decision-making on how to proceed. In some cases it is unclear exactly how much damage to a women's fertility will result, as the diagnosis itself may not be clear. In other cases where the diagnosis is known, the initially planned treatment may have a reassuring fertility prognosis, but if the first-line treatment fails, second-line therapies may be more detrimental, and the timeframe to start these may be very short, potentially precluding FP at that point. This can make counselling women in these scenarios challenging. Providing information that conveys potential consequences of either proceeding with FP or not may assist women with decision-making and reduce future regret. Women are relying on their FP clinicians to provide information from different viewpoints to help them make as well-informed decisions as possible.

Pearl #7: - **FP patients should know that even if they choose not to undergo FP treatment before cancer treatment, they have other options for family building and/or follow up care.**

Case 7a: - Talia is a 34-year-old BRCA1 carrier who had a bilateral mastectomy and chemotherapy for an invasive left breast cancer 2 years ago. She decided against FP prior to her treatment but did check her anti-mullerian hormone (AMH) level pretreatment. She is returning now for an assessment of her ovarian reserve and to discuss her options for conceiving.

Case 7b: - Raven is 23 years old who recently completed successful treatment for leukemia, which included chemotherapy, total body irradiation, and a stem cell transplant. She was too ill prior to her cancer treatment to undergo FP. She is coming to discuss her future options for family building.

Many women will either choose to forego FP or be unable to have FP due to timing or medical indications. It is often very helpful, therefore, to remind women of what options they may have in the future, even if FP is not done. For example, many women will still have some ovarian function after chemotherapy, and they may retain some ability to conceive, although they may have lower cycle fecundity than age-matched controls. Similarly, assessing baseline ovarian reserve before and after cancer treatment can provide some measure to women as to how significantly their fertility has been compromised. This can be useful for counselling around how soon to proceed with conception attempts and via which methods (i.e., unassisted vs. assisted reproductive technologies [ART]). Moreover, it is imperative that all options for family building be discussed at the initial FP visit. This includes oocyte donation, gestational carriage, adoption, and child-free living. For some same-sex female couples, the other female partner may decide to conceive instead, providing an alternate method of having a family. It is important to ensure that women understand that not proceeding with FP does not preclude their ability to have a family but rather that their path to achieve a family may or may not be as they originally envisioned.

Pearl #8: - **FP patients want information about how FP treatment and timing may or may not impact their cancer prognosis.**

Case 8a: - Tasha is a 32-year-old woman diagnosed with an estrogen receptor/progesterone receptor (ER/PR)-positive breast cancer. After discussing the option of controlled ovarian stimulation and oocyte retrieval, Tasha expresses significant concern about the use of hormones given her receptor status. She is also very nervous about a future pregnancy and fears it might increase her risk of cancer recurrence.

Case 8b: - Noel has been diagnosed with non-Hodgkin lymphoma. Her oncologist has indicated that a wait of 3 weeks for a FP cycle before starting treatments is reasonable. Noel is conflicted and worries that this delay may make her cancer treatment ineffective and increase her risk of death.

There is considerable worry amongst women with hormone-sensitive cancers about the effects of hormonal treatments for FP and future pregnancy with respect to their cancer prognosis. Similarly, women may worry that delaying cancer treatment to undergo FP will worsen their cancer prognosis. It is helpful to inform women that controlled ovarian stimulation (COS) causes temporary supraphysiologic hormone levels and to describe the possible effects this may have on hormone-responsive cancers (which are very minimal, if any) [4, 5]. Even more important is to discuss how aromatase inhibitors such as letrozole can be used in conjunction with COS to minimize any theoretic risks [6]. One such protocol is for women to use oral letrozole 5 mg daily from the start of COS continuing until 2 weeks after oocyte retrieval [7]. With respect to the safety of pregnancy after cancer, current available research suggests that pregnancy after cancer does not cause or increase the risk of recurrence, even after breast cancer [8]. It is also important to counsel patients that rates of congenital anomalies are no higher in children born to those who have previously undergone potentially mutagenic cancer treatment [9].

24

Pearl #9: - FP patients have unique psychosocial issues beyond those seen in patients who are actively trying to conceive.

Case 9a: - Omotola is 19 years old and considering FP in the setting of a recent diagnosis of cervical cancer. Her prognosis is relatively poor. Her parents attend the FP consultation with her. They are strongly encouraging Omotola to have FP, but she does not seem as enthusiastic.

Case 9b: - Barika is 24 years old, has bilateral ovarian cancer, and was recently married. She feels significant pressure from her community to be fertile and have a large family. She worries that FP may not be possible given her tumors. She is also worried that if she cannot do FP and cannot have children in the future, her husband will leave her. Donor oocytes and adoption are not readily accepted in her culture, so these are not an option for her. She is desperate to have FP done.

Some young women may not have thought about having children. However, family members, especially parents, who may have a strong interest in grandchildren, or who simply believe that desire for children may come at a later age, can sometimes appear to pressure their relative into having FP. In other cases, there may be cultural or religious expectations of what it means to be a woman, a wife, or a mother, and failing to meet these expectations can have significant social harm to a woman or her family. Recognize that motivations to undergo FP are diverse, some of which may not be apparent to you as the clinician at the outset. Frequently women will not disclose if they are feeling pressure from others to undergo FP, and although it might be helpful to ask these questions, this can lead to challenges in the therapeutic relationship between the clinician and the woman and/or her family. It is essential that women not feel forced into doing FP by their care providers; rather, it is our role to provide information to allow women to make informed choices about their care.

Pearl #10: - FP patients may benefit from financial assistance programs available in your area.

Case 10: - Svetlana is a new immigrant and has been diagnosed with breast cancer. She has seen you for consideration of FP, and wishes to proceed, but mentions how she and her husband are not working at the moment and that they cannot afford to pay for FP at this time. She asks if there are any organizations that might provide financial assistance to them.

The absolute costs associated with various forms of FP are often significant but will vary among regions and countries. Some regions provide coverage for fertility preservation, while others have mandates for insurance coverage of these treatments. In other areas, no coverage exists. Many countries have other non-governmental/insurance organizations which may provide financial compensation to women undergoing FP or can provide no or low-cost medications. It is disheartening as a care provider to have women who may be excellent candidates for FP but who are unable to undergo FP due to financial limitations. Therefore, it is imperative that clinicians offering FP be knowledgeable about local resources available to their patients.

24.2 Conclusion

Above we have highlighted some key things to remember as a new FP clinician, with specific examples from our past experiences. These issues are the most complicated part of providing FP care, as they are often more complex and challenging than what is encountered with infertility patients. However, proceeding with a cycle of oocyte or embryo cryopreservation for an FP patient is very similar to any other infertility treatment cycle. We strongly feel that with a little practice and preparation, every clinician can provide excellent FP care and should not shy away from offering this very important option to women in need.

Review Questions and Answers

Q1. What reproductive goals need to be considered when discussing fertility preservation?

A1. Both short- and long-term goals.

Q2. Name some scenarios where fertility preservation may not be possible.

A2. Woman is too ill, cannot tolerate the sedation or logistics of an oocyte retrieval, or risk of performing on oocyte retrieval is too high.

Q3. Name some options for family building if women do not undergo fertility preservation.

A3. Normal conception, ART with autologous oocytes, use of donor oocytes, adoption, gestational carrier (if applicable).

Q4. Are financial resources available to assist women with fertility preservation?

A4. Yes, but these vary by region. It is important to be familiar with the local resources available.

References

1. Davies C, Pan H, Godwin J, Gray R, Arriagada R, Raina V, et al. Long-term effects of continuing adjuvant tamoxifen to 10 years versus stopping at 5 years after diagnosis of oestrogen receptor-positive breast cancer: ATLAS, a randomised trial. Lancet. 2013;381(9869):805–16.
2. Early Breast Cancer Trialists' Collaborative Group (EBCTCG), Davies C, Godwin J, Gray R, Clarke M, Cutter D, et al. Relevance of breast cancer hormone receptors and other factors to the efficacy of adjuvant tamoxifen: patient-level meta-analysis of randomised trials. Lancet. 2011;378(9793):771–84.
3. Pagani O, Ruggeri M, Manunta S, Saunders C, Peccatori F, Cardoso F, et al. Pregnancy after breast cancer: are young patients willing to participate in clinical studies? Breast. 2015;24(3):201–7.
4. Gennari A, Costa M, Puntoni M, Paleari L, De Censi A, Sormani MP, et al. Breast cancer incidence after hormonal treatments for infertility: systematic review and meta-analysis of population-based studies. Breast Cancer Res Treat. 2015;150(2):405–13.
5. Brinton LA, Scoccia B, Moghissi KS, Westhoff CL, Niwa S, Ruggieri D, et al. Long-term relationship of ovulation-stimulating drugs to breast cancer risk. Cancer Epidemiol Biomark Prev. 2014;23(4):584–93.
6. Oktay K, Turan V, Bedoschi G, Pacheco FS, Moy F. Fertility preservation success subsequent to concurrent aromatase inhibitor treatment and ovarian stimulation in women with breast cancer. J Clin Oncol. 2015;33(22):2424–9.
7. Oktay K, Hourvitz A, Sahin G, Oktem O, Safro B, Cil A, et al. Letrozole reduces estrogen and gonadotropin exposure in women with breast cancer undergoing ovarian stimulation before chemotherapy. J Clin Endocrinol Metabol. 2006;91(10):3885–90.
8. Lambertini M, Kroman N, Ameye L, Cordoba O, Pinto A, Benedetti G, et al. Long-term safety of pregnancy following breast cancer according to estrogen receptor status. J Natl Cancer Inst. 2017;31(6):458.
9. Signorello LB, Mulvihill JJ, Green DM, Munro HM, Stovall M, Weathers RE, et al. Congenital anomalies in the children of cancer survivors: a report from the childhood cancer survivor study. J Clin Oncol. 2012;30(3):239–45.

The Birds and the Bees and the Bank: Talking with Families About Future Fertility Amidst a Cancer Diagnosis

Gwendolyn P. Quinn, Caprice Knapp, and Devin Murphy

T. K. Woodruff et al. (eds.), *Textbook of Oncofertility Research and Practice*,
https://doi.org/10.1007/978-3-030-02868-8_25

Key Points
- Fertility is a key quality of life issues for AYA with cancer.
- Communicating about fertility and preservation options improves patient's future quality of life.
- Oncology providers may be uncomfortable discussing fertility and reproductive health with AYA.
- Parents and teens often disagree about fertility issues.

25.1 Introduction

Talking with teens about reproductive health issues can be awkward and uncomfortable. Talking with families about a cancer diagnosis, treatment, and prognosis can be devastating and traumatic. Talking about reproductive health and a cancer diagnosis at the same time, with teens and their parents, confounds these overwhelming emotions.

25.2 Why Is There a Communication Gap in Oncofertility?

When parents learn their child has cancer, or when a patient hears the word "cancer," often nothing else is heard after that point. It is common for the parents and/or patient to forget much of what was told to them during the initial conversation in which the cancer diagnosis was disclosed. Additionally, the shock and devastation of the diagnosis may put parents and the patient in an emotional state where they are incapable of making a decision or choosing a treatment regimen [1, 2]. Often parents look to health-care providers to make important decisions for them or to guide them toward information that will aid in decision-making.

Unfortunately, there are decisions that need to be made around the time of diagnosis and prior to treatment that can impact the future health-related quality of life (HRQOL) for the teen cancer patient. Loss of fertility is an expected long term sequela of many cancer chemotherapy and radiation treatments. The exact odds of temporary or permanent infertility for teens are unknown and depend on the age of the patient, the cancer type and stage, and the treatment type and duration [3, 4]. Several national organizations, including the American Society of Clinical Oncology [4], the American Society for Reproductive Medicine [5], and the American Academy of Pediatrics [6], advise clinicians to discuss fertility issues with *all* cancer patients of childbearing age and refer interested patients to a reproductive endocrinologist (REI) or infertility specialist prior to their first cancer-related treatment. Discussing fertility and preservation of fertility (e.g., banking of sperm, oocytes, embryos, or gonadal tissue) prior to the first cancer-related treatment provides the best opportunity and the most options for ensuring biological children in the future. However, even among those cancer patients who choose to pursue fertility preservation prior to treatment, having a biological child in the future is never guaranteed.

Several studies of adult survivors of childhood cancer show that fertility is their most prevalent concern, resulting in not only a physical late effect but a psychological late effect [7, 8]. The fertility status of survivors is not well known [3, 9], and some studies indicate that survivors may be unaware they may have impaired fertility because of their cancer treatment [10, 11]. Other research reports that some survivors believed they were permanently sterile and then unintentionally became pregnant or impregnated their partner [12–14].

Poor communication on the topic of fertility and reproductive health at the time of a cancer diagnosis is understandable for a multitude of reasons. First, the priority for all involved is treating the cancer, and so it is possible that discussions about reproductive health and fertility simply do not occur during this crisis. Second, adolescent patients and family members may "shut down" after receiving a cancer diagnosis and may not absorb subsequent information about treatment options, schedules, and expectations, let alone information on future reproductive capacity. Third, oncology health-care providers may not feel comfortable discussing reproductive health issues with teen cancer patients, especially younger-aged teens and teens whose parents are present in the room with them. Compounding their own personal discomfort, these providers may not have training in communicating about reproductive health with adolescent patients who are still treated in a pediatric setting and may not feel comfortable discussing an issue outside their area of expertise. Fourth, there may not be an institutional infrastructure, system, or process in place to support referrals to a local REI, and in some cases, no such specialist may exist within the oncology health-care system or even the state [15, 16]. Finally, physicians may attempt to discuss reproductive health issues with the patient and/or parents, and one or both parties may decline the information, believing it is not important at a time when treating the cancer is their only priority.

There are resources in place to assist health-care providers with communication [▶ myoncofertility.org; ▶ fertilityscout.org ▶ livestrong.org] and developing a referral system within their health-care institution [17, 18]. Despite these resources, little is known about the best way for oncology health-care providers to provide information to families and patients that facilitates information sharing and the decision-making process. While education materials are usually recommended to improve health literacy and patient understanding of a health-care issue, recent studies suggest that in the area of reproductive health, these materials are often not distributed [19–21]. Designing tailored educational materials that match the information needs of the population and the protocols and guidelines of the institution regarding fertility and referrals is especially recommended [22–25].

It is important to note that distributing educational materials alone is usually insufficient to guide parents and patients on the path of informed decision-making about future fertility and options for fertility preservation/banking. The reality is that some adolescent patients may not fully understand basic human reproduction or may not have thought about their future parenting goals. Additionally, parents may not have had the opportunity or desire to discuss reproductive health issues or their children's desires for parenthood, particularly with younger children.

25.3 What Is Important to Young Cancer Patients and Their Families?

While several recent studies have systematically assessed the reproductive concerns and preferences of adolescent and young adult (AYA) cancer patients, only a handful have focused exclusively on the teen population [26–30]. Females have been studied more often than males, and adolescents in particular are an important understudied group as they represent the majority of childhood cancer patients [31]. Despite the prevalence of more studies on females with cancer, a recent systematic review noted male patients were more likely to receive information about sexual health/infertility than females [32].

HRQOL assessment tools are commonly used in the adolescent cancer population to measure physical, psychological, social, and cognitive domains that can predict and track outcomes in clinical trials, as well as highlight the need for a variety of health-care services [33]. HRQOL tools can also be used for research and evaluation purposes. Though HRQOL assessments are intended to be completed by the patients themselves, there are settings, particularly in child and adolescent populations, in which patients cannot complete them due to illness, age, cognitive impairments, or extreme fatigue [34]. In these cases, parents may serve as the proxy patient; however, parent reports of their child's HRQOL should be noted as a secondary outcome and not identified as the patient's own words due to the incongruence of many parent-proxy reports [33, 35, 36]. Other studies and practice settings have even used assessment tools with adolescent populations that are designed for and by adults, further limiting the accuracy of the results [37, 38].

Using parents as proxy reporters in HRQOL assessments and discussions about their child's fertility concerns may lead to an ineffective use of resources, as health-care workers attempt to meet the needs of both the parent and adolescent. It was once thought that parents should be the only reporters of their children's HRQOL [39], but now adolescents' unique health perceptions are being recognized as important [35, 40].

Current HRQOL instruments for both adult and adolescent cancer patients lack comprehensive assessments of reproductive concerns. Wenzel developed a stand-alone 14-item Reproductive Concerns Scale (RCS) in 2005 to assess a variety of reproductive concerns of adult female cancer survivors [41]. The RCS was validated using adult female healthy controls with a high internal consistency among survivors (Cronbach's alpha coefficient = 0.91) [41]. No parallel measure currently exists for adolescent oncology patients.

25.4 How Can We Improve Communication About Oncofertility?

A systematic review by Trevena et al. on communicating with patients about evidence suggests that communication tools that are interactive increase patient understanding [42]. Recent studies have examined decision aids for oncofertility. One study examined a self-help web-based intervention to alleviate fertility-related distress. Results showed feasibility in decreasing fertility-related distress among men and women aged 19–43 [43]. Another US-based group designed a website-based decision aid for young women with cancer. Stakeholder assessment showed the decision aid improved knowledge and was regarded favorably [44]. An additional component of the website was an interactive values clarification exercise.

Improved understanding of communication needs and tailored intervention is the use of values clarification exercises. These exercises can be particularly relevant for patients if the evidence to be assessed or the uptake of a service requires individual decision-making. A values clarification exercise or values clarification tool (VCT) is often used in environments in which a common shared vision or purpose is required, the goal of which may be to develop the common vision, define roles, or develop long-range plans. Similarly, a values clarification exercise can aid patients and family members to define values and beliefs, especially those that influence behavior. This clarification can lead to decisions that are reflective of beliefs and goals, rather than hypothetical situations or spontaneous thoughts, which are often elicited in stressful or fearful situations [45–48]. Dismantling barriers to decision-making and identifying gaps between what a patient believes or values and the behaviors that are actually exhibited are a key component of resolving decisional conflict [49]. While not a decision aid, a values clarification tool is a precursor or priming tool for future decision-making.

VCTs can also be used with parents and partners of AYA with cancer. In these cases it is important to examine the impact the tool had on the decision-making process and the perception of the user regarding the quality of the decision. Studies of oncofertility-related decision-making have, importantly, evaluated the decision process; two recent studies suggest negative emotions of the patient and lack of provider support for decision have an adverse effect of decision quality [30, 50].

Based on our pilot study findings, we believe the best use of the RCS-Teen HRQOL instrument is as a VCT, administered to adolescent teens and parents under the guidance of a social worker, nurse, psychologist, or child life specialist (◘ Fig. 25.1). VCTs have specific advantages over HRQOL assessments. HRQOL instruments measure the responder's perceptions by utilizing a norm-based scoring method, such as comparing the respondent's scores of fatigue or pain to the average person in order to determine the "normalcy" of the patient's issues. It would not be in the adolescent oncology patients' best interest to score their concerns about fertility against the general population because adolescent oncology patients have unique concerns that the general population does not, and there is currently no data on healthy adolescents' concerns about fertility and reproduction to be used for comparison.

VCTs have a dual purpose in benefiting both the adolescent and administrator, whether that person is a researcher, social worker, or psychologist. The open-ended statements of the VCT encourage the patient/parent and administrator to begin a dialogue so that the patient/parent may *process* the idea of having children first and then consider their feelings about possibly not being able to have children in the future. This allows the administrator to accurately assess the patient's concerns and develop approaches to educate the patient on her risk as well as risk-reducing options. Our experience with the RCS-Teen showed that a teen's initial reaction to the first few statements was not consistent with their reaction to later statements. For example, with item 3, "I would like to have a baby one day," the majority of the teens said "I guess so" or "Maybe, it's not a big deal." However, by the time the interviewer read the items talking about blame, their responses became less ambiguous, and as they began to process the idea of first wanting children and then thinking about not being able to have them, their responses were emotional and led to more concrete statements such as "I've wanted to be a mother my whole life" or "I might not be able to find a husband if I can't have kids." This delay in providing clear statements may be due to many factors, including difficulty thinking about the future, fear of having "one more thing wrong" that

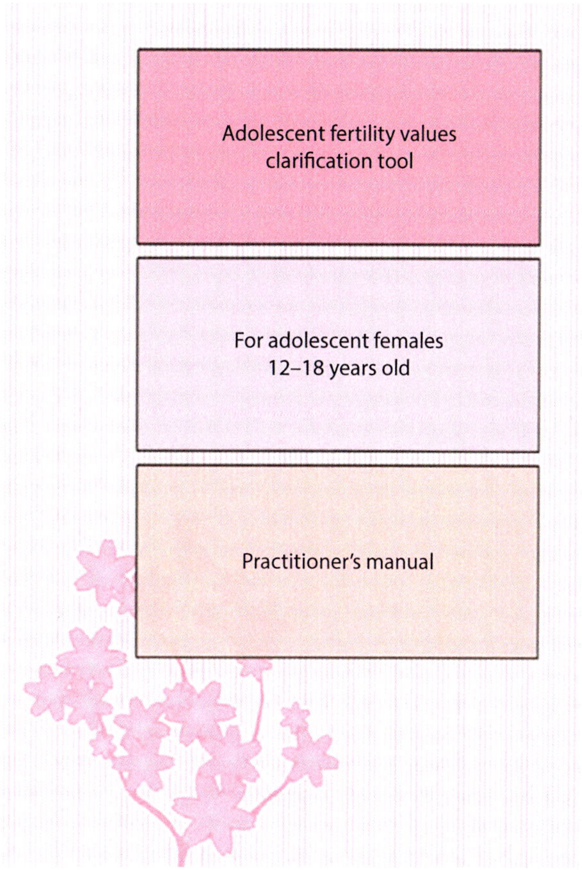

Fig. 25.1 Adolescent fertility values clarification tool

needs to be addressed, disinterest in the topic, or the inability to immediately process the idea that goals for the future, which may be 10 or 20 years ahead and may be impacted by decisions they make at the present time. The order of the items in the RCS-Teen is also important to minimize distress and reduce risk of psychological harm to the teen. Coping strategies, resiliency, and familial support may not be known at the time of test administration. Allowing patients to process the concepts of infertility, their own values, and their own desire for control through a safe and private discussion can empower the adolescent to take an active role in achieving future goals related to biological children.

25.5 Conclusions

Adolescents, whether diagnosed with cancer or healthy, have clear expectations for biological parenthood in the future. However, barriers to discussions and lack of comprehensive assessment tools too often prevent these expectations from being realized, expressed, or taken seriously. Discussions regarding adolescents' values and goals for parenting in the future should be encouraged with patients and their parents prior to beginning cancer treatment. The VCT can be a particularly useful tool in the clinical setting to begin this dialogue.

Acknowledgments This work was supported by the Oncofertility Consortium NIH/NICHD 5UL1DE019587.

Review Questions and Answers

Q1. There are no tools available to help AYA make fertility decisions. True or False?

A1. False

Q2. Most oncology providers are well trained in AYA reproductive health. True or False?

A2. False

Q3. The reproductive concerns scale was designed for male teens. True or False?

A3. False

Q4. AYA patients often "shut down" after receiving a cancer diagnosis. True or False?

A4. True

References

1. Brock DW, Wartman SA. When competent patients make irrational choices. N Engl J Med. 1990;322:1595–9.
2. Levi RB, et al. Diagnosis, disclosure, and informed consent: learning from parents of children with cancer. J Pediatr Hematol Oncol. 2000;22:3–12.
3. Byrne J, et al. Effects of treatment on fertility in long-term survivors of childhood or adolescent cancer. N Engl J Med. 1987;317:1315–21.
4. Oktay K, Harvey BE, Partridge AH, Quinn GP, Reinecke J, Taylor HS, Hamish Wallace W, Wang ET, Loren AW. Fertility preservation in patients with cancer: ASCO clinical practice guideline update. J Clin Oncol. 2018;36(19):1994–2001. https://doi.org/10.1200/JCO.2018.78.1914.
5. Ethics Committee of the American Society for Reproductive Medicine. Fertility preservation and reproduction in patients facing gonadotoxic therapies: a committee opinion. Fertil Steril. 2013;100(5):1224–31.
6. Fallat ME, Hutter J, American Academy of Pediatrics Committee on Bioethics, American Academy of Pediatrics Section on Hematology/Oncology, American Academy of Pediatrics Section on Surgery. Preservation of fertility in pediatric and adolescent patients with cancer. Pediatrics. 2008;121:e1461–9.
7. Edge B, Holmes D, Makin G. Sperm banking in adolescent cancer patients. Arch Dis Child. 2006;91:149–52.
8. Soliman H, Agresta SV. Current issues in adolescent and young adult cancer survivorship. Cancer Control. 2008;15:55–62.
9. Byrne J, et al. Fertility of long-term male survivors of acute lymphoblastic leukemia diagnosed during childhood. Pediatr Blood Cancer. 2004;42:364–72.
10. Zebrack BJ, et al. Fertility issues for young adult survivors of childhood cancer. Psychooncology. 2004;13:689–99.
11. Chapple A, et al. Fertility issues: the perceptions and experiences of young men recently diagnosed and treated for cancer. J Adolesc Health. 2007;40:69–75.
12. Oosterhuis BE, et al. Concerns about infertility risks among pediatric oncology patients and their parents. Pediatr Blood Cancer. 2008;50:85–9.
13. de Wildt SN, Taguchi N, Koren G. Unintended pregnancy during radiotherapy for cancer. Nat Clin Pract Oncol. 2009;6:175–8.
14. Antypas C, et al. Fetal dose evaluation during breast cancer radiotherapy. Int J Radiat Oncol Biol Phys. 1998;40:995–9.
15. Fertile Hope. Fertility resource guide. Austin: Fertile Hope; 2011. http://www.fertilehope.org/tool-bar/referral-guide.cfm. Accessed 20 July 2011.
16. Letourneau JM, et al. A changing perspective: improving access to fertility preservation. Nat Rev Clin Oncol. 2011;8:56–60.
17. Quinn GP, et al. Developing a referral system for fertility preservation among patients with newly diagnosed cancer. J Natl Compr Cancer Netw. 2011;9:1219–25.
18. Peavey M, Arian S, Gibbons W, Lu K, Gershenson D, Woodard T. On-site fertility preservation services for adolescents and young adults in a comprehensive cancer center. J Adolesc Young Adult Oncol. 2017;6(2):229–34. https://doi.org/10.1089/jayao.2016.0057.. Epub 2016 Nov 15. PMID: 27845854 [PubMed – indexed for MEDLINE] Free PMC Article.
19. Quinn GP, et al. Oncologists' use of patient educational materials about cancer and fertility preservation. Psychooncology. 2011; https://doi.org/10.1002/pon.2022.
20. Schover LR, et al. Knowledge and experience regarding cancer, infertility, and sperm banking in younger male survivors. J Clin Oncol. 2002;20:1880–9.
21. Quinn GP, et al. Discussion of fertility preservation with newly diagnosed patients: oncologists' views. J Cancer Surviv. 2007;1:146–55.
22. Willock J, Grogan S. Involving families in the production of patient information literature. Prof Nurse. 1998;13:351–4.
23. Cushen N, South J, Kruppa S. Patients as teachers: the patient's role in improving cancer services. Prof Nurse. 2004;19:395–9.
24. Wizowski L, Harper T, Hutchings T. Writing health information for patients and families: a guide to creating patient education materials that are easy to read, understand and use. Hamilton: Hamilton Health Sciences; 2005.
25. Nagel K, et al. Using plain language skills to create an educational brochure about sperm banking for adolescent and young adult males with cancer. J Pediatr Oncol Nurs. 2008;25:220–6.
26. Crawshaw M, et al. Male and female experiences of having fertility matters raised alongside a cancer diagnosis during the teenage and young adult years. Eur J Cancer Care. 2009;18:381–90.
27. Crawshaw M, Sloper P. A qualitative study of the experiences of teenagers and young adults when faced with possible or actual fertility impairment following cancer treatment, Executive summary. York: University of York; 2006.
28. Zarnegar S, Gosiengfiao Y, Rademaker A, Casey R, Albritton KH. Recall of fertility discussion by adolescent female cancer patients: a survey-based pilot study. J Adolesc Young Adult Oncol. 2018;7(2):249–53. https://doi.org/10.1089/jayao.2017.0079.. Epub 2017 Oct 23. PMID: 29058500 [PubMed – in process].

29. Benedict C, Thom B, Friedman DN, Pottenger E, Raghunathan N, Kelvin JF. Fertility information needs and concerns post-treatment contribute to lowered quality of life among young adult female cancer survivors. Support Care Cancer. 2018;26(7):2209–15. https://doi.org/10.1007/s00520-017-4006 z.. Epub 2018 Feb 1. PMID: 29387996 [PubMed - in process].
30. Melo C, Fonseca A, Moura-Ramos M, Almeida-Santos T, Canavarro MC. Female cancer patients' perceptions of the fertility preservation decision-making process: an exploratory prospective study. J Psychosoc Oncol. 2018;36(3):364–81. https://doi.org/10.1080/07347332.2018.1436629.. Epub 2018 Mar 20. PMID: 29558339 [PubMed - in process].
31. Bleyer A, et al. Trailblazers in adolescent and young adult oncology. J Adolesc Young Adult Oncol. 2011; 1:13–8.
32. Logan S, Perz J, Ussher JM, Peate M, Anazodo A. A systematic review of patient oncofertility support needs in reproductive cancer patients aged 14 to 45 years of age. Psycho-Oncology. 2018;27:401–9. https://doi.org/10.1002/pon.4502.
33. Varni JW, Burwinkle TM, Lane M. Health-related quality of life measurement in pediatric clinical practice: an appraisal and precept for future research and application. Health Qual Life Outcomes. 2005;3:1–9.
34. Palmer SN, et al. The PedsQL™ brain tumor module: initial reliability and validity. Pediatr Blood Cancer. 2007;49:287–93.
35. Levi RB, Drotar D. Health-related quality of life in childhood cancer: discrepancy in parent–child reports. Int J Cancer. 1999;83:58–64.
36. Klosky JL, Simmons JL, Russell KM, Foster RH, Sabbatini GM, Canavera KE, et al. Fertility as a priority among at-risk adolescent males newly diagnosed with cancer and their parents. Support Care Cancer. 2015;23(2):333–41.
37. Lewandowski AS, Toliver-Sokol M, Palermo TM. Evidence-based review of subjective pediatric sleep measures. J Pediatr Psychol. 2011;36:780–93.
38. Vitale MG, et al. Assessment of quality of life in adolescent patients with orthopaedic problems: are adult measures appropriate? J Pediatr Orthop. 2001;21:622–8.
39. Strong P. The ceremonial order of the clinic: parents, doctors, and medical bureaucracies. London: Routledge & Kegan Paul Books; 1979.
40. Perrin JM, MacLean WE, Perrin EC. Parental perceptions of health status and psychologic adjustment of children with asthma. Pediatrics. 1989;83:26–30.
41. Wenzel L, et al. Defining and measuring reproductive concerns of female cancer survivors. J Natl Cancer Inst Monogr. 2005;2005:94–8.
42. Trevena LJ, et al. A systematic review on communicating with patients about evidence. J Eval Clin Pract. 2006;12:13–23.
43. Wiklander M, Strandquist J, Obol CM, Eriksson LE, Winterling J, Rodriguez-Wallberg KA, Sjögren Fugl-Meyer K, Ahlgren J, Ljungman P, Lampic C, Wettergren L. Feasibility of a self-help web-based intervention targeting young cancer patients with sexual problems and fertility distress. Support Care Cancer. 2017;25(12):3675–82. https://doi.org/10.1007/s00520 017-3793-6.. Epub 2017 July 18.
44. Woodard TL, Hoffman AS, Crocker LC, Holman DA, Hoffman DB, Ma J, Bassett RL Jr, Leal VB, Volk RJ. Patient-centred decision counselling for women at risk of cancer-related infertility: a protocol for a comparative effectiveness cluster randomised trial. BMJ Open. 2018;8(2):e019994. https://doi.org/10.1136/bmjopen-2017-019994.
45. Manley K. Organisational culture and consultant nurse outcomes: part 2. Nurse outcomes. Nurs Stand. 2000;14:34–9.
46. Manley K. A conceptual framework for advanced practice: an action research project operationalizing an advanced practitioner/consultant nurse role. J Clin Nurs. 1997;6:179–90.
47. Manley K, McCormack B. Practice development: purpose, methodology, facilitation and evaluation. Nurs Crit Care. 2003;8:22–9.
48. Warfield C. Nursing development unit: developing a new philosophy in the NDU. Nurs Stand. 1990;4:27–30.
49. Guimond P, et al. Validation of a tool to assess health practitioners' decision support and communication skills. Patient Educ Couns. 2003;50:235–45.
50. Koizumi T, Nara K, Hashimoto T, Takamizawa S, Sugimoto K, Suzuki N, Morimoto Y. Influence of negative emotional expressions on the outcomes of shared decision making during oncofertility consultations in Japan. J Adolesc Young Adult Oncol. 2018;7(4):504–8. https://doi.org/10.1089/jayao.2017.0108.. Epub 2018 July 23.

Patient and Family Tools to Aid in Education and Decision-Making About Oncofertility

Gwendolyn P. Quinn, Susan Thomas Vadaparampil, Ivana Sehovic-Neff, and Marla L. Clayman

T. K. Woodruff et al. (eds.), *Textbook of Oncofertility Research and Practice*,
https://doi.org/10.1007/978-3-030-02868-8_26

Key Points
- Adolescent and Young Adult (AYA) patients may not focus on late effects.
- AYA patients may need priming for decision-making about fertility and presentation at diagnosis.
- There are typically three components to decision-making: risk appraisal, information integration, and long-term consideration.
- AYA decision-making may be facilitated by value clarification tools and decision aids.

26.1 Introduction

When an adolescent or young adult (AYA) patient is facing cancer treatment, potential loss of fertility may not be the first thing on his or her mind. Patients often describe their immediate concern is "getting rid of the cancer" or wondering if they will survive. While these concerns are normal, addressing fertility preservation prior to the initiation of cancer treatment provides the most optimal options and opportunity for success. The majority of female AYA patients, based on recent literature, choose not to take steps to preserve fertility, but overwhelmingly appreciate being informed about potential loss of fertility [1]. The reasons for not using fertility preservation among females include financial costs, lack of a male partner, unwillingness to use donor sperm, and the perception of an inability to delay treatment [2, 3]. About 50% of AYA males chose to bank sperm prior to cancer treatment, and those who do not often report feelings of regret and remorse [4]. Males also report appreciation for the information, yet are more likely to recall they had not thought about and/or were embarrassed to discuss sperm banking and future children with their parents or healthcare professional.

How does a cancer patient make a decision about whether or not to pursue fertility preservation? The risk of potential fertility loss should be conveyed to patients by oncologists early in treatment planning, as suggested by the American Society for Clinical Oncology (ASCO). When the oncologist is uncertain about the threat to fertility or what options may be available to the patient, ASCO also recommends that a referral be made to a reproductive endocrinologist or infertility specialist. However, receiving the medical information regarding potential fertility loss is just one component of the decision-making process. Decisions about fertility preservation may be considered to have three components: risk appraisal, information integration, and long-term consideration.

In one component, the patient must appraise and comprehend the amount of risk associated with pursuing fertility preservation options. These risks may be cancer-related, such as the effect of treatment delay on cancer outcomes, as well as risks associated with the fertility preservation options themselves. The risk may also be psychological: how will the patient feel if she becomes infertile and did not take steps to preserve her fertility? It is also possible that for newer and more experimental options, patients may have to contend with an unknown likelihood of success. Based on this appraisal, the patient must decide if these risks and uncertain benefits are acceptable. To make these decisions, the patient must also consider present and future desire for a biological child. Added to this is the consideration of the patients' perception of mortality in light of the diagnosis and whether a limited life span has an impact on decisions about having a biological child. However, people tend to be poor forecasters of what they will want in the future [5]; this is especially true of teens and adolescents. A second component, which may occur concomitant with other decision-making processes, involves assessing information about the fertility preservation options, the medical procedures, the costs for the procedure and storage, the patient's current relationship status, health status, and religious, ethical, or moral concerns about these options. Steps one and two may not happen in a linear fashion and a patient may move back and forth between these components in the decision-making process.

The third component is one which is often not considered until years later, but we suggest it should be considered at the same time as the other two components. This component relates to retrieving the stored sperm, embryo, oocytes, or tissue. How will the patient feel about using assisted reproductive technology (ART) to become a parent? When will a patient be assessed for return of fertility post-treatment? If the patient regains fertility, will he or she continue to store gametes or embryos? How will long-term storage be financed? For men this may mean their female partner becomes the patient when stored sperm requires the use of ART for insemination. For women this may mean decisions about how long to store embryos, what to do with unused oocytes, or asking a partner to parent a child born from donor sperm or eggs. Thinking about these issues at the time of making fertility preservation decisions can be seen as analogous to the need to begin survivorship planning at the time of diagnosis.

The issues for decision-making in fertility preservation among cancer patients are complex and intricate. Unfortunately, tools and decision aids to support patients in this process are limited. Decision support tools and decision-making strategies may be useful for the healthcare professional or researcher working with AYA cancer patients.

The criteria for what constitutes a patient decision aid are quite specific. According to the International Patient Decision Aid Standards (IPDAS) Collaboration, a decision aid prepares a patient for decision-making by doing three things: (1) providing facts about the patient's condition, options, and features; (2) helping people to clarifying their values (the features that matter most to them); and (3) helping people share their values with their healthcare practitioner and others. The IPDAS has developed a set of criteria to determine the quality of patient decision aids. A "users' checklist" summarizes the standards that determine whether or not a decision aid is a source of reliable health information that can help in decision-making [6]. The values clarification process may be particularly important with respect to fertility preservation, as there may be uncertainty surrounding disease outcome and survival as well as uncertainty about the success of fertility preservation techniques themselves (Fig. 26.1).

While the IPDAS provides recommended criteria for patient decision aids, the Ottawa Decision Support Framework (ODSF) offers a three-step process for a strategy to address the conflict experienced by patient in the medical decision-making process. Using concepts and theories from general psychology, social psychology, decision analysis, decisional conflict, values, social support, and self-efficacy, the ODSF is an

IPDAS patient decision aid checklist for users

I. Content: Does the patient decision aid ...

Provide information about options in sufficient detail for decision making?

- ☐ describe the health condition 2.1
- ☐ list the options 2.2
- ☐ list the options of doing nothing 2.3
- ☐ describe the natural course without options 2.4
- ☐ describe procedures 2.5
- ☐ describe positive features [benefits] 2.6
- ☐ describe negative features of options [harms / side effects / disadvantages] 2.7
- ☐ include chances of positive / negative outcomes 2.8

Additional items for tests

- ☐ describe what test is designed to measure 2.9
- ☐ include chances of true positive, true negative, false positive, false negative test results 2.10
- ☐ describe possible next steps based on test result 2.11
- ☐ include chances the disease is found with / without screening 2.12
- ☐ describe detection / treatment that would never have caused problems if one was not screened 2.13

Present probabilities of outcomes in an unbiased and understandable way?

- ☐ use event rates specifying the population and time period 3.1
- ☐ compare outcome probabilities using the same denominator, time period, scale 3.2, 3.3, 3.6
- ☐ describe uncertainty around probabilities 3.4
- ☐ use visual diagrams 3.5
- ☐ use multiple methods to view probabilities [words, numbers diagrams] 3.7
- ☐ allows the patient to select a way of viewing probabilities [words, numbers, diagrams] 3.8
- ☐ allow patient to view probabilities based on their own situation [e.g. age] 3.9
- ☐ place probabilities in context of other events 3.10
- ☐ use both positive and negative frames [e.g. showing both survival and death rates] 3.13

include methods for clarifying and expressing patients' values?

- ☐ describe the procedures and outcomes to help patients imagine what it is like to experience their physical, emotional, social effects 4.1
- ☐ ask patients to consider which positive and negative features matter most 4.2
- ☐ suggest ways for patients to share what matters most with others 4.3

include structured guidance in deliberation and communication?

- ☐ provide steps to make a decision 6.1
- ☐ suggest ways to talk about the decision with a health professional 6.2
- ☐ include tools [worksheet, question list] to discuss options with others 6.3

Fig. 26.1 IPDAS patient decision aid checklist. (Permission from Anton Saarimaki, OHRI)

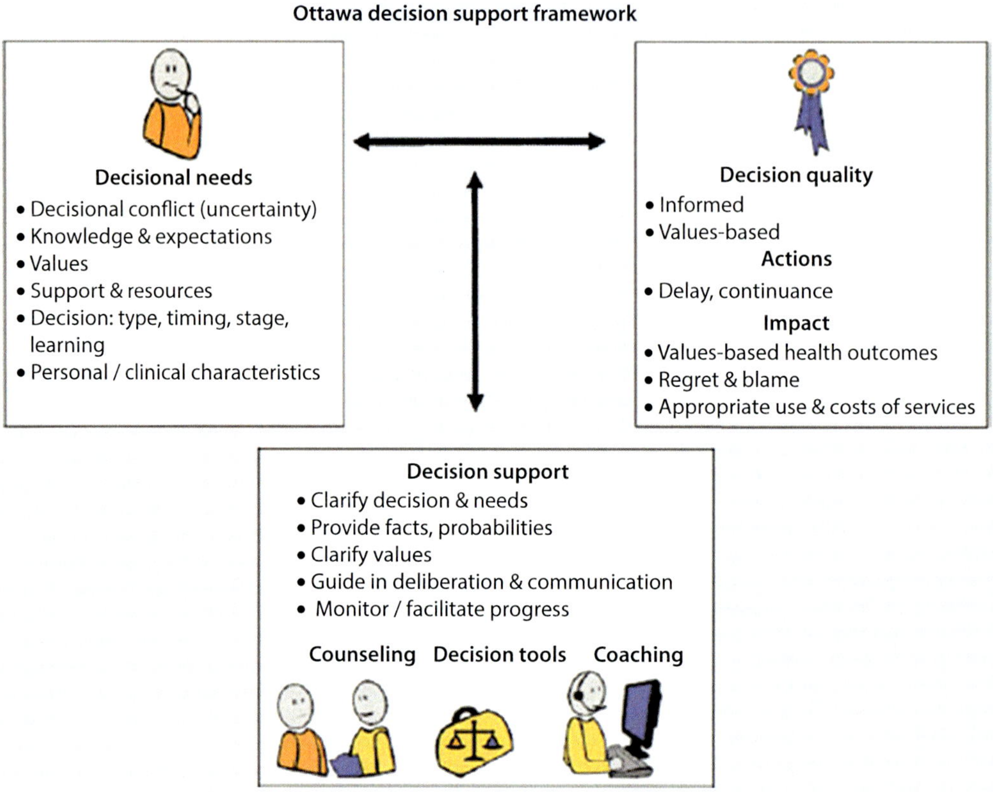

Fig. 26.2 Ottawa decision support framework. (Permission from Anton Saarimaki, OHRI)

26

evidence-based theory for guiding patients in making health decisions [7, 8]. The three-step process assesses patient and practitioner determinants of decisions to identify decision support needs; provides decision support tailored to patient needs; and evaluates the decision-making process and outcomes (Fig. 26.2).

While IPDAS and ODSF provide structure for the design and development of patient decision aids and decision support strategies, Learner Verification (LV) is a framework that helps ensure the materials developed (e.g., decision aids, decision support strategies) are suitable for the intended audience and better matched to patients' learning needs [9]. LV provides an excellent framework for the health communication challenge of developing materials with effective messaging [10]. LV is rooted in information processing theory, focusing on the persuasiveness of a health message and provides a systematic process for assessing the intended messages of a decision aid or educational materials [10]. Specific components of LV are typically assessed with the target audience (the specific group for whom the material is intended, e.g., AYA cancer patients considering fertility preservation). These components include Attractiveness, Comprehension, Cultural Acceptability, Self-efficacy, and Persuasion (4). LV is a quality control process and technique that helps ensure materials are suitable for the intended audience and better matched to patients' learning needs [9] (Table 26.1) (Fig 26.3).

26.2 Examples of Oncofertility-Related Educational Materials and Decision Aids

As another chapter in this volume will present provider-oriented decision support, this section focuses on patient and family-oriented educational tools and decision aids. Institutions and

Table 26.1 Elements of learner verification assessed in study brochure

Elements of learner verification assessed	Questions from interview guide
Attraction (does the material appeal to the target audience?)	What about the appearance of this brochure intrigued you?
	If you were sent this brochure in the mail, would you want to read it to find out more about breast cancer?
Comprehension (does the target audience understand the material?)	Tell me in your own words what you think the purpose of this brochure is?
	Did this brochure help you to understand the purpose of genetic testing?
	Are there any risks in your family that would make you want to have genetic testing?
Self-efficacy (does the target audience feel the message is doable for them?	After reading this brochure, would you want to participate in this study? (probes: If you wanted to participate would you be able to?)
	Did this brochure help you to understand why genetic testing is important to African American women with breast cancer?
Did this brochure help you to understand why genetic testing is important to African American women with breast cancer?	How do feel about the phrase "Women of Color"? (probes: Do you think most African American women would feel the same way?; do you think there is another term that African American women identify with?)
	Is there anything in this brochure that makes you feel uncomfortable about genetic testing?
	Do you relate to any of the women in this brochure?
Persuasion (does the message convince the target audience to take action?)	If you received this brochure in the mail, would you want to have a genetic test for *BRCA*?
	Do you think your family and friends might have genetic counseling/testing if they received this brochure?

Permission from Dr. Susan Vadaparampil, MCC

healthcare professionals may wish to create their own educational materials or decision aids based on knowledge of their own patients or their institutions' policies, guideline, and resources. The following is a list of existing tools and strategies related to oncofertility that may serve as a guide for developing practice-specific tools. Practitioners may also choose to use these materials or modify them as allowed and applicable.

26.2.1 Oncofertility Website [11]

The Oncofertility Consortium maintains a website that has both provider and patient-oriented content. Patient and provider content can be found at ► http://www.savemyfertility.org. In addition to information about fertility preservation, these resources include risk tables and information about how to discuss fertility with your patient and/or provider (Fig. 26.4).

26.2.2 Web-Based Decision Aid [12]

This collaborative project between a reproductive endocrinologist, clinical psychologist, and oncology expert involves an interactive, web-based decision aid designed to be used in concert with fertility preservation counseling. The goal of the

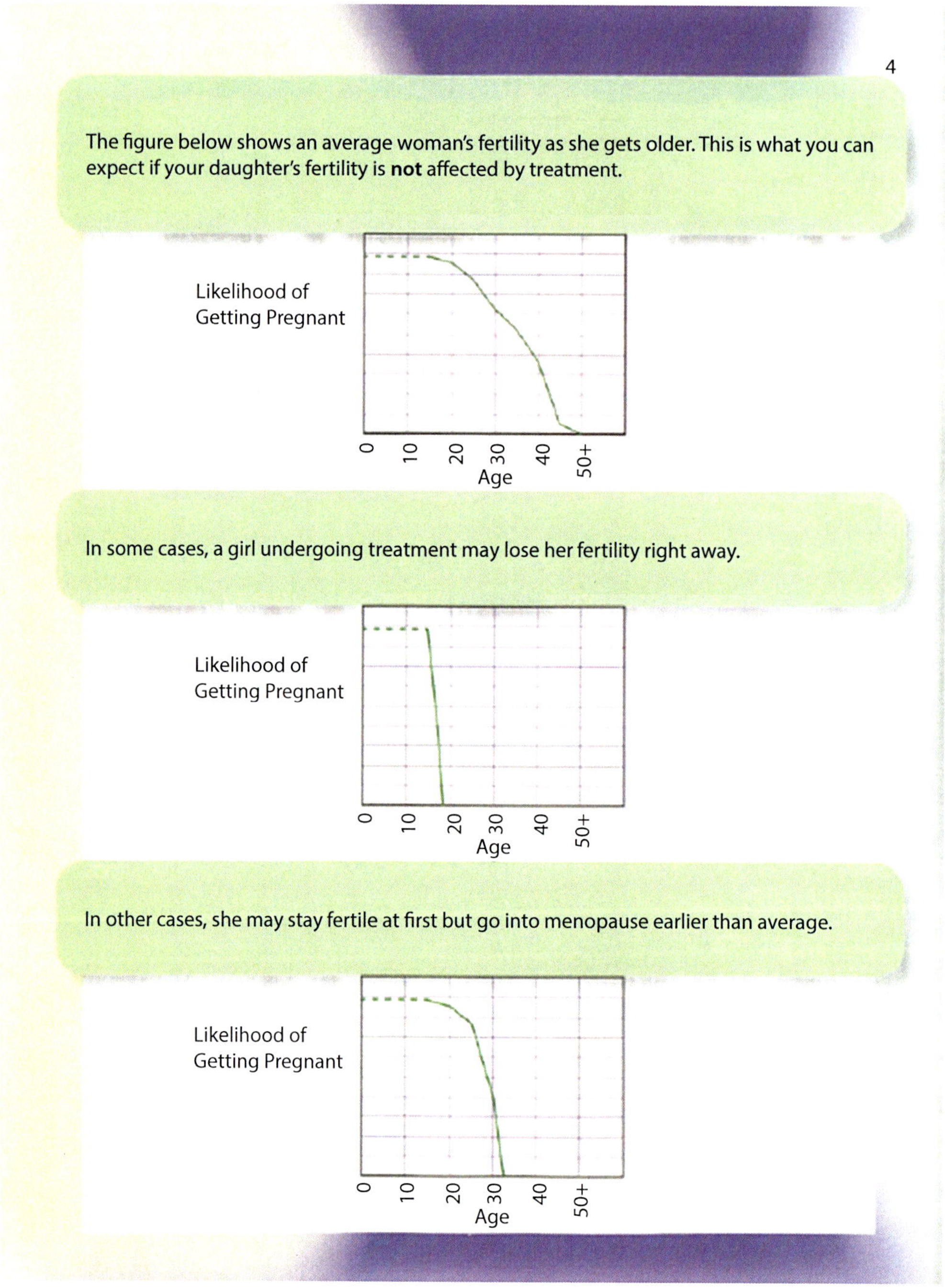

Fig. 26.3 ▶ FertileHope.org Website. (Adapted from LIVESTRONG Fertility Website. Permission from LIVESTRONG)

decision aid is to develop and make available a web-based tool that could be used for patients who do not have easy access to a full fertility preservation consultation with a reproductive endocrinologist (Fig. 26.5).

26.2.3 "A Young Person's Guide to Cancer and Fertility": Male and Female Brochure [13]

The majority of patient information on FP was designed by and for adults, and may not be

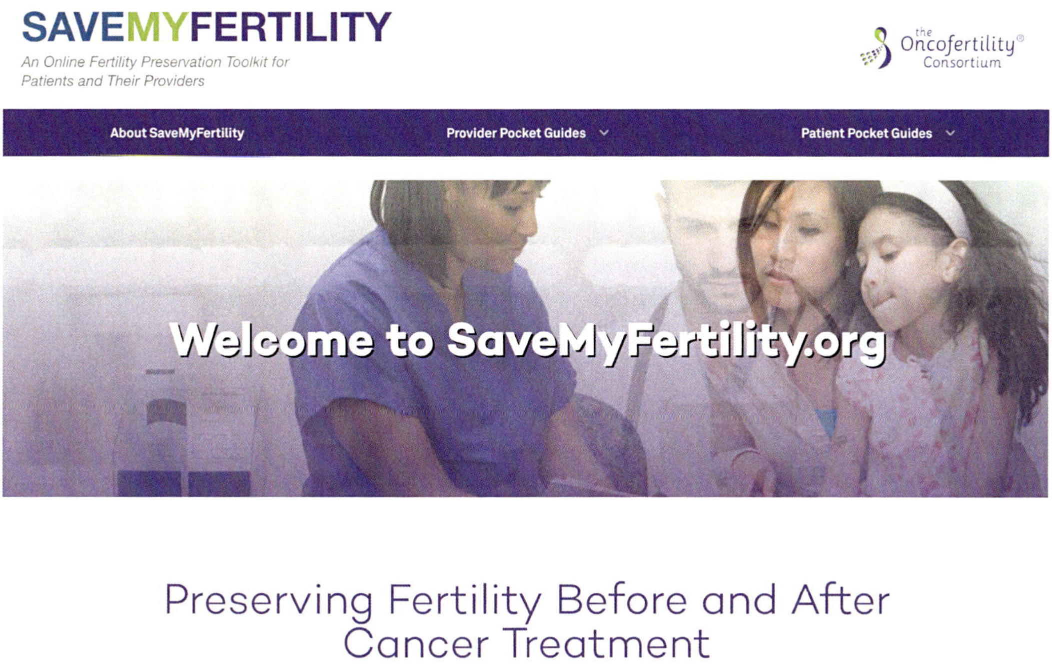

Fig. 26.4 ► SaveMyFertility.org Website. (Permission from Dr. Teresa Woodruff, NW)

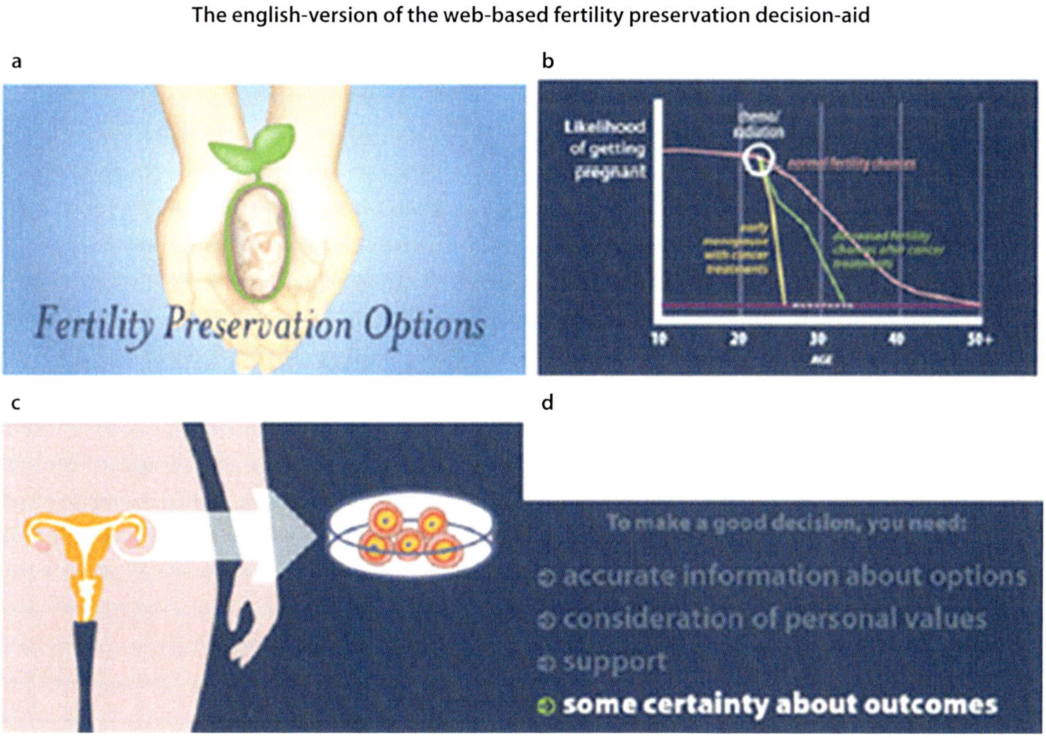

Fig. 26.5 Web-based fertility preservation decision aid. Screen shots from english version of the fertility preservation decision aid. **a** Intro screen. **b** Graphic demonstration about age and fertility. **c** Animation about IVF egg removal. **d** Review of decision-making strategies. (Permission from Dr. Jennifer Mersereau, UNC)

appropriate for pediatric populations. These brochures were developed for a specific children's hospital after a review of available literature and existing educational materials. First, the research team designed a preliminary brochure outlining cancer-related infertility and the options available for pediatric patients. Due to the vast differences between female and male fertility issues and options, a separate male and female brochure was developed. The brochures were tested with three groups (patients and survivors aged 12–21 (N = 7), their parents (N = 11), and healthcare providers (N = 6)). The final brochures were revised based on majority feedback and feasibility (◘ Fig. 26.6).

26.2.4 Fertility-Related Choices: A Decision Aid for Younger Women with Early Breast Cancer [14]

This is a booklet for young women who have recently been diagnosed with early breast cancer. As chemotherapy and hormonal therapy may decrease fertility and reduce the chance of having children in the future, the information provided here is designed to help women decide which, if any, of the available fertility options are of interest to them. This booklet was specifically designed for the following patient characteristics: recently diagnosed with early breast cancer and reproductive age (having regular periods and no menopausal symptoms), and thinking of starting a family or having more children in the future (◘ Fig. 26.7).

26.2.5 Adolescent Fertility Values Clarification Tool [15, 16]

This tool was designed to provide healthcare providers with a platform for discussing the impact of cancer treatment on future fertility with adolescent females. It discusses the preservation options and provides an approach for allowing the teen to consider her knowledge, desire, and value of parenthood. Since this is a tool, and not an instrument, there is no scoring guide. The tool will help practitioners assess the patient's values and understanding of fertility in relation to the cancer diagnosis and treatment plan. The tool provides examples of common coping techniques used by teens during the piloting and testing of the instrument (◘ Fig. 26.8).

26.2.6 Learning About Cancer and Fertility: A Guide for Parents of Young Girls [17]

This decision aid was designed for parents of young girls diagnosed with cancer. Through interviews with parents (N = 20), the developers chose to develop a paper-based tool that acknowledges parents' focus on their child's survival than future fertility. The decision aid explains that some cancer treatments can affect their daughter's fertility in both short and long term and there may be decisions parents can make to preserve their daughter's fertility. Due to the age of the patients whose parents are the target of this decision aid, experimental options are also described. The focus of the tool is not just for making fertility preservation decisions but also serves as a guide to give parents information that will help them talk with their child's healthcare team now and in the future as she grows (◘ Fig. 26.9).

This is not a comprehensive list of all tools and materials available on the topic of fertility preservation among AYA populations but serves as a sample of those that were developed using multidisciplinary teams and a scientific approach. It is important for healthcare providers and researchers to explore decision aids and educational strategies that may improve the understanding of fertility preservation and its limitations. Healthcare professionals may consider which of these existing tools is appropriate for the institution and the population or if tailored tools should be developed based on unique characteristics of the patient population. Cancer survivors value the ability to make an informed decision about their future fertility preservation options. While decision aids, tools, and strategies are not a replacement for a discussion with a medical professional, they can assist patients and survivors as they explore their choices.

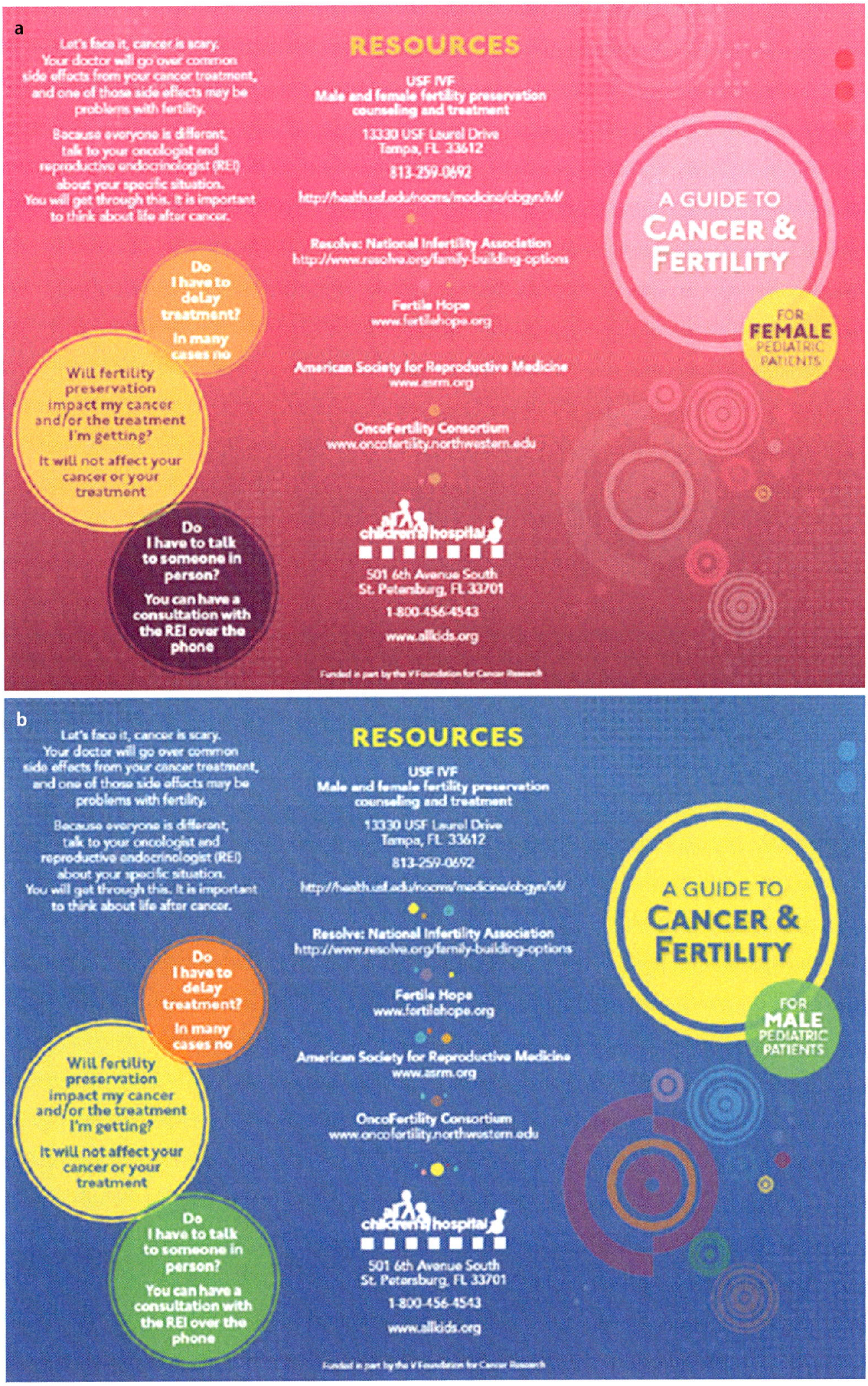

Fig. 26.6 (**a**, **b**) A guide to cancer and fertility for female pediatric patients, a guide to cancer and fertility for male pediatric patients. ► https://www.bcna.org.au/media/3685/bcn1189_fertility_booklet_2016_online.pdf. (Permission from Dr. Gwendolyn Quinn, NYU)

26

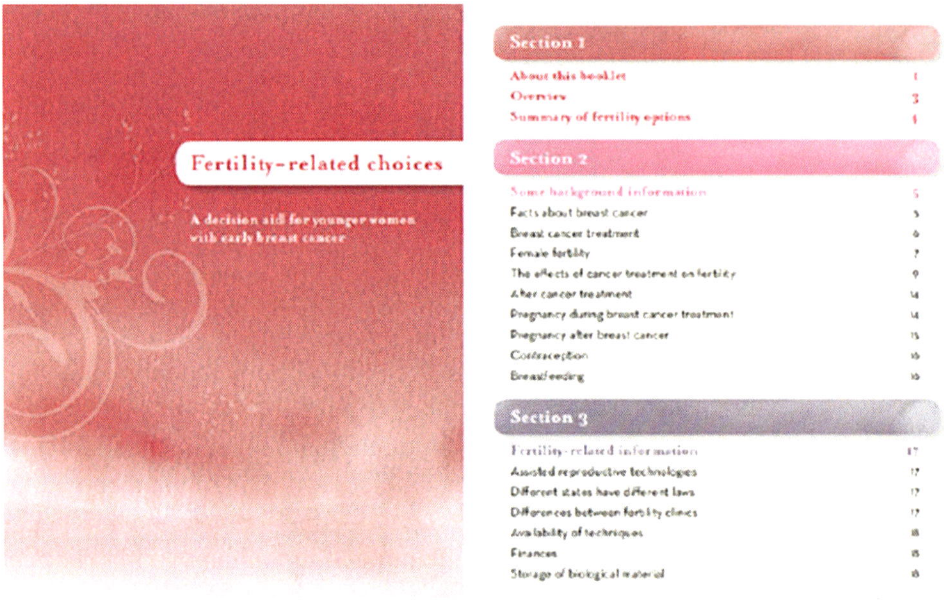

Fig. 26.7 Fertility-related choices: a decision aid for younger women with early breast cancer. (Permission from Dr. Michelle Peate, UNSW)

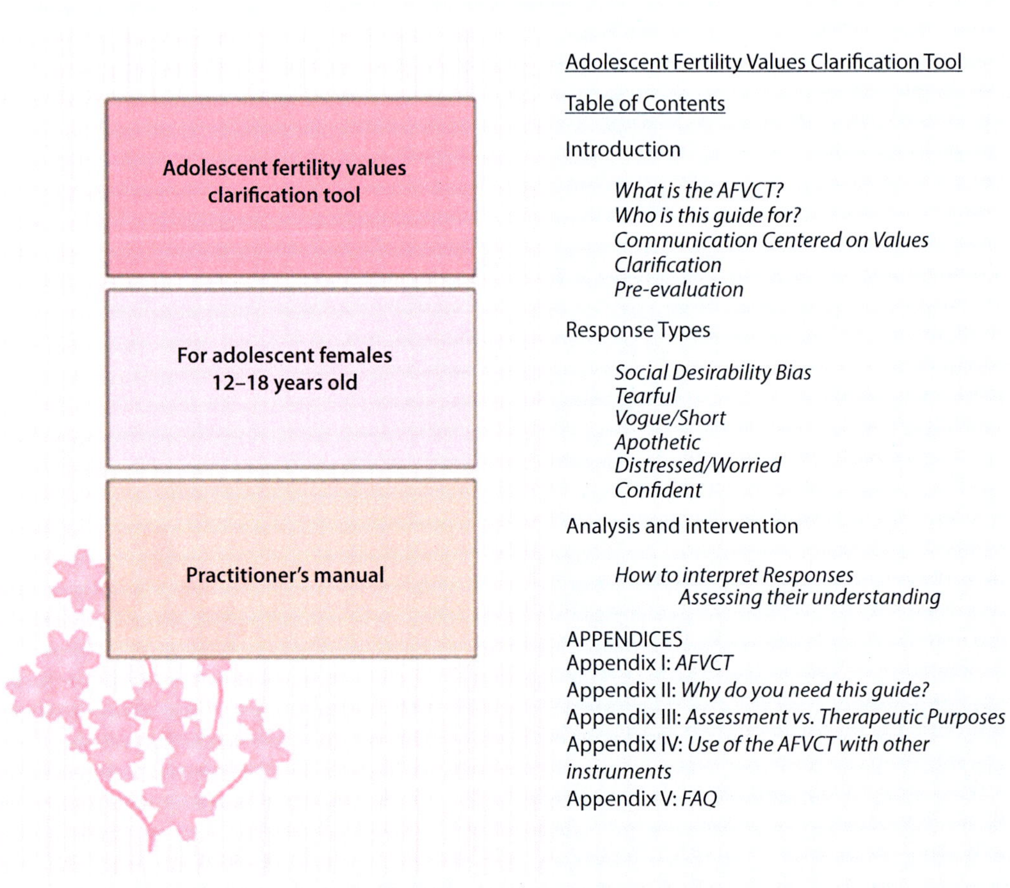

Fig. 26.8 Adolescent fertility values clarification tool. (Permission from Dr. Gwendolyn Quinn, NYU)

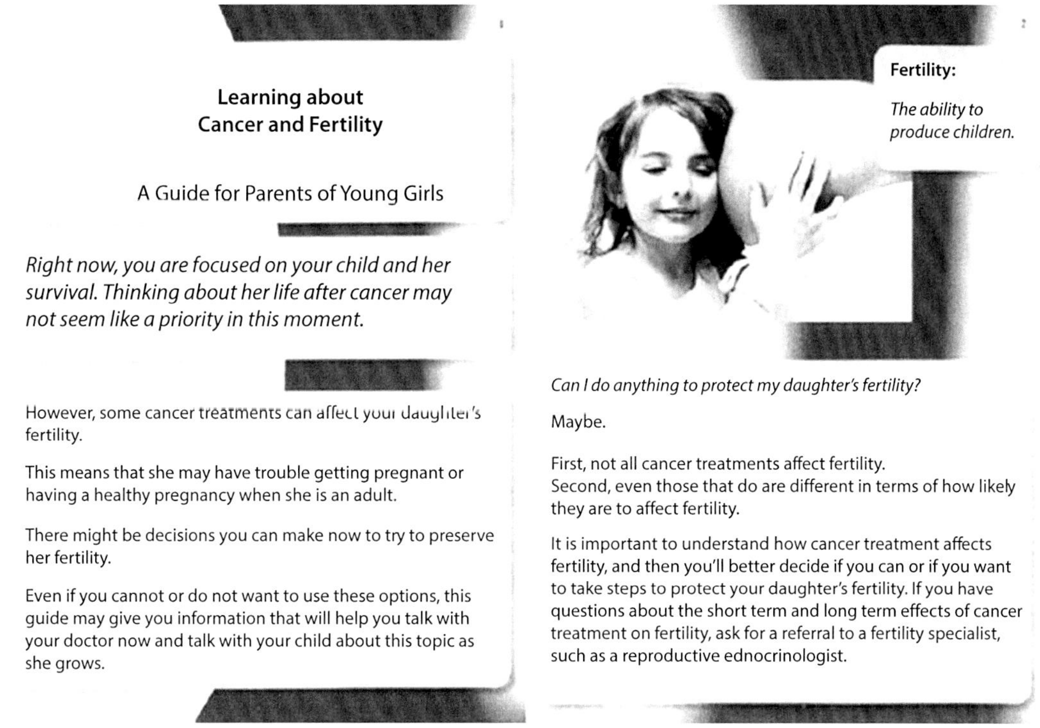

Learning about Cancer and Fertility

A Guide for Parents of Young Girls

Right now, you are focused on your child and her survival. Thinking about her life after cancer may not seem like a priority in this moment.

However, some cancer treatments can affect your daughter's fertility.

This means that she may have trouble getting pregnant or having a healthy pregnancy when she is an adult.

There might be decisions you can make now to try to preserve her fertility.

Even if you cannot or do not want to use these options, this guide may give you information that will help you talk with your doctor now and talk with your child about this topic as she grows.

Fertility:

The ability to produce children.

Can I do anything to protect my daughter's fertility?

Maybe.

First, not all cancer treatments affect fertility.
Second, even those that do are different in terms of how likely they are to affect fertility.

It is important to understand how cancer treatment affects fertility, and then you'll better decide if you can or if you want to take steps to protect your daughter's fertility. If you have questions about the short term and long term effects of cancer treatment on fertility, ask for a referral to a fertility specialist, such as a reproductive ednocrinologist.

Fig. 26.9 Learning about cancer and fertility: a guide for parents of young girls. (Permission from Dr. Marla Clayman, AIR)

Review Questions and Answers

Q1. What are the three components of decision-making?

A1. Risk appraisal, information integration, and long-term consideration.

Q2. What are the three ways decision aids can assist patients?

A2. Provide facts, clarify values, and share values with the provider.

Q3. What is learner verification?

A3. A framework for assessing health education materials.

References

1. Peddie V, Porter M, Barbour R, et al. Factors affecting decision making about fertility preservation after cancer diagnosis: a qualitative study. BJOG. 2012; 119:1049–57.
2. Yee S, Abrol K, McDonald M, et al. Addressing oncofertility needs: views of female cancer patients in fertility preservation. J Psychosoc Oncol. 2012;30(3):331–46.
3. Quinn GP, Vadaparampil ST, Jacobsen PB, et al. Frozen hope: fertility preservation for women with cancer. J Midwifery Womens Health. 2010;55(2):175–80.
4. Knapp CA, Quinn GP, Murphy DM. Assessing the reproductive concerns of children and adolescents with cancer: challenges and potential solutions. J Adolesc Young Adult Oncol. 2011;1(1):31–5.
5. Quinn GP, Murphy DM, Knapp CA, et al. Who decides? Decision making and fertility preservation in teens with cancer: a review of the literature. J Adolesc Health. 2011;49(4):337–46.
6. IPDAS. Criteria for judging the quality of patient aids. 2005. Retrieved from http://www.ipdas.ohri.ca/IPDAS_checklist.pdf.
7. O'Connor AM. Ottawa decision support framework to address decisional conflict. 2006. Retrieved from http://decisionaid.ohri.ca/docs/develop/ODSF.pdf.
8. O'Connor AM, Stacey D, Jacobsen MJ. Ottawa decision support tutorial: improving practitioners' decision support skills Ottawa Hospital Research Institute: patient decision aids. 2011. Retrieved from https://decisionaid.ohri.ca/ODST/pdfs/ODST.pdf.
9. Doak LG, Doak CC, Meade CD. Strategies to improve cancer education materials. Oncol Nurs Forum. 1996; 23(8):1305–12.
10. Vadaparampil ST, Quinn GP, Gjyshi A, et al. Development of a brochure for increasing awareness of inherited

breast cancer in black women. Genet Test Mol Biomark. 2011;15(1–2):59–67.
11. SaveMyFertility.org. The oncofertility consortium. 2018. Retrieved on 4 September 2018 savemyfertilityorg.
12. Web-based fertility preservation decision-aid: fertility preservation options. Available at Oncofertilitydecision.org. Please contact author for more information: Mersereau JE: jennifer_mersereau@med.unc.edu.
13. Murphy D, Sawczyn KK, Quinn GP. Using a patient-centered approach to develop a fertility preservation brochure for pediatric oncology patients: a pilot study. J Pediatr Adolesc Gynecol. 2012;25(2):114–21.
14. Peate M, Meiser B, Cheah BC, et al. Making hard choices easier: a prospective, multicentre study to assess the efficacy of a fertility-related decision aid in young women with early-stage breast cancer. Br J Cancer. 2012;106:1053–61.
15. Quinn GP, Murphy D, Wang H, et al. Having cancer does not change wanting a baby: healthy adolescent girls' perceptions of cancer-related infertility. J Adolesc Health. 2012;52(2):164–9.
16. Quinn G, Knapp C, Murphy D. Congruence of reproductive concerns among adolescents with cancer and their parents. Pediatrics. 2012;129:930–6.
17. Clayman ML. Learning about cancer and fertility: a guide for parents of young girls. Unpublished work 2012; please contact author for more information: m-clayman@nrthwestern.edu.

Establishing Insurance Coverage for Iatrogenic Infertility

Joyce D. Reinecke, Nanette Elster, Joseph Letourneau, and Meghan Bowman-Curci

T. K. Woodruff et al. (eds.), *Textbook of Oncofertility Research and Practice*,
https://doi.org/10.1007/978-3-030-02868-8_27

Key Points
- Fertility preservation is essential to a significant number of patients who undergo potentially sterilizing medical treatment.
- The cost of fertility preservation treatment, and the concomitant lack of insurance for these services, is a significant barrier for patients.
- Many arguments support insurance coverage for fertility preservation, including: bioethical principles, policy principles, financial offsets, and improved patient outcome.
- There are several potential avenues for implementation of insurance coverage, including: voluntary adoption of coverage by insurers, administrative changes, and legislation.

27.1 Introduction

In this chapter, we discuss the need for and current state of fertility preservation insurance coverage in the United States. Our discussion will be limited to the situation in which an individual is diagnosed with a medical condition for which they must undergo certain treatments that threaten their fertility. When infertility arises as a side effect of a necessary medical treatment, this is referred to as iatrogenic infertility.

27.2 Who Needs Fertility Preservation?

27.2.1 Population

In the United States this year, an estimated 1,735,350 people will receive a cancer diagnosis. Approximately 8.8% of these patients – 152,711 people – will be in their "reproductive years" – meaning under 45 years [1]. The most significant sub-population at risk is breast cancer patients, approximately 25% of whom are diagnosed in this age range [2]. Even pediatric patients who have not yet entered puberty are at risk of reproductive damage, depending on the diagnosis and extent of their cancer treatment [3, 4].

In addition to cancer patients, individuals with particular autoimmune diseases like rheumatoid or psoriatic arthritis, systemic lupus erythematosus, and certain non-malignant hematologic diseases like thalassemia or sickle cell anemia may require chemotherapy and/or bone marrow transplants that place them at risk for iatrogenic infertility [5, 6]. Emerging populations who seek fertility preservation also include transgender patients who may wish to protect their future ability to have genetic offspring before undergoing hormone therapy or transition surgery [7, 8]; and individuals who have hereditary cancer syndromes like BRCA who may desire egg banking prior to prophylactic measures such as oophorectomy to reduce their future risk of developing cancer [9, 10].

27.2.2 Level and Scope of the Risk

Because the risk of iatrogenic infertility usually stems from the treatment for cancer rather than from the cancer itself, most, but not all, cancer patients face some level of risk. Predicting the nature and extent of damage for individual patients is difficult because many factors influence outcome, including patient age, dose and type of chemotherapy, dose and location of radiation, and underlying individual biology [1].

Moreover, while a patient's initial treatment may pose only a limited risk of infertility, lack of response or recurrence may alter the treatment plan and result in a sudden escalation of risk. For example, a young patient with Hodgkin lymphoma undergoing first line chemotherapy with Adriamycin® (doxorubicin), Bleomycin, Vinblastine, and Dacarbazine (ABVD), faces only a small risk of premature ovarian failure, and may therefore refrain from undertaking fertility preservation measures [11]. However, if the patient's cancer is resistant, or she suffers a relapse, her chemotherapy regimen may shift to include more gonadotoxic alkylating agents, or she may need to undergo high-dose chemotherapy and radiation prior to a stem cell transplant. Under these circumstances, the risk of infertility from treatment would drastically increase, often without an opportunity for fertility preservation.

27.2.3 Demand for Services

In the decade since Teresa Woodruff coined the term "oncofertility," [12] the demand for fertility preservation services is burgeoning. This demand has been driven by advances in cancer treatment that have dramatically improved survival, coupled with significant advances in reproductive technologies that allow for quicker, more efficacious fertility interventions [13]. The emergence of vitrification as a method of oocyte freezing and the subsequent recognition of egg freezing as "non-investigational" by the American Society for Reproductive Medicine (ASRM) in 2012 [14] has been particularly instrumental in making fertility preservation a truly viable option for female cancer patients. In addition to these medical advances, demographic and cultural changes have also driven demand for fertility preservation. In the United States, the trend toward delayed marriage and childbearing [15] means that more cancer patients are being diagnosed before they have begun or completed their family building. At the same time, now 40 years after the birth of Louise Brown [16], the acceptance of the use of reproductive technology is at an all-time high [17]. A recent study showed that the majority of the population approves of egg freezing, with the strongest support – 89% – for its use in fertility preservation by cancer patients [18].

27.3 Why Do Patients Need Insurance Coverage?

While the demand for fertility preservation grows, access to these services remains limited. Numerous studies, based on patient and provider feedback, have identified cost as the single greatest obstacle preventing cancer patients from obtaining desired fertility preservation services [19–21]. Treatments such as sperm banking and egg banking are expensive, and without insurance coverage, many patients are simply unable to pay for these procedures. Typically, sperm banking can be done for a few hundred dollars [22], but egg freezing is significantly more expensive. A 2017 survey found the average nationwide cost for one cycle of egg freezing, including procedures and medications, was approximately $16,000 [23].

For young people facing a new cancer diagnosis, the cost of fertility preservation is often coupled with other financial pressures, including any uncovered portions of cancer treatment itself as well as a potential loss of income due to their illness. Recent articles have detailed the significant financial strain that a cancer diagnosis can cause, even giving the phenomenon a name – "cancer-related financial toxicity" or CRFT [24– 27]. CRFT is highest for young adult cancer patients who typically have more debt and lower incomes; these cancer patients have two to five times the bankruptcy rates of older cancer patients [24–27]. According to the 2015 Millennial Money Survey [28], 75% of Americans in their 20s earned under $50,000.00 a year; they also had less than $7000 in savings and over $36,000 in student loan debt. Given this financial reality, many young adult patients without insurance coverage are forced to forego fertility preservation.

> When I was diagnosed, I was given less than a week to discuss my options with my husband, a newly arrived immigrant from West Africa, whose culture marks marriage with the ability to expand the family tree. We met with a fertility specialist who told us that we would need to begin immediately – and come up with $15,000 in cash by the next day. We were told that fertility preservation was not part of my health care plan's coverage. The process was disorganized and left me feeling that I did not have a choice. I now have to watch as chemotherapy drugs are pumped into my body, knowing that they are killing my cancer, but could be destroying my chances of having a child. I can say with all sincerity that is what keeps me up at night.
> –Victoria D., 25, Hodgkin Lymphoma, (testimony given in support of California SB 172, April 26, 2017)

27.4 Why Should Coverage Be Provided?

In addition to the personal stories of patients who would benefit from this type of coverage, there are many arguments that support coverage for fertility preservation for the broad population of individuals facing iatrogenic infertility.

27.4.1 Bioethical Bases for Coverage

There is a strong ethical argument for insurance coverage for fertility preservation, based on traditional principles of autonomy, beneficence, nonmaleficence, and justice [29].

Autonomy refers to the idea that individuals should be able to make health care decisions that align with their personal goals and values. For patients who desire genetic offspring but are facing iatrogenic infertility, autonomy supports the ability to pursue fertility preservation. If an individual undergoes medical treatment that results in iatrogenic infertility without the choice to pursue fertility preservation, then his or her autonomy has not been respected. The principle of autonomy extends to children, supporting what Joel Feinberg calls a child's right to an "open future." "[The child's right] while . . . still a child is to have future options kept open until [the child] is a fully formed, self-determining adult capable of deciding among them" [30].

Beneficence and nonmaleficence refer, respectively, to doing good and avoiding harm. Iatrogenic infertility inherently differs from infertility that occurs spontaneously, either due to natural aging, as the direct result of an underlying medical condition, or due to unknown etiology. The nature of this causation imposes a duty to cover the remedy for this harm. Typically, when a medical treatment causes collateral damage, interventions to address that damage are covered as part of the treatment [31, 32]. For example, wigs, prosthetics, and antiemetics are generally covered benefits that are viewed as an integral part of cancer care [33]. This duty to redress an unintended harm of treatment is consistent with the basic bioethical medical tenet "do no harm" as described by bioethicist Lisa Campo-Engelstein [33].

In addition, numerous studies have suggested that inaccessibility of fertility preservation services may worsen medical outcomes [34–36]. Unresolved fertility concerns are correlated with higher rates of depression and lower quality of life in cancer survivors [34–36]. Fertility concerns have been shown to be a factor in treatment decision-making for approximately one-third of pre-menopausal breast cancer patients [37]. Some of these patients would opt for potentially less-effective treatment regimens if they were less gonadotoxic. Newer research indicates that significant numbers of young breast cancer patients will avoid or compromise necessary medical treatment such as tamoxifen because of overriding reproductive goals [38]. Patients who cannot pay for fertility preservation services may compromise their health or deviate from their recommended cancer treatment due to their desire to have genetic children. Improved access to fertility preservation could alleviate this need.

Finally, the principle of justice – treating people in comparable circumstances similarly – is paramount to the argument for fertility preservation coverage for iatrogenic infertility. Social justice suggests that "all groups and individuals [are] entitled equally to important rights . . ." [29] Sixteen states now require insurance coverage for the treatment and diagnosis of infertility [39]. The provision of infertility services for individuals with infertility resulting from physiologic or medical causes, but denying access to the same services for individuals with iatrogenic infertility, is inherently inequitable and unjust. This distinction is frequently made because coverage may be restricted to individuals who cannot conceive after 6 or 12 months of actively trying to get pregnant. The injustice of denying a patient access to benefits that are already covered as a part of her health plan because she is *going to be* rendered infertile rather than *is* infertile is demonstrated in this excerpt from a final internal adverse benefit denial:

> You asked for coverage of retrieving and freezing your eggs. You asked for this because you have cancer and will start chemotherapy. You may want to get pregnant in the future. We looked at your . . . health plan benefits. This type of treatment is not covered unless you have been trying to get pregnant for 12 months . . . That was not . . .the case for you. . . . The service is therefore not covered . . .[i]t would be covered if you are infertile after your chemotherapy [40]. (Final decision from United Healthcare to J.H., 34 year old breast cancer patient. February 1, 2018)

The absurdity of this logic – that the patient must wait to access covered benefits until a time that such treatments would be substantially less effective or entirely ineffective – underscores the inherent injustice in the current predominant structure defining the scope of standard infertility coverage. Moreover, different patient populations suffer disproportionally for this lack of coverage. For example, the cost of fertility preservation for women is approximately 30 times higher than it is for men, thereby establishing a significant gender disparity in access to care [41].

For all these reasons, provision of coverage for iatrogenic infertility is an ethical imperative.

27.4.2 Policy Bases for Coverage

In addition to the ethical bases for coverage, fertility preservation should be covered because it meets the standard threshold elements for coverage – "medical necessity" and "standard of care."

A prerequisite to health insurance coverage in the United States is a finding that a particular service or procedure is *medically necessary*. Any services that are not "medically necessary" generally fall outside the scope of coverage. Thus, categorization of fertility preservation services for iatrogenic infertility as "medically necessary" is a crucial first step in positioning those services as worthy of coverage. Unfortunately, how and who makes this determination is often unclear. The vagueness of the term is addressed by Professor Daniel Skinner:

> In the United States, the concept of "medical necessity" continues to serve as the primary gatekeeper for the utilization of health care services. [It is used] to distinguish not only necessary from unnecessary care but also medical from cosmetic, experimental, elective . . .[to] ensur[e] that patients receive treatment that is appropriate and medically indicated while also controlling costs. At the same time, the concept's meaning remains elusive [42].

As Professor Skinner notes, identifying what is *not* medically necessary is often easier – that which is "cosmetic, experimental" or "elective," – than what is clearly included in the definition. The American Medical Association (the "AMA") defines medical necessity as:

> Health care services or products that a prudent physician would provide to a patient for the purpose of preventing, diagnosing or treating an illness, injury, disease or its symptoms in a manner that is: (a) in accordance with generally accepted standards of medical practice; (b) clinically appropriate in terms of type, frequency, extent, site, and duration; and (c) not primarily for the economic benefit of the health plans and purchasers or for the convenience of the patient, treating physician, or other health care provider [43].

Infertility services are often viewed as "elective," a label that continues to shield insurers from paying for treatment. Although the AMA in June 2017 adopted the World Health Organization's conception of infertility as a "disease," [44] currently only 16 states have laws concerning insurance coverage for infertility diagnosis or treatment [39], and these laws vary widely in scope. Only eight states required coverage for in vitro fertilization (IVF), and even these have significant prerequisites to coverage that would make access to fertility preservation difficult, if not impossible [39]. Cancer patients are uniquely rendered infertile because they must accept sterilizing medical treatment to combat their disease and preserve their life. They have no rational choice under these circumstances to reject curative treatments to spare their gametes or their reproductive organs. The immediacy of the decision-making required in this circumstance further obviates the "electiveness" of this choice. Under these complex circumstances, a patient's ability to effectively research, consider, and select their reproductive options, and to grasp the long-term implications of those choices, is severely curtailed.

A second facet in the definition of medical necessity is the requirement that the procedures or interventions for which coverage is being sought represent "standard of care," meaning they are recognized and accepted as appropriate by practitioners in the field. All of the relevant oncology and reproductive medicine societies, most notably the American Society of Clinical Oncology (ASCO) and the ASRM, have formal guidelines supporting fertility preservation for iatrogenic infertility as part of the standard of care for cancer treatment in age-eligible, at-risk patients [45–47]. The existence of the ASCO [45] and ASRM [46] guidelines as evidence of the standard of care has been critical to findings of medical necessity in several external medical reviews in California and Illinois. These reviews uniformly concluded that coverage was wrongly denied to cancer patients who needed emergency fertility preservation services [48]. In addition, a California Health Benefits Review Program Report (CHBRP) noted that specific procedures such as sperm, egg, and embryo cryopreservation represent the "standard of care" for fertility preservation for cancer patients [49].

27

27.4.3 Financial Arguments for Coverage

As discussed above, the cost of fertility preservation services are high for the individual patient [50]. These costs are the basis for resistance to coverage by the insurance industry. The primary purpose of insurance from the perspective of the individual who purchases it is to offset the financial risk of an unforeseen medical treatment. Insurance is tool to amortize that risk across a population, thereby minimizing any individual's cost. Independent analyses done in states where coverage bills have been considered estimate that costs of covering standard fertility preservation services would range from a low of one cent per member per month ($0.01 PMPM) [41] to a high of $0.10–$0.24 PMPM [51].

The extremely low cost of adding this benefit is a direct function of both the low eligibility and the low utilization rates for fertility preservation services. Eligibility rates are low because the number of newly diagnosed cancer patients aged 45 and under, in the population at large, is very low. In the United States, the annual incidence of cancer in individuals under 45 years is 43.9 in 100,000, amounting to approximately 150,000 age-eligible patients in 2018. Of these, approximately 10,000 will be pediatric cases [1]. Given current technology, these pre-pubertal patients could only preserve fertility using experimental techniques, which would not be covered. Even among all "eligible" patients, utilization rates for fertility preservation will never approach 100%. Some patients will not receive gonadotoxic or fertility-impairing treatments; some will have already completed their family building; some may not have enough time or may be too sick to undergo such treatments; some may have religious or personal opposition to using assisted reproductive technology; and some may not be concerned about loss of future fertility or genetic parenthood. Actual utilization rates are difficult to obtain because coverage is uncommon, and insurers who do provide this coverage do not share their data. Published estimates for maximum utilization (derived from actual use by patients with private coverage) range from 16.7% to 33% for female patients and from 34.8% to 43.8% for male patients [49, 51, 52].

The estimated cost of coverage, in addition to being objectively low, is also miniscule as compared to total cancer care costs. In addition, there are offsets that could potentially reduce the net cost of fertility preservation services. As previously mentioned, numerous studies have identified unrelated medical benefits for cancer patients who undergo fertility preservation, such as improved quality of life and reduced levels of psychological distress [34–36, 53]. While the value of improved mental health outcomes has not been quantified, it is logical to infer it may reduce the need for medical and/or psychological services as well as increased productivity. Additional cost savings may be generated through the achievement of better medical outcomes in young adult patients who, once their fertility concerns are met, may better adhere to prescribed cancer treatment recommendations. As previously described, young breast cancer patients have been reported to defer or abandon prescribed tamoxifen treatment due to overriding concerns about fertility [38]. These voluntary deviations from treatment may increase the risk of preventable cancer recurrence, which itself may increase the costs of cancer care. The average cost of treating early stage breast cancer over the first 24 months after diagnosis has been estimated at $71,909; the average cost of treating stage IV breast cancer over that same time period was $182,655 [54]. Because direct cancer treatment costs are generally covered, these increased expenses would be borne by insurers.

27.5 How Can Coverage Be Pursued?

Insurance coverage can be established in a variety of ways. Insurers can choose to provide coverage for particular procedures and include these benefits in their policies. Alternatively, legislators can pass laws requiring insurers to cover or to offer coverage for certain services. Finally, administrative or regulatory changes can add or clarify coverage parameters and policies. Any of these mechanisms or a combination of approaches can be used to pursue coverage for fertility preservation for those facing iatrogenic infertility.

27.5.1 Voluntary Coverage for Fertility Preservation

To our knowledge, the first insurance provider to voluntarily add coverage for fertility preservation

8. Administration of Infertility Benefits

As of October 1, 2009 for new sales and upon renewal for existing accounts, we are updating the administration of infertility benefits. In addition to providing coverage to diagnose and treat infertility for healthy members who have not been able to conceive or produce conception during a period of one year. Blue Cross Blue Shield of Massachusetts may approve coverage for infertility services in two other situations. First, when a member has been diagnosed with cancer and is expected to become infertile after treatment. Second, coverage may be approved when a healthy member is age 35 or older and has not been able to conceive or produce conception during a period of six months. Prior-authorization requirements are in effect and remain the same for these services.

Please note that additional information regarding the administration of infertility benefits is available in Blue Cross Blue Shield of Massachusetts' medical policy.

Fig. 27.1 The first insurance provider to voluntarily add coverage for fertility preservation procedures for cancer patients was Blue Cross Blue Shield of Massachusetts, which did so in 2009

procedures for cancer patients was Blue Cross Blue Shield of Massachusetts [55], which did so in 2009 (Fig. 27.1). As a result of an initiative developed by Fertile Hope and undertaken by the Livestrong Foundation in 2010, 3 additional commercial insurers and more than 35 self-insured companies added fertility preservation coverage for those facing iatrogenic infertility, resulting in coverage for approximately 7 million people [55, 56]. Over the past few years, many large companies have started to provide egg freezing coverage as part of a push to expand their "family-friendly" benefits to recruit young talent. While these benefits were primarily intended to provide egg freezing for young women concerned about natural ovarian aging, they nonetheless extend coverage to individuals with iatrogenic infertility as well [57, 58]. Recently, the Veteran's Health Administration has also chosen to cover fertility preservation due to a medical need, including for at-risk cancer patients. In June 2017, they issued a directive clarifying their coverage of infertility benefits [59]. It expressly stated that:

> Gamete cryopreservation (sperm or oocytes) is allowable when it is determined by appropriate health care professionals that the care is needed to promote, preserve, or restore the health of the individual and is in accord with generally accepted standards of medical practice (e.g., for oncofertility with cryopreservation of gametes to preserve fertility prior to cancer treatment which would ordinarily render the patient permanently sterile) [59].

27.5.2 Legislating Coverage

Attempts to impose coverage for fertility preservation procedures for cancer patients through legislative means began as early as 2002. A bill introduced in New Jersey sought coverage for egg freezing for women who were facing possible infertility due to chemotherapy or radiation treatments for cancer [60]. The bill would have expanded the state's existing infertility mandate which required coverage for the diagnosis and treatment of infertility, to also include the prevention of infertility, and it added oocyte freezing for cancer patients to the list of specifically included procedures [61]. The bill was introduced every session from 2002 to 2013, but never moved out of committee. Over the past decade, similar bills have been introduced in several states to require that insurers cover the costs of fertility preservation for cancer patients at risk for iatrogenic infertility, with no success until recently.

In 2017, two states – Connecticut and Rhode Island – passed legislation mandating fertility preservation coverage for iatrogenic infertility [62, 63]. Both already had existing laws requiring insurers to cover infertility treatment, including IVF [62, 63]. The Connecticut bill was signed into law on June 20, 2017, making Connecticut the first state in the country to require that certain insurers provide coverage for patients facing iatrogenic infertility. The bill was originally introduced in 2014 by Representative Matt Lesser, a cancer survivor, as a stand-alone fertility preservation bill, and it would have only provided coverage for cancer patients who were at least 18 years old and who had not yet started cancer treatment. The bill was reintroduced in every subsequent year, ultimately passing in 2017. The final version was very different from the original bill. Instead of adding a separate clause for fertility preservation coverage to the state's infertility coverage law, it changed the statutory definition of "infertility" itself. That definition, which had been codified as a result of the 2005 infertility coverage mandate [64], was altered in a few ways. First, the words "presumably healthy" were stricken from the existing law; second, an exception to the functional definition of infertility as a year of unsuccessful attempts at pregnancy was created for the case of "medical necessity."

> For purposes of this section, "infertility" means the condition of an individual who is unable to conceive or produce conception or sustain a successful pregnancy during a one-year period *or such treatment is medically necessary*. (emphasis added)

Two weeks later, Rhode Island became the second state to require fertility preservation coverage [65]. The Rhode Island bill [63, 65] also amended an existing state infertility coverage mandate, but did so by inserting more specific language: "for standard fertility preservation services when a medically necessary medical treatment may directly or indirectly cause iatrogenic infertility to a covered person" [63]. The Rhode Island bill took effect immediately, and the state's only fertility clinic has already witnessed a significant increase in the number of patients seeking fertility preservation [66].

On the heels of the successes in 2017, numerous additional states either introduced or reintroduced bills requiring FP coverage (Table 27.1). Some of these bills only addressed medically needed fertility preservation, and some were broader bills that sought to also establish coverage for IVF [63, 67]. Two states – Maryland [67] and Illinois [68] – saw FP-only coverage signed into law. Like Connecticut and Rhode Island, Maryland and Illinois already had IVF coverage laws in place; Maryland was, in fact, the first state in the country to require IVF coverage [69]. Delaware also passed a bill, but its law [70] mandated coverage not only for fertility preservation, but also for the treatment of infertility itself, including for IVF. This broad legislation was the first new IVF mandate signed into law in over a decade [64]. The last infertility mandate that included IVF coverage was passed in Connecticut in 2005 [64]. At the time of this writing, one additional FP coverage bill is still pending in New Jersey [71, 72].

While these recent legislative victories will make fertility preservation available to thousands of cancer patients, there are still many limitations inherent to these laws, and to some of the proposed bills, should they pass in the future. One significant limitation is that these state laws only affect certain subsets of insurance. For example, they do not reach private self-insured plans that are governed by a federal law, the Employee Retirement Income Security Act (ERISA) [73]. In 2016, approximately 58% of workers receive their health insurance through employer-based, self-insured plans [74], so this represents a sizable portion of insured Americans. In addition, only Illinois' law affects its state Medicaid plan; coverage in other states leaves out many of the patients who can least afford and most need this coverage [74]. Beyond restricting coverage obligations to certain types of insurers, the scope of the coverage may be further constricted by additional limits. For example, particularly where fertility preservation coverage is structured to modify existing infertility mandates, restrictions concerning age limits, religious exemptions, or cycle restrictions, could be applied to fertility preservation benefits [75]. Further, the language of some of the proposed bills limits coverage to individuals with a diagnosis of cancer, thereby excluding those facing iatrogenic infertility from treatment for other diseases or conditions. These bills even place additional inclusion criteria on cancer patients, such as a requirement that cancer treatment has not yet been initiated, and lower and upper age bounds. These parameters would reduce patient eligibility for coverage, and their purpose should be considered carefully before adoption. At least one state has concluded that age restrictions for infertility coverage violate the Affordable Care Act's (ACA) nondiscrimination clause, and lifetime cycle caps may be viewed as illegitimate preexisting-condition exclusions in contravention of Health Insurance Portability and Accountability Act (HIPAA) [76].

27.5.3 Administrative Recognition of Coverage

Generally, states are responsible for regulating insurance sold within their state. They can implement

Table 27.1 Fertility preservation coverage legislation 2017–2018

State	Bill	Status	Coverage	Details
CT	HB7124	Signed into law 6/20/17	"Medically necessary" treatments	Amended existing infertility law; changed statutory definition of "infertility" to include "medical necessary" treatment
RI	S0821A & H6170A	Signed into law 7/05/17	FP	Amended existing IVF mandate to add standard FP services if necessary medical treatment may cause iatrogenic infertility
MD	SB271 & HB908	Signed into law 5/18/18	FP	Standard FP services if necessary medical treatment may cause iatrogenic infertility; large groups only
DC	SB139	Signed into law 6/30/18	Infertility, including IVF+FP	New infertility mandate, includes coverage for specified treatments including IVF and FP. Does not include state employees or Medicaid recipients
IL	HB2617	Signed into law 8/27/18	FP	Standard FP services if necessary medical treatment may cause iatrogenic infertility; broad coverage including state employees and Medicaid recipients
NJ	A3150 & S2133	Pending	FP	IVF mandated was updated in 2017; FP to be added in 2018
AZ	SB1149	Intro in Senate; Inactive	Infertility, including IVF+FP	IVF mandate; specific procedures listed; includes FP
CA	SB172	Heard in Sen. Health Cmte; Inactive	FP	Standard FP services if necessary medical treatment may cause iatrogenic infertility
HI	HB2669	Heard in House HHS Cmte; Inactive	FP (cancer only)	Oocyte and sperm cryopreservation. Limits: adult patients who have not started treatment; one cycle
KY	SB95	Passed Senate; Inactive	FP	Standard FP services if necessary medical treatment may cause iatrogenic infertility; one year of storage; Limit: one cycle
LA	HB698	Hearings in House; sent to Cmte on Approps for reconsideration; Inactive	FP (cancer only)	Coverage for embryo, oocyte, and sperm cryopreservation; limited to 18–40 years old; dx of cancer only; has not started cancer treatment. Limit: one cycle
MS	HB1198	Died in Cmte; Failed	IVF+FP (iatrogenic)	IVF mandate; specific procedures listed; includes FP
MO	HB2388	Referred to House Judiciary Cmte; Inactive	FP (cancer only)	Coverage for embryo, oocyte, and sperm cryopreservation; limited to 18–40 years old; dx of cancer only; has not started cancer treatment. Limit: one cycle
NY	A02646A & S3148 (S8441b)	Different versions passed in Assembly & House; Inactive	IVF+FP (iatrogenic)	Update existing infertility mandate to include IVF and fertility preservation for iatrogenic infertility
	S7163 & A10660	Sent to Cmte in both chambers; Inactive	FP (cancer only)	Coverage for standard fertility treatment when a necessary cancer treatment may directly or indirectly cause iatrogenic infertility
VT	H629	Referred to Cmte on Healthcare; Inactive	FP (cancer only)	Coverage for embryo, oocyte, and sperm cryopreservation; limited to 18–40 years old; dx of cancer only; has not started cancer treatment. Limit: one cycle

27

and/or enforce rules and regulations about all aspects of coverage that insurers must abide by to participate in the market. In the state of California, along with the Department of Insurance, the Department of Managed Healthcare (DMHC) is the primary agency for regulating insurers within the managed healthcare system; it oversees the insurers of some 25 million Californians. The DMHC has an online, external appeals process whereby individuals may request an independent medical review (IMR) when they feel they have wrongly been denied coverage for a medical service or procedure. Within the past year, four IMRs in California have been issued finding fertility preservation prior to potentially sterilizing cancer treatment should have been covered [77]. One decision, on behalf of a breast cancer patient in her 30s is excerpted here:

> *Nature of Statutory Criteria/Case Summary*: An enrollee has requested reimbursement for fertility preservation services . . . enrollee . . . has a history of breast cancer. *Findings*: The physician reviewer found that there is support in the medical literature for the services at issue. With current technology, sperm and embryo as well as oocyte cryopreservation, are considered standard practice and are widely available. In this case, treatment options were considered that included chemotherapy. Because of the unpredictable nature of a cancer diagnosis and future treatments, the American Society of Clinical Oncology and the American Society for Reproductive Medicine guidelines recommend immediate fertility treatment so that the opportunity is not lost and cancer treatment is not delayed. Such treatment is considered the standard of care by these societies. . . . [I]n order to preserve this patient's fertility, it was medically necessary for this patient to undergo fertility sparing treatment. *Final Result*: Health Plan's denial should be overturned [78].

The other three IMRs contained virtually the same language and all ruled in favor of the cancer patients [77]. Based on the consistency of these outcomes and the underlying rationale of the decisions, the DMHC has now recognized fertility preservation for those facing iatrogenic infertility as covered benefit per se; with access to that benefit turning on medical facts of the individual case [66]. Its position relies, in part, on the Knox-Keene Health Care Service Plan Act of 1975 which provides that all medically necessary "basic healthcare services" must be covered. Significantly, the broad categories of "basic healthcare services" do not include expressly include infertility procedures or treatments, and California has not mandated infertility coverage (only that such services be "offered"). Coverage for fertility preservation procedures arises not from a specifically delineated infertility benefit, but rather from the patient's medical need to protect their genetic material due to cancer treatment that will expose them to possible reproductive harm [79]. The DMHC's position on medically needed fertility preservation coverage was recently elucidated in written response to a patient complaint:

> Your EOC [Evidence of Coverage] lists specific services that are not covered for the treatment of infertility. . . . However, the services for which you seek reimbursement are intended to preserve a person's ability to have children before undergoing medical treatment that may cause infertility. These are *basic healthcare services* (emphasis added) that require coverage under California health plan law. (Letter from DMHC to V.F., 39-year-old ovarian cancer patient. June 5, 2018)

This recognition that fertility preservation coverage is not dependent on the presence of broader infertility coverage is consistent with and analogous to the rationale for the coverage of reconstructive surgery – also a remedy for an iatrogenic harm – in the breast cancer context [80, 81]. While this particular mechanism for redress is unique to California, under the ACA, all states must have external review procedures for insurance appeals. This means that similar arguments for coverage can be made elsewhere, even when a "final" internal denial has been issued by an insurer.

27.6 Conclusion

Fertility preservation for iatrogenic infertility is a medically necessary, non-elective intervention to prevent potential reproductive damage and/or sterility for cancer patients and for others who must submit to required – often life-saving – medical treatments. Numerous rationales for requiring insurance coverage for these procedures exist and are starting to be acknowledged. The recent succession of state legislation, coupled with administrative recognition for this coverage reflects an emerging and welcome trend to recognize patients' right to protect their reproductive ability.

Review Questions and Answers

Q1. True or False? Cost is the most common reason cancer patients cannot access fertility preservation services.

A1. True

Q2. To date, all except the following states have insurance coverage for fertility preservation services for cancer patients *except*:
(a) CT
(b) NY
(c) RI
(d) MD

A2. (b)

Q3. Explain why if fertility preservation services were covered by insurance, the cost would be minimal.

A3. The extremely low cost of adding this benefit is a direct function of both the low eligibility and the low utilization rates for these services. Eligibility rates are low because the number of newly diagnosed cancer patients aged 45 and under, in the population at large, is very low. Utilization rates would be low considering several factors. Some patients will not receive gonadotoxic or fertility-impairing treatments; some will have already completed their family building; some may not have enough time or may be too sick to opt-in to such treatments; some may have religious or personal opposition to using assisted reproductive technology; and some may not be interested in or concerned about their future fertility or genetic parenthood.

Q4. True or False? One of the limitations of the current fertility preservation legislation is that many of the bills passed do not affect Medicaid plans, leaving out many of the patients who can least afford and most need this coverage.

A4. True

References

1. Center for Disease Control and Prevention. United States cancer statistics: data visualizations. https://gis.cdc.gov/Cancer/USCS/DataViz.html, https://www.cancer.gov/about-cancer/treatment/side-effects/fertility-women, https://www.cancer.gov/about-cancer/treatment/side-effects/fertility-men. Published 2017. Accessed 8 June 2018.
2. National Cancer Institute. Cancer stat facts: female breast cancer. https://seer.cancer.gov/statfacts/html/breast.html. Published 2014. Accessed 14 July 2018.
3. Green DM, Kawashima T, Stovall M, et al. Fertility of male survivors of childhood cancer: a report from the Childhood Cancer Survivor Study. J Clin Onocol. 2010;28(2):332–9.
4. Green DM, Kawashima T, Stovall M, et al. Fertility of female survivors of childhood cancer: a report from the childhood cancer survivor study. J Clin Onocol. 2009;27(16):332–9.
5. Katsifis GETA. Ovarian failure in systemic lupus erythematosus patients treated with pulsed intravenous cyclophosphamide. Lupus. 2004;13:673–8.
6. Rovoa T, Passweg J, Heim D, Meyer-Monard S, Holzgreve W. Spermatogenesis in long term survivors after allogenic hematopoietic stem cell transplantation is associated with age, time interval since transplantation, and apparently absence of chronic GVHD. Blood. 2006;108(3):1100.
7. Nahata L, Bowman-Curci M, Quinn GP. Exploring fertility preservation intentions among transgender youth. J Adolesc Health. 2018;62(2):123–5.
8. Chen D, Simons L, Johnson EK, et al. Fertility preservation for transgender adolescents. J Adolesc Health. 2017;61(1):120–3.
9. Dean M, Rauscher EA. "It was an Emotional Baby": previvors' family planning decision-making styles about hereditary breast and ovarian cancer risk. J Genet Couns. 2017;26(6):1301–13.
10. Insogna IG, Ginsburg ES. PAH. Fertility preservation in BRCA carriers: special considerations. In: Managing BRCA mutation carriers. Cham: Springer; 2017. p. 171–86.
11. van der Kaaij M, Heutte N, Meijnders P, Abeilard-Lemoisson E, et al. Premature ovarian failure and fertility in long-term survivors of Hodgkin's lymphoma: a European Organisation for Research and Treatment of Cancer Lymphoma Group and Groupe d'Étude des Lymphomes de l'Adulte Cohort study. J Clin Onocol. 2012;30(3):291–9.

12. Woodruff TK. The emergence of a new interdiscipline: oncofertility. In: Oncofertility fertility preservation for cancer survivors. Cham: Springer; 2007. p. 3–11.
13. Walsh SK, Ginsburg ES, Lehmann LS, Partridge AH. Oncofertility: fertile ground for conflict between patient autonomy and medical values. Oncologist. 2017;22(7):860–3.
14. American Society for Reproductive Medicine. Recommendations for gamete and embryo donation: a committee opinion. Fertil Steril. 2012;99(1):47–62.
15. Center for Disease and Prevention. Mean age of mothers is on the rise: United States, 2000–2014. https://www.cdc.gov/nchs/products/databriefs/db232.htm. Published 2016.
16. History. World's first test tube baby born. https://www.history.com/this-day-in-history/worlds-first-test-tube-baby-born. Published 2010.
17. Fortin C, Abele S. Increased length of awareness of assisted reproductive technologies fosters positive attitudes and acceptance among women. Int J Fertil Steril. 2016;9(4):452–64.
18. Lewis EI, Missmer SA, Farland LV, Ginsburg ES. Public support in the United States for elective oocyte cryopreservation. Fertil Steril. 2016;106(5):1183–9.
19. Quinn GP, Vadaparampil ST, Bell-Ellison BA, Gwede CK, Albrecht TL. Patient–physician communication barriers regarding fertility preservation among newly diagnosed cancer patients. Soc Sci Med. 2008;66(3):784–9.
20. Schover LR. Patient attitudes toward fertility preservation. Pediatr Blood Cancer. 2009;53(2):281–4.
21. Rashedi AS, de Roo SF, Ataman LM, et al. Survey of fertility preservation options available to patients with cancer around the globe. J Glob Oncol. 2017;4:1–16.
22. American Cancer Society. Preserving fertility in men with cancer. https://www.cancer.org/treatment/treatments-and-side-effects/physical-side-effects/fertility-and-sexual-side-effects/fertility-and-men-with-cancer/preserving-fertility-in-men.html. Published 2016. Accessed 31 July 2018.
23. FertilityIQ. The costs of egg freezing. https://www.fertilityiq.com/egg-freezing/the-costs-of-egg-freezing. Published 2017. Accessed 14 July 2018.
24. Bona K, Lynch DM, Ramsey S, et al. Cancer-related financial toxicity and its pervasive effects on patients and families: solving a national health and economic crisis hiding in plain sight. 2018. https://familyreach.org/wp-content/uploads/2018/02/february_wp_final.pdf.
25. Zafar YS, Peppercorn JM, Schrag D, et al. The financial toxicity of cancer treatment: a pilot study assessing out-of-pocket expenses and the insured cancer patient's experience. Oncologist. 2013;18(4):381–90.
26. Zafar YS. Financial toxicity of cancer care: it's time to intervene. J Natl Cancer Inst. 2016;108(5):djv370.
27. Carrera PM, Kantarjian HM, Blinder VS. The financial burden and distress of patients with cancer: understanding and stepping-up action on the financial toxicity of cancer treatment. CA A J Cancer Clin. 2018; 68(2):153–65.
28. Weliver D. The 2015 Millennial Money Survey: how much do 20-somethings earn and save? https://www.moneyunder30.com/20-somethings-money-survey. Published 2015.
29. Beauchamp TL, Childress JF. Principles of biomedical ethics. New York: Oxford University Press; 2009.
30. Aiken W, LaFollette H. Whose child? Children's rights, parental authority, and state power. Totowa: Rowman and Littlefield. p. 1980.
31. Frith H, Harcourt D, Fussell A. Anticipating an altered appearance: women undergoing chemotherapy treatment for breast cancer. Eur J Oncol Nurs. 2007;11(5):385–91.
32. Stevens LA, McGrath MH, Druss RG, Kister SJ, Gump FE, Forde KA. The psychological impact of immediate breast reconstruction for women with early breast cancer. Plast Reconstr Surg. 1984;73(4):69–628.
33. Campo-Engelstein L. Insurance coverage for cancer treatment-induced conditions: comparing fertility preservation technology and breast reconstructive surgery. DePaul Law Rev. 2012;61(3):849–60.
34. Benedict C, Shuk E, Ford JS. Fertility issues in adolescent and young adult cancer survivors. J Adolesc Young Adult Oncol. 2016;5(1):48–57.
35. Gonçalves V, Sehovic I, Quinn G. Childbearing attitudes and decisions of young breast cancer survivors: a systematic review. Hum Reprod. 2014;20(2):279–92.
36. Howard-Anderson J, Ganz PA, Bower JE, Stanton AL. Quality of life, fertility concerns, and behavioral health outcomes in younger breast cancer survivors: a systematic review. J Natl Cancer Inst. 2012;104(5): 386–405.
37. Partridge AH, Gelber S, Peppercorn J, Sampson E, Knudsen K, Laufer M, Rosenberg R, Przypyszny M, Rein A, Winer EP. Web-based survey of fertility issues in young women with breast cancer. J Clin Oncol. 2004;22(20):4174–83.
38. Jeruss JS, Partridge AH. Use of tamoxifen by young women is influenced by fertility concerns. J Natl Cancer Inst. 2015;107(10):djv202.
39. Resolve. Infertility coverage by state. https://resolve.org/what-are-my-options/insurance-coverage/infertility-coverage-state/. Published 2018. Accessed 1 Aug 2018.
40. United Healthcare. Personal communication, February 1, 2018.
41. California Health Benefits Review Program (CHBRP). Analysis of assembly bill 219: health care coverage: cancer treatment. Oakland: CHBRP; 2013.
42. Skinner D. Defining medical necessity under the patient protection and affordable care act. Public Adm Rev. 2013;73(1):49–59.
43. American Medical Association. Statement of the American Medical Association to the Institute of Medicine's Committee on Determination of Essential Health Benefits. Washington, DC: AMA; 2011.
44. SART. AMA adopts ASRM sponsored resolution to designate infertility a disease.
45. Oktay K, Harvey BE, Partridge A, et al. Fertility preservation in patients with cancer: ASCO clinical practice guideline update. J Clin Onocol. 2018. https://doi.org/10.1200/JCO.2018.78.1914.
46. American Society of Reproductive Medicine. Fertility preservation and reproduction in patients facing gonadotoxic therapies: a committee opinion. Fertil Steril. 2013;100(5):1224–31.

47. Association AM. Oncofertility and fertility preservation treatment. http://www.ama-assn.org/ama/pub/news/news/2013/2013-06-17-new-ama-policies-annual-meeting.page. Published 2013.
48. California Department of Managed Healthcare. Internal Medical Review Decision, Reference ID: EI11-12274. Internal Medical Review Decision, Reference ID: EI11-12274. http://wpso.dmhc.ca.gov/imr.
49. California health benefits review program report, analysis of California Senate Bill 172 fertility preservation: a report to the 2017–2018 California State Legislature. 26.
50. Alliance for Fertility Preservation. How much does fertility preservation cost? http://www.alliancefor fertilitypreservation.org/costs/paying-for-treaments. Accessed 15 Aug 2018.
51. Novak D, Bender K. Annual mandate report: coverage for fertility preservation for iatrogenic infertility. 2017.
52. Klosky JL, et al. Prevalence and predictors of sperm banking in adolescents newly diagnosed with cancer: examination of adolescent, parent, and provider factors influencing fertility preservation outcomes. J Clin Onocol. 2017;35(34):3830–6.
53. Letourneau JM, Ebbel EE, Katz PP, et al. Pretreatment fertility counseling and fertility preservation improve quality of life in reproductive age women with cancer. Cancer. 2012;118(6):1710–7.
54. Blumen H, Fitch K, Polkus V. Comparison of treatment costs for breast cancer, by tumor stage and type of service. Am Health Drug Benefits. 2016;9(1):23–32.
55. Blue Cross Blue Shield of Massachusetts. Product portfolio and benefit design updates. 2009. https://www.bluecrossma.com/bluelinks-for-brokers/pdf/enews/06-2009/product-portfolio-and-benefit-design-update.pdf.
56. Hayes-Lattin B. Insurance coverage for fertility preservation – what can we do? In: Oncofertility Consortium Conference. Chicago; 2015.
57. Tran M. Apple and Facebook offer to freeze eggs for female employees. The Guardian. https://www.theguardian.com/technology/2014/oct/15/apple-facebook-offer-freeze-eggs-female-employees. Published 2014.
58. Hall G. These tech companies pay for egg-freezing as an employee benefit. Silicon Val Bus J. https://www.theguardian.com/technology/2014/oct/15/apple-facebook-offer-freeze-eggs-female-employees. Published 2017.
59. Veterans Health Administration. Infertility evaluation and treatment: veterans health directive 1332. Washington, DC: Veterans Health Administratio; 2017.
60. State of New Jersey. Senate Bill 1423. 2002. https://www.njleg.state.nj.us/2002/Bills/S1500/1423_I1.PDF.
61. State of New Jersey. Group health insurance policy to provide coverage for treatment of infertility, NJ Rev Stat § 17B:27-46.1x. 2013.
62. State of Connecticut. An act requiring health insurance coverage for fertility preservation for insureds diagnosed with cancer: HB 7124. 2017. https://www.cga.ct.gov/2017/TOB/h/2017HB-05968-R01-HB.htm.
63. State of Rhode Island. An act relating to insurance-coverage for infertility, § 27-20-20 A. 2017.
64. State of Connecticut. An act requiring health insurance coverage for fertility preservation for insureds diagnosed with cancer: HB 7124. 2005.
65. Arditi L. RI requires coverage for 'fertility preservation' by private insurers. Providence J. http://www.providencejournal.com/news/20170801/ri-requires-coverage-for-fertility-preservation-by-private-insurers. Published 2017.
66. California Department of Managed Health Care Staff. Private communication. 2018.
67. State of Maryland. Health insurance – coverage of fertility preservation procedures for iatrogenic infertility, HB 908. 2018.
68. Insurance CD-Fertility Preservation: HB 2617. 2018.
69. State of Maryland. Maryland Insurance Code Ann §15–810. 2000.
70. State of Delaware. An act to amend title 18 of the Delaware code relating to insurance coverage for obstetrical and gynecological services: Senate Bill 139. 2018. https://legis.delaware.gov/BillDetail?LegislationId=26219.
71. State of New Jersey. An act concerning health benefits coverage for fertility preservation services under certain health insurance plans and supplementing various parts of statutory law, Assembly Bill 3150. 2018.
72. State of New Jersey. An act concerning health benefits coverage for fertility preservation services under certain health insurance plans and supplementing various parts of statutory law, Senate Bill 2133. 2018.
73. Employee Retirement Income Security Act of 1974. 1974.
74. Employee Benefit Research Institute. ERISA preemption: implications for health reform and coverage. https://www.ebri.org/publications/ib/index.cfm?fa=ibDisp&content_id=3879. Published 2008. Accessed 20 Aug 2018.
75. Wade K. Health insurance coverage for infertility treatment and procedures—Conn. Gen. Stat. § 38a-509 and § 38a-536. 2015. http://www.ct.gov/cid/lib/cid/BulletinHC-104-InfertilityTreatmentandProcedures.pdf.
76. State of Connecticut Insurance Department. Health insurance coverage for infertility treatment and procedures—Conn. Gen. Stat. § 38a-509 and § 38a-536. 2015. http://www.ct.gov/cid/lib/cid/BulletinHC-104-InfertilityTreatmentandProcedures.pdf.
77. California Department of Managed Healthcare. Internal Medical Review Decision, References IDs: MN17-26855; MN17-27049; MN17-26920; MN17-2718.
78. California Department of Managed Healthcare. Internal Medical Review, Reference ID: MN17-27186.
79. American Society of Reproductive Medicine. California Department of Managed Health Care determines fertility preservation is a covered benefit under existing law. ASRM Bull. 2018;20(3).
80. Walter JR, Shuai X, Woodruff TK. A call for fertility preservation coverage for breast cancer patients: the cost of consistency. J Natl Cancer Ins. 2017;109(5). https://doi.org/10.1093/jnci/djx006.
81. Cardozo ER, Huber J, Stuckey AR, Alvero RJ. Mandating coverage for fertility preservation – a step in the right direction. New Engl J Med. 2017;377:1607–9.

Ethical and Legal Considerations in Oncofertility

Contents

Legal Issues in Oncofertility Treatment

Susan L. Crockin

The author would like to thank her former student, Jennifer Madrid, JD, for her invaluable assistance in preparing this chapter.

T. K. Woodruff et al. (eds.), *Textbook of Oncofertility Research and Practice*,
https://doi.org/10.1007/978-3-030-02868-8_28

28

Key Points

- Informed consent and dispositional contracts are separate, critical legal protections for fertility preservation patients undergoing assisted reproduction.
- State laws vary and impact both access to cryopreserved genetic material and parent-child status in any posthumous reproduction.
- Laws mandating coverage for fertility preservation for oncofertility patients are expanding.
- Third-party reproduction in the form of surrogacy and gamete donation is a legally complex and ever-changing family building option that requires current, experienced, objective and jurisdictionally specific legal guidance.

28.1 Introduction

With advances in cancer treatments dramatically improving survival rates for children, adolescents and young adults (AYA), and child-bearing age cancer patients, fertility preservation has become an increasingly relevant consideration and integral aspect of treatment plans, as this book attests. Studies show that oncology patients want to discuss fertility preservation as part of their treatment plans, and the American Society of Clinical Oncology (ASCO) guidelines recommend addressing the possibility of infertility as early as possible and before treatment starts [1]. In recent years, In Vitro Fertilization (IVF) and other Assisted Reproductive Technologies (ART) have significantly expanded the number of available fertility preservation options and concomitant legal issues. Current standard of care for fertility preservation for post-pubescent males and females involves preservation of sperm and eggs, with the latter requiring an IVF procedure [1]. For pre-pubescent males and females, still experimental protocols offer the possibility of ovarian or testicular tissue cryopreservation with potential future thaw, maturation, fertilization, and implantation of resulting IVF embryos. This chapter explores the legal issues attendant to currently available, experimental, and future potential fertility preservation protocols.

While any medical procedure can raise legal and ethical issues, fertility preservation raises a number of unique legal issues given its implications for reproductive and future parentage rights. What techniques, on whom, and requiring whose informed consent; who has the right to access and use any cryopreserved genetic material in the future in the event of divorce or death; and the legal relationships created from any such use, are some of the most significant and novel of those issues [2].

For patients who are coupled, a decision to create and cryopreserve embryos with both partners' genetic material inextricably links two individuals to one another's reproductive future. Men have long been able to avoid these legal vulnerabilities through cryopreserving sperm in lieu of embryos. Recent advances in cryopreserving eggs may offer women the ability to avoid these legal vulnerabilities as well. For any fertility preservation patient, there will be the risk that their stored material may not produce a future pregnancy, or may be lost, damaged, or destroyed, thus depriving them of their opportunity to create a biologically linked family and potentially leading them to utilize donor gametes. Since gametes or embryos can be, and in some instances have been, cryopreserved for over 20 years [3], a child may be born from a patient's genetic material long after his or her death, presenting novel legal questions of posthumous reproduction and posthumous parentage [4].

Minor patients incapable of giving legal informed consent raise more unique legal issues over their future reproductive potential and the need for specific protocols to address them. Two central tenets of informed consent law are that a medical procedure requires informed consent and must offer the patient a potential benefit [5]. In pediatric cases, except for those whom the law deems "mature minors," a legal parent or guardian must give consent for the child (with the child giving "assent" to the treatment if capable of doing so), and, while there is some variation in applicable legal theories, any such consent needs to be clearly for the minor patient's own anticipated benefit [6].

Finally, third-party ART may be necessary for some patients who desire a biological child but who, despite undergoing fertility preservation measures, may be unable to carry a pregnancy or use their own gametes. Third parties may include a genetic (traditional) surrogate or gestational surrogate carrier, and/or sperm, egg or embryo donors. Each of those possibilities gives rise to a variety of legal issues for patients and providers.

This chapter highlights the unique legal issues surrounding fertility preservation, including: legal issues of informed consent and autonomy; embryo disputes; current, relevant legislation and case law surrounding access to insurance coverage for fertility preservation; posthumous reproduction; and third-party reproduction.

28.2 Fertility Preservation for Adult Patients

28.2.1 Men

For most post-pubertal males, fertility preservation is relatively simple, time efficient, and effective. Sperm can typically be obtained without the need for invasive procedures, or creating embryos, as sperm has been successfully cryopreserved for decades. As such, standard protocols for sperm retrieval and storage will typically not delay or impact treatment, and avoid the legal vulnerabilities attendant to creating and later being able to use embryos, as discussed infra. To the extent obtaining sperm need not involve a medical procedure or medical facility, there may also be limitations on the applicability of health law.

28.2.2 Women

For females, fertility preservation is inherently more complicated, both medically and legally, since egg retrieval requires medical stimulation and retrieval procedures and, before recent advances in egg freezing through vitrification, routinely involved fertilization (from a male partner or donor) and creation of embryos for cryopreservation. For oncofertility patients, although the stimulation protocol may be altered and the time line reduced, effective fertility preservation can still potentially delay or impact their cancer treatment. Compared to sperm retrieval, this oocyte or embryo banking is physically invasive, time-consuming, and costly (see the following section for emerging state laws mandating insurance for this procedure).

In 2012, the American Society for Reproductive Medicine (ASRM) removed the "experimental" label from oocyte cryopreservation technology, finding that there is "good evidence that fertilization and pregnancy rates are similar to IVF...with fresh oocytes when vitrified/warmed oocytes are used." [7] Notwithstanding that categorization, for a number of years prior to 2012, oocyte cryopreservation had been done with some regularity in a number of IVF programs [8]. Currently, whether all oocytes are cryopreserved without fertilization, or whether all or some are first fertilized to create embryos, may partly depend on the expertise and experience of the specific IVF physician, embryologist, and lab [9]. From a legal perspective, egg freezing puts females on equal footing with males, allowing them to control their individual future fertility and avoid disputes over who controls IVF cryopreserved embryos. For pre-pubescent females, ovarian tissue cryopreservation, while currently considered experimental, may be the only viable option for attempting fertility preservation [10]. According to ASCO guidelines, "the field of ovarian tissue cryopreservation is advancing quickly and may evolve to become standard therapy in the future." [1]

28.3 State Legislation Mandating Insurance Coverage of Fertility Preservation

Since 2017, five states have passed laws mandating insurance coverage of fertility preservation procedures for patients potentially facing iatrogenic infertility. Connecticut, Rhode Island, Illnois and Maryland expanded existing infertility mandates. Delaware enacted a new law mandating coverage for both infertility and fertility preservation, including storage costs [11]. These laws each have certain specific caveats and exclusions that are beyond the scope of this overview, and patients and providers should carefully review their state's requirements. As of publication time, two additional states have pending fertility preservation legislation, and eight others have inactive legislation.[1]

1 As of press time, IL passed its law Aug. 2019, NJ has pending active fertility preservation legislation, and AZ, CA, HI, KY, LA, MS, MO, NY and VT have inactive pending bills (see ► http://www.allianceforfertility-preservation.org/advocacy/state-legislation for more information).

In June 2017, Connecticut became the first state to enact legislation on fertility preservation coverage [12]. The law removes from the mandate's statutory definition of infertility the words "a presumably healthy" (from "the condition of a presumably healthy individual who is unable to conceive or produce conception or sustain a successful pregnancy during a 1-year period") and adds additional language "or such treatment is medically necessary," so that infertility is now defined as, "the condition of an individual who is unable to conceive or produce conception or sustain a successful pregnancy during a one-year period or such treatment is medically necessary,"[2] which presumably includes iatrogenic infertility due to impending cancer treatment.

Rhode Island amended its existing infertility mandate that private insurers must offer coverage for infertility treatments to also include coverage "...for standard fertility preservation services when a medically necessary medical treatment may directly or indirectly cause iatrogenic infertility to a covered person." [13] "Standard fertility preservation services" are defined in the statute as the established medical practices and professional guidelines published by ASRM, ASCO, or other reputable medical organizations [13]. As such, covered services may expand if and as professional recommendations and guidelines are updated.

In May 2018, Maryland became the third state to expand its infertility mandate, effective January 1, 2019. The law includes a requirement that insurers provide coverage for standard fertility preservation services, excluding any storage costs, when medically necessary due to the risk of iatrogenic infertility [14].

Delaware passed new legislation in June 2018 mandating coverage for both general infertility and fertility preservation services for patients facing iatrogenic fertility (including the cost of storing sperm, eggs, embryos, and tissue), making it the 16th state in the nation to mandate some form of insurance coverage for infertility treatment and the 4th requiring such coverage for fertility preservation services [15].

2 For an illustration of the changes made to the CT infertility mandate, see the CT General assembly website at ▸ https://www.cga.ct.gov/2017/lcoamd/pdf/2017LCO07854-R00-AMD.PDF.

These legislative examples, as well as ASCO's 2018 "key recommendations," may provide helpful support to advocates looking to expand mandatory access to fertility preservation [1].

28.4 Informed Consent: Unique Issues for Fertility Preservation

As a general legal and ethical principle, physicians must obtain a competent adult patient's informed consent prior to performing any medical treatment, otherwise any treatment would result in the physician committing a battery under common law [16]. IVF patients routinely provide informed consent prior to undergoing gamete retrieval, embryo creation, fertility preservation via cryopreservation of gametes and/or embryos, and the transfer or implantation of any such genetic material [17]. In some states, such as California, failure to obtain required consent or unauthorized use of genetic material can expose a physician to criminal penalties as well as potential civil, tort liability [18]. The issue of informed consent for minor patients presents a more complex legal and ethical analysis that will be discussed separately below in ▸ Sect. 28.3 of this chapter.

Assisted reproduction or ART raises unique legal issues for all patients because of the singular nature of reproductive tissue and its potential to create a new life, as well as the possibility that two patients may have reproductive tissue inseparably preserved in an IVF pre-implantation embryo. For oncofertility patients, informed consent for fertility preservation treatment raises additional issues as to the relative risks and benefits of various options, including clinic specific v. national data as to freezing embryos and gametes, unique dispositional options and legal impact for the patient or any surviving partner or other designated individual, as well as the risks and benefits of any delay in cancer treatment [19].

28.5 Informed Consent Law v. Contract Law

Both ART treatments and disposition of genetic material resulting from those treatments continue to be a rapidly evolving area of medicine and law. Informed consent documents for treatment and cryopreservation of reproductive tissue may or may not include future dispositional choices for cryopreserved gametes and embryos. Increasingly, future dispositional choices are being treated by medical programs, professional guidelines (and their model documents), storage facilities, patients, and courts as an integrally related, but distinct, matter, addressed in separate dispositional agreements and interpreted under the law of contracts rather than informed consent [20]. The legal distinction between informed consent prior to performing a medical procedure on a patient and obtaining a patient's authorization as to how his or her gametes or embryos may, or may not, be used in the future, has been the subject of litigation and the characterization of those documents, as discussed below, may be legally determinative. Use of donor sperm or eggs to create embryos adds further legal complexities. In the context of fertility preservation immediately prior to cancer treatment, the issues are obviously heightened since the sole purpose of the medical procedure may be to make genetic material available for future procreative use.

Both statutory and case law is developing around this distinction. California has enacted legislation mandating that healthcare providers offering fertility treatment provide patients with a form setting forth advanced written directives for embryo disposition, including certain minimum options under a variety of scenarios [21]. SART has created (and continues to update) model documents for its professional members, which include separate informed consent documents to treatment and dispositional agreements for genetic material to be customized in accordance with state law as recommended by local state legal counsel [22].

Counseling a patient as to his or her options for disposition of gametes or embryos, separate from the medical treatment, can be as much legal as medical in nature, and clinics referring for, or engaging in, fertility preservation practices would be prudent to recommend patients also obtain legal counseling prior to completing any clinic's dispositional agreement to better understand the critical legal implications of their options and choices. For embryo cryopreservation, it also may be advisable for coupled patients to obtain separate legal counseling, and/or create additional legal documents, to help address any potential future conflicts of interest or relatively different rights to conjoined genetic material. Although time is often of the essence, and any such recommendations may not be followed, offering and documenting them would be both a cautious and protective practice.

28.6 Legal Embryo Disputes

Embryo-related legal disputes have arisen in a number of contexts in the United States[3]: between divorcing couples over frozen embryos (created with both patients' own genetic material, and thus each is a progenitor, or with donor sperm or eggs); surrounding posthumous reproduction where a surviving progenitor, non-progenitor partner, or another family member is seeking to use a deceased's genetic material, as well as the legal status of any posthumously born child; and in a myriad of scenarios involving mix-ups and loss or damage to embryos and gametes. This section highlights illustrative court cases in some of these areas most relevant to patients facing iatrogenic infertility and considering fertility preservation. It is important to note that, with one exception involving posthumous reproduction, the United States Supreme Court has never addressed these issues, so the cases discussed in this chapter only have precedential value, or apply, in their own state and serve solely as advisory guidance in other jurisdictions.

The trend in over 20 appellate cases over the past 25 years has generally been to favor the progenitor who does not want embryos used to procreate over the wishes of the other, at least where there is no specific agreement to the contrary (with the clinic or otherwise) [23]. Where there are signed consent forms or legal agreements, however, the outcomes and legal theories supporting them have varied. These cases highlight both the importance of clear documentation and evidence of intent consistent with applicable state law, and the reality that cryopreserving gametes

3 Embryo and gamete losses, mix-ups, or damage cases are beyond the scope of this chapter; however, it should be noted that in the event of any such cases, the measure of damages for oncofertility patients who cannot readily replace any lost, damaged, discarded, or misused genetic material is likely to be higher than other scenarios. Both reported cases and damages amounts are difficult to identify since most cases are resolved through confidential settlement agreements.

instead of embryos would alleviate the dependency and vulnerability of patients to their former partners under future circumstances.

In 1992, the first, seminal case of *Davis v. Davis*, was decided by the Tennessee Supreme Court. *Davis* addressed a divorcing couple's disagreement over embryo disposition where the wife first sought to use, and ultimately to donate to another couple, remaining cryopreserved embryos contrary to the husband's wishes [24]. Because the parties had not entered into a dispositional agreement at the clinic, the court performed a balancing test based on each individual's constitutional right to privacy. The court found that the burden of unwanted genetic parenthood for the husband outweighed the wife's interest in allowing another couple to use the embryos, and, in the absence of an agreement to the contrary, his right not to procreate should trump her right to procreate [25]. The court took note that the wife had the capacity to have genetic children through IVF if she so chose [25].

Since 1992, a myriad of appellate courts have applied a variety of legal rationales to come to similar outcomes under their state law [26]. One often cited case is *A.Z. v. B.Z.*, where the Massachusetts Supreme Court, that state's highest court, found that even though a former married couple had signed several agreements with their IVF program stating the wife would be given the embryos if the couple "separated", any agreement that resulted in forced parentage was void as against public policy [27]. The New Jersey Supreme Court followed and cited *A.Z.* in the case of *J.B. v. M.B.*, allowing an ex-wife to veto her husband's desire to donate their unused embryos [28]. Interestingly, that court noted that even if *legal* parentage would be transferred to the recipients, forcing unwanted *biological* parentage would be an unfair burden on the woman [29].

Not surprisingly, a number of embryo disputes involve cancer survivors, since patients who still have a future opportunity to have biological children would likely choose to produce more gametes or embryos rather than embark on protracted, expensive, and uncertain court battles. Although few appellate courts have done so, some lower courts have expressed sympathy toward a cancer survivor with only "last chance embryos" and, at least absent signed documents opposing such an outcome, have granted use over a former partner's objections. The following cases illustrate courts' varying approaches and the critical role enforceable agreements can play.

A 2012 Pennsylvania trial court in *Reber v. Reiss* sided with an ex-wife who had undergone IVF with her then husband for purposes of fertility preservation prior to commencing cancer treatment and afterward wished to use the embryos despite her former husband wanting them destroyed [30]. The couple had not signed the section of the consent form at the IVF clinic that addressed how the embryos would be handled in the event of divorce, so the court balanced the interests of both parties as done in *Davis v. Davis* and *J.B. v. M.B* [31]. The court distinguished its case on the grounds that the wife likely had no ability to become a biological parent without using the embryos, finding that her interest in procreation outweighed her ex-husband's interest in avoiding procreation, and also noted that Pennsylvania public policy did not prohibit forced biological parenthood under the specific circumstances of the case [32].

In 2015, the intermediate, Appellate Court of Illinois decided *Szafranski v. Dunston*. The case involved an unmarried couple who had been together only a short time, the woman was significantly older than the man, and the couple had undergone IVF as a means of fertility preservation prior to her undergoing treatment for lymphoma which was expected to render her infertile [33]. The clinic's consent form did not specify embryo disposition elections in the event the couple separated, with the clinic instead believing that matter was a distinct legal issue beyond the scope of a standard informed consent form that needed to be detailed in a separate document prepared by an attorney [34]. The court found that there was an enforceable *oral* contract between the parties that the woman could use the embryos for procreation without limitation, including if they were no longer a couple, and without the man's consent at the time of use [35]. Although noting that a balancing test was moot in light of its finding of an advance oral agreement regarding embryo disposition, the court nonetheless concluded that the woman's interest in using embryos created specifically for the purpose of preserving her ability to have a biological child and representing her only possibility for achieving that goal outweighed any subsequently expressed interest her ex-partner had in preventing her from using them [36].

A 2015 California trial court case, *Findley v. Lee,* illustrates the impact of a carefully crafted dispositional agreement, properly executed in accordance with applicable state law. That court found conclusive a clinic's dispositional agreement (distinct from its informed consent related to the IVF procedures) in which the couple clearly agreed the embryos would be destroyed in the event of a divorce, even though the IVF was undertaken because of a breast cancer diagnosis in an effort to preserve fertility [37]. That court carefully reviewed California's requirements for a legal contract, found that the clinic's form was drafted in accordance with the requirements of California Health and Safety Code Section 125315 enacted for the purpose of regulating IVF clinics' dispositional agreements, and thus was enforceable as a valid contract [37].

There have been some legislative efforts to clarify embryo use and parentage. The 2017 Uniform Parentage Act (UPA 2017) is a nonbinding, model law which state legislatures may choose to enact in its entirety or in part. Washington and Vermont have adopted it and several other states are considering as of press time.[4] UPA 2017 addresses situations where a person may enter into reproductive treatment and later change his or her mind about proceeding. It states that a person who initially consents to participate in assisted reproduction with the intent of parenting a resulting child may withdraw consent before a pregnancy is achieved through an embryo transfer procedure [38] and that he or she will no longer be deemed the future-conceived child's parent [39]. Because UPA 2017 was drafted as a model family law it does not address under what circumstances the remaining intended parent may or may not use the genetic material.

Legislation enacted in 2018 in Arizona throws into question whether even a clear dispositional agreement will be honored. That law, which may be subject to challenge under constitutional principles [40], explicitly gives a divorce court the authority to provide embryos to "the spouse who intends to allow" them to "develop to birth," regardless of any prior consents or agreements [41]. The law does not address parentage or best interests of any resulting child, and should prove problematic for Arizona clinics and patients who wish to respectively offer and provide their own, deliberate, dispositional choices as to future procreation. The law was enacted in reaction to a lawsuit in which a female cancer survivor lost her court case to use cryopreserved embryos where she and her ex-husband had agreed such use would require their mutual consent [42]. The statute may not have the intended effect since it favors whichever progenitor is more likely to bring the embryos to life, an argument any healthy former partner can make. The law provides yet another example of why storing gametes individually may better protect individual procreative autonomy.

28.7 Posthumous Reproduction

ART and posthumous reproduction raise unique legal issues. This section will review posthumous access to, and use of, gametes or embryos of a deceased, and the legal status of any child resulting from those gametes or embryos. Beyond the scope of this chapter are legal issues presented by requests to *extract* gametes from dead or comatose patients in the absence of explicit prior consent or instructions from those individuals.

28.7.1 Access

For any surviving spouse, partner, or other third party seeking to use a deceased's genetic material for procreative purposes, having the deceased's clear, prior authorization during their life in a legally recognized, memorialized dispositional agreement which clearly reflects their intentions, will provide the best assurance of the genetic material being used in accordance with those expressed wishes, as the cases below illustrate. A 2018 ASRM Ethics Committee opinion suggests that, absent explicit instructions, medical providers may wish to abide by a surviving partner's request for access but not those from others, family or otherwise [43]. Those few state courts that have been presented with the issue have emphasized the importance of the deceased having

4 UPA 2017 has been adopted in whole or in part by Washington state and Vermont, is under consideration in several state legislatures and in April, 2018 was endorsed unanimously by the National Child Support Enforcement Association [NCSEA], Resolution Endorsing Uniform Parentage Act (2017), 4/26/18; for text, information, and updates see ► http://www.uniformlaws.org/.

provided, or at a minimum evidenced, such authorization during life, as the following cases illustrate.

In 2008, the California Court of Appeal refused a widow's request to use her deceased husband's stored sperm from previous IVF attempts, instead honoring his intent as indicated by his choice in what the court referred to as a clinic "consent agreement" that his sperm sample be destroyed upon his death [44]. The Court also noted that because the deceased was the only progenitor, as the sperm had not been used to create embryos, only he had "an interest, in the nature of ownership, to the extent that he had decisionmaking authority as to the use of his sperm for reproduction" and that the wife's procreative autonomy was therefore not implicated in destroying the sperm [45].

The Court quoted and followed a 1993 California Court of Appeal ruling, *Hecht v. Superior Court,* where the court ruled that a deceased's intent regarding use of his sperm for procreative purposes controlled in the disposition of his frozen sperm after death, thus allowing his girlfriend to use his sperm for posthumous reproduction, against his adult children's wishes [46]. The agreement the decedent had signed at the sperm bank authorized his sperm samples to be released to his girlfriend [47]. Further, his will named her as executor of his estate and reiterated that she could use the sperm samples for procreation after his death if she so wished [47]. Before committing suicide, he wrote a note to his two adult children indicating the possibility, and his hope, that his current girlfriend would bear his child posthumously [48]. The court found that in light of the decedent being the proper decision-maker in regards to his sperm's use, the Superior Court had abused its discretion in ordering the destruction of the sperm samples, and further noted that posthumous insemination did not violate public policy and should not be prohibited on that basis [49].

28.7.2 Legal Parent-Child Status

Another significant legal issue in posthumous reproduction is the resulting child's legal status, specifically whether they are legally considered the child of the deceased, and thus entitled to survivorship benefits under federal law. Starting in 2002, a number of courts confronted such claims of parentage, resulting in contradictory decisions in accordance with different states' laws, and in 2012, the US Supreme Court agreed to take a case, *Astrue v. Capato*, to attempt to reconcile these discrepancies [50].

In *Astrue*, the Supreme Court answered the question of whether a posthumously conceived child should be legally recognized as the child of a deceased for purposes of Social Security survivor's benefit entitlements. The Court ruled that these federal benefits flow to legally recognized dependents, as determined by state intestacy law [51]. The decision thus leaves to individual states, rather than creating a federal standard, the issue of whether or not a child conceived or born posthumously from the genetic material of a deceased domiciliary of that state will be considered a legal child of the decedent, eligible to inherit and consequently, entitled to receive federal Social Security benefits [52].

State intestacy variations will therefore continue, as illustrated by two cases from neighboring states with different outcomes. In 2002, the Massachusetts Supreme Judicial Court found in *Woodward v. Commissioner of Social Security* that a claimant must prove three elements (assuming the claim is filed timely): (1) a genetic relationship between the child and the decedent; (2) the decedent unequivocally consented not only to posthumous reproduction; but also to (3) supporting the resulting child [53]. The court noted the deceased's silence or ambiguous consent to posthumous reproduction was insufficient, and that freezing gametes during life did not constitute implied consent to procreating posthumously [54]. In 2007, the Supreme Court of New Hampshire came to a different conclusion, finding that "surviving issue" in the state's intestacy statute refers only to children "alive" or "in existence" at the time of the decedent's death, thus excluding by definition any posthumously conceived children, regardless of the deceased's consent to posthumous reproduction and intent to be deemed the parent of the resulting child [55].

Some state legislatures,[5] and UPA 2017, have offered clear guidance on this question, with UPA 2017 stating that a decedent may be considered a

5 *See Astrue v. Capato*, 566 U.S. 541, 555 (2012) for examples of state statutes addressing inheritance rights for children conceived posthumously.

parent when: (1) gametes or embryos are transferred after death where the deceased either consented on the record to posthumous assisted reproduction with the intent of being considered a parent or this intent is established by clear and convincing evidence; (2) the embryos are transferred within 36 months postmortem; or (3) the child is born within 45 months of the decedent's death [56].

28.8 Third Party Reproduction as Affecting Oncofertility/Fertility Preservation Patients

Third-party assisted reproduction refers to family building techniques that include genetic or gestational contributions from individuals who are not intended parents, including sperm, egg, or embryo donors, and genetic or gestational surrogates, and may offer a path to parenthood for some oncofertility patients. While this section highlights legal issues specifically pertinent to third-party assisted reproduction for fertility preservation patients, this is a legally complex, often extremely costly, and constantly changing assortment of family building options. In addition to specific ART law, it can involve health, contract, insurance, conflicts and choice of law, and for international arrangements, additional and nuanced immigration, citizenship, and health insurance laws. Because both ART-related legislation and case law are extremely fluid and state specific, references to any laws in this section should be considered illustrative, rather than exhaustive and should always be confirmed for current accuracy and applicability. Those recommending or considering these options can find in-depth legal analysis of third-party family building options in numerous articles, and scholarly and other resources, and will also want to carefully investigate any potential options to help ensure patients are working with appropriately licensed, independent, ethical, and experienced professionals.

28.8.1 Surrogacy

Surrogacy may be an option for female cancer survivors who cannot carry a pregnancy, especially for those with previously cryopreserved gametes or embryos. This discussion focuses on gestational surrogacy, the more legally secure and widely acceptable form of surrogacy, rather than genetic (also known as traditional) surrogacy. In gestational surrogacy, the gestational surrogate, also known as a gestational carrier, undergoes an IVF embryo transfer, not using her own egg, and thus is not directly genetically related to the resulting child. The embryo is either genetically that of one or both of the intended parents as progenitors, or may have been donated or formed using donor egg and/or donor sperm. Gestational surrogacy is governed by individual state laws, which vary dramatically across the country. There is a growing trend in state laws toward recognizing gestational surrogacy arrangements as consistent with public policy, and recognizing the intended parents as the legal parents of the child from or close to the time of birth, at least where the arrangements are carried out in accordance with legal protections established by applicable state statutory or case law [57].

Typically, states permitting gestational surrogacy arrangements will have a legal framework both for structuring contracts, and for a legal process to ensure legal parentage upon the child's birth and ideally have the intended, legal parents' names appear on the child's initial birth certificate [57].[6] The agreements may have statutorily required components: as one example, UPA 2017 includes minimum age requirements for surrogates, at least one live birth for a surrogate, independent legal counsel for each party, agreement as to number of embryos to transfer, provisions and criteria for any possible selective reduction or termination, autonomy around pregnancy decision-making for the surrogate, and clear compensation that avoids any suggestion of illegal baby buying or selling [39].

Laws addressing parentage orders usually involve a court order and judgment of parentage effective upon the birth of the child, or variation thereof [39], although in some states, such as Illinois, there may be an administrative process eliminating the need to obtain a court

6 Examples of states with such legislation include: CA, CT (only as to birth certificates), DC, IL, ME, NJ, NV, WA; examples of states with similar frameworks developed through judicial decisions rather than legislation, include MA, CT (only as to agreements) and, to a less comprehensive extent, PA.

judgment [58]. States also vary as to whether or not at least one of the intended parents must be genetically related to the child by providing either eggs or sperm.[7]

A few states still prohibit compensated surrogacy, such as Michigan and New York, or otherwise have laws making the state undesirable for pursuing gestational surrogacy arrangements.[8] Both New Jersey and the District of Columbia had long prohibited compensated surrogacy, but in 2018 both enacted legislation recognizing compensated surrogacy arrangements [59]. New York has had legislation introduced and debated for over 7 years, with a 2018 bill pending as of publication time which would allow compensated surrogacy [60]. Interstate arrangements are common, but can be legally complex, especially where intended parents from "surrogacy unfriendly" states work with a gestational carrier who resides in a "surrogacy friendly" state in accordance with those laws, necessitating experienced ART legal counsel to ensure what are applicable laws and how to comply with them to protect vulnerable parties.

Both the laws and practices surrounding gestational surrogacy are complex and constantly changing, and medical providers should recommend their patients consult experienced ART attorneys specializing in, or knowledgeable about, surrogacy in the relevant jurisdictions to understand the nuances of this option. To complicate matters, in some states, statutory and common law may be silent on the subject of surrogacy, neither establishing a legal framework for pursuing such arrangements nor prohibiting them [57]. International surrogacy exponentially increases these complexities, and requires sophisticated knowledge and advice of not only current surrogacy law, but immigration and citizenship laws.

Would-be parents via surrogacy will also want to be vigilant and informed as to the potential for conflicts of interest among ART professionals, as well as the availability or nonavailability of insurance for related healthcare expenses, and possible protections such as third-party escrow accounts to hopefully protect the extraordinary costs and expenses that can be associated with this family-building option. Experienced ART attorneys licensed in the appropriate state, states, or countries should have the requisite knowledge, skill, and professional independence to structure and negotiate, with independent counsel for each party a legally compliant and well-thought-out contract to minimize the vulnerabilities that can surround the surrogacy process, to counsel as to expenses and minimizing financial risks, and to advise their clients where and how a surrogacy arrangement may be entered into as legally secure as possible for all parties involved, including the resulting child [61].

28.8.2 Donor Sperm

For male cancer survivors who are not able to produce or store sperm before treatment, sperm donation remains an option as it does for female cancer survivors without fertile male partners. Unlike egg banks, sperm banks with cryopreserved sperm have been commercially available for many decades. As such, the majority of states have long had laws, largely based on earlier versions of the UPA, that clarify a sperm donor is not a parent [62]. Most of these statutes, however, are limited to protecting the paternity rights of the recipient male, and predate IVF and cryopreservation. As such, few address newer standards of care such as

7 Some examples include IL, HI, KS, MA and NC. However, every surrogacy case, even within a state, can be very fact and circumstance-specific, and parties should consult with experienced legal counsel before proceeding.

8 Michigan Surrogate Parenting Act, § 722.857(2) (1988), "A person other than an unemancipated minor female or a female diagnosed as being intellectually disabled or as having a mental illness or developmental disability who enters into, induces, arranges, procures, or otherwise assists in the formation of a contract described in subsection (1) is guilty of a felony punishable by a fine of not more than $50,000.00 or imprisonment for not more than 5 years, or both."; N.Y. Dom. Rel. § 123, "No person or other entity shall knowingly request, accept, receive, pay or give any fee, compensation or other remuneration, directly or indirectly, in connection with any surrogate parenting contract, or induce, arrange or otherwise assist in arranging a surrogate parenting contract for a fee, compensation or other remuneration, except for (a) payments in connection with the adoption of a child permitted by ▸ subdivision six of section three hundred seventy-four of the social services law and disclosed pursuant to ▸ subdivision eight of section one hundred fifteen of this chapter; or (b) payments for reasonable and actual medical fees and hospital expenses for artificial insemination or in vitro fertilization services incurred by the mother in connection with the birth of the child."

counseling or rights to cryopreserved sperm or embryos made with them. For some, family members may be an option to consider as a donor. As with known egg donors, both medical and mental health evaluation and/or counseling should be utilized and are best practices [63]. To ensure all parties understand their roles and obligations, and to clarify legal parentage of the intended parents and the lack of parentage for the donor, a legal agreement is strongly recommended, and in many instances required, by ART clinics.

28.8.3 Donor Eggs

Given the relative newness of egg donation and even more recently cryopreserved egg banking, there are fewer statutes explicitly addressing the legal status of egg donors, banked donor eggs, or embryos created from donated eggs. In approximately 14 states[9], and in UPA 2017 [64], laws seek to clarify the legal parent-child status of children born via egg donation, and the non-parental status of egg donors. Very little law exists in the United States on whether a donor has a right to change their mind over donated but as yet unused and unfertilized, cryopreserved eggs or sperm. One unusual example can be found in the New York reproductive tissue bank regulations, which explicitly require that donors' informed consent include, "a statement that the reproductive tissue donor has the right to withdraw his/her consent to donation up until such time that a specific recipient has begun an assisted reproduction cycle in reliance on the availability of tissue from that donor." [65] What constitutes reliance, or how far such a regulation extends when a New York donor's frozen gametes may be shipped and used in other states is not addressed.

Egg donors may be family, friends, or commercially matched donors through medical programs, donor recruiting or coordinating programs (sometimes referred to as "agencies" although there are currently no licensing requirements), or increasingly through egg banks with an inventory of frozen eggs. Medical and mental health evaluation for the donor, psychoeducational counseling for recipients, and executing documents that "define or limit their rights and duties as to any offspring" are all part of the applicable professional guidelines [66]. For matched donors and recipients, including commercially matched, family and friends, a legal agreement with independent counsel for each party may be most protective and help avoid later disputes [61]. With previously frozen, banked eggs, without a direct link between donors and intended parents, however, there is no opportunity for such an agreement.

Egg donation costs may vary depending on multiple factors, and no general figures can be reliable. Obviously, unpaid donors such as family and friends will avoid the costs of donor compensation, but medical evaluations and testing, medication, and other costs are still significant. Many matching programs and egg banks have websites where current and updated estimated costs can be found. While much media attention, and criticism, has surrounded the potential for compensation to be coercive or unduly influential, the reality is that those who are close to an intended parent such as a family member or friend, can feel pressured or be emotionally reluctant, to undertake this process, and mental health screening, independent legal counsel and an agreement are professionally recommended protections for all parties [61].

28.9 Minors

With the remarkable advances in cancer therapies, most children and adolescents diagnosed with cancer now survive their cancer [67]. Survivors may be faced with damage to the reproductive system and resulting impaired fertility [68]. For post-pubertal minors, gametes can be cryopreserved using the same means as adults, with females undergoing hormone stimulation to produce multiple eggs for extraction, and resultant time delays for the start of treatment [68] have been significantly reduced in recent years. For pre-pubertal patients, cryopreservation of gonadal tissue may be attempted; although still considered experimental, as noted above, ovarian tissue cryopreservation is advancing quickly and may become standard therapy in the future [69].

The United States Constitution protects the right to procreate [70], although this does not necessarily equate to a right to access medical treat-

9 While the number is likely to increase as states consider adopting UPA 2017 in whole or in part, current states with statutes clarifying an egg donor is not a parent include: CA, CO, CT, FL, LA, ND, NY, OK, OR, TX, UT, VA, WA, WY.

ment to aid in procreation. In general, a minor's right to access birth control without the need for parental consent is recognized by the majority of states [71]. The US Supreme Court has also recognized minors' rights not to be forced to carry a pregnancy by a parent or guardian, and the US Supreme Court has recognized judicial review procedures to protect minors if their parents refuse to consent to, or a minor is unwilling to involve her parents in, an abortion she seeks [72].

Several legal, and intertwined ethical, issues arise in the context of fertility preservation for minor patients, including their capacity to legally consent and whether the offered fertility preservation procedure offers them a realistic, potential benefit [73]. For minor patients whose prognosis for survival is either extremely poor or whose only treatment option may be experimental, such as cryopreservation of gonadal tissue, the potential benefit, a core principle of informed consent law, may be speculative [5]. Yet, given rapid and anticipated developments in fertility preservation treatment options and ART generally, it may be reasonable to assume cryopreserved tissue or other experimental options will become the future standard of care by the time these patients reach child-bearing age.

Since generally, minors are not considered legally competent, they cannot give or withhold consent to medical treatment but must rely on their parents or guardians to legally consent to such treatment by proxy. In such cases, while "assent" by the minor child is often sought, it is not legally sufficient to consent to treatment [74]. Under the "mature minor doctrine," many states have statutes that allow minors, on a finding of sufficient maturity, to give legally effective consent to medical treatment.[10] However, these statutes may require that minors have attained a certain minimum age and may be applicable only to specific treatments, therefore not necessarily pertaining to the fertility preservation context described herein. For mature minors, however, the recognition of relatively broad authority to make decisions about their reproductive health noted above should support their ability to make fertility preservation decisions in the oncofertility context

Parental consent in the context of fertility preservation can raise unique concerns since a choice to preserve fertility may provide a potential benefit for the parent but not the child if the child does not survive treatment. Parental decisionmaking in healthcare in general follows one of two possible standards. The first requires parents to make a decision that is in the best interests of the child [75]. While a parent may decide that it is in their child's best interest to undergo fertility preservation treatment to produce gametes for the child's future procreative use, that would not include a decision to preserve their child's gametes for their own potential use should their child not survive his or her cancer treatment. Alternatively, the "substituted decisionmaking" standard would require the decisionmaker to attempt to determine what the patient would have chosen if competent, taking into consideration their previous or known behavior, wishes, values, and goals, and make a decision based on that information [76]. Applying this standard to minors has been criticized, as decisionmakers can merely speculate as to what a child would do if he or she was an adult, since the child has never been legally competent [77]. Moreover, parents may be strongly influenced by their beliefs or hopes for what their child would do if he or she were legally capable of giving consent [77]. In the context of assisted reproduction options, a parent might feel their child would want to donate or provide his or her own gametes to the parent for their own use or otherwise. [11] [78].

10 *See, e.g.*, ALA. CODE §22-8-4 to 6 (authorizing minors at least 14 years old to consent to any medical treatment; authorizing all minors to consent to treatment related to pregnancy, sexually transmitted diseases, as well as chemical dependency); CAL. FAMILY CODE §6920–§6929 (authorizing minors at least 15 years old to consent to most medical treatment; authorizing minors at least 12 years old to consent to certain treatments for mental health, substance abuse, as well as the diagnosis and treatment of rape and of communicable diseases); MD. CODE ANN., HEALTH-GEN. §20-101-104, (authorizing minors at least 17 years old to consent to treatment of substance abuse, sexually transmitted diseases, pregnancy, contraception, and rape exams; authorizing minors at least 16 years old to consent to treatment of mental or emotional issues).

11 For an example of such a parental request for an incompetent, adult patient, see Greer et al., "Case 21-2010: A Request for Retrieval of Oocytes from a 36-Year-Old Woman with Anoxic Brain Injury." N Engl J Med 2010;363:276-83. The author has been involved in several such requests on behalf of minors and incompetent adults that were resolved without reported or published litigation.

Because of such concerns, it has been the author's position in developing protocols with various IVF programs that to avoid this issue and potential pressure, protocols for cryopreserving minors' gametes should not include a dispositional option for donating unused gametes to third parties for procreation, a common option for adult patients. Assuming survival, minor patients have the option to update their forms upon reaching maturity to include all dispositional options available to adults. In addition, and while there is no reported law on this question, a conservative approach to further respect the procreative autonomy of minor patients would also preclude parents or guardians from consenting to destroying or donating to medical research their child's reproductive tissue, except in the event of the minor's death.

Finally, whether parental failure to *preserve* a minor's reproductive capabilities could be compared to active sterilization prohibited by the Constitution is unknown, including whether a future court faced with such a case might define an obligation on the part of parents or healthcare providers to preserve fertility in minor children facing iatrogenic infertility [73]. If and when certain techniques for preserving fertility in children become the standard of care, this legal obligation might become a more likely possibility.

28.10 Conclusion

Given the swift pace of medical advances in both cancer treatment and reproductive medicine, it will be a continuing challenge for the law to keep pace with the myriad of legal aspects they engender. This chapter provides a snapshot-in-time, and can neither predict future changes or exhaustively address all the nuanced legal aspects of fertility preservation. Clinicians and patients will do well to recognize that, as possible treatment and family-building options expand, standards of care are likely to change and the law will undoubtedly need to keep pace.

For the present time, a few legal principles can be articulated. First, it seems advisable for patients – single or partnered and post-pubescent minors as well as adults – to cryopreserve gametes rather than embryos, at least where clinics have demonstrated proficiency in both. Second, consents should be up-to-date, reviewed regularly, and adhere to current applicable state law. Third, legal agreements as contracts may be more protective of patients' choices than informed consents for both the disposition of their cryopreserved genetic material and posthumous reproduction, and such documents should also be reviewed regularly and adhere to current applicable law. Fourth, third-party ART presents both exciting and legally complex opportunities to expand family building and should be approached with caution and appropriate professional guidance. Fifth, the processes of obtaining legal informed consent to medical treatment for minors and adults may each require distinct protocols. Sixth, documented recommendations that patients consult with independent, experienced legal professionals in many of these scenarios would be protective of all involved. Lastly, medical advances will continue to both offer exciting new possibilities for future biological parentage and at the same time challenge existing legal protections and frameworks, necessitating continued vigilance by both oncology and fertility providers.

Review Questions and Answers

? Q1. What are the key differences in informed consent and contracts and the role each plays in assisted reproduction?

✓ A1. Increasingly, embryo or gamete disposition decisions are viewed as contractual decisions, and agreements recorded between two patients may be more protective of their choices, and less likely to be subject to a change of mind, than a traditional informed consent process and document.

? Q2. How is fertility preservation legally different for minor than adult patients?

✓ A2. Given minors' general lack of capacity to legally consent, parental consent must be limited to the minor patient's best interests and protocols should offer more limited posthumous options than adults.

28

Q3. How should oncofertility patients considering surrogacy or other third-party assisted reproduction be counseled?

A3. Given the complexities and variability inherent in this process; physicians should stress the importance of patients relying on experienced, ethical, objective, and jurisdictionally appropriate legal professionals, recognizing that international arrangements add increased uncertainties around immigration, citizenship, genetic make-up, and health costs.

Q4. Legally, how can the consent process for adult fertility preservation patients be enhanced?

A4. Given advances in egg freezing, moving counseling and informed consent from couples counseling and consenting around embryo freezing, to individual counseling, decisionmaking, and consenting around the relative legal and medical advantages of freezing embryos or gametes will enhance future family-building protections.

References

1. Oktay K, et al. Fertility preservation in patients with cancer: ASCO clinical practice guideline update. J Clin Oncol. 2018;36(19):1994–2001. https://doi.org/10.1200/JCO.2018.78.1914. Epub 2018 Apr 5.
2. Crockin S, Jones HW Jr. Legal conceptions: the evolving law and policy of assisted reproductive technologies. Baltimore: Johns Hopkins University Press; 2010.
3. Zhang S. A woman gave birth from an embryo frozen for 24 years. The Atlantic. 2017 Dec 21.
4. Crockin S, Jones HW Jr. Legal conceptions: the evolving law and policy of assisted reproductive technologies. Baltimore: Johns Hopkins University Press; 2010. p. 20–73275–300.
5. Beauchamp T, Childress J. Principles of biomedical ethics. 7th ed. Nova York: Oxford University Press; 2013.
6. Robbennolt J. Advancing the rights of children and adolescents to be altruistic: bone marrow donation by minors. J Law Health. 1995;9:213218–21; *Bonner v. Moran*, 126 F.2d 121, 123 (D.C. Cir. 1941).
7. ASRM. Practice committee, mature oocyte cryopreservation: a guideline. Fertil Steril. 2013;99, 37(1)
8. Argyle CE, Harper JC, Davies MC. Oocyte cryopreservation: where are we now? Hum Reprod Update. 2016;22(4):440.
9. Noyes N, Boldt J, Nagy ZP. Oocyte cryopreservation: is it time to remove its experimental label? J Assist Reprod Genet. 2010;27:69.
10. ASRM. Practice committee, ovarian tissue cryopreservation: a committee opinion. Fertil Steril. 2014;101(5):1237.
11. Del. Code tit. 18 §§ 3342(i), 3556(i).
12. Conn. Gen. Stat. §§ 38a-509, 38a-536.
13. R.I. Gen. Laws §§ 27-18-30, 27-19-23, 27-20-20, 27-41-33.
14. Md. Code, Ins., § 15-810.1.
15. Del. Code Ann. tit. 18 §§ 3342(i), 3556(i).
16. Faden R, Beauchamp T. A history and theory of informed consent. New York: Oxford University Press; 1986. p. 119–20.
17. ASRM. Practice committee, revised minimum standards for practices offering assisted reproductive technologies: a committee opinion. Fertil Steril. 2014; 102(3):682.
18. Cal. Pen. Code § 367g.
19. ASRM. Ethics committee, fertility preservation and reproduction in patients facing gonadotoxic therapies: a committee opinion. Fertil Steril. 2013;100(5):1224.
20. *Findley v. Lee*, No. FDI-13-780539, 2016 WL 270083 (Cal. Super. Ct. January 11, 2016) (final divorce judgment on reserved issues entered July 26, 2016); *McQueen v. Gadberry*, 507 S.W.3d 127 (Mo. Ct. App. 2016).
21. Cal. Health & Safety Code § 125315.
22. www.asrm.org (section accessible only to professional members).
23. Crockin S. The "embryo" wars: at the epicenter of science, law, religion, and politics. Fam Law Q. 2005; 39:599.
24. *Davis v. Davis*, 842 S.W.2d 588 (Tenn. 1992).
25. *Davis v. Davis*, 842 S.W.2d 604 (Tenn. 1992).
26. Crockin S, Jones HW Jr. Legal conceptions: the evolving law and policy of assisted reproductive technologies. Baltimore: Johns Hopkins University Press; 2010. p. 20–73.
27. *A.Z. v. B.Z.*, 725 N.E.2d 1051 (Mass. 2000).
28. *J.B. v. M.B.*, 783 A.2d 707 (N.J. 2001).
29. *J.B. v. M.B.*, 783 A.2d 717 (N.J. 2001).
30. *Reber v. Reiss*, 42 A. 3d 1131 (Pa. Super. Ct. 2012).
31. *Reber v. Reiss*, 42 A. 3d 1136 (Pa. Super. Ct. 2012).
32. *Reber v. Reiss*, 42 A. 3d 1142 (Pa. Super. Ct. 2012).
33. *Szafranksi v. Dunston*, 34 N.E.3d 1132 (Ill. App. 2015).
34. *Szafranksi v. Dunston*, 34 N.E.3d 1144 (Ill. App. 2015).
35. *Szafranksi v. Dunston*, 34 N.E.3d 1148-53 (Ill. App. 2015).
36. *Szafranksi v. Dunston*, 34 N.E.3d 1161-63 (Ill. App. 2015).
37. *Findley v. Lee, No. FDI-13-780539,* 2016 WL 270083 (Cal. Super. Ct. January 11, 2016), (final divorce judgment on reserved issues entered July 26, 2016).
38. Model Uniform Parentage Act §707(a) (2017).

39. Model Uniform Parentage Act §707(b) (2017).
40. Cohen G, Adashi E. Personhood and the three branches of government. New Eng J Med. 2018;378:2453. https://doi.org/10.1056/NEJMp1801940.
41. Ariz. Rev. Stat. § 25-318.03(A).
42. Alltucker K. Cancer survivor battling ex-husband ordered to destroy embryos. Azcentral. 1 Sept 2017. https://www.azcentral.com/story/news/local/arizona-health/2017/08/31/cancer-battling-arizona-woman-ex-husband-ordered-donate-fertilized-embryos/617118001/.
43. ASRM. Ethics committee, posthumous retrieval and use of gametes or embryos: an ethics committee opinion. Fertil Steril. 2018;110(1):45.
44. *Estate of Kievernagel*, 166 Cal. App. 4th 1024 (2008).
45. *Estate of Kievernagel*, 166 Cal. App. 4th 1032–3 (2008) (citing *Hecht v. Superior Court*, 16 Cal. App. 4th 836, 850) (1993)).
46. *Hecht v. Superior Court*, 16 Cal. App. 4th 836 (1993).
47. *Hecht v. Superior Court*, 16 Cal. App. 4th 840 (1993).
48. *Hecht v. Superior Court*, 16 Cal. App. 4th 841 (1993).
49. *Hecht v. Superior Court*, 16 Cal. App. 4th 858–9 (1993).
50. *Astrue v. Capato*, 566 U.S. 541 (2012).
51. *Astrue v. Capato*, 566 U.S. 556 (2012).
52. *Astrue v. Capato*, 566 U.S. 558–9 (2012).
53. *Woodward v. Comm'r of Soc. Sec.*, 435 Mass. 536, 552 (2002).
54. *Woodward v. Comm'r of Soc. Sec.*, 435 Mass. 536, 552–3 (2002).
55. *Eng Khabbaz v. Comm'r, Soc. Sec. Admin.*, 930 A.2d.1180 (N.H. 2007).
56. Model Uniform Parentage Act §708(b) (2017).
57. https://www.creativefamilyconnections.com/us-surrogacy-law-map/.
58. 750 Ill. Comp. Stat. § 47/1, et seq. (Gestational Surrogacy Act).
59. New Jersey Gestational Carrier Agreement Act, 2018 N.J. Sess. Law Serv. Ch. 18 (SENATE 482) (WEST); D.C. Code § 16-406.
60. N.Y. S.B. S17A (introduced 2017–2018 legislative session) (currently in committee).
61. Crockin S, Debele G. Ethical issues in assisted reproduction. J Am Acad Matrimonial Attorneys. 2015;27: 289–357, at. 320–1.
62. Crockin S, Jones HW Jr. Legal conceptions: the evolving law and policy of assisted reproductive technologies. Baltimore: Johns Hopkins University Press; 2010. p. 132–87.
63. ASRM. Practice committee, recommendations for gamete and embryo donation: a committee opinion. Fertil Steril. 2013;99(1):47.
64. Model Uniform Parentage Act §702 (2017).
65. N.Y. Comp. Codes R. & Regs, §§ 52-8.7, 52-8.8 (2000).
66. ASRM. Practice committee, recommendations for gamete and embryo donation: a committee opinion. Fertil Steril. 2013;99(1):47; ASRM. Ethics committee, interests, obligations, and rights in gamete donation: a committee opinion. Fertil Steril. 2014;102(3):675.
67. Crockin S. Legal issues related to parenthood after cancer. JNCI Monogr. 2005;2005(34):111.
68. Levine J. Preserving fertility in children and adolescents with cancer. Children (Basel). 2014;1(2):166.
69. Davi L, Goel S. Fertility preservation through gonadal cryopreservation. Reprod Med Biol. 2016;15(4):235.
70. *Skinner v. Oklahoma, ex rel. Williamson*, 316 U.S. 535 (1942).
71. An Overview of Minors' Consent Law. https://www.guttmacher.org/state-policy/explore/overview-minors-consent-law. Accessed 10 July 2018.
72. E.g., *Bellotti v. Baird*, 443 U.S. 622 (1979) (as to abortion).
73. Dolin G, Roberts D, Rodriguez L, Woodruff T. Medical hope, legal pitfalls: potential legal issues in the emerging field of oncofertility. In: Oncofertility: ethical, legal, social and medical perspectives. New York: Springer; 2010. p. 109–32.
74. American Association of Paediatricians Committee on Bioethics. Informed consent, parental permission, and assent in pediatric practice. Pediatrics. 1995;95:314. Available at http://pediatrics.aappublications.org/content/pediatrics/95/2/314.full.pdf.
75. Robbennolt J. Advancing the rights of children and adolescents to be altruistic: bone marrow donation by minors. J Law Health. 1995;9:213222–3.
76. Robbennolt J. Advancing the rights of children and adolescents to be altruistic: bone marrow donation by minors. J Law Health. 1995;9, 213221–2
77. Robbennolt J. Advancing the rights of children and adolescents to be altruistic: bone marrow donation by minors. J Law Health. 1995;9:213226.
78. Greer DM, et al. Case 21–2010: a request for retrieval of oocytes from a 36-year-old woman with anoxic brain injury. N Engl J Med. 2010;363:276–83.

Adoption in the Cancer Setting

Jessica R. Gorman, Adam S. DuVall, and Brandon Hayes-Lattin

T. K. Woodruff et al. (eds.), *Textbook of Oncofertility Research and Practice*,
https://doi.org/10.1007/978-3-030-02868-8_29

Key Points

- Adoption is a family building option for cancer survivors who want to have a child, but are infertile or choose not to have a biological child.
- Many young adult cancer survivors report an interest in adoption, but do not receive information about adoption from their healthcare teams.
- Barriers to pursuing adoption include high financial cost, challenges navigating widely variable adoption processes and regulations, and uncertainty about whether they would be perceived as a good candidate by adoption agencies.
- Oncology and reproductive health teams can support their cancer survivor patients by providing culturally sensitive education and counseling to help them make informed decisions and prepare for the potential complexities and challenges of pursuing adoption.

29

29.1 Introduction

Many cancer survivors wish to have children, and may choose to pursue adoption because they are unable to have biological children or because it is their preference. While adoption is often part of a broader discussion about family-building after cancer, there is limited research on cancer survivors' interest in, and concerns about, adoption. There is evidence that many young adult cancer survivors want to learn more about adoption. In one survey, 44% of survivors expressed a need for information about adoption services [1]. Another study reported that over 60% of female cancer survivors would adopt if they were unable to have biological children [2]. Among reproductive-aged women in the general population, 25–40% say that they have ever considered adoption [3, 4], although only about 20% of them take steps to adopt [4]. In a survey of female cancer survivors 18–35 years of age, 81.6% (95% CI 75.7–87.6) reported that they would consider adoption compared to 40.3% (95% CI 40.3–40.3) of women in the general population [5]. In this same survey, only 44.2% of the sample reported that they would have considered adoption before their cancer diagnosis, suggesting an increase in willingness to consider adoption after cancer.

Many reproductive-aged cancer survivors may consider adoption a more viable option than biological parenthood for a number of reasons, including the potential impact of pregnancy and hormones on their personal health, infertility as a result of their cancer treatment, and concerns about the health of biological children born after cancer and cancer treatment [2, 6, 7]. Other factors that may influence decisions about pursuing adoption include the desire to avoid additional invasive medical treatments, the expense of fertility preservation and/or assisted reproductive technology (ART), being a poor candidate for ART, cultural and religious values, and perceived societal benefit [8, 9].

29.2 Concerns and Barriers to Adoption

Despite interest in adoption, research indicates that survivors also have concerns. In a survey of 163 female cancer survivors age 18–35 years, 85% of cancer survivors reported at least one concern about adoption. The most common concerns were preference for biological child (48%), expense (48%), worry about not being perceived as a good candidate by adoption agencies (41%), needing more information (39%), and worry about personal health negatively impacting their ability to raise a child (25%). Other concerns included the health of the adopted child (20%), possible legal problems (20%), and the time and effort required to adopt (16%) [5]. There is also variation in the way infertility and adoption are viewed by people from different racial, ethnic, cultural, and socioeconomic groups, which could impact support for, and decisions about, pursuing adoption [9]. Survivors who are considering their family-building options would benefit from culturally sensitive communication with their healthcare providers regarding the process and cost of adoption.

There is also evidence of system-level barriers to adoption and discrimination against cancer survivors navigating the adoption process. In a pilot survey of 7 adoption specialists, 6 international adoption agencies, and 11 cancer organizations, all of the adoption agencies reported that many countries view a history of cancer as a contraindication to adoption. Furthermore, all of the adoption specialists reported that many birth parents would be afraid to place their child with a cancer survivor [10]. A qualitative study involving nurse interviews of adoption agencies about the adoption process for cancer survivors identified several potential barriers, including high cost (typically $20,000–$30,000), requirements for physician letters attesting to the health of the adopting parent, and significant wait times. The study also reported that a candidate's medical history may or may not be shared with birth mothers, and that this history could influence her decisions in selecting adoptive parents [11]. An analysis of domestic and international adoption agencies found various types of discrimination in the adoption process for people with medical conditions such as cancer at state, national, and international levels. While there is no specific legislation prohibiting cancer survivors from adoption in the United States, this analysis identified wide variability in the way that states and adoption agencies make decisions about placing children, which often put cancer survivors at a disadvantage [12].

29.3 Quality of Life Implications

There may be significant quality of life implications of whether and how parenthood is achieved after cancer. In a study of long-term female cancer survivors who wanted a child at the time of their diagnosis, those who remained childless were most distressed about infertility and had more infertility-related traumatic symptoms than those who had biological children. Those with non-biological children (i.e., those not genetically related to the mother) were less distressed than those without children, but more distressed than those with biological children [13]. Adoption may not always be possible, which could result in additional trauma from unsuccessful adoption, in addition to cancer diagnosis and infertility. However, the transition to parenthood after adoption may be easier for cancer survivors than the general population [14].

29.4 Considerations for Healthcare Teams

While adoption is a rare event with multiple influencing factors and challenges, it may be an even more complex process and decision for those with a history of cancer. As such, it is important for healthcare teams to be prepared to discuss adoption with their patients, particularly the challenges and complexities of this process, while also taking into consideration cultural and religious values that could impact perceptions about family-building and adoption [9–11]. Adoption is briefly mentioned in the American Society of Clinical Oncology guidelines on fertility preservation for patients with cancer, but no specific recommendations or details on discussions about adoption are provided [15]. Typically, survivors must be cancer free for 5 years before pursuing adoption, although this may vary by adoption agency and circumstance. All potential adoptive parents must undertake an extensive home study by a social worker or other professional, who will visit the home and conduct interviews with the potential adoptive parents. This process can take 6 months or more to complete, before applicants are approved for adoption. The home study also includes a medical form, which may ask if potential adoptive parents have had a life-threatening disease such as cancer. The process requires doctors to complete a form detailing diagnosis, treatment, and prognosis, and possibly to provide a detailed letter. Patients and healthcare professionals can access general information about adoption from The National Infertility Association [19] and Academy of Adoption and Assisted Reproduction Attorneys [20].

Because of significant differences between adoption processes, regulations, and resources in different states and countries, there is a need for oncology and reproductive healthcare teams, including physicians, nurses, social workers, and other allied health professionals, to be able to access and share resources and information relevant to their cancer survivor patients. The American Society of Reproductive Medicine has patient materials on adoption considerations [16], the Oncofertility Consortium maintains a list of Cancer Friendly Adoption Agencies [17], and Fertile Action offers information and resources about adoption on their website [18].

Healthcare teams may also contact local adoption agencies for resources and information. However, there remains a need for curated educational materials for cancer survivors and clinical guidelines on when and with whom to discuss this option.

29.5 Conclusions

Many cancer survivors are interested in learning more about adoption as a family-building option. However, they also express concerns about adoption and face financial and system level barriers. Oncology and reproductive health teams can support their cancer survivor patients by providing culturally sensitive education and counseling to help them make informed decisions and prepare for and navigate the potential complexities and challenges of pursuing adoption. There are some resources available, but more detailed guidance for healthcare providers to facilitate culturally sensitive, patient-centered communication and recommendations regarding adoption would be beneficial.

Review Questions and Answers

Q1. Name one concern that cancer survivors have expressed about adoption.
- (a) Cost
- (b) Lack of information
- (c) Worry about not being perceived as a good candidate
- (d) Personal health concerns about raising a child
- (e) Preference for a biological child
- (f) Possible legal problems
- (g) Time and effort to adopt
- (h) All of the above

A1. (h)

Q2. Are adoption processes and regulations consistent across agencies, states, and nations?

A2. No

Q3. Must all cancer survivors undertake an extensive home study process before pursuing adoption?

A3. Yes

Q4. Name one resource relevant to cancer survivors interested in finding out more about adoption.
- (a) American Society of Reproductive Medicine
- (b) Oncofertility Consortium
- (c) Fertile Action
- (d) The National Infertility Association
- (e) Academy of Adoption and Assisted Reproduction Attorneys
- (f) All of the above

A4. (f)

References

1. Zebrack B. Information and service needs for young adult cancer patients. Support Care Cancer Off J Multinatl Assoc Support Care Cancer. 2008;16(12):1353–60.
2. Schover LR, Rybicki LA, Martin BA, Bringelsen KA. Having children after cancer. A pilot survey of survivors' attitudes and experiences. Cancer. 1999;86(4):697–709.
3. Chandra A, Abma J, Maza P, Bachrach C. Adoption, adoption seeking, and relinquishment for adoption in the United States. Adv Data. 1999;306(306):1–16.
4. Van Laningham JL, Scheuble LK, Johnson DR. Social factors predicting women's consideration of adoption. Mich Fam Rev. 2012;16(1):1–21.
5. Gorman JR, Whitcomb BW, Standridge D, Malcarne VL, Romero SA, Roberts SA, Su HI. Adoption consideration and concerns among young adult female cancer survivors. J Cancer Survivorship Res Pract. 2017;11(1):149–57.
6. Gorman JR, Bailey S, Pierce JP, Su HI. How do you feel about fertility and parenthood? The voices of young female cancer survivors. J Cancer Survivorship Res Pract. 2012;6(2):200–9.
7. Goncalves V, Sehovic I, Quinn G. Childbearing attitudes and decisions of young breast cancer survivors: a systematic review. Hum Reprod Updat. 2014;20(2):279–92.
8. Horowitz JE. Non-traditional family building planning. In: Quinn GP, Vadaparampil S, editors. Reproductive health and cancer in adolescents and young adults. 2012/01/03 ed. New York: Springer Science+Business Media; 2012. p. 115–30.
9. Jenkins RL. Ensuring access to education and services on infertility for the underserved. J Natl Cancer Inst Monogr. 2005;34:101–3.

10. Rosen A. Third-party reproduction and adoption in cancer patients. J Natl Cancer Inst Monogr. 2005;34: 91–3.
11. Quinn GP, Zebrack BJ, Sehovic I, Bowman ML, Vadaparampil ST. Adoption and cancer survivors: findings from a learning activity for oncology nurses. Cancer. 2015;121(17):2993–3000.
12. Gardino SL, Russell AE, Woodruff TK. Adoption after cancer: adoption agency attitudes and perspectives on the potential to parent post-cancer. Cancer Treat Res. 2010;156:153–70.
13. Canada AL, Schover LR. The psychosocial impact of interrupted childbearing in long-term female cancer survivors. Psychooncology. 2012;21(2):134–43.
14. Brodzinsky D. A stress and coping model of adoption adjustment. In: Brodzinsky D, Schechter M, editors. Psychology of adoption. New York: Oxford University Press; 1990. p. 3–24.
15. Loren AW, Mangu PB, Beck LN, Brennan L, Magdalinski AJ, Partridge AH, Quinn G, Wallace WH, Oktay K, American Society of Clinical O. Fertility preservation for patients with cancer: American Society of Clinical Oncology clinical practice guideline update. J Clin Oncol Off J Am Soc Clin Oncol. 2013;31(19):2500–10.
16. American Society of Reproductive Medicine. Adoption: where to start and what to think about. Available from: https://www.asrm.org/topics/topics-index/adoption/.
17. Oncofertility Consortium. Cancer friendly adoption agencies. 2018. Available from: https://oncofertility.northwestern.edu/files/documents/cancer-friendly-adoption-agencies.
18. Fertile Action. Adoption. 2018. Available from: http://www.fertileaction.org/learning-center/parenthood-after-cancer/adoption/.
19. The National Infertility Association. Adoption. 2018. Available from: https://resolve.org/what-are-my-options/adoption/.
20. Academy of Adoption and Assisted Reproduction Attorneys. Adoption. 2018. Available from: https://adoptionart.org/adoption.

Common Ethical Issues in Oncofertility

Lisa Campo-Engelstein

An earlier version of this paper titled "Addressing the Three Most Frequently Asked Questions of a Bioethicist in an Oncofertility Setting" was published in Oncofertility Medical Practice, *eds. T.K. Woodruff and C. Gracia (2012).*

T. K. Woodruff et al. (eds.), *Textbook of Oncofertility Research and Practice*,
https://doi.org/10.1007/978-3-030-02868-8_30

Key Points
- Whereas age and prognosis may sometimes be ethically relevant factors in who should be offered fertility preservation, marital status, sexual orientation, and gender identity should not.
- The author argues that fertility preservation should be covered by insurance because other iatrogenic conditions already are.
- Healthcare professionals should discuss fertility preservation with patients, regardless of their financial circumstances.
- Disputes over frozen reproductive material can be minimized, and even prevented, if people have written documentation of their wishes before undergoing fertility preservation and if people freeze gametes rather than embryos.

30.1 Introduction

The goal of this chapter is to examine some of the ethical concerns that arise in the interdisciplinary field of oncofertility. Specifically, I will address three commonly asked ethical questions: (1) Who should be offered fertility preservation? (2) Who should pay for fertility preservation? and (3) How should disputes over frozen gametes, embryos, and gonadal tissue (collectively referred to as reproductive material) be resolved and prevented? Unfortunately, there are not always easy and universal answers to these questions. As with other aspects of patient care, we need to consider each patient and make a case-by-case judgment.

30.2 Who Should Be Offered Fertility Preservation?

30.2.1 Age

Offering medical treatment to minors raises a number of ethical concerns—too many to consider here—so instead, I will focus on the ethical concerns specific to fertility preservation. If a girl has reached puberty, then it is feasible for her to undergo controlled ovarian hyperstimulation with hormones to produce mature eggs for cryopreservation or "banking." However, some girls may not yet be emotionally mature to handle the medical procedure of egg removal. For example, the vaginal ultrasounds necessary to identify mature oocytes for retrieval may be traumatic to a girl who is not sexually active and/or has not yet had a gynecological visit. In addition to emotional issues, there is also a concern about health risks, particularly those associated with ovarian hyperstimulation, in someone so young.

If a boy has reached puberty, then sperm banking is a relatively easy and established method of fertility preservation. Yet, some postpubertal boys may not have experience masturbating or have not been able to achieve orgasm. Discussing masturbation can be difficult and awkward, as most boys will probably be embarrassed, especially if their parents are present. Parents too can often feel embarrassed and may not be comfortable discussing their son's sexuality. Depending on their cultural and religious beliefs, the parents may believe masturbation is a sin or that sexual behavior in teenagers and/or unmarried individuals should not be encouraged.

For prepubertal girls and boys, the only fertility preservation option available is gonadal tissue (or whole organ) banking. This option is considered experimental and thus should be discussed with caution and under IRB approval. Although surgical removal of the gonads is a low-risk procedure, some may be concerned about exposing children with cancer to yet another treatment, especially one that is experimental and addresses with a quality of life issue that probably will not affect the children for at least a decade. Yet, others argue that children have a right to an open future and that in order to uphold their future reproductive autonomy, we should preserve their fertility [33].

In addition to concerns about offering fertility preservation to those on the younger end of the age spectrum, there are also concerns about fertility preservation for those on the older end of the age spectrum. For most adult women, fertility begins to decrease in their 30s and significantly declines after age 37 [12, 15]. Some fertility clinics refuse to provide infertility treatment to women over 40 using their own eggs because the success rate is so low [20]. In order to maintain consistency and to avoid futile treatment, healthcare providers should follow the guidelines set out by the American Society for Reproductive Medicine (ASRM) regarding age [15]. Since men do not experience the equivalent of menopause, they are able to reproduce throughout their lifetimes; however, studies have shown that the probability of infertility [12] and the risk of certain diseases in children increases with age for men as well [18, 30]. Additionally, the mere fact that they are able to reproduce does not mean that they should. Some have argued that there should be age restrictions not just for women but also for men when it comes to assisted reproductive technology due to concerns surrounding life expectancy, overall health, finances, etc. [9].

30.2.2 Prognosis

Fertility preservation for patients with a poor prognosis raises a host of ethical issues. Providers may worry that discussing fertility preservation will give patients false hope about their prognosis. In other words, these patients may feel their providers deceived them by mentioning fertility preservation, leading them to believe that their prognosis is not as bad as they originally thought. Yet, at the same time, pursuing fertility preservation may be a source of hope and happiness for patients during difficult times. It may furnish them with mental and physical strength [36], making them even more motivated to survive for the sake of their potential future children. Additionally, these patients, and their families, may feel a degree of inner peace knowing that part of their lives will continue on in the reproductive material even if they are never used [27, 34].

Nevertheless, some may argue that, despite any personal and emotional benefits they may experience, offering patients with a poor prognosis fertility preservation options is an unjust allocation of resources. From a utilitarian perspective, it does not make sense to devote resources to patients who will likely not benefit from them. Put differently, resources should be allocated to those who have a high probability of a positive outcome, which means individuals with a poor prognosis should be placed lower on the priority list for receiving fertility preservation resources than individuals with a good prognosis.

On the other hand, if we take a deontological (duty-based, individual rights) approach, providers have a duty to care for their patients. Not offering fertility preservation to all of their patients, including those with a poor prognosis, may be seen as diminishing patient autonomy. According to this view, providers should be more concerned with the needs and rights of their individual patients than with social justice (i.e., fair allocation of resources).

30.2.3 Marital Status

Some providers have been reluctant to treat single individuals suffering from infertility [2, 35]. Additionally, many insurance companies and state laws mandating insurance coverage of infertility treatment limit these services to married couples and, furthermore, require that only the gametes of the couple be used (i.e., donor gametes are prohibited) [4]. In the case of fertility preservation, denying patients this service does not make sense since many of them are minors and not legally permitted to be married or they are young adults who may see marriage as something they are not yet ready for, but they would like in the future. Fertility preservation is inherently forward-looking; that is, its purpose is to take the necessary precautions in order to ensure options (namely, genetic parenthood) later on in life. Denying patients fertility preservation because they are unmarried at the time they seek treatment fails to recognize the future-oriented nature of fertility preservation treatment and that patients' marital status may change by the time they decide to use their reproductive material.

Even if individuals seeking fertility preservation state that they plan on raising future children in a single-parent household, this is not sufficient justification to deny them fertility preservation. There is an increasing social acceptance of single parenthood and various family formations [32]. Furthermore, there is empirical evidence showing that children raised in single-parent households are not necessarily disadvantaged compared to children in two parent households [3, 38]. ASRM states that denying assistive technologies based on marital status is unethical [2].

30.2.4 Sexual Orientation and Gender Identity

Like marital status, some providers may be uncomfortable treating LGBTQ (lesbian, gay, bisexual, transgender, and queer) individuals for infertility treatments [2, 35]. Additionally, some providers may not offer fertility preservation to LGBTQ individuals because they assume they will not be interested in it. This assumption rests on a dominant heteronormative and cissexist norm that only certain people (i.e. heterosexual and cisgender people) are interested in reproduction and furthermore will be good parents. However, there is evidence that LGBTQ individuals are interested in becoming parents [10] and are successful parents [5]. Fertility preservation in transgender individuals may raise some unique challenges (e.g., exacerbating gender dysphoria, gametes not "matching" gender identity) [16]. However, these challenges should not be grounds to deny fertility preservation to transgender individuals. Indeed, ASRM asserts that refusing to provide assisted reproductive technologies to individuals in the LGBTQ community is unjustified [1, 2].

30.3 Who Should Pay for Fertility Preservation?

As I have argued elsewhere, I believe insurance companies should cover fertility preservation for cancer patients [6, 7]. One of the strongest reasons is that insurance typically covers treatment for other iatrogenic conditions resulting from cancer treatment, including treatment that may otherwise be considered elective for conditions that "naturally" occur. For example, breast reconstructive surgery is covered by insurance when breast asymmetry (the extreme is the loss or lack of an entire breast) is iatrogenic but rarely when it is naturally occurring. The Women's Health and Cancer Rights Act of 1998 [39] institutionalizes the medical realm's responsibility for iatrogenic harms by mandating that private health insurance companies cover the costs of breast reconstruction surgery if they cover the costs of mastectomy. As such, breast reconstruction surgery following mastectomy is coded as a cancer treatment rather than as an elective treatment. In contrast, it is highly unlikely that insurance companies will cover breast surgery to produce symmetrical breasts for a woman born with only one breast (an extremely remote or even unheard of phenomenon) or, as is more common, asymmetrical breasts.

The reason for this differential treatment can be partially explained by the harm principle and causal responsibility: if healthcare professionals cause harm—a violation of Hippocratic Oath—then the medical profession as a whole must assume responsibility for alleviating this harm. Thus, if a woman has breast asymmetry or only one breast due to mastectomy (a medical procedure), the health insurance company should cover the expense of "fixing" her breast(s). Assuming there are no morally significant differences between breast surgery and fertility preservation—a claim I support in my previous works [6, 7]—insurance companies' failure to cover fertility preservation is unjustified. In other words, for the sake of consistency and fairness, insurance companies should treat fertility preservation as a treatment for an iatrogenic condition (infertility) caused by cancer treatment.

Assuming insurance companies will not, or will only partially, pay for fertility preservation, how can healthcare providers help individuals afford fertility preservation? One option is not to charge patients for the services received; however, this may not be within providers' control, as hospitals and reproductive material storage facilities, for example, may still charge fees even if the provider does not. Furthermore, many of these services are quite expensive, and forgoing payment may be a financial hardship for providers. Another option is for providers to point their patients to external resources that provide financial assistance for fertility preservation procedures. LIVESTRONG, for instance, offers aid to cancer patients who would like to pursue fertility preservation but are limited financially [26]. Providers can also refer their patients to institutions that offer discounted services, such as Northwestern University [37].

Even with financial assistance and a reduced price, the cost of fertility preservation procedures may still be prohibitive for some patients. Moreover, the cost of these procedures does not include storage fees and later use of reproductive material. Given that patients may have to undergo numerous attempts in order to achieve a pregnancy, it is not surprising that the average cost of a live birth baby using assisted reproductive technology is much higher than the average price for a cycle of IVF: $41,132 versus $12,513 [11]. Some providers may be concerned that discussing fertility preservation with patients who they know cannot afford it may be seen by their patients as cruel or callous.

Yet, there are several reasons why providers should always discuss fertility preservation, regardless of their patients' (presumed) financial circumstances. Providers are not privy to their patients' financial status, so determinations they make about whether patients can or cannot afford fertility preservation are, at best, estimated guesses. Even if patients disclose their financial circumstances to their providers, providers should not make value judgments regarding how patients should spend their money (e.g., spending funds on fertility preservation rather than a much-needed new car), as such judgments may preclude them from enumerating all of the patients' options. Additionally, providers may not be aware of external funds patients may receive from family members or others who have a stake in their health and the possibility of their future reproduction. That it may be difficult and upsetting for patients to learn about fertility preservation options even though they most likely cannot afford them should not affect the providers' decision to discuss those options. Giving bad news is an inherent aspect of the medical profession. While providers may struggle with sharing bad news with patients, it is essential that they do so in order to provide good care. Thus, in order to treat patients fairly and to provide the best care for all patients, providers should not let patients' finances determine what options are presented.

A final reason why providers should always discuss fertility preservation is because guidelines issued by the American Society for Clinical Oncology state that they should: "As part of education and informed consent before cancer therapy, oncologists should address the possibility of infertility with patients treated during their reproductive years and be prepared to discuss possible fertility preservation options or refer appropriate and interested patients to specialists" [25] (p2917)."

30.4 How Should Disputes over Reproductive Material Be Resolved and Prevented?

Under the law, gametes and embryos are often classified as a type of quasi-property [21, 23], and people whose genetic material the gametes or embryos contain are generally the ones who control their use and are responsible for them. Gametes and embryos can be bequeathed to others upon death as part of one's estate [22]. Unlike most other Western countries, the USA permits the sale of gametes. Given this legal understanding, disputes over reproductive material may have to be resolved in court if bioethics consultants or others cannot first help resolve the matter. Unfortunately, it is not possible to predict the outcome of these court cases because there is no set precedent in this matter and individual judges have ruled quite differently in similar cases [13, 19, 24].

The USA does not permit the same degree of commodification of organs as it does gametes and embryos. Organs are not viewed as property; thus, they cannot be bought and sold [8, 29]. However, donors can have some say in how their organs are allocated (e.g., a brother choosing to donate his kidney to his sister). Because gonadal tissue does not fit neatly into either of the two existing legal categories for body organs/cells/systems transplantation—organs or gametes/embryos—there is no legal precedent upon which to draw in disputes over ownership. As I have argued elsewhere, gonadal tissue should be legally classified similar to gametes/embryos because gonads are not currently regulated by the United Network for Organ Sharing and because gonads, unlike other organs but like gametes, can lead to pregnancy [8].

It is best to try to prevent disputes over reproductive material in the first place rather than deal with them after they have occurred. There are at least two ways to minimize or avoid such disputes. First is to encourage individuals to freeze their gametes or gonadal tissue rather than creating and freezing embryos. Before 2012, egg freezing was considered an experimental technology [28], so many women chose to freeze embryos rather than eggs. Today, however, both egg and sperm freezing are considered established technologies, so there is no medical reason for women to have to create embryos instead of freezing eggs. Determining who should have control over reproductive material that contains just one person's genes is much easier than when reproductive material contains a mix of two people's genes. Second, according to professional society guidelines, providers, fertility clinics, and storage facilities should ensure that patient's document their wishes regarding their reproductive material should their circumstances change (e.g., divorce, death, incapacitation) [14, 31]. While written documentation, such as a will or advance directive, of one's wishes will not always prevent disputes, both the healthcare system and the legal system typically rely on them when disputes arise [17, 22].

30.4.1 Minors

30

Lastly, it is important to recognize the special category of minors to prevent disputes between children and their parents. Given that reproductive material technically belongs to the child, parents should not be allowed to use or discard their child's reproductive material before the child turns 18. Upon reaching legal adulthood, parents should relinquish all rights to the reproductive material, and it should be reclassified as the "property" of the child turned adult. If a minor child passes away, the child's reproductive material should be immediately destroyed or donated to science. Parents should not have the option of using their child's reproductive material for reproductive purposes. Indeed, there is consensus in the medical community that posthumous reproduction by minor children should be prohibited.

30.5 Conclusion

In this chapter, I have raised and addressed three common ethical questions in oncofertility, yet there are clearly many additional ethical issues. Those working in the field of oncofertility, especially bioethicists, should strive not only to address these current ethical issues but also to predict future ethical issues and work to mitigate, prevent, or find solutions for them. It is also important for clinicians to understand the ethical issues and anticipate these questions and work closely with bioethicists to address their patients' concerns about fertility preservation options.

Acknowledgments This work was supported by the Oncofertility Consortium NIH/NICHD 5UL1DE019587.

Review Questions and Answers

Q1. Circle all of the following that may be ethically relevant factors in decisions about who should be offered fertility preservation.
- (a) Age
- (b) Prognosis
- (c) Marital status
- (d) Sexual orientation
- (e) Gender identity

A1. (a) and (b)

Q2. Why does the author argue that fertility preservation should be covered by insurance?
- (a) It is too expensive for people to afford it out-of-pocket.
- (b) Other iatrogenic conditions resulting from cancer treatment are already covered by insurance.
- (c) It is considered a medically indicated procedure.
- (d) All of the above.

A2. (b)

Q3. Healthcare professionals should discuss fertility preservation with patients, regardless of their financial circumstances. True or False?

A3. True

Q4. How can disputes over frozen reproductive materials be minimized and prevented?
- (a) Providing written documentation before freezing materials.
- (b) Freezing gametes rather than embryos.
- (c) Both (a) and (b).
- (d) Neither (a) nor (b).

A4. (c)

References

1. Access to fertility services by transgender persons: an ethics committee opinion. Fertil Steril. 2015;104(5):1111–5. https://doi.org/10.1016/j.fertnstert.2015.08.021
2. Access to fertility treatment by gays, lesbians, and unmarried persons: a committee opinion. Fertil Steril. 2013;100(6):1524–7. https://doi.org/10.1016/j.fertnstert.2013.08.042
3. Amato PR, Patterson S, Beattie B. Single-parent households and children's educational achievement: a state-level analysis. Soc Sci Res. 2015;53:191–202. https://doi.org/10.1016/j.ssresearch.2015.05.012.
4. Basco D, Campo-Engelstein L, Rodriguez S. Insuring against infertility: expanding state infertility mandates to include fertility preservation technology for cancer patients. J Law Med Ethics. 2010;38(4):832–9. https://doi.org/10.1111/j.1748-720X.2010.00536.x.
5. Bos HMW, Balen FV, Boom DCVD. Lesbian families and family functioning: an overview. Patient Educ Couns. 2005;59(3):263–75. https://doi.org/10.1016/j.pec.2004.10.006.
6. Campo-Engelstein L. Consistency in insurance coverage for iatrogenic conditions resulting from cancer treatment including fertility preservation. J Clin Oncol. 2010a;28(8):1284–6. JCO.2009.25.6883 [pii]. https://doi.org/10.1200/JCO.2009.25.6883.
7. Campo-Engelstein L. For the sake of consistency and fairness: why insurance companies should cover fertility preservation treatment for iatrogenic infertility. Cancer Treat Res. 2010b;156:381–8. https://doi.org/10.1007/978-1-4419-6518-9_29.
8. Campo-Engelstein L. Gametes or organs? How should we legally classify ovaries used for transplantation in the USA? J Med Ethics. 2011;37(3):166–70. jme.2010.038588 [pii]. https://doi.org/10.1136/jme.2010.038588.
9. Caplan AL, Patrizio P. Are you ever too old to have a baby? The ethical challenges of older women using infertility services. Semin Reprod Med. 2010;28(4):281–6. https://doi.org/10.1055/s-0030-1255175.
10. Center PR. A survey of LGBT Americans. Washington, DC: Pew Research Center; 2013.
11. Chambers GM, Sullivan EA, Ishihara O, Chapman MG, Adamson GD. The economic impact of assisted reproductive technology: a review of selected developed countries. Fertil Steril. 2009;91(6):2281–94. S0015-0282(09)00873-5 [pii]. https://doi.org/10.1016/j.fertnstert.2009.04.029.
12. Dunson DB, Baird DD, Colombo B. Increased infertility with age in men and women. Obstet Gynecol. 2004;103(1):51–6. https://doi.org/10.1097/01.AOG.0000100153.24061.45. 103/1/51 [pii]
13. Elster NR. Assisted reproductive technologies: contracts, consents, and controversies. Am J Fam Law. 2005;18(4):193–9.
14. Ethics Committee of the American Society for Reproductive Medicine. Posthumous collection and use of reproductive tissue: a committee opinion. Fertil Steril. 2013;99(7):1842–5. https://doi.org/10.1016/j.fertnstert.2013.02.022.
15. Female age-related fertility decline. Committee Opinion No. 589. Fertil Steril. 2014;101(3):633–4. https://doi.org/10.1016/j.fertnstert.2013.12.032.
16. Finlayson C, Johnson EK, Chen D, Dabrowski E, Gosiengfiao Y, Campo-Engelstein L, Rosoklija I, Jacobson J, Shnorhavorian M, Pavone ME, Moravek MB, Bonifacio HJ, Simons L, Hudson J, Fechner PY, Gomez-Lobo V, Kadakia R, Shurba A, Rowell E, Woodruff TK. Proceedings of the working group session on fertility preservation for individuals with gender and sex diversity. Transgender Health. 2016;1(1):99–107.
17. Forman DL. Embryo disposition and divorce: why clinic consent forms are not the answer. J Am Acad Matrimonial Lawyers. 2011;24:57-105.
18. Frans E, McGrath J, Sandin S, Lichtenstein P, Reichenberg A, Langstrom N, Hultman C. Advanced paternal and grand paternal age and schizophrenia: a three-generation perspective. Schizophr Res. 2011;133:120–4.
19. Fuselier BM. The trouble with putting all of your eggs in one basket: using a property rights model to resolve disputes over cryopreserved pre-embryos. Tex J Civ Lib Civ Rights. 2009;14(2):143–91.
20. Garrido N, Bellver J, Remohi J, Simon C, Pellicer A. Cumulative live-birth rates per total number of embryos needed to reach newborn in consecutive in vitro fertilization (IVF) cycles: a new approach to measuring the likelihood of IVF success. Fertil Steril. 2011;96(1):40–6. S0015-0282(11)00763-1 [pii]. https://doi.org/10.1016/j.fertnstert.2011.05.008.
21. Hardcastle R. Law and the human body: property rights, ownership and control. North America: Hart Publishing; 2007.
22. Hecht v. Superior Court CAt, 59 Cal.Rptr. 222 (2d Dist. 1996).
23. Howell SD. The frozen embryo: scholarly theories, case law, and proposed state regulation. DePaul J Health Care Law. 2013;14(3):407-440.
24. Kindregan CP, Snyder SH. Clarifying the law of ART: the new American Bar association model act governing assisted reproductive technology. Fam Law Q. 2008;42(2):203–29.
25. Lee SJ, Schover LR, Partridge AH, Patrizio P, Wallace WH, Hagerty K, Beck LN, Brennan LV, Oktay K. American Society of Clinical Oncology recommendations on fertility preservation in cancer patients. J Clin Oncol. 2006;24(18):2917–31. https://doi.org/10.1200/JCO.2006.06.5888.
26. LIVESTRONG LIVESTRONG Fertility. https://www.livestrong.org/we-can-help/livestrong-fertility. Accessed 4 Feb 2018.
27. Maltaris T, Boehm D, Dittrich R, Seufert R, Koelbl H. Reproduction beyond cancer: a message of hope for young women. Gynecol Oncol. 2006;103(3):1109–21. https://doi.org/10.1016/j.ygyno.2006.08.003.
28. Mature oocyte cryopreservation: a guideline. Fertil Steril. 2013;99(1):37–43. https://doi.org/10.1016/j.fertnstert.2012.09.028
29. National Organ Transplantation Act U.
30. Parner E, Baron-Cohen S, Lauritsen M, Jorgensen M, Schieve L, Yeargin-Allsopp M, Obel C. Parental age and autism spectrum disorders. Ann Epidemiol. 2012;22(3):143–50.

31. Pennings G, de Wert G, Shenfield F, Cohen J, Devroey P, Tarlatzis B. ESHRE task force on ethics and law 11: posthumous assisted reproduction. Hum Reprod. 2006;21(12):3050–3. https://doi.org/10.1093/humrep/del287.
32. Pew Research Center. The decline of marriage and rise of new families. Washington, DC; 2010.
33. Quinn GP, Stearsman DK, Campo-Engelstein L, Murphy D. Preserving the right to future children: an ethical case analysis. Am J Bioeth. 2012;12(6):38–43. https://doi.org/10.1080/15265161.2012.673688.
34. Quinn GP, Vadaparampil ST, Jacobsen PB, Knapp C, Keefe DL, Bell GE. Frozen hope: fertility preservation for women with cancer. J Midwifery Womens Health. 2010;55(2):175–80. https://doi.org/10.1016/j.jmwh.2009.07.009.
35. Robinson BE. Birds do it. Bees do it. So why not sigle women and lesbians? Bioethics. 1997;11(3&4):217–27.
36. Saito K, Suzuki K, Iwasaki A, Yumura Y, Kubota Y. Sperm cryopreservation before cancer chemotherapy helps in the emotional battle against cancer. Cancer. 2005;104(3):521–4. https://doi.org/10.1002/cncr.21185.
37. Smith K. Cost of fertility preservation treatment at Northwestern University; 2018.
38. Waldfogel J, Craigie T-A, Brooks-Gunn J. Fragile families and child wellbeing. Future Child/Cent Future Child David Lucile Packard Found. 2010;20(2):87–112.
39. Women's Health and Cancer Rights Act (WHCRA). The center for consumer information & insurance oversight U.S. Centers for Medicare & Medicaid Services.

The Importance of Disclosure for Sexual and Gender Minorities in Oncofertility Cases

Gwendolyn P. Quinn, Christina Tamargo, Matthew B. Schabath, Amani Sampson, and Susan Thomas Vadaparampil

T. K. Woodruff et al. (eds.), *Textbook of Oncofertility Research and Practice*,
https://doi.org/10.1007/978-3-030-02868-8_31

Key Points
- Collecting sexual orientation and gender identity are important aspects of quality care.
- The LGBTQ community experiences stigma in society and healthcare.
- LGBTQ patients with cancer are interested in having families.
- Providers should not assume patients are cisgender or heterosexual.

» Laura 33 years old, is seeing oncologist Dr. Smith to discuss results of her recent biopsy. Dr. Smith has reviewed Laura's social and medical history, which includes a previous benign biopsy for testicular cancer and says, "Your name is Laura? That's an unusual name for a guy." The patient responds, "I identify as female and chose the name Laura." Dr. Smith, uncertain of how to respond, proceeds to explain the cancer diagnosis. "You have colorectal cancer and your treatment will include both alkylating agents and radiation. This type of treatment can render you sterile but that is probably not a concern with folks like you. "Laura responds, "Why would you say that? I've always wanted to have children." Dr. Smith, still uncertain how to address his patient says "I'm going to call my nurse in here to talk to you; her son is gay and she knows more about this stuff than I do." Laura, reeling from the cancer diagnosis, is crying and says with anger "I'm not gay, I'm transgender, and I am still a human being."

31.1 Introduction

The lesbian, gay, bisexual, transsexual/transgender, and queer/questioning (LGBTQ) population is an understudied and underserved community often referred to as sexual and gender minorities [1]. The labels "lesbian, gay, and bisexual" refer to sexual orientation [2, 3]. The term "transgender" refers to a gender identity where an individual does not identify with the sex assigned to him or her at birth (i.e., biological sex) [2, 3]. The labels "queer" and "questioning" may be used to refer to either sexual orientation or gender identity [4, 5]. There are several other terms associated with this community (e.g., "gender fluid, genderqueer, two-spirit") as well as nomenclature used within these groups that is typically not acceptable to be used by nonmembers (e.g., "dyke") [6, 7]. It is estimated that 3–12% of the US population identifies as gay, lesbian, or bisexual and 1–3% are transgender [8].

Each of the subpopulations under the term sexual and gender minorities is likely to be unique, with varied health risk factors, communication preferences, and medical and social histories [4, 9]. It is common for all LGBTQ communities to perceive discrimination and lack of acceptance by society in general and in the healthcare setting in particular [4]. Several recent studies have identified that LGBTQ patients avoid preventive healthcare due to fear of perceived discrimination or because they cannot find an LGBTQ-friendly provider [1, 10–16]. LGBTQ individuals experience a variety of health disparities including higher rates of suicide attempts, higher prevalence of mental health issues, and increased risk for certain cancers [17–22].

31.2 LGBTQ Populations and Cancer

Because LGBTQ status is not collected in national surveys and registries [23], at present there are limited published data on cancer rates in LGBTQ populations [19, 24, 25]. As such, the cancer burden among the community is not known despite researchers utilizing novel approaches to estimate prevalence, density, incidence, and mortality of cancer among sexual minorities [26–29]. A recent review by Quinn et al. [19] synthesized the current literature on seven cancer sites that may disproportionately affect LGBTQ populations, specifically cancers of the anus, breast, uterine cervix, colon, endometrium, lung, and prostate. The authors noted that cancer health disparities in the LGBTQ community are likely attributed to multiple elements including social and economic factors, lower rates of access to healthcare and screening, and higher rates of risk factors and deleterious behaviors [19].

31.3 Disclosure of Gender Identity and Sexual Orientation in Healthcare

The increased risk for cancer among LGBTQ individuals are further exacerbated by nondisclosure of gender identity and sexual orientation by patients and failure to inquire by providers, which can lead to failure to screen, diagnose, or treat important medical problems [30–36]. The American Academy of Pediatrics, the American Medical Association, and the Society for Adolescent Health and Medicine all recommend providers discuss sexuality with all adolescents and offer nonjudgmental communication about sexual orientation [33, 37–39]. Patient disclosure of sexual orientation is associated with increased patient satisfaction and improved quality of care [33]. The majority of studies on LGBTQ disclosure have focused on older adults. Quinn et al. [40] surveyed 632 LGBTQ individuals, with a mean age of 58, about experiences with healthcare providers and reported 67% always or often disclosed their status to their provider. Further, less than 10% had ever experienced discrimination in a healthcare setting [40]. In a study of 291 LGBT patients with cancer, with a mean age of 62, 79% reported disclosing their identity to their cancer provider; 34% reported making this disclosure to correct a heteronormative assumption [32].

Very little is known about LGBTQ youth, especially those with cancer and their healthcare experiences [19, 24, 25, 33, 41–43]. The limited data that are available suggest younger sexual minorities may be less likely to disclose their sexual orientation or gender identity preferences to a healthcare provider [9]. A study of LGBTQ 18- to 23-year-olds without cancer found only 13% had disclosed to a provider [33]. This finding is particularly important given the documented reproductive health needs and concerns regarding infertility and fertility experienced by adolescent and young adult (AYA) oncology patients [44–52]. The vast majority of studies focused on AYA concerns in these areas have not included assessments of sexual orientation and/or gender identity. The remainder of this chapter provides an overview of the potential unique concerns related to fertility.

31.4 Discussion of Fertility Considerations for LGBTQ AYA Cancer Patients

AYAs with cancer may experience permanent or temporary infertility [53–57]. The risk of infertility depends on a variety of factors such as cancer type, stage, chemotherapy regimen and dose, use of endocrine therapy, radiation site and dose, surgical site, and/or use of bone marrow or stem cell transplantation [58–67]. There are several excellent reviews that discuss these factors in greater detail [68–73]. Generally, younger patients are less likely to experience infertility [66, 67]. The American Society of Clinical Oncology (ASCO), the National Comprehensive Cancer Network (NCCN), and the American Academy of Pediatrics (AAP) have all issued guidelines urging oncology healthcare providers to discuss infertility risk and fertility options with AYA patients and to refer them to fertility specialists [58, 74, 75]. ASCO and NCCN guidelines also suggest further reproductive health discussions such as the use of contraception and referrals to genetic counselors in the case of familial cancer syndromes [58, 75].

However, studies suggest these discussions are either not occurring, as evidenced by lack of documentation in the medial record, or not recalled by AYA patients, as shown in retrospective studies of cancer survivors' satisfaction with and recall of discussion of fertility with oncology healthcare providers [76–80]. Several recent studies recognized that discussions with a healthcare provider about fertility risk, regardless of whether preservation methods were used, were associated with higher quality of life (QoL) and less regret than patients who did not report such discussions [51, 76, 81–84].

LGBTQ AYAs with a cancer diagnosis face the same serious threats to QoL due to temporary or permanent fertility issues as heterosexual and gender-aligned AYA [68, 71, 85–89]. Impaired fertility can have a ripple effect on other QoL issues such as romantic partnering, body image, and sexuality [71, 86]. Although this has not been empirically validated in populations with cancer, surveys and case studies of men and women with infertility issues suggest a relationship between poor self-image and the inability to procreate/produce biological children [90–92]. Although many AYAs have strong ideas about having children in their future, equal numbers may not have seriously thought about it, and may not consider it unless a healthcare provider brings it up [45, 46, 79, 93–100].

Available studies suggest that sexual and gender minority AYAs with cancer are likely to be interested in discussion of fertility preservation at similar rates as heterosexual and gender-aligned patients. T'Sjoen [87] reported that prior to initiating cross-sex hormones, some transgender persons elect to preserve fertility so that a future biological child may be possible. Wierckx [88] interviewed 50 transsexual men to identify reproductive wishes; 54% desired children and 37% had considered banking sperm prior to beginning cross-sex hormones. A single case study of a 33-year-old gay man with prostate cancer identified that fertility was a key issue in making his treatment choices [89].

While discussing risks of infertility and fertility preservation (FP) options is important for this population, it is also important to consider the unique psychosocial and developmental issues of LGBTQ AYAs diagnosed with cancer. Unique experiences and considerations of LGBTQ individuals may cause them to have different desires regarding future childbearing and thus FP. For example, one transgender male-to-female child desired to have children in the future, but not with the sperm that could have been stored from her male body [101]. Given such situations, it may be useful for healthcare providers to focus on more diverse family building options, rather than solely on biological parenting – for example, surrogacy and adoption may be of interest to LGBTQ individuals like this child.

Multiple studies of AYA cancer patients and survivors have identified several reasons why discussions about fertility and reproductive health do not take place with newly diagnosed patients. These reasons include the severity of the cancer diagnosis, a provider's discomfort or lack of knowledge on the topic, and a perception that a patient is not interested in fertility if he or she does not initiate a conversation about it [46, 79, 93, 94, 98–100]. To date, there have been very limited studies on LGBTQ AYAs with cancer and their fertility concerns, their childbearing intentions, or oncology healthcare providers' attitudes toward recommending fertility preservation to these patients. One of the first studies assessing oncologists' knowledge of the need to discuss fertility risks with patients identified many would not recommend sperm banking to a gay male patient [98]. It is not clear from this study if the perception is that gay male patients are perceived to be uninterested in having children, or if a value judgment is being made that this population should not have children.

31.5 Availability of and Challenges to Accessing FP and Biological Parenting Options for LGBTQ AYA Patients

For LGBTQ patients who wish to pursue FP options, it is important to consider the unique challenges that they may face. The American College of Obstetricians and Gynecologists (ACOG) acknowledges that lesbian and bisexual women experience barriers in the healthcare system due to concerns about confidentiality, need to disclose, and fear of discrimination [102]. ACOG urges providers to consider that any patient, even one who is pregnant, may be a lesbian or bisexual woman [102]. ACOG also sees refusal to provide reproductive health services to same-sex couples or transgender individuals as a form of discrimination [102–104]. The European Society for Health Reproduction Ethics (ESHRE) also stresses that denying any group access to assisted reproduction "cannot be reconciled with a human rights perspective" [105]. Yet, a recent study showed sexual minority women seek fertility services at half the rate of heterosexual women [106]. However, Grover et al. [107] report the number of same-sex male couples seeking reproductive health services has had a 21-fold increase since 2003. Yager et al. [108] report that lesbian and bisexual women trying to conceive perceive reduced lack of support and heterosexism in fertility healthcare systems.

A survey of 41 transgender men who had become pregnant showed 36 (88%) achieved this pregnancy through their own oocytes despite having used testosterone prior to the pregnancy. Only half of the men reported receiving prenatal care, and all subjects reported low levels of provider knowledge of transgender health. However, what the study also reveals is that many transgender men who have transitioned socially, and in some case medically, still desire a biological child [109].

However, studies of healthcare providers suggest some bias in dealing with LGBTQ patients. A study of Canadian providers showed 11% did not offer sperm banking to gay men [99]. A study of nine transgender individuals living in Canada who attempted to use ART reported all had a negative experience with providers [110]. A US study of obstetrics and gynecology providers revealed 14%

would not suggest ART to women in same-sex relationships or unmarried women [111]. In a 2012 analysis of the websites of US fertility clinics, 11% of clinics did not accept lesbian and single women, and only 10% of all clinic websites had an explicit nondiscrimination disclosure [112]. Several legal studies have examined the juxtaposition between a provider's right not to provide medical care that he or she deems contrary to moral values or conscientious refusal, and discrimination in the context of reproductive medicine [113–117]. The AMA guidelines, however, state, "Physicians cannot refuse to care for patients based on race, gender, sexual orientation, gender identity or any other criteria that would constitute invidious discrimination" [118], nor can they discriminate against patients with infectious diseases [119].

Ongoing advances in assisted reproductive technology (ART) such as uterine transplants for successful pregnancy will continue to raise new ethical issues about the ability for transgender females to carry a pregnancy. For example, Murphy [120] explored this ethical conundrum in a recent commentary and concluded that there are no strong arguments to preclude either the state from developing a line of research to explore the medical feasibility of this or for a transgender woman to pursue a uterine transplant with the goal of carrying a pregnancy.

31.6 Policy and Practice

Institutional policies and practices as well as healthcare providers' verbal and nonverbal communication provide a foundation for AYA LGBTQ patients to disclose their status [30, 121, 122]. Implementing systems-level approaches to routinely collecting relevant information for LGBTQ populations can provide an important starting point to facilitate optimal care [30, 122]. However, health intake forms with binary categories of gender and sexual orientation may dissuade patients from providing this important piece of their social and medical history. Inclusive health forms allow patients to use their own language to describe their gender, romantic relationship, and sexual history [30]. For example, the *Fenway Guide to Lesbian, Gay, Bisexual, and Transgender Health* suggests providers should consider the possibility that "every new patient may have any gender identity or sexual orientation or engage in any sexual behavior: avoid making assumptions based on stereotypes or generalizing from your own experience" [123]. As shown in ◘ Table 31.1, taking a sexual history can involve multiple questions that may be different than most providers learned in medical school [4, 124, 125]. ◘ Table 31.1 provides suggestions for taking a

◘ Table 31.1 Suggested sexual health history questions for face-to-face interview

Partners	Are you having sex with women only, men only, or both (if both, ask the next question twice – once for male partners and once for female partners)?
Practices and past history of STDs	What kinds of sex are you having (e.g., oral sex, vaginal sex, anal sex, sharing sex toys)?
For transgender patients, younger patients, and women who have sex with women, for example, you may find that open-ended questions are preferred and may bring you more accurate information	What do you do to protect yourself from HIV and STDs? When was the last time you had unprotected sex?
Protection from STDs	In the past year, have you had anal sex (penis in the anus/rear end)? Vaginal sex (penis in the vagina)? Oral sex (mouth on penis, vagina, or anus)?
Choose questions based on the sex of partners	Do you use condoms, never, sometimes, or always, when you have (insert type) sex?

Adapted from the Fenway Institute [121]

Table 31.2 Dos and don'ts in taking a sexual history

Do begin with a statement explaining that you ask these questions of all your patients and that the questions are vital to the patient's overall health	*Don't* make assumptions about past, current, or future sexual behavior
Do avoid language that presumes heterosexuality	*Don't* assume that a person who identifies as lesbian or gay has never had an opposite-sex partner
Do check yourself for judgmental facial expressions, body language, and tone of speech	*Don't* assume that an LGBTQ person does not have (or lacks the desire to have) children or has never been pregnant
Do be prepared to answer questions about STI and HIV transmission risk for various sexual activities relevant to LGBTQ people	–
Do note that transgender individuals, men who have sex with men, and those who engage in high-risk sexual activities are at increased risk for contracting HIV and certain STIs	–
Do screen and treat according to the CDC guidelines (▶ www.cdc.gov/std/treatment)	–
Do realize that although STIs are less common among lesbians, clinicians should still screen all women for STI risk, regardless of sexual orientation. The more sexual partners a woman has (female or male), the greater her risk. Bacterial vaginosis may be more common in women who have sex with women than in the general population	–
Do consider the overall health of patients who present with sexual functioning concerns, including their psychological status, physical wellness, and relationship health	–

Makadon et al. [123]

31

sexual history. Table 31.2 offers considerations for healthcare providers when asking these questions such as examining your own values and being aware of nonverbal body language.

The Joint Commission, the Centers for Disease Control and Prevention (CDC), and the Institute of Medicine (IOM) all recommend sexual orientation, and gender identity should be collected in patient medical records [5, 126–129]. CDC and IOM further recommend the aggregation of these data to ensure these populations are represented in clinical research and to reduce health disparities in the population [5, 129]. Figure 31.1 below provides sample wording for the collection of sexual orientation and gender identity on a medical form.

31.7 Conclusion

Healthcare providers in the oncology care setting are increasingly called to understand the unique needs of, and provide care to, a diverse patient population [19, 130]. While great strides have been made over the last decade with respect to cultural competence, there is a growing awareness that diversity spans beyond minority groups solely based on race and ethnicity and includes sexual and gender minority groups that have long been marginalized in the US healthcare system. Our review specifically discusses the challenges of AYA LGBTQ patients in the context of cancer-related infertility and fertility preservation. However, many of the issues and considerations that we

Please provide the following information so that providers and staff may address you correctly and bill for services correctly.

a. Name on Insurance or Legal Government Records: ____________________

b. Preferred name/Nickname (if different): ____________________

c. What is your current gender identity (check all that apply):
Male   Female   Transgender Male/Trans Man/FTM
Transgender Female/Trans Woman/ MTF   Genderqueer
Additional Category, please specify: ____________________
Decline to Answer

d. What sex were you assigned at birth_on your original birth certificate (check one)
Male   Female   Decline to Answer

e. What sex is listed on your health insurance of government records
Male   Female

f. What gender pronoun do you prefer (he, she, they, zie etc): ____________________

g. Do you think of yourself as:
Lesbian   Gay   Homosexual
Straight or heterosexual   Bisexual   Something else ________
Don't know

Fig. 31.1 Sample language for a medical form. (Makadon et al. [123])

have discussed as well as the suggestions we provide can be used to more broadly impact and improve healthcare for sexual and gender minority groups.

Review Questions and Answers

Q1. Individuals in the LGBTQ community aren't interested in having biological families. (True or False)

A1. False.

Q2. What are some of the health disparities faced by the LGBTQ community?

A2. Higher rates of suicide attempts, higher prevalence of mental health issues, and increased risk for certain cancers.

Q3. What do inclusive health forms do differently to assess sexual orientation and gender identity?

A3. Allow patients to use their own language to describe themselves outside of binary categories.

Q4. Patient disclosure of sexual orientation is associated with greater patient discomfort. (True or False)

A4. False.

References

1. Fredriksen-Goldsen KI, Kim HJ, Barkan SE, Muraco A, Hoy-Ellis CP. Health disparities among lesbian, gay, and bisexual older adults: results from a population-based study. Am J Public Health. 2013;103(10):1802–9. Pubmed Central PMCID: Pmc3770805, Epub 2013/06/15. eng.

2. Spectrum Center. LGBT terms and definitions [internet]. Ann Arbor: Spectrum Center; 2015. [cited 2015 Jul 20], Available from: http://internationalspectrum.umich.edu/life/definitions.
3. Johnson CV, Mimiaga MJ, Bradford J. Health care issues among lesbian, gay, bisexual, transgender and intersex (LGBTI) populations in the United States: introduction. J Homosex. 2008;54(3):213–24. Epub 2008/10/02. eng.
4. Institute of Medicine. The health of lesbian, gay, bisexual, and transgender people: building a foundation for better understanding. Washington, DC: National Academies Press; 2011.
5. Institute of Medicine. Collecting sexual orientation and gender identity data in electronic health records. Washington, DC: National Academies Press; 2013.
6. UC Berkeley Gender Equity Resource Center. Definition of terms [Internet]. Berkeley: UC Berkeley Gender Equity Resource Center. p. c2014. [updated 2013 Jul; cited 2015 Jul 21]. Available from: http://geneq.berkeley.edu/lgbt_resources_definiton_of_terms.
7. Gender and Sexuality Center. LGBT vocab 101 [Internet]. Northfield: Gender and Sexuality Center; [date unknown] [updated 2014 May 27; cited 2015 Jul 21]. Available from: https://apps.carleton.edu/campus/gsc/students/ally/lgbtvocab/.
8. Gates GJ. How many people are lesbian, gay, bisexual, and transgender? Los Angeles: The Williams Institute, University of California, Los Angeles School of Law; 2011.
9. Durso LE, Meyer IH. Patterns and predictors of disclosure of sexual orientation to healthcare providers among lesbians, gay men, and bisexuals. Sex Res Soc Policy. 2013;10(1):35–42.
10. Hart SL, Bowen DJ. Sexual orientation and intentions to obtain breast cancer screening. J Women's Health (Larchmt). 2009;18(2):177–85. Pubmed Central PMCID: Pmc2945722, Epub 2009/02/03. eng.
11. Tracy JK, Lydecker AD, Ireland L. Barriers to cervical cancer screening among lesbians. J Women's Health (Larchmt). 2010;19(2):229–37. Pubmed Central PMCID: Pmc2834453, Epub 2010/01/26. eng.
12. Tracy JK, Schluterman NH, Greenberg DR. Understanding cervical cancer screening among lesbians: a national survey. BMC Public Health. 2013;13:442. Pubmed Central PMCID: Pmc3693978, Epub 2013/05/07. eng.
13. Newman PA, Roberts KJ, Masongsong E, Wiley DJ. Anal cancer screening: barriers and facilitators among ethnically diverse gay, bisexual, transgender, and other men who have sex with men. J Gay Lesbian Soc Serv. 2008;20(4):328–53. Pubmed Central PMCID: Pmc3002049, Epub 2008/10/01. Eng.
14. Potter J, Peitzmeier SM, Bernstein I, Reisner SL, Alizaga NM, Agenor M, et al. Cervical cancer screening for patients on the female-to-male spectrum: a narrative review and guide for clinicians. J Gen Intern Med. 2015;30(12):1857–64. Epub 2015/07/15. Eng.
15. Lutz AR. Screening for asymptomatic extragenital gonorrhea and chlamydia in men who have sex with men: significance, recommendations, and options for overcoming barriers to testing. LGBT Health. 2015;2(1):27–34.
16. Dodge B, Van Der Pol B, Rosenberger JG, Reece M, Roth AM, Herbenick D, et al. Field collection of rectal samples for sexually transmitted infection diagnostics among men who have sex with men. Int J STD AIDS. 2010;21(4):260–4. Epub 2010/04/10. eng.
17. McKay B. Lesbian, gay, bisexual, and transgender health issues, disparities, and information resources. Med Ref Serv Q. 2011;30(4):393–401. Epub 2011/11/02. eng.
18. National Alliance on Mental Illness. Mental health issues among gay, lesbian, bisexual, and transgender (GLBT) people [Internet]. Arlington: National Alliance on Mental Illness Multicultural Action Center; 2007. [cited 2015 Jul 21]. Available from: http://www.nami.org/Content/ContentGroups/Multicultural_Support1/Fact_Sheets1/GLBT_Mental_Health_07.pdf.
19. Quinn GP, Sanchez JA, Sutton SK, Vadaparampil ST, Nguyen GT, Green BL, et al. Cancer and lesbian, gay, bisexual, transgender/transsexual, and queer/questioning (LGBTQ) populations. CA Cancer J Clin. 2015;65:384.
20. Almeida J, Johnson RM, Corliss HL, Molnar BE, Azrael D. Emotional distress among LGBT youth: the influence of perceived discrimination based on sexual orientation. J Youth Adolesc. 2009;38(7):1001–14. Pubmed Central PMCID: Pmc3707280, Epub 2009/07/29. eng.
21. Burgess D, Tran A, Lee R, van Ryn M. Effects of perceived discrimination on mental health and mental health services utilization among gay, lesbian, bisexual and transgender persons. J LGBT Health Res. 2007;3(4):1–14. Epub 2008/12/02. eng.
22. National Institutes of Health. Plans for advancing LGBT health research [Internet]. Bethesda: U.S. Department of Health and Human Services; 2013. [updated 2013 Jan 4; cited 2015 Jul 21]. Available from: http://nih.gov/about/director/01032013_lgbt_plan.htm.
23. Margolies L. Bisexual women and breast cancer [internet]. Santa Monica: National LGBT Cancer Network; c2015 [updated 2013 Oct 7; cited 2015 Jul 21]. Available from: http://cancer-network.org/cancer_information/bisexuals_and_cancer/bisexual_women_and_breast_cancer.php.
24. Brown JP, Tracy JK. Lesbians and cancer: an overlooked health disparity. Cancer Causes Control. 2008;19(10):1009–20.
25. NIH LGBT Research Coordinating Committee. Consideration of the institute of medicine (IOM) report on the health of lesbian, gay, bisexual, and transgender (LGBT) individuals. Washington, DC: National Institutes of Health; 2013.
26. Boehmer U, Miao X, Maxwell NI, Ozonoff A. Sexual minority population density and incidence of lung, colorectal and female breast cancer in California. BMJ Open. 2014;4(3):e004461. Pubmed Central PMCID: Pmc3975738, Epub 2014/03/29. eng.
27. Boehmer U, Miao X, Ozonoff A. Cancer survivorship and sexual orientation. Cancer. 2011;117(16):3796–804. Epub 2011/05/11. eng.
28. Boehmer U, Ozonoff A, Miao X. An ecological analysis of colorectal cancer incidence and mortality: differ-

ences by sexual orientation. BMC Cancer. 2011;11:400. Pubmed Central PMCID: Pmc3188512, Epub 2011/09/23. eng.
29. Boehmer U, Ozonoff A, Miao X. An ecological approach to examine lung cancer disparities due to sexual orientation. Public Health. 2012;126(7):605–12. Pubmed Central PMCID: Pmc3389196, Epub 2012/05/15. eng.
30. Quinn GP, Schabath MB, Sanchez JA, Sutton SK, Green BL. The importance of disclosure: lesbian, gay, bisexual, transgender/transsexual, queer/questioning, and intersex individuals and the cancer continuum. Cancer. 2015;121(8):1160–3.
31. Dahan R, Feldman R, Hermoni D. Is patients' sexual orientation a blind spot of family physicians? J Homosex. 2008;55(3):524–32. Epub 2008/12/02. eng.
32. Kamen CS, Smith-Stoner M, Heckler CE, Flannery M, Margolies L, editors. Social support, self-rated health, and lesbian, gay, bisexual, and transgender identity disclosure to cancer care providers. Oncol Nurs Forum. 2015;42(1):44–51: NIH Public Access.
33. Meckler GD, Elliott MN, Kanouse DE, Beals KP, Schuster MA. Nondisclosure of sexual orientation to a physician among a sample of gay, lesbian, and bisexual youth. Arch Pediatr Adolesc Med. 2006;160(12):1248–54.
34. Bjorkman M, Malterud K. Being lesbian–does the doctor need to know? A qualitative study about the significance of disclosure in general practice. Scand J Prim Health Care. 2007;25(1):58–62.
35. Boehmer U, Case P. Physicians don't ask, sometimes patients tell. Cancer. 2004;101(8):1882–9.
36. Johnson MJ, Nemeth LS. Addressing health disparities of lesbian and bisexual women: a grounded theory study. Womens Health Issues. 2014;24(6):635–40.
37. American Medical Association. AMA policy regarding sexual orientation [Internet]. Chicago: American Medical Association; c1995–2015 [cited 2015 Jul 22]. Available from: http://www.ama-assn.org/ama/pub/about-ama/our-people/member-groups-sections/glbt-advisory-committee/ama-policy-regarding-sexual-orientation.page.
38. Frankowski BL. Sexual orientation and adolescents. Pediatrics. 2004;113(6):1827–32. Epub 2004/06/03. eng.
39. Society for Adolescent Health and Medicine. Recommendations for promoting the health and well-being of lesbian, gay, bisexual, and transgender adolescents: a position paper of the Society for Adolescent Health and Medicine. J Adolesc Health. 2013; 52(4):506–10. Epub 2013/03/26. eng.
40. Quinn GP, Sutton SK, Winfield B, Breen S, Canales J, Shetty G, et al. Lesbian, gay, bisexual, transgender, queer/questioning (LGBTQ) perceptions and health care experiences. J Gay Lesbian Soc Serv. 2015;27(2):246–61.
41. Fisher CB, Mustanski B. Reducing health disparities and enhancing the responsible conduct of research involving LGBT youth. Hast Cent Rep. 2014;44(Suppl 4):S28–31. Epub 2014/09/19. eng.
42. Mayer KH, Bradford JB, Makadon HJ, Stall R, Goldhammer H, Landers S. Sexual and gender minority health: what we know and what needs to be done. Am J Public Health. 2008;98(6):989–95.
43. Mustanski B. Future directions in research on sexual minority adolescent mental, behavioral, and sexual health. J Clin Child Adolesc Psychol. 2015;44(1):204–19. Pubmed Central PMCID: Pmc4314941, Epub 2015/01/13. eng.
44. Carter J, Penson R, Barakat R, Wenzel L. Contemporary quality of life issues affecting gynecologic cancer survivors. Hematol Oncol Clin North Am. 2012; 26(1):169–94.
45. Partridge AH, Gelber S, Peppercorn J, Sampson E, Knudsen K, Laufer M, et al. Web-based survey of fertility issues in young women with breast cancer. J Clin Oncol. 2004;22(20):4174–83.
46. Schover LR. Patient attitudes toward fertility preservation. Pediatr Blood Cancer. 2009;53(2):281–4.
47. Howard-Anderson J, Ganz PA, Bower JE, Stanton AL. Quality of life, fertility concerns, and behavioral health outcomes in younger breast cancer survivors: a systematic review. J Natl Cancer Inst. 2012; 104(5):386–405.
48. Bleyer A, Barr R, Hayes-Lattin B, Thomas D, Ellis C, Anderson B, et al. The distinctive biology of cancer in adolescents and young adults. Nat Rev Cancer. 2008;8(4):288–98.
49. Levine J, Canada A, Stern CJ. Fertility preservation in adolescents and young adults with cancer. J Clin Oncol. 2010;28(32):4831–41.
50. Canada AL, Schover LR. The psychosocial impact of interrupted childbearing in long-term female cancer survivors. Psychooncology. 2012;21(2):134–43. Pubmed Central PMCID: 3123665.
51. Letourneau JM, Ebbel EE, Katz PP, Katz A, Ai WZ, Chien AJ, et al. Pretreatment fertility counseling and fertility preservation improve quality of life in reproductive age women with cancer. Cancer. 2012;118(6):1710–7. Pubmed Central PMCID: 3235264.
52. Gorman JR, Usita PM, Madlensky L, Pierce JP. Young breast cancer survivors: their perspectives on treatment decisions and fertility concerns. Cancer Nurs. 2011;34(1):32–40. Pubmed Central PMCID: 2980796.
53. Bahadur G. Fertility issues for cancer patients. Mol Cell Endocrinol. 2000;169(1–2):117–22. Epub 2001/01/13. eng.
54. Padron OF, Sharma RK, Thomas AJ Jr, Agarwal A. Effects of cancer on spermatozoa quality after cryopreservation: a 12-year experience. Fertil Steril. 1997;67(2):326–31. Epub 1997/02/01. eng.
55. Drasga RE, Einhorn LH, Williams SD, Patel DN, Stevens EE. Fertility after chemotherapy for testicular cancer. J Clin Oncol. 1983;1(3):179–83. Epub 1983/03/01. eng.
56. Carter J, Rowland K, Chi D, Brown C, Abu-Rustum N, Castiel M, et al. Gynecologic cancer treatment and the impact of cancer-related infertility. Gynecol Oncol. 2005;97(1):90–5. Epub 2005/03/26. eng.
57. Crawshaw M, Sloper P. A qualitative study of the experiences of teenagers and young adults when faced with possible or actual fertility impairment following cancer treatment. York: Department of Social Policy and Social Work, University of York; 2006.

58. Loren AW, Mangu PB, Beck LN, Brennan L, Magdalinski AJ, Partridge AH, et al. Fertility preservation for patients with cancer: American Society of Clinical Oncology clinical practice guideline update. J Clin Oncol. 2013;31(19):2500–10. Epub 2013/05/30. eng.
59. Gracia CR, Sammel MD, Freeman E, Prewitt M, Carlson C, Ray A, et al. Impact of cancer therapies on ovarian reserve. Fertil Steril. 2012;97(1):134–40.e1. Pubmed Central PMCID: Pmc4005036. Epub 2011/12/06. eng.
60. Critchley HO, Wallace WH. Impact of cancer treatment on uterine function. J Natl Cancer Inst Monogr. 2005;34:64–8. Epub 2005/03/24. eng.
61. Littley MD, Shalet SM, Beardwell CG, Ahmed SR, Applegate G, Sutton ML. Hypopituitarism following external radiotherapy for pituitary tumours in adults. Q J Med. 1989;70(262):145–60. Epub 1989/02/01. eng.
62. Su HI, Sammel MD, Velders L, Horn M, Stankiewicz C, Matro J, et al. Association of cyclophosphamide drug-metabolizing enzyme polymorphisms and chemotherapy-related ovarian failure in breast cancer survivors. Fertil Steril. 2010;94(2):645–54. Pubmed Central PMCID: Pmc2891284, Epub 2009/04/21. eng.
63. van Dorp W, van den Heuvel-Eibrink MM, Stolk L, Pieters R, Uitterlinden AG, Visser JA, et al. Genetic variation may modify ovarian reserve in female childhood cancer survivors. Hum Reprod. 2013;28(4):1069–76. Epub 2013/01/31. eng.
64. American Cancer Society. Fertility and women with cancer [internet]. Atlanta: American Cancer Society; 2013. [cited 2015 Jul 22]. Available from: http://www.cancer.org/acs/groups/cid/documents/webcontent/acspc-041244-pdf.pdf.
65. LIVESTRONG. LIVESTRONG Fertility [Internet]. Austin: LIVESTRONG; c2014 [cited 2015 Jul 22]. Available from: http://assets.livestrong.org/we-can-help/LIVESTRONG-Fertility-Brochure.pdf.
66. Cancer.net. Fertility Concerns and Preservation for Men [Internet]. [place unknown]: American Society of Clinical Oncology; c2005–2015 [cited 2015 Jul 22]. Available from: http://www.cancer.net/coping-and-emotions/sexual-and-reproductive-health/fertility-concerns-and-preservation-men.
67. Cancer.net. Fertility Concerns and Preservation for Women [Internet]. [place unknown]: American Society of Clinical Oncology; c2005–2015 [cited 2015 Jul 22]. Available from: http://www.cancer.net/coping-and-emotions/sexual-and-reproductive-health/fertility-concerns-and-preservation-women.
68. Levine JM, Kelvin JF, Quinn GP, Gracia CR. Infertility in reproductive-age female cancer survivors. Cancer. 2015;121(10):1532–9. Epub 2015/02/05. eng.
69. Hulvat MC, Jeruss JS. Maintaining fertility in young women with breast cancer. Curr Treat Options in Oncol. 2009;10(5–6):308–17. Pubmed Central PMCID: Pmc2908234, Epub 2010/03/20. eng.
70. Duffy C, Allen S. Medical and psychosocial aspects of fertility after cancer. Cancer J. 2009;15(1):27–33. Pubmed Central PMCID: Pmc2719717, Epub 2009/02/07. eng.
71. Goldfarb S, Mulhall J, Nelson C, Kelvin J, Dickler M, Carter J. Sexual and reproductive health in cancer survivors. Semin Oncol. 2013;40(6):726–44. Epub 2013/12/18. eng.
72. Tournaye H, Dohle GR, Barratt CL. Fertility preservation in men with cancer. Lancet. 2014;384(9950):1295–301. Epub 2014/10/07. eng.
73. Ginsberg JP. Educational paper: the effect of cancer therapy on fertility, the assessment of fertility and fertility preservation options for pediatric patients. Eur J Pediatr. 2011;170(6):703–8. Epub 2010/12/04. eng.
74. Fallat ME, Hutter J. Preservation of fertility in pediatric and adolescent patients with cancer. Pediatrics. 2008;121(5):e1461–9. Epub 2008/05/03. eng.
75. Coccia P, Pappo A, Altman J, Bhatia S, Borges V, Borinstein S, et al. The NCCN adolescent and young adult (AYA) oncology clinical practice guideline, version 2.2015 [internet]. Cold Spring Harbor: Harborside Press, LLC; 2015. [cited 2015 Jul 22]. Available from: http://www.nccn.org/professionals/physician_gls/pdf/aya.pdf.
76. Quinn GP, Block RG, Clayman ML, Kelvin J, Arvey SR, Lee JH, et al. If you did not document it, it did not happen: rates of documentation of discussion of infertility risk in adolescent and young adult oncology patients' medical records. J Oncol Pract. 2015;11(2):137–44. Epub 2015/01/01. eng.
77. Vadaparampil ST, Quinn GP. Improving communication between oncologists and reproductive specialists to promote timely referral of patients with cancer. J Oncol Pract. 2013;9(6):300–2. Epub 2013/08/15. eng.
78. Banerjee R, Tsiapali E. Occurrence and recall rates of fertility discussions with young breast cancer patients. Support Care Cancer. 2015;24(1):163–71. Epub 2015/05/15. eng.
79. Quinn GP, Vadaparampil ST, Lee JH, Jacobsen PB, Bepler G, Lancaster J, et al. Physician referral for fertility preservation in oncology patients: a national study of practice behaviors. J Clin Oncol. 2009;27(35):5952–7. Epub 2009/10/15. eng.
80. Yeomanson DJ, Morgan S, Pacey AA. Discussing fertility preservation at the time of cancer diagnosis: dissatisfaction of young females. Pediatr Blood Cancer. 2013;60(12):1996–2000. Epub 2013/07/10. eng.
81. Partridge AH, Gelber S, Peppercorn J, Ginsburg E, Sampson E, Rosenberg R, et al. Fertility and menopausal outcomes in young breast cancer survivors. Clin Breast Cancer. 2008;8(1):65–9. Epub 2008/05/27. eng.
82. Bastings L, Baysal O, Beerendonk CC, IntHout J, Traas MA, Verhaak CM, et al. Deciding about fertility preservation after specialist counselling. Hum Reprod. 2014;29(8):1721–9. Epub 2014/06/12. eng.
83. Wilkes S, Coulson S, Crosland A, Rubin G, Stewart J. Experience of fertility preservation among younger people diagnosed with cancer. Hum Fertil (Camb). 2010;13(3):151–8. Epub 2010/09/21. eng.
84. Jeruss JS, Woodruff TK. Preservation of fertility in patients with cancer. N Engl J Med. 2009;360(9):902–11. Pubmed Central PMCID: Pmc2927217, Epub 2009/02/28. eng.

85. Rowan K. Fertility preservation during treatment is a growing issue for women. J Natl Cancer Inst. 2010;102(5):294–6. Epub 2010/02/23. eng.
86. Murphy D, Klosky JL, Reed DR, Termuhlen AM, Shannon SV, Quinn GP. The importance of assessing priorities of reproductive health concerns among adolescent and young adult patients with cancer. Cancer. 2015;121(15):2529–36. Epub 2015/06/05. eng.
87. T'Sjoen G, Van Caenegem E, Wierckx K. Transgenderism and reproduction. Curr Opin Endocrinol Diabetes Obes. 2013;20(6):575–9.
88. Wierckx K, Van Caenegem E, Pennings G, Elaut E, Dedecker D, Van de Peer F, et al. Reproductive wish in transsexual men. Hum Reprod. 2012;27(2):483–7.
89. Santillo VM. Prostate cancer diagnosis and treatment of a 33-year-old gay man. J Gay Lesbian Ment Health. 2005;9(1–2):155–71.
90. [author unknown]. New survey finds infertility delivers a serious blow to self-esteem [Internet]. Whitehouse Station: PR Newswire; 2010 [cited 2015 Jul 24]. Available from: http://www.prnewswire.com/news-releases/new-survey-finds-infertility-delivers-a-serious-blow-to-self-esteem-82242177.html.
91. Faramarzi M, Pasha H, Esmailzadeh S, Kheirkhah F, Hajian-Tilaki K, Salmalian H. A survey of correlation infertility self-efficacy with behavioral health scales in infertile women. Health (N Y). 2014;6(10):943.
92. Wischmann T, Schilling K, Toth B, Rosner S, Strowitzki T, Wohlfarth K, et al. Sexuality, self-esteem and partnership quality in infertile women and men. Geburtshilfe Frauenheilkd. 2014;74(8):759–63. Pubmed Central PMCID: Pmc4153818, Epub 2014/09/16. Eng.
93. Jukkala AM, Azuero A, McNees P, Bates GW, Meneses K. Self-assessed knowledge of treatment and fertility preservation in young women with breast cancer. Fertil Steril. 2010;94(6):2396–8. Epub 2010/05/08. eng.
94. Oosterhuis BE, Goodwin T, Kiernan M, Hudson MM, Dahl GV. Concerns about infertility risks among pediatric oncology patients and their parents. Pediatr Blood Cancer. 2008;50(1):85–9. Epub 2007/05/22. eng.
95. Burns KC, Boudreau C, Panepinto JA. Attitudes regarding fertility preservation in female adolescent cancer patients. J Pediatr Hematol Oncol. 2006;28(6):350–4. Epub 2006/06/24. eng.
96. Maltaris T, Seufert R, Fischl F, Schaffrath M, Pollow K, Koelbl H, et al. The effect of cancer treatment on female fertility and strategies for preserving fertility. Eur J Obstet Gynecol Reprod Biol. 2007;130(2):148–55. Epub 2006/09/19. eng.
97. Klock SC, Zhang JX, Kazer RR. Fertility preservation for female cancer patients: early clinical experience. Fertil Steril. 2010;94(1):149–55. Epub 2009/05/02. eng.
98. Schover LR, Brey K, Lichtin A, Lipshultz LI, Jeha S. Oncologists' attitudes and practices regarding banking sperm before cancer treatment. J Clin Oncol. 2002;20(7):1890–7. Epub 2002/03/29. eng.
99. Achille MA, Rosberger Z, Robitaille R, Lebel S, Gouin JP, Bultz BD, et al. Facilitators and obstacles to sperm banking in young men receiving gonadotoxic chemotherapy for cancer: the perspective of survivors and health care professionals. Hum Reprod. 2006;21(12):3206–16. Epub 2006/08/05. eng.
100. Quinn GP, Vadaparampil ST, Gwede CK, Miree C, King LM, Clayton HB, et al. Discussion of fertility preservation with newly diagnosed patients: oncologists' views. J Cancer Surviv. 2007;1(2):146–55. Epub 2008/07/24. eng.
101. Navasky M, O'Connor K. Growing up trans [television broadcast]. FRONTLINE. Boston: Public Broadcasting Service; 2015.
102. ACOG Committee on Health Care for Underserved Women. ACOG Committee opinion no. 525: health care for lesbians and bisexual women. Obstet Gynecol. 2012;119(5):1077.
103. ACOG Committee on Health Care for Underserved Women. Committee opinion no. 512: health care for transgender individuals. Obstet Gynecol. 2011; 118(6):1454–8. Epub 2011/11/23. eng.
104. American College of Obstetricians Gynecologists. ACOG Committee Opinion No. 385 November 2007: the limits of conscientious refusal in reproductive medicine. Obstet Gynecol. 2007;110(5):1203.
105. De Wert G, Dondorp W, Shenfield F, Barri P, Devroey P, Diedrich K, et al. ESHRE task force on ethics and Law 23: medically assisted reproduction in singles, lesbian and gay couples, and transsexual people. Hum Reprod. 2014;29(9):1859–65.
106. Blanchfield BV, Patterson CJ. Racial and sexual minority women's receipt of medical assistance to become pregnant. Health Psychol. 2015;34(6):571.
107. Grover SA, Shmorgun Z, Moskovtsev SI, Baratz A, Librach CL. Assisted reproduction in a cohort of same-sex male couples and single men. Reprod BioMed Online. 2013;27(2):217–21.
108. Yager C, Brennan D, Steele LS, Epstein R, Ross LE. Challenges and mental health experiences of lesbian and bisexual women who are trying to conceive. Health Soc Work. 2010;35(3):191–200.
109. Light AD, Obedin-Maliver J, Sevelius JM, Kerns JL. Transgender men who experienced pregnancy after female-to-male gender transitioning. Obstet Gynecol. 2014;124(6):1120–7.
110. James-Abra S, Tarasoff L, Epstein R, Anderson S, Marvel S, Steele L, et al. Trans people's experiences with assisted reproduction services: a qualitative study. Hum Reprod. 2015;30(6):1365–74.
111. Lawrence RE, Rasinski KA, Yoon JD, Curlin FA. Obstetrician–gynecologists' beliefs about assisted reproductive technologies. Obstet Gynecol. 2010;116(1): 127–35.
112. Johnson KM. Excluding lesbian and single women? An analysis of US fertility clinic websites. Womens Stud Int Forum. 2012;35(5):394–402.
113. Lumpkin CA. Does a pharmacist have the right to refuse to fill a prescription for birth control. Univ Miami Law Rev. 2005;60:105.
114. Smearman CA. Drawing the line: the legal, ethical and public policy implications of refusal clauses for pharmacists. Ariz Law Rev. 2006;48:469.

115. Storrow RF. Medical conscience and the policing of parenthood. William Mary J Women Law. 2009; 16:369.
116. Dickens B. Legal protection and limits of conscientious objection: when conscientious objection is unethical. Med Law. 2009;28(2):337.
117. Langlois N. Life-sustaining treatment law: a model for balancing a woman's reproductive rights with a pharmacist's conscientious objection. BCL Rev. 2005;47:815.
118. American Medical Association. Opinion 9.12 – Patient-physician relationship: respect for law and human rights [Internet]. Chicago: American Medical Association; c1995–2015 [updated 2008 Jun; cited 2015 Jul 23]. Available from: http://www.ama-assn.org/ama/pub/physician-resources/medical-ethics/code-medical-ethics/opinion912.page.
119. American Medical Association. Opinion 2.23 – HIV testing [internet]. Chicago: American Medical Association; 2010. [cited 2015 Jul 23]. Available from: http://www.ama-assn.org/ama/pub/physician-resources/medical-ethics/code-medical-ethics/opinion223.page.
120. Murphy TF. Assisted gestation and transgender women. Bioethics. 2015;29(6):389–97. Epub 2014/12/17. eng.
121. The Fenway Institute. Asking patients questions about sexual orientation and gender identity in clinical settings: a study in four health centers. Boston: The Fenway Institute and the Center for American Progress; 2013.
122. Makadon HJ. Ending LGBT invisibility in health care: the first step in ensuring equitable care. Cleve Clin J Med. 2011;78(4):220–4.
123. Makadon HJ, Mayer KH, Potter J, Goldhammer H. The Fenway guide to lesbian, gay, bisexual, and transgender health. 2nd ed. Philadelphia: ACP Press; 2015.
124. White W, Brenman S, Paradis E, Goldsmith ES, Lunn MR, Obedin-Maliver J, et al. Lesbian, gay, bisexual, and transgender patient care: medical students' preparedness and comfort. Teach Learn Med. 2015;27(3):254–63. Epub 2015/07/15. eng.
125. Sequeira GM, Chakraborti C, Panunti BA. Integrating lesbian, gay, bisexual, and transgender (LGBT) content into undergraduate medical school curricula: a qualitative study. Ochsner J. 2012;12(4):379–82. Pubmed Central PMCID: Pmc3527869, Epub 2012/12/26. eng.
126. Cahill S, Makadon H. Sexual orientation and gender identity data collection in clinical settings and in electronic health records: a key to ending LGBT health disparities. LGBT Health. 2014;1(1):34–41.
127. The Joint Commission. Advancing effective communication, cultural competence, and patient- and family-centered care for the lesbian, gay, bisexual, and transgender (LGBT) community: a field guide. Oak Brook; 2011.
128. Institute of Medicine Board on the Health of Select Populations. The national academies collection: reports funded by National Institutes of Health. Collecting sexual orientation and gender identity data in electronic health records: workshop summary. Washington, DC: National Academies Press (US); 2013.
129. Ward BW, Dahlhamer JM, Galinsky AM, Joestl SS. Sexual orientation and health among U.S. adults: national health interview survey, 2013. Natl Health Stat Rep. 2014;15(77):1–10. Epub 2014/07/16. eng.
130. Davey MP, Waite R, Nunez A, Nino A, Kissil K. A snapshot of patients' perceptions of oncology providers' cultural competence. J Cancer Educ. 2014;29(4):657–64. Epub 2014/02/08. eng.

Ethics of Posthumous Reproduction

Lisa Campo-Engelstein

T. K. Woodruff et al. (eds.), *Textbook of Oncofertility Research and Practice*,
https://doi.org/10.1007/978-3-030-02868-8_32

Key Points
- Posthumous assisted reproduction raises justice concerns about access, cost, and the legal rights of posthumously conceived children
- It is important to consider the benefits and harms of posthumous assisted reproduction for the deceased, the surviving partner, the surviving family, and posthumously conceived children
- Written consent regarding posthumous assisted reproduction is the best method for ensuring that the autonomy of the deceased is upheld
- Spouse or partner request for posthumous assisted reproduction is the least ethically contentious since the couple had a joint reproductive project

32

32.1 Introduction

Cryopreservation of gametes is becoming more common with individuals choosing to freeze their gametes before cancer treatment, gender-affirming treatment, and military deployment or in anticipation of age-related infertility. Additionally, there are more than 620,000 frozen embryos in storage in the United States [6], many of which were created by heterosexual couples as part of infertility treatment. Given the growing number of frozen gametes and embryos, the question arises of what should be done with them when the people who froze them die. One option is posthumous assisted reproduction (PAR), which involves using assisted reproductive technologies (ART) to conceive a child after one of the genetic parents has died.

For individuals who have not already frozen gametes or embryos, PAR is still possible, but posthumous gamete retrieval is required. Postmortem gamete retrieval typically occurs when there is an unexpected event (e.g., accident, sudden illness) leading to the death or imminent death of an individual [4]. For example, the first reported case of posthumous sperm procurement took place in 1980 when a 30-year-old man was in a car accident and was declared brain-dead [23]. The vast majority of postmortem gamete retrieval cases involve men, and one of the first, if not the first, cases of postmortem egg retrieval was not until 2011 [24]. There are a few reasons for this gender disparity in postmortem gamete retrieval. First, whereas posthumous sperm retrieval is a relatively easy and fast procedure (it usually needs to occur within 24 hours of death), posthumous egg retrieval is more medically complicated, and it can take a couple of weeks to hyperstimulate the ovaries and collect mature eggs. Second, in a heterosexual couple, if the male partner dies, the female partner can carry the pregnancy. If the female partner dies, the male partner would need to use a gestational surrogate, which creates additional legal, ethical, and financial considerations. Third, empirical studies show that men are more willing than women to approve of their partner using their gametes posthumously to conceive a child [5, 8]. This difference may be explained by dominant gender norms, such as the cultural expectation that women are the primary caregivers of children.

Both types of PAR – those involving already frozen gametes or embryos and those requiring postmortem gamete retrieval – raise a host of ethical issues. In this chapter, I will explore the ethics of PAR based on the core ethical principles. Then I will examine who should be permitted to request PAR. I will draw heavily on the guidelines issued by the ethics committees of the American Society for Reproductive Medicine (ASRM) and the European Society of Human Reproduction and Embryology (ESHRE).

32.2 Bioethical Principles

32.2.1 Justice

The ethical principle of justice demands that we be fair to the wider community in terms of the consequences of an action, especially ensuring that risks and benefits are equally distributed. One justice concern is that PAR is not equally accessible to all people. PAR is illegal in certain countries, such as Sweden, France, Germany, Canada, and some states in Australia, even if the deceased has given consent [2]. In countries where it is legal, its availability depends upon the institution. Furthermore, since ART, including PAR, are often not covered by insurance in the United States, PAR may only be within reach of individuals who are wealthier and/or have insurance coverage for ART. A different financial concern with PAR is that it may not be the best use of limited healthcare resources, particularly when more basic healthcare needs are not met [16].

Another justice concern is that children who are posthumously conceived are sometimes treated differently under the law, especially regarding inheritance. Laws on inheritance vary by country and also by state in the United States. In 2012, the US Supreme Court ruled unanimously in *Astrue v. Capato* that whether posthumously conceived children were entitled to Social Security benefits should be based on state law [1]. Some claim it is unfair that children would receive fewer rights due to the method or time of their conception. ESHRE recommends that posthumously conceived children should be legally recognized as the child of the deceased parent and be able to receive inheritance rights [17].

32.2.2 Beneficence/Nonmaleficence

Beneficence is the ethical principle to promote good and nonmaleficence is the ethical principle to prevent harm. When considering the potential benefits and harms, we should consider the deceased, the surviving partner and family of the deceased, and the potential future child.

Knowing that PAR is possible may give peace of mind to people who freeze their gametes, particularly those who face life-threatening situations such as cancer or military deployment. Yet, as I will discuss in more depth in the next section, if we do not know the wishes of the deceased and we proceed with PAR, we risk the harm of violating the autonomy of the deceased. Furthermore, if the deceased has not already frozen reproductive material, then gamete retrieval is required and this may be seen as a violation of bodily integrity [7]. Additionally, we can question whether "retrieving sperm from a dying or dead man would be in his own interests, as there is no direct benefit for him, while there is the possibility for harm" [16] (p. 147).

PAR may ease the pain and suffering of the surviving partner and family of the deceased. Both ASRM and ESHRE recommend a waiting period and counseling before surviving partners and family seek PAR to avoid hasty decisions made out of grief. The majority of people who request sperm retrieval following the death of a partner do not end up using the sperm for PAR [17]. The use of PAR can be contentious and can cause disagreements within families. For instance, Bill Kane froze his sperm and bequeathed it to his girlfriend, Deborah Hecht. After Kane died, his adult children from a previous relationship took Hecht to court to prevent her from using their father's sperm. Because Kane had provided explicit written documentation that he wanted Hecht to use his sperm, the court ruled in Hecht's favor [12].

There are ethical concerns that PAR may harm potential future children. One concern is that the child will likely be raised in a single-parent household. In response to this concern, ESHRE argues "even if single parenthood has a negative effect on health and well-being of the child, it is unlikely that this effect is of such magnitude that it jeopardizes the reasonable welfare of the child" [17] (p. 3051). Another concern is that posthumously conceived children will feel stigmatized and may suffer psychological stress. There is also the worry that the child will be seen as "commemorative" or as a "symbolic replacement of the deceased" [17] (p. 3052). There is no empirical evidence, however, to suggest that these concerns are a reality. Moreover, it seems reasonable to assume that posthumously conceived children are deeply wanted and may be cherished by the surviving family of their deceased parent.

32.2.3 Autonomy

Autonomy is the ethical principle that we should respect the personal decisions of individuals. One of the biggest ethical concerns with PAR is whether deceased individuals consented to or would agree with the use of their gametes posthumously. As John Robertson asserts, "If a person becomes a parent after death without his consent his reproductive autonomy is altered" [13] (p. 434). For many people, genetic reproduction is a deeply personal and private decision, one that they want to make for themselves and without interference from others. While there does not exist a positive right to reproduction – a right to receive assistance in having a child – in the United States, there is a negative right to reproduction – a right to avoid procreation. For example, when heterosexual couples disagree about how to handle embryos that contain both of their genetic material, courts typically find in favor of the individual who does not want to reproduce [14]. These rulings show that the US legal system generally prioritizes the negative right to reproduce over the positive right to reproduce. Furthermore, the importance of the negative right to reproduction is also present in Europe, as ESHRE states regarding PAR: "Because of the special value of autonomy in the context of reproduction, an opting-in system is preferred to an opting-out system" [17] (p. 3051). In short, the worry with PAR is that we may violate the autonomy of the deceased by using their genetic material without their permission.

When individuals are alive and have decision-making capacity, it is easy to know what their wishes are and to follow them. However, when individuals lose capacity or are deceased, it can be challenging to determine what they would want done in a given situation. While some have claimed that the dead no longer have any interests [22], most agree that "it is considered disrespectful toward the dead to do things to their bodies to which they would have objected when alive" [25] (p. 743). In other words, even after people are deceased, we still have an obligation to uphold their autonomy as best as we can. To do this, we first turn to forms of explicit consent, such as written documentation (e.g., advance directives) or verbal consent given to healthcare providers. If they are not available, then we rely on inferred consent by asking the proxy and loved ones of the deceased individuals to ascertain what their wishes would be [25].

When the deceased has provided written consent for PAR, both the ASRM and ESHRE find it ethically justifiable[1] since we are respecting reproductive autonomy of the deceased. Ideally, individuals who freeze their gametes or gonadal tissue in anticipation of future infertility (e.g., due to cancer treatment, gender-affirming treatments, or age-related infertility) and heterosexual couples who create embryos (e.g., as part of infertility treatment) should provide written documentation outlining what they would like to happen to their gametes or embryos when they die. Specifically, they should state whether they would approve of posthumous reproduction and if so, under what circumstances. ASRM and ESHRE both recommend that conversations and consent for PAR be included in the informed consent process of cryopreserving reproductive material.

While there is a general consensus that PAR is ethical when the deceased has written consent, there is more ambiguity in the case where the deceased does not have any written documentation. Professional societies disagree: ESHRE claims that PAR is only permissible when "written consent has been given by the deceased person" [17] (p. 3050), whereas ASRM allows for the possibility of PAR-based on inferred consent, stating "in the absence of written documentation from the decedent, programs open to considering requests for posthumous gamete procurement or reproduction should only do so when such requests are initiated by the surviving spouse or life partner" [7] (p. 1842).

How can we follow the deceased's wishes if there is no documentation? When patients do not have capacity, the protocol is to appoint a healthcare proxy, generally a partner/spouse, parent, adult child, or another family member. The same can be done for cases involving PAR. Proxies should use the substituted judgment standard, which means relying on the known values, preferences, and beliefs of the deceased to make decisions that are mostly likely what the deceased would make in that situation. Yet relying on a proxy in the case of PAR may be problematic because "[i]n some cases, the only evidence of their [the deceased's] wishes will be the testimony of a person bearing an apparent conflict of interest, namely the one who wishes to use the deceased's sperm or eggs to reproduce" [7] (p. 1844).

It is important to note that evidence that people wanted to reproduce while living, including freezing reproductive material, does not necessarily mean that they would agree to PAR. According to ESHRE, "[t]he presence of cryostored gametes or embryos shows that a parental project existed, but it does not demonstrate that the deceased accepted the continuation of the project after his or her death" [17] (p. 3051). A significant reason why many people have children is because of the relationship they will have with their child; since no such relationship exists in posthumous reproduction, people may reject it. Furthermore, some people may oppose PAR because they are concerned about having their child raised in a single-

1 Some other conditions have to be met as well for these societies to find PAR ethically justifiable.

parent household or worry that their child will feel "wronged or stigmatized" [17] (p. 3051). A study by Nakhuda et al. found a minority of heterosexual couples who are actively trying to have children through ART were not in favor of PAR; specifically, 22% of respondents opposed or were undecided about PAR, and 25% of couples disagreed about PAR [15].

Overall, however, the majority of individuals using ART and individuals in the general population find PAR acceptable. The vast majority (approximately 78%) of couples in the Nakhuda et al. study would consent to PAR [15]. Other research examining heterosexual couples using or who have already used ART echo these results. For instance, Côté et al. looked at PAR in heterosexual couples who had frozen embryos and found that 61.8% of women and 73.5% of men would allow their partners to use their frozen embryos after their death [5]. The American public mostly looks favorably on PAR: a study by Barton et al. showed that almost 50% of respondents support PAR in both women and men [3], a study by Hans and Frey found that around two thirds of respondents agree with PAR [10], and a study by Hans and Dooley concluded that, depending upon the circumstances, between half to three quarters of respondents were in favor of PAR [9].

In the absence of written documentation, are these studies coupled with evidence from loved ones that a particular person would have agreed to PAR sufficient to allow PAR? Many people, especially young people, do not complete advanced directives [19] and in the case of a sudden, unexpected adverse event, there may not be time to obtain written consent. If an entire family is in agreement that an incapacitated or deceased person would support PAR, then "the insistence on prior written consent may seem unreasonable or even cruel" [7] (p. 1844). Some bioethicists have argued in favor of presumed consent for PAR, claiming that the consent of the deceased should not be the primary focus; rather, we should consider the welfare of the partner and the prospective child as our main ethical concern [26]. Israel follows a presumed consent model "based on the assumption that a man who lived in a loving relationship with a woman would want her to have his genetic child after his death even if he never had the opportunity formally to express such a desire" [20] (p. 6).

In the case of minors who have cryopreserved reproductive material, there is a consensus that PAR is not ethically acceptable because minors are not able to consent, as they lack decision-making capacity and certain legal rights due to their age. We typically understand reproductive material as "belonging" to the individual or individuals whose genetic material it contains. When parents or guardians consent to having their children's reproductive material banked, they are doing so to secure their children's future reproductive autonomy, not so that they can use this material themselves.

32.2.4 Who Requests PAR?

If the deceased has left written documentation about their preferences regarding PAR, both ASRM and ESHRE support following the wishes of the deceased. However, if the deceased did not leave written documentation, the question then arises who should be able to request it and to use the gametes or embryos. ASRM asserts that, in the absence of written documentation, the surviving spouse or partner is the only one who should be able to request and use the deceased's gametes or embryos because the spouse or partner and the deceased had an existing joint parental project. Partner requests for PAR is acceptable since it allows one partner to continue that project after the death of the other. ESHRE finds partner requests for PAR the least ethically problematic for the same reason as ASRM.

The importance of this joint reproductive project is why ASRM finds PAR "less compelling" for single individuals than for partnered individuals. Given the increasing acceptance of single parenthood and various family formations [18], some may claim that it is possible for a single individual to have a reproductive project with another person who is not a spouse or partner. Also, some may be concerned that by focusing so heavily on the fact that the reproductive project is joint, ASRM is prioritizing heteronormative nuclear family formations and discounting the importance of the reproductive project for single individuals.

ASRM's opposition to parental requests for PAR also centers on the idea of a joint reproductive project: "In the case of a surviving parent, no joint reproductive project can ever be said to have existed. Nor do the desires of the parents give them any ethical claim to their child's gametes" [7]

(p. 1844). Here, again, some may object to the assumption that a reproductive project can only exist within a couple. Furthermore, one could argue that the genetic parents of the deceased could also have some claim in the genetic material of their child. In Israel, parental requests for PAR "are becoming more and more accepted, building on the same logic that the family lineage or perpetuation of the blood line does not end with one's death" [11] (p. 26). All of the parental requests in Israel that have been permitted have involved an arrangement in which a single woman who did not know the deceased used his sperm and planned to raise any resulting children by herself while allowing a relationship between the children and the genetic grandparents. The Israeli courts have approved of these arrangements, calling them a "harmonious coming together of the interests of all parties involved" [21]. Part of the reason why these arrangements may be more ethically permissible is because the parents of the deceased are not raising their genetic grandchildren themselves, but rather are establishing a more "traditional" grandparent/grandchild relationship.

Whereas the arrangement in Israel involves parental requests for PAR, ESHRE also discusses PAR outside of partner and parental requests. This type of third-party request would most likely involve the donation of already existing frozen reproductive material to anonymous recipients interested in using them for reproduction. Some members of the ESHRE task force believe that "posthumous reproduction outside the initial parental project to be justified on the conditions that donors consent to this broad use and that all safety measures usually applicable to gametes or embryos donation are respected" [17] (p. 3051).

32.3 Conclusion

In this chapter, I have provided an overview of some of the pertinent ethical issues raised by PAR. As reproductive technologies continue to become more common and advance, ethical dilemmas surrounding PAR may change and become more frequent. It is important to continue to examine these ethical issues in this rapidly developing field.

Review Questions and Answers

Q1. Posthumous assisted reproduction raises which of the following justice concerns?
- (a) Posthumous assisted reproduction is not equally accessible to all people.
- (b) Posthumous assisted reproduction may not be the best use of limited healthcare resources.
- (c) Children who are posthumously conceived are sometimes treated differently under the law.
- (d) All of the above.

A1. (d)

Q2. When weighing the benefits and harms of posthumous assisted reproduction, we should consider
- (a) The deceased
- (b) The surviving partner
- (c) The surviving family
- (d) Posthumously conceived children
- (e) All of the above.

A2. (e)

Q3. What is the best way to ensure that the autonomy of the deceased is upheld regarding posthumous assisted reproduction?
- (a) Written consent
- (b) Implied consent
- (c) The word of the surviving partner or family
- (d) The autonomy of the deceased cannot be violated

A3. (a)

Q4. Spouse or partner request for posthumous assisted reproduction is the least ethically contentious since the couple had a joint reproductive project. True or False?

A4. True

References

1. Astrue v. Capato_566 US. 2012.
2. Bahm SM, Karkazis K, Magnus D. A content analysis of posthumous sperm procurement protocols with considerations for developing an institutional policy. Fertil Steril. 2013;100(3):839–43. https://doi.org/10.1016/j.fertnstert.2013.05.002.
3. Barton SE, Correia KF, Shalev S, Missmer SA, Lehmann LS, Shah DK, Ginsburg ES. Population-based study of attitudes toward posthumous reproduction. Fertil Steril. 2012;98(3):735–740.e735. https://doi.org/10.1016/j.fertnstert.2012.05.044.
4. Clarke J. Dying to be mommy: using intentional parenthood as a proxy for consent in posthumous egg retrieval cases. Mich St L Rev. 2012;2012:1331.
5. Côté S, Affdal A-O, Kadoch I-J, Hamet P, Ravitsky V. Posthumous reproduction with surplus in vitro fertilization embryos: a study exploring users' choices. Fertil Steril. 2014;102(5):1410–5. https://doi.org/10.1016/j.fertnstert.2014.07.1202.
6. Embryo Adoption. U.S. Department of Health & Human Services, Office of Population Affairs. 2017.
7. Ethics Committee of the American Society for Reproductive Medicine. Posthumous collection and use of reproductive tissue: a committee opinion. Fertil Steril. 2013;99(7):1842–5. https://doi.org/10.1016/j.fertnstert.2013.02.022.
8. Hans JD. Posthumous gamete retrieval and reproduction: would the deceased spouse consent? Soc Sci Med. 2014;119:10–7. https://doi.org/10.1016/j.socscimed.2014.08.010.
9. Hans JD, Dooley B. Attitudes toward making babies ... with a deceased partner's cryopreserved gametes. Death Stud. 2014;38(6–10):571–81. https://doi.org/10.1080/07481187.2013.809033.
10. Hans JD, Frey LM. American attitudes in context: posthumous use of cryopreserved gametes. J Clin Res Bioethics. 2013;4(S1).
11. Hashiloni-Dolev Y, Schicktanz S. A cross-cultural analysis of posthumous reproduction: the significance of the gender and margins-of-life perspectives. Reprod Biomed Soc Online. 2017;4(Supplement C):21–32. https://doi.org/10.1016/j.rbms.2017.03.003.
12. Hecht v. Superior Court CAt, 59 Cal.Rptr. 222 (2d Dist. 1996).
13. Hostiuc S, Curca CG. Informed consent in posthumous sperm procurement. Arch Gynecol Obstet. 2010;282(4):433–8. https://doi.org/10.1007/s00404-010-1475-4.
14. J.B. v. M.B. 783 A.2d 707 (N.J. 2001).
15. Nakhuda GS, Wang JG, Sauer MV. Posthumous assisted reproduction: a survey of attitudes of couples seeking fertility treatment and the degree of agreement between intimate partners. Fertil Steril. 2011;96(6):1463–1466.e1461. https://doi.org/10.1016/j.fertnstert.2011.09.018.
16. Panagiotopoulou N, Karavolos S. "Let me keep my dead husband's sperm": ethical issues in posthumous reproduction. J Clin Ethics. 2015;26(2):143–51.
17. Pennings G, de Wert G, Shenfield F, Cohen J, Devroey P, Tarlatzis B. ESHRE task force on ethics and law 11: posthumous assisted reproduction. Hum Reprod. 2006;21(12):3050–3. https://doi.org/10.1093/humrep/del287.
18. Pew Research Center. The decline of marriage and rise of new families. Washington, DC: Pew Research Center; 2010.
19. Rao JK, Anderson LA, Lin F-C, Laux JP. Completion of advance directives among U.S. consumers. Am J Prev Med. 2014;46(1):65–70. https://doi.org/10.1016/j.amepre.2013.09.008.
20. Ravitsky V. Posthumous reproduction guidelines in Israel. Hast Cent Rep. 2004;34(2):6–7.
21. Rimon-Greenspan H, Ravitsky V. New frontiers in posthumous reproduction. Bionews. 2013;709.
22. Robertson JA. Posthumous reproduction. In: Kempers RD, Cohen J, Haney AF, et al., editors. Fertility and reproductive medicine. New York: Elsevier Science; 1998. p. 255–9.
23. Rothman CM. A method for obtaining viable sperm in the postmortem state. Fertil Steril. 1980;34(5):512.
24. Sherwood H. Israeli family can freeze eggs of daughter killed in road accident. The Guardian. 2011 August 8.
25. Strong C, Gingrich JR, Kutteh WH. Ethics of postmortem sperm retrieval: ethics of sperm retrieval after death or persistent vegetative state. Hum Reprod. 2000;15(4):739–45. https://doi.org/10.1093/humrep/15.4.739.
26. Tremellen K, Savulescu J. A discussion supporting presumed consent for posthumous sperm procurement and conception. Reprod Biomed Online. 2015;30(1):6–13. https://doi.org/10.1016/j.rbmo.2014.10.001.

Basic Science Advances in Oncofertility

Contents

Fertility Preservation and Restoration in Pediatric Males

Maxwell E. Edmonds, Kyle E. Orwig, and Robert E. Brannigan

T. K. Woodruff et al. (eds.), *Textbook of Oncofertility Research and Practice*,
https://doi.org/10.1007/978-3-030-02868-8_33

Key Points
- The greater majority of childhood cancer patients survive beyond 5 years.
- The full extent of a patient's diagnosis, and management plan, should be considered when assessing their risk for subsequent infertility.
- All pediatric male patients, moreover all patients with testes, who possess a potentially fertility-impairing health condition or management plan, should be consulted with options for fertility preservation. This includes sperm cryopreservation for those that can provide sperm, and testicular tissue cryopreservation (TTC) for those who are unable to provide sperm.
- All fertility patients should have their future fertility discussed with their legal guardian, and pubertal-aged patients should be involved in the discussion when they are able, especially older teenagers.
- If a medical team is uncomfortable in managing a cancer patient's fertility and endocrine health, they should refer the patient to a competent outside team or institution.
- Several investigational methods are currently in the research pipeline to develop future technologies for pediatric fertility preservation and restoration.

33

33.1 Introduction

Oncofertility in pediatric and adolescent male patients is particularly challenging and poses additional barriers beyond those present in restoring and protecting the fertility of adults. Boys become fertile as they progress through puberty and do not possess fertility-competent gametes beforehand. Only during and after puberty does spermatogenesis initiate (approximately 13 years of age for the average male). Before this age, humans do not possess mature spermatozoa or other haploid sperm capable of fertilization with an ovum. This becomes an especially challenging scenario for pediatric patients faced with fertility-diminishing health conditions and/or fertility-sacrificing therapies. The golden standard of male fertility preservation has long been, and still is, sperm cryopreservation. However, sperm cryopreservation is not applicable to pediatric male patients, leaving this specific cohort of patients in a clinical scenario without many options. Currently, there are no clinically proven methods to restore fertility for prepubertal male patients; however, immature testicular tissue cryopreservation from prepubertal boys is an accepted investigational technique that might one day enable future fertility restoration. In this chapter, we will cover the methods currently under investigation for future fertility preservation and restoration, and briefly explore the many potential methods in the research pipeline that might one day become available for this particularly at-risk cohort of fertility patients.

33.2 Clinical Need/Epidemiology

Survivorship of childhood cancer has drastically increased in the past several decades, so much so that the current 5-year survival estimate for a US childhood cancer patient exceeds 84% [25]. Increasing with the number of childhood cancer survivors is an increasing number of chronic health complications that result from or present with a cancer diagnosis and its therapy. The St. Jude Lifetime Cohort Study (LCS) has estimated that as many as 99.9% of childhood cancer survivors in their cohort possess a cancer or treatment-associated chronic condition by middle age; this list of conditions includes gonadotoxicity, stressing the need to trail blaze effective guidelines for pediatric fertility preservation [9].

The risk of future infertility for childhood cancer survivors is influenced by several considerations. These include treatment regimen (chemotherapy and/or radiation therapy), chemotherapy type, total dosage, cancer type, malignancy location, and surgery. The St. Jude LCS estimates that childhood cancer survivors are approximately 50% less likely to achieve a pregnancy as their siblings who have not had a cancer diagnosis [20, 55]. As such, it is incredibly important to understand that prepubertal age is *not* a protective state for the fertility of pediatric cancer patients. An obligatory step in the cancer and fertility management of a boy patient is estimating their risk for resulting oligospermia or azoospermia as an adult. Beginning with chemotherapy, there are two common methods for quantifying the cumulative dosage of alkylating chemotherapy. The first is the cyclophosphamide equivalent dose (CED), which ranges from 1 to 20,000 mg/m^2, and the summed alkylating agent dose score, which ranges from 0 to 12 [51]. CED is the most commonly used measure, with scores greater than 7500 mg/m^2 associated with the highest risk of infertility; overall CED scores negatively correlate with sperm concentration in long-term childhood cancer survivors [21]. Among the alkylating agents commonly used, high doses of cyclophosphamide and procarbazine are particularly associated with subsequent azoospermia [3, 20, 24, 42]. Cisplatin and ifosfamide have also been associated with oligospermia and azoospermia after pediatric cancer therapy. When considering non-alkylating chemotherapy, vincristine, vinblastine, and actinomycin appear to not have detrimental effects on spermatogenesis [3]. However, bleomycin has had conflicting reports of azoospermia after childhood therapy with some studies reporting fertility into adulthood for surviving pediatric patients and others reporting lasting azoospermia [52, 55]. In terms of radiation therapy, the seminiferous epithelium, most pertinently germ cells, is exquisitely sensitive to radiation exposure, with doses as low as 0.1–0.2 Gy causing lasting oligospermia and azoospermia. Turning to endocrine function of the testis, Leydig cells are much more resistant to radiation exposure compared with germ cells; however, at 20 Gy and above, pediatric male patients exhibit Leydig cell dysfunction [46, 48]. This can impact their future pubertal transition, requiring the need for hormone replacement therapy. Radiation therapy targeted at other locations external to the testes can also result in infertility and endocrine dysfunction. Cranial radiation specifically can result in pituitary and hypothalamus damage, causing a hypogonadotropic hypogonadism (also termed central or secondary hypogonadism) by removing the higher centers of the HPG axis. While hormone supplementation can be highly effective in these patients, it is important to know that childhood cancer patients with brain neoplasms are often concurrently taking systemic gonadotoxic chemotherapy along with cranial radiation [54]. Lastly, patients who require removal of testicular tissue due to a local tumor or neoplasm might later present with oligospermia or azoospermia, and patients undergoing retroperitoneal lymph node removal, extirpative pelvic surgery, or pelvic radiation can lose future sexual function due to damage of the nervous system pathways responsible for ejaculation and therefore will become reliant upon assisted reproductive technologies (ART) for their future fertility [16, 50]. The full extent of a patient's diagnosis, and management plan, should be considered when assessing their risk for subsequent infertility.

33.3 Management of Pediatric Oncofertility

Surveys have demonstrated that many US oncologists and healthcare staff report feeling underprepared to manage cases of fertility preservation or underinformed on current fertility preservation options and ARTs [1, 8, 41]. However, both the American Society of Clinical Oncology (ASCO) and the American Society for Reproductive Medicine (ASRM) highly encourage that healthcare teams refer to subspecialists at other institutions in the circumstance that they feel unprepared to manage fertility preservation themselves [36]. Despite these recommendations, in the 2011 SPARE study, a survey of over 200 US healthcare providers, the greater majority of whom were pediatric oncologists, it was identified that over 80% of responders utilize ASCO recommendations in their clinical decision-making 50% of the time or less [29]. This is disconcerting when placed in context to the preferences and concerns expressed about fertility preservation by childhood male cancer survivors and their parents. For both patients and parents, regret has been shown to be the largest concern when reflecting on their cancer management experiences [49]. Beyond pediatric cancer patients, pediatric patients with other etiologies of infertility (i.e., Klinefelter's, hypogonadism with anosmia) or need for fertility preservation include patients with differences in sexual development, transgender/transsexual patients, and patients who are gender-nonconforming [13, 26, 28]. Regardless of identity, pediatric and adolescent patients born with testes should be fully considered for fertility preservation and hormonal health prognosis when facing a potentially gonadotoxic insult, condition, or therapy.

The ASRM emphasizes that both physicians and parents can and should act to preserve the fertility of pediatric patients [40]. Unfortunately, clinical options for prepubertal males are limited to testicular tissue cryopreservation (TTC), which is still considered investigational. Nevertheless, barriers to accessing TTC, or alternative routes of sperm acquisition for cryopreservation for pubertal-aged patients, should not be allowed. All patients should have their future fertility discussed with their legal guardian, and pubertal-aged patients should be involved in the discussion when they are able, especially teenagers. Methods that can be pursued to obtain a semen or sperm sample for pubertal-aged patients include, masturbation, vibratory stimulation, electro-ejaculation, and surgical testicular sperm extraction (TESE and onco-TESE) [10]. In a patient for whom a semen or sperm sample is not able to be collected (i.e., prepubertal boys), the only remaining option is testicular biopsy and TTC, in hopes that technologies will be created in the future that will allow clinicians to access and mature the spermatogonial stem cells within the cryopreserved testicular tissue of their patients.

Clearly there is still much work to be done in improving the clinical options available for the fertility preservation of pediatric male patients. Nevertheless, just as pediatric survivorship is on the rise, so are developing research protocols working towards creating future methods of fertility preservation and restoration for these patients. If there is a take-away lesson to this chapter, it is that all pediatric male patients, moreover all patients with testes, who possess a potentially fertility-impairing health condition or management plan, should be consulted with options for fertility preservation, including sperm cryopreservation for those that can provide sperm, and TTC for those who are unable to provide sperm. Our goal in the Oncofertility Consortium is that TTC will become commonplace throughout the United States, and the world, when managing the fertility of pediatric patients. We are likely to see new technologies released in the next decade that will enable the restoration of fertility using these cryopreserved cells and tissues.

33

33.4 Testicular Tissue Cryopreservation and Experimental ARTs

TTC is the forefront clinical option for prepubertal male fertility patients. Even neonatal testicular tissues possess spermatogonial stem cells (SSC), and given the opportunity to mature, these SSCs can replenish full spermatogenesis within the seminiferous epithelium of the testis [11, 17]. Cryopreserved testicular tissues contain this important cell population, as well as all other cell types native to the testis. We will recommend here that testicular tissues are cryopreserved instead of cellular suspensions. Cryopreserved tissues are potentially useful for all experimental ARTs in the research pipeline currently, whereas cellular suspensions are applicable to only a portion of experimental methods. Testicular tissue biopsy has been observed to be safe and without ill-effects and is a quick procedure with little-to-no delay in subsequent therapy and postoperative morbidity [18, 19, 56]. However, late term effects of testicular tissue biopsy need further study to rule out all possible comorbidities. Furthermore, we will briefly identify critical areas in need of further investigation and future clinical guidelines to make TTC an evidence-driven practice for prepubertal fertility management. These include (i) how much testis tissue should be cryopreserved and how much should be left inside the patient (this is particularly relevant for young patients with very small testes or those with trauma to the testes) and (ii) best practices for tissue cryopreservation and warming (i.e., controlled slow-freezing vs. vitrification).

Current basic and translational science investigations are focusing upon the utilization of cryopreserved testis for experimental fertility preservation methods (future ARTs). These methods include SSC transplantation, testicular tissue transplantation, *ex vivo* tissue maturation, *in vitro* spermatogenesis, and induced pluripotent stem cell (iPS cell)-derived germ cell therapy. For further reading into recent developments of these technologies, we recommend the following reviews which cover these topics in detail [17, 27, 53]. The present status of developing techniques for *ex vivo* testicular tissue culture and *in vitro* spermatogenesis is the subject of the remainder of this chapter.

33.5 Testicular Organ Culture

Attempts at complete *in vitro* spermatogenesis have largely been unsuccessful in mammals, with a few successes in lower animal models (i.e., fish species) [23], and *ex vivo* spermatogenesis in rodents [45]. Most investigators agree that somatic support is essential for the *ex vivo* maintenance of germ cells and spermatogenesis, and therefore, many groups have taken to the investigation of testicular tissue maturation *ex vivo* [59]. The technique of testicular organ culture was first revived by Takehiko Ogawa at Yokohama University in Japan [45]. Briefly, this technique involves neonatal murine testis pieces being cultured upon agarose gel "stands" at an air-liquid interface, with the cultured tissue providing for maintenance of early germ cell populations, and germ cell differentiation up until fertility-competent pachytene round spermatids [30]. Since Ogawa's seminal paper, other groups have also successfully cultured neonatal and fetal rodent testicular tissue in this fashion, both in attempts to optimize media and culture conditions for long-term culture, and in initial pilot experiments investigating this method's utility as an *in vitro* model for toxicology studies [44, 47]. Of these reports, most authors agree that knockout serum replacement, a protein source in the culture medium, is crucial for germ cell maintenance and that this might be due to its high lipid and bovine serum albumin content [35, 37, 43]. The Ogawa laboratory has recently published a "chemically defined" medium comparison between various protein and lipid sources with and without reproductive hormones and metabolic factors [37]. However, replication of their conclusions by other groups and translation of their protocols to human tissues will be needed, in order to further the field. Within human testis organ culture attempts, far minimal results comparatively to rodent models have been achieved. While there are two reports on *ex vivo* cultured human seminiferous tubules recapitulating spermatogenesis, most human attempts have resulted in diminishing germ cell numbers and somatic cell dysfunction [12, 15]. The most successful reports to-date of pre-pubertal human testis culture are by De Michele et al., who were able to culture prepubertal human tissues for upwards of 139 days. Their results demonstrated the maturation of Sertoli cells, and the attainment of haploid germ cells as denoted by immunohistochemistry; however, spermatogonia quickly diminished in number within the first couple weeks of their culture system [14, 15]. The most successful reports of *in vitro* cultured testicular tissue comes again from the Ogawa group, in which they use a microfluidic culture system to dramatically increase the viability of cultured testis explants for long-term culture, increasing the proportion of long-term cultured tubules populated by haploid germ cells by greater than 30% over standard organ culture methods [31, 32]. Between culture medium and microphysiologic devices, hopefully further advances in human testis culture and maturation will be achieved within the near future.

33.6 *In Vitro* Spermatogenesis

While much work is left to be done in the human model, the collective work in *ex vivo* culture highlights the necessity of an intact somatic testis architecture in supporting spermatogenesis *in vitro*. Several groups have attempted 2D *in vitro* differentiation of germ cells utilizing multiple cell types and media-based protocols; however, much is left to be desired in this line of investigation, namely, the establishment of a somatic cell population (i.e., seminiferous epithelium) supportive of SSC maintenance and differentiation. Tissue engineering and biomaterial approaches to recreate the testicular architecture have seen a resurgence in the past few years. Before 2013 when Yokonishi et al. of the Ogawa group successfully created seminiferous tubules by culturing a testicular cell pellet at a gas-liquid interface, *de novo* testicular tissue had only been achieved through the transplantation of cell "pellets" under the skin of immunocompromised mice [57]. In the past year, this work has been expanded to the canine model while also using Matrigel hydrogel encapsulation to aid the grafting process [33]. These transplants organized to form tubules with germ cells, but without full spermatogenesis. However, this line of investigation is paving the way for auto-transplantation as a clinical option of fertility preservation for male patients. Additionally, entirely *in vitro* tissues have been created within fish, murine, and nonhuman primate models upon adherent 2D culture using gelatin (fish) and 3D suspension-based (nonadherent) culture frameworks (all three models) [4, 23, 34]. Suspension culture models have best mimicked the somatic testicular architecture, along with expansion of germ cells. However, nonhuman primate experiments have thus far not induced spermatogenesis progression (through meiosis), only spermatogonial expansion. Moving to human experiments, scaffold instruction of *de novo* tissue development has been investigated. Biomechanical scaffolds have been generated and characterized using human testicular extracellular matrix (ECM) by Baert et al. [5–7]. Recent papers from this group demonstrated the formation of human testis micro-tissues (herein termed organoids) upon a human testis ECM scaffold. While these organoids did not recapitulate the full testicular architecture (they did not possess compartmentalization of cell types or tubulogenesis), they did possess spermatogonia and secreted testosterone and inhibin B endocrine products. However, Baert et al. were not convinced the scaffold provided a benefit in testicular tissue or organoid formation. Experiments from a separate group, testing porcine spermatogonial stem cells across multiple ECM varieties, have suggested that laminin is the most important environmental protein for undifferentiated germ cell expansion [38]. To date, our knowledge of the microenvironmental cues necessary for testis culture outside the body remain ill-defined and are one of the primary challenges in the progression of *in vitro* based experimental ART techniques.

Other groups have had greater success using ECM-based hydrogels for *de novo* tissue formation. Matrigel has surfaced as a highly useful ECM for modeling testicular tissue. Several authors have investigated Matrigel as a media additive to recreate rodent testicular tissue in adherent culture [22, 58]. These attempts have not resulted in comparable testis architecture as afforded by 3D approaches; however, they do sustain all major cell types. The most impressive recreation of testicular architecture to date has been published by Alves-Lopes et al. [2]. In a novel three-layer gradient (3-LGS) Matrigel organoid system, neonatal rat testicular cells efficiently reformed testicular organoids *in vitro*, and exhibited proliferating germ cells, a functional blood-testis barrier, and responded to retinoic acid and TNF and RA inhibitors as would testes *in vivo*. Returning to human experiments, solubilized human testis ECM was used in the creation of human testicular organoids by Pendergraft et al. [39]. Created in hanging drop culture, these organoids contained all major testis cell types sourced from immortalized adult testis cells, grew in size over 3 weeks of culture, and demonstrated an upregulation of post-meiotic germ cell gene transcription over the culture period. Yet, the challenge of creating a tubule-mimetic lumen remains in this and all human models. Nevertheless, Pendergraft's model was also amenable to cryopreservation by slow freezing and vitrification and responded to chemotherapy (cisplatin and etoposide), with LC50 values significantly greater than comparable 2D cultures, demonstrating the future research and clinical utility that an optimized human testicular organoid approach would provide. Even more promising results should be expected with the use of prepubertal tissues, which confer more robust organoid modeling across many tissue types. Between biomaterial scaffolds, decellularized human testis ECM, and microfluidic culture systems, engineered human testicular constructs may become both a clinically useful tool for the study and alleviation of male reproductive disease and infertility.

33.7 Conclusions

Fertility preservation and restoration for pediatric males and individuals with testicular tissue is a challenging clinical area with opportunities for standardization in clinical management and innovation practice that will have a significant impact on the lives of many patients. Despite the current challenges and limitations in current options for fertility preservation, all pediatric patients with testes should be given a fertility consult when facing a fertility-sacrificing diagnosis and/or therapy. In the setting of cancer diagnosis and therapy, CED and radiation location and dose should be assessed prior to beginning therapy, as a mechanism for determining patients at high risk for subsequent oligospermia and azoospermia. In the event that a clinical team feels unprepared to adequately provide for the fertility and endocrine management of a patient, the patient should be referred to an outside institution. Sperm cryopreservation is the gold standard of fertility preservation, and TTC provides an investigational mechanism for preserving the fertility for patients who cannot offer a sperm sample for cryopreservation. Both sperm cryopreservation and TTC fertility preservation techniques come with minimal-to-zero risk to the patient and minimal delay of subsequent therapy for a malignancy. With many tissue maturation, transplantation, *in vitro* spermatogenesis, and stem cell-based therapies currently in the pipeline, utilization of cryopreserved testicular tissue should see success at the bench and translation into the clinic in the near future.

Review Questions and Answers

Q1. Which of the following persons should be counseled on fertility preservation?
- (a) Pediatric cancer patients
- (b) Klinefelters patients
- (c) Hypogonadal patients
- (d) Patients with trauma to the gonads, pelvis, or genitalia
- (e) Stem cell transplantation patients
- (f) Patients with differences in sexual development
- (g) Transgender patients
- (h) All of the above

A1. (h)

Q2. What is the most common fertility management concern for pediatric cancer patients and their parents, upon reflection after their cancer management?
- (a) Time
- (b) Cost
- (c) Regret
- (d) Discussing sex and family planning

A2. (c)

Q3. Which of the following are useful tools to determine a patient's risk of developing iatrogenic oligospermia or azoospermia?
- (a) Cyclophosphamide equivalent dosage
- (b) Serum cortisol
- (c) Summed alkylating agent dose score
- (d) (a) and (c)
- (e) All of the above

A3. (d)

Q4. What clinical option(s) is(are) there for fertility preservation of pediatric males and pediatric individuals with testes?
- (a) Sperm banking
- (b) IVF
- (c) None, only investigational immature testicular cryopreservation

A4. (c)

Q5. What new approaches are currently in the pipeline for developing *in vitro* spermatogenesis?
- (a) Biomaterial scaffolds
- (b) Decellularized extracellular matrix
- (c) Microfluidic culture systems
- (d) Spermatogonial stem cell culture and transplantation
- (e) All the above

A5. (e)

References

1. Adams E, Hill E, Watson E. Fertility preservation in cancer survivors: a national survey of oncologists' current knowledge, practice and attitudes. Br J Cancer. 2013; 108(8):1602–15. https://doi.org/10.1038/bjc.2013.139.
2. Alves-Lopes JP, Soder O, Stukenborg JB. Testicular organoid generation by a novel in vitro three-layer gradient system. Biomaterials. 2017;130:76–89. https://doi.org/10.1016/j.biomaterials.2017.03.025.
3. Aubier F, Flamant F, Brauner R, Caillaud JM, Chaussain JM, Lemerle J. Male gonadal function after chemotherapy for solid tumors in childhood. J Clin Oncol. 1989;7(3):304–9. https://doi.org/10.1200/JCO.1989.7.3.304.
4. Azizi H, Skutella T, Shahverdi A. Generation of mouse spermatogonial stem-cell-colonies in a non-adherent culture. Cell J. 2017;19(2):238–49. https://doi.org/10.22074/cellj.2016.4184.
5. Baert Y, De Kock J, Alves-Lopes JP, Soder O, Stukenborg JB, Goossens E. Primary human testicular cells self-organize into organoids with testicular properties. Stem Cell Rep. 2017a;8(1):30–8. https://doi.org/10.1016/j.stemcr.2016.11.012.
6. Baert Y, Rombaut C, Goossens E. Scaffold-based and scaffold-free testicular organoids from primary human testicular cells. Methods Mol Biol. 2017b. https://doi.org/10.1007/7651_2017_48.
7. Baert Y, Stukenborg JB, Landreh M, De Kock J, Jornvall H, Soder O, Goossens E. Derivation and characterization of a cytocompatible scaffold from human testis. Hum Reprod. 2015;30(2):256–67. https://doi.org/10.1093/humrep/deu330.
8. Banerjee R, Tsiapali E. Occurrence and recall rates of fertility discussions with young breast cancer patients. Support Care Cancer. 2016;24(1):163–71. https://doi.org/10.1007/s00520-015-2758-x.
9. Bhakta N, Liu Q, Ness KK, Baassiri M, Eissa H, Yeo F, Chemaitilly W, Ehrhardt MJ, Bass J, Bishop MW, Shelton K, Lu L, Huang S, Li Z, Caron E, Lanctot J, Howell C, Folse T, Joshi V, Green DM, Mulrooney DA, Armstrong GT, Krull KR, Brinkman TM, Khan RB, Srivastava DK, Hudson MM, Yasui Y, Robison LL. The cumulative burden of surviving childhood cancer: an initial report from the St Jude Lifetime Cohort Study (SJLIFE). Lancet. 2017;390(10112):2569–82. https://doi.org/10.1016/S0140-6736(17)31610-0.

10. Brannigan RE. Fertility preservation in adult male cancer patients. Cancer Treat Res. 2007;138:28–49.
11. Burns KC, Hoefgen H, Strine A, Dasgupta R. Fertility preservation options in pediatric and adolescent patients with cancer. Cancer. 2018. https://doi.org/10.1002/cncr.31255.
12. Chapin RE, Winton T, Nowland W, Danis N, Kumpf S, Johnson K, Coburn A, Stukenborg JB. Lost in translation: the search for an in vitro screen for spermatogenic toxicity. Birth Defects Res B Dev Reprod Toxicol. 2016; 107(6):225–42. https://doi.org/10.1002/bdrb.21188.
13. Chen D, Matson M, Macapagal K, Johnson EK, Rosoklija I, Finlayson C, Fisher CB, Mustanski B. Attitudes toward fertility and reproductive health among transgender and gender-nonconforming adolescents. J Adolesc Health. 2018. https://doi.org/10.1016/j.jadohealth.2017.11.306.
14. de Michele F, Poels J, Weerens L, Petit C, Evrard Z, Ambroise J, Gruson D, Wyns C. Preserved seminiferous tubule integrity with spermatogonial survival and induction of Sertoli and Leydig cell maturation after long-term organotypic culture of prepubertal human testicular tissue. Hum Reprod. 2017;32(1):32–45. https://doi.org/10.1093/humrep/dew300.
15. De Michele F, Poels J, Vermeulen M, Ambroise J, Gruson D, Guiot Y, Wyns C. Haploid germ cells generated in organotypic culture of testicular tissue from prepubertal boys. Front. Physiol. 2018; 9:1413. https://doi.org/10.3389/fphys.2018.01413.
16. Fode M, Krogh-Jespersen S, Brackett NL, Ohl DA, Lynne CM, Sonksen J. Male sexual dysfunction and infertility associated with neurological disorders. Asian J Androl. 2012;14(1):61–8. https://doi.org/10.1038/aja.2011.70.
17. Gassei K, Orwig KE. Experimental methods to preserve male fertility and treat male factor infertility. Fertil Steril. 2016;105(2):256–66. https://doi.org/10.1016/j.fertnstert.2015.12.020.
18. Ginsberg JP, Carlson CA, Lin K, Hobbie WL, Wigo E, Wu X, Brinster RL, Kolon TF. An experimental protocol for fertility preservation in prepubertal boys recently diagnosed with cancer: a report of acceptability and safety. Hum Reprod. 2010;25(1):37–41. https://doi.org/10.1093/humrep/dep371.
19. Ginsberg JP, Li Y, Carlson CA, Gracia CR, Hobbie WL, Miller VA, Mulhall J, Shnorhavorian M, Brinster RL, Kolon TF. Testicular tissue cryopreservation in prepubertal male children: an analysis of parental decision-making. Pediatr Blood Cancer. 2014;61(9):1673–8. https://doi.org/10.1002/pbc.25078.
20. Green DM, Kawashima T, Stovall M, Leisenring W, Sklar CA, Mertens AC, Donaldson SS, Byrne J, Robison LL. Fertility of male survivors of childhood cancer: a report from the childhood Cancer survivor study. J Clin Oncol. 2010;28(2):332–9. https://doi.org/10.1200/JCO.2009.24.9037.
21. Green DM, Nolan VG, Goodman PJ, Whitton JA, Srivastava D, Leisenring WM, Neglia JP, Sklar CA, Kaste SC, Hudson MM, Diller LR, Stovall M, Donaldson SS, Robison LL. The cyclophosphamide equivalent dose as an approach for quantifying alkylating agent exposure: a report from the Childhood Cancer Survivor Study. Pediatr Blood Cancer. 2014;61(1):53–67. https://doi.org/10.1002/pbc.24679.
22. Harris S, Shubin SP, Wegner S, Van Ness K, Green F, Hong SW, Faustman EM. The presence of macrophages and inflammatory responses in an in vitro testicular co-culture model of male reproductive development enhance relevance to in vivo conditions. Toxicol In Vitro. 2016;36:210–5. https://doi.org/10.1016/j.tiv.2016.08.003.
23. Higaki S, Shimada M, Kawamoto K, Todo T, Kawasaki T, Tooyama I, Fujioka Y, Sakai N, Takada T. In vitro differentiation of fertile sperm from cryopreserved spermatogonia of the endangered endemic cyprinid honmoroko (*Gnathopogon caerulescens*). Sci Rep. 2017;7:42852. https://doi.org/10.1038/srep42852.
24. Hobbie WL, Ginsberg JP, Ogle SK, Carlson CA, Meadows AT. Fertility in males treated for Hodgkins disease with COPP/ABV hybrid. Pediatr Blood Cancer. 2005; 44(2):193–6. https://doi.org/10.1002/pbc.20172.
25. Howlader N, Noone AM, Krapcho M, Miller D, Bishop K, Kosary CL, Yu M, Ruhl J, Tatalovich Z, Mariotto A, Lewis DR, Chen HS, Feuer EJ, Cronin KA. SEER cancer statistics review, 1975–2014 (trans: National Cancer Institute). posted to the SEER web site, April 2017 edn., Bethesda; 2017.
26. Johnson EK, Chen D, Gordon EJ, Rosoklija I, Holl JL, Finlayson C. Fertility-related care for gender and sex diverse Individuals: a provider needs-assessment survey. Transgend Health. 2016;1(1):197–201. https://doi.org/10.1089/trgh.2016.0030.
27. Johnson EK, Finlayson C, Rowell EE, Gosiengfiao Y, Pavone ME, Lockart B, Orwig KE, Brannigan RE, Woodruff TK. Fertility preservation for pediatric patients: current state and future possibilities. J Urol. 2017a;198(1):186–94. https://doi.org/10.1016/j.juro.2016.09.159.
28. Johnson EK, Rosoklija I, Shurba A, D'Oro A, Gordon EJ, Chen D, Finlayson C, Holl JL. Future fertility for individuals with differences of sex development: parent attitudes and perspectives about decision-making. J Pediatr Urol. 2017b;13(4):402–13. https://doi.org/10.1016/j.jpurol.2017.06.002.
29. Kohler TS, Kondapalli LA, Shah A, Chan S, Woodruff TK, Brannigan RE. Results from the survey for preservation of adolescent reproduction (SPARE) study: gender disparity in delivery of fertility preservation message to adolescents with cancer. J Assist Reprod Genet. 2011;28(3):269–77. https://doi.org/10.1007/s10815-010-9504-6.
30. Kojima K, Sato T, Naruse Y, Ogawa T. Spermatogenesis in explanted fetal mouse testis tissues. Biol Reprod. 2016. https://doi.org/10.1095/biolreprod.116.140277.
31. Komeya M, Hayashi K, Nakamura H, Yamanaka H, Sanjo H, Kojima K, Sato T, Yao M, Kimura H, Fujii T, Ogawa T. Pumpless microfluidic system driven by hydrostatic pressure induces and maintains mouse spermatogenesis in vitro. Sci Rep. 2017;7(1):15459. https://doi.org/10.1038/s41598-017-15799-3.
32. Komeya M, Kimura H, Nakamura H, Yokonishi T, Sato T, Kojima K, Hayashi K, Katagiri K, Yamanaka H, Sanjo H, Yao M, Kamimura S, Inoue K, Ogonuki N, Ogura A, Fujii T, Ogawa T. Long-term ex vivo maintenance of testis tissues producing fertile sperm in a microfluidic device. Sci Rep. 2016;6:21472. https://doi.org/10.1038/srep21472.
33. Lee KH, Lee WY, Kim DH, Lee SH, Do JT, Park C, Kim JH, Choi YS, Song H. Vitrified canine testicular cells allow

the formation of spermatogonial stem cells and seminiferous tubules following their xenotransplantation into nude mice. Sci Rep. 2016;6:21919. https://doi.org/10.1038/srep21919.
34. Lin ZY, Hikabe O, Suzuki S, Hirano T, Siomi H, Sasaki E, Imamura M, Okano H. Sphere-formation culture of testicular germ cells in the common marmoset, a small New World monkey. Primates. 2016;57(1):129–35. https://doi.org/10.1007/s10329-015-0500-4.
35. Liu F, Cai C, Wu X, Cheng Y, Lin T, Wei G, He D. Effect of KnockOut serum replacement on germ cell development of immature testis tissue culture. Theriogenology. 2016;85(2):193–9. https://doi.org/10.1016/j.theriogenology.2015.09.012.
36. Loren AW, Mangu PB, Beck LN, Brennan L, Magdalinski AJ, Partridge AH, Quinn G, Wallace WH, Oktay K, American Society of Clinical O. Fertility preservation for patients with cancer: American Society of Clinical Oncology clinical practice guideline update. J Clin Oncol. 2013;31(19):2500–10. https://doi.org/10.1200/JCO.2013.49.2678.
37. Nakamura N, Merry GE, Inselman AL, Sloper DT, Del Valle PL, Sato T, Ogawa T, Hansen DK. Evaluation of culture time and media in an in vitro testis organ culture system. Birth Defects Res. 2017;109(7):465–74. https://doi.org/10.1002/bdr2.1002.
38. Park MH, Park JE, Kim MS, Lee KY, Hwang JY, Yun JI, Choi JH, Lee E, Lee ST. Effects of extracellular matrix protein-derived signaling on the maintenance of the undifferentiated state of Spermatogonial stem cells from porcine neonatal testis. Asian-Australas J Anim Sci. 2016;29(10):1398–406. https://doi.org/10.5713/ajas.15.0856.
39. Pendergraft SS, Sadri-Ardekani H, Atala A, Bishop CE. Three-dimensional testicular organoid: a novel tool for the study of human spermatogenesis and gonadotoxicity in vitro. Biol Reprod. 2017;96(3):720–32. https://doi.org/10.1095/biolreprod.116.143446.
40. Practice Committee of American Society for Reproductive M. Fertility preservation in patients undergoing gonadotoxic therapy or gonadectomy: a committee opinion. Fertil Steril. 2013;100(5):1214–23. https://doi.org/10.1016/j.fertnstert.2013.08.012.
41. Quinn GP, Vadaparampil ST, Lee JH, Jacobsen PB, Bepler G, Lancaster J, Keefe DL, Albrecht TL. Physician referral for fertility preservation in oncology patients: a national study of practice behaviors. J Clin Oncol. 2009;27(35):5952–7. https://doi.org/10.1200/JCO.2009.23.0250.
42. Relander T, Cavallin-Stahl E, Garwicz S, Olsson AM, Willen M. Gonadal and sexual function in men treated for childhood cancer. Med Pediatr Oncol. 2000;35(1):52–63.
43. Rondanino C, Maouche A, Dumont L, Oblette A, Rives N. Establishment, maintenance and functional integrity of the blood-testis barrier in organotypic cultures of fresh and frozen/thawed prepubertal mouse testes. Mol Hum Reprod. 2017;23(5):304–20. https://doi.org/10.1093/molehr/gax017.
44. Rwigemera A, Joao F, Delbes G. Fetal testis organ culture reproduces the dynamics of epigenetic reprogramming in rat gonocytes. Epigenetics Chromatin. 2017;10:19. https://doi.org/10.1186/s13072-017-0127-3.
45. Sato T, Katagiri K, Gohbara A, Inoue K, Ogonuki N, Ogura A, Kubota Y, Ogawa T. In vitro production of functional sperm in cultured neonatal mouse testes. Nature. 2011;471(7339):504–7. https://doi.org/10.1038/nature09850.
46. Shalet SM, Tsatsoulis A, Whitehead E, Read G. Vulnerability of the human Leydig cell to radiation damage is dependent upon age. J Endocrinol. 1989;120(1):161–5.
47. Smart E, Lopes F, Rice S, Nagy B, Anderson RA, Mitchell RT, Spears N. Chemotherapy drugs cyclophosphamide, cisplatin and doxorubicin induce germ cell loss in an in vitro model of the prepubertal testis. Sci Rep. 2018;8(1):1773. https://doi.org/10.1038/s41598-018-19761-9.
48. Speiser B, Rubin P, Casarett G. Aspermia following lower truncal irradiation in Hodgkin's disease. Cancer. 1973;32(3):692–8.
49. Stein DM, Victorson DE, Choy JT, Waimey KE, Pearman TP, Smith K, Dreyfuss J, Kinahan KE, Sadhwani D, Woodruff TK, Brannigan RE. Fertility preservation preferences and perspectives among adult male survivors of pediatric cancer and their parents. J Adolesc Young Adult Oncol. 2014;3(2):75–82. https://doi.org/10.1089/jayao.2014.0007.
50. Sullivan JF, Stember DS, Deveci S, Akin-Olugbade Y, Mulhall JP. Ejaculation profiles of men following radiation therapy for prostate cancer. J Sex Med. 2013;10(5):1410–6. https://doi.org/10.1111/jsm.12101.
51. Tucker MA, Meadows AT, Boice JD Jr, Stovall M, Oberlin O, Stone BJ, Birch J, Voute PA, Hoover RN, Fraumeni JF Jr. Leukemia after therapy with alkylating agents for childhood cancer. J Natl Cancer Inst. 1987;78(3):459–64.
52. van der Kaaij MA, Heutte N, Le Stang N, Raemaekers JM, Simons AH, Carde P, Noordijk EM, Ferme C, Thomas J, Eghbali H, Kluin-Nelemans HC, Henry-Amar M, European Organisation for R, Treatment of Cancer ELG, Groupe d'Etude des Lymphomes de lA. Gonadal function in males after chemotherapy for early-stage Hodgkin's lymphoma treated in four subsequent trials by the European Organisation for Research and Treatment of Cancer: EORTC Lymphoma Group and the Groupe d'Etude des Lymphomes de l'Adulte. J Clin Oncol. 2007;25(19):2825–32. https://doi.org/10.1200/JCO.2006.10.2020.
53. Vermeulen M, Poels J, de Michele F, des Rieux A, Wyns C. Restoring fertility with cryopreserved prepubertal testicular tissue: perspectives with hydrogel encapsulation, nanotechnology, and bioengineered scaffolds. Ann Biomed Eng. 2017. https://doi.org/10.1007/s10439-017-1789-5.
54. Vern-Gross TZ, Bradley JA, Rotondo RL, Indelicato DJ. Fertility in childhood cancer survivors following cranial irradiation for primary central nervous system and skull base tumors. Radiother Oncol. 2015;117(2):195–205. https://doi.org/10.1016/j.radonc.2015.10.001.
55. Wasilewski-Masker K, Seidel KD, Leisenring W, Mertens AC, Shnorhavorian M, Ritenour CW, Stovall M, Green DM, Sklar CA, Armstrong GT, Robison LL, Meacham LR. Male infertility in long-term survivors of pediatric cancer: a report from the childhood cancer survivor study. J Cancer Surviv. 2014;8(3):437–47. https://doi.org/10.1007/s11764-014-0354-6.

56. Wyns C, Curaba M, Petit S, Vanabelle B, Laurent P, Wese JF, Donnez J. Management of fertility preservation in prepubertal patients: 5 years' experience at the Catholic University of Louvain. Hum Reprod. 2011;26(4):737–47. https://doi.org/10.1093/humrep/deq387.
57. Yokonishi T, Sato T, Katagiri K, Komeya M, Kubota Y, Ogawa T. In vitro reconstruction of mouse seminiferous tubules supporting germ cell differentiation. Biol Reprod. 2013. https://doi.org/10.1095/biolreprod.113.108613.
58. Zhang X, Wang L, Zhang X, Ren L, Shi W, Tian Y, Zhu J, Zhang T. The use of KnockOut serum replacement (KSR) in three dimensional rat testicular cells co-culture model: an improved male reproductive toxicity testing system. Food Chem Toxicol. 2017;106(Pt A):487–95. https://doi.org/10.1016/j.fct.2017.05.001.
59. Zhou Q, Wang M, Yuang Y, Zhao X-Y, Sha J, Zhou Q. Complete meiosis from embryonic stem cell-derived germ cells in vitro. Cell Stem Cell. 2016;18:1–11.

Uterus Transplantation

Mats Brännström and Jana Pittman

Financial support and sponsorship: Jane and Dan Olsson Foundation for Science

T. K. Woodruff et al. (eds.), *Textbook of Oncofertility Research and Practice*,
https://doi.org/10.1007/978-3-030-02868-8_34

Key Points

- In 2014, proof of uterus transplantation as a treatment for absolute uterine factor infertility was achieved in Sweden, after the birth of the first live baby post UTx.
- The successful clinical application of UTx in humans was preceded by extensive preclinical animal-based studies. This is in line with the IDEAL recommendations for introduction of surgical innovations.
- Uterine harvesting from live donors included bilateral dissection of vascular pedicles comprising the uterine vessels along with segments of the anterior division of the internal iliac arteries and segments of the internal iliac veins. After back-table preparations, the donor vascular pedicles were anastomosed end-to-side to the recipient external iliac vessels.
- Immunosuppression after UTx is only required short term (usually <5 years) compared to other solid-organ transplants, thereby lessening long-term side effects. However, women with a history of malignancy should be at least 5 years post treatment before UTx is considered.

34.1 Introduction

Absolute uterine factor infertility (AUFI) was the last major infertility etiology without a solution, until uterus transplantation (UTx) was established as proof of concept in 2014 [1]. Women with previous malignancies are included in the infertility subgroup of AUFI, with a total estimated prevalence of around 20,000 fertile aged women in a population of 100 million [2]. The existence of AUFI may result from absence of the uterus, as after hysterectomy for uterine or cervical malignancy, or in presence of a non-functional uterus, as after pelvic or total body irradiation to cure malignancy. Thus, UTx can be considered as a fertility-restoring procedure in these women with infertility secondary to cancer treatment.

Non-malignant causes of AUFI refer to congenital absence of the uterus (MRKH syndrome), uterine malformations, severe intrauterine adhesions, and hysterectomy for benign indications (inoperable/large leiomyoma, obstetric hemorrhage due to invasive placentation, or uterine atony).

Over the past 20 years, there have been numerous research initiatives undertaken in the field of UTx. Initial experiments were conducted in rodents and later moved onto large domestic species. Finally, non-human primate models were introduced as a last step in the preparations toward human UTx. The evolution of this new procedure, from basic animal studies toward clinical application, follows the IDEAL recommendations for introduction of surgical innovations [3].

34.2 Animal Research in UTx

In the rodent UTx models, the deceased donor (DD) concept was utilized and tested since parts of the vital arteries (aorta/common iliac arteries) were harvested alongside the uterine graft, in order to obtain vessels of a size that would enable vascular anastomoses. There was no need for immunosuppression, as using inbred rodent strains made it attainable to perform syngeneic transplantation. A key advantage of this approach was that potential immunosuppression-related effects did not confound results, enabling surgical technique to be evaluated in isolation.

In the larger animal models and non-human primate models, both the DD and living donor (LD) concepts were utilized. The DD concept was exclusively for allogeneic UTx in these animals. Thus, the LD concept was evaluated in these larger animal models both by autologous UTx, to study isolated effects of surgery, and by allogeneic UTx, to examine the impact of surgical stress and graft rejection.

34.2.1 Rodent Models

The mouse UTx model utilized the DD concept in a syngeneic setting, with blood flow through caval-caval and aortic-aortic vascular anastomoses, the uterus heterotopically transplanted, and the native uterus remaining in situ [4]. Transfer was completed by trans-myometrial approach using donor embryos. Pregnancy rate per uterus was similar in the transplanted uteri and the native control uteri with offspring being of normal birth weight [4]. Growth trajectory during the initial months followed the typical curves, and normal fertility was seen. No studies exist on fertility after allogeneic UTx in the mouse.

In the larger rat, also with the DD concept, the uterus was positioned orthotopically with anastomoses end-to-side on the common iliac vessels. In syngeneic UTx, the pregnancy rate was similar in UTx rats as in controls, with no difference in pups per pregnancy [5]. Growth trajectory was comparable in offspring from animals of the UTx group and the sham group. The first report of fertility after allogeneic UTx was in the rat, utilizing two strains with discordance in two major histocompatibility sites and immunosuppression with tacrolimus to prevent rejection [6]. Pregnancy rate was equal between the UTx group and the control group. A second study involved Lewis donors and Piebald-Virol-Glaxo recipients and tacrolimus treatment [7]. The pregnancy rate was 50% in the UTx group and 70–80% in the two sham-operated control groups. Birth weights of offspring after allogeneic UTx under tacrolimus immunosuppression and growth trajectory were similar to controls [7].

34.2.2 Sheep Models

Autologous UTx was initially used to demonstrate fertility in sheep, with uterine-tubal-ovarian transplantation and anastomoses of the uterine artery, utero-ovarian vein, and the ovarian artery to the external iliac vessels [8]. Pregnancy was achieved with spontaneous mating 3 months after UTx, and 60% of mated animals later delivered offspring of normal weight.

The allogeneic sheep UTx, exploring the LD concept, used bilateral end-to-end anastomosis of the uterine arteries and veins [9]. Embryo transfer was performed in five ewes, and three became pregnant. One pregnancy resulted in a live birth via cesarean section [9]. This birth is the only documented live birth from a large animal undergoing allogeneic UTx.

34.2.3 Non-human Primate Model

The only offspring after non-human primate UTx was after an autologous procedure in the cynomolgus macaque [10]. The uterus, with the uterine artery and the deep uterine vein, was anastomosed bilaterally end-to-side to the external iliac arteries and veins. Total surgical duration was 13.5 hours. Pregnancy occurred after three menstrual cycles and timed mating. A partial placental abruption occurred on gestational day 143, and a cesarean section was performed with delivery of a live offspring.

34.2.4 Cervical Cancer: Presenting UTx and First UTx Mother to Be Transplanted

The oncofertility concept has been central in the development of UTx. The initial notion of UTx to restore fertility was originally presented to our team by a patient who underwent radical hysterectomy for stage 2b cervical cancer. This occurred in Australia in 1998, the same year that the first-hand transplantation was carried out under the leadership of Australian and French doctors. Thus, the notion of transplanting not only lifesaving organs, but also those that would enhance quality of life, was discussed extensively in the media. Prior to the surgery, the patient was informed that the ability to become pregnant and deliver a child would be lost after hysterectomy, but that her ovaries would be preserved. A gestational surrogacy arrangement would be possible in the future if she would desire her own genetic offspring. However, this was not an option for the patient as she wished to experience her own pregnancy and did not agree with the concept of her fetus developing inside the uterus of another woman who would assume the medical risks associated with pregnancy and childbirth. She therefore suggested the idea of a uterine transplant using the uterus of her mother or older sister. After several months of thorough discussions, our team decided to start an animal-based research project to assess the feasibility of UTx in the human.

It took more than a decade to optimize and safeguard the UTx procedure using meticulous research in rodents and large animals, including non-human primates as described above. Finally, in 2013, the Swedish UTx trial was initiated with ethical approval and permission from the hospital to perform up to ten LD UTx procedures. After initial recruitment and screening, nine eligible patients were selected [11], eight had congenital absence of the uterus (MRKH syndrome) and one had undergone hysterectomy because of cervical cancer at age 25. Although all patients were eager to participate in the trial, the woman with the history of cervical cancer was the only one who volunteered to undergo the first UTx. Having previously undergone extensive surgery with radical hysterectomy and pelvic lymph node dissection, she was unafraid of undergoing a second major surgery, even though the surgical procedure was unfamiliar to the operative team in the human setting. The patient's mother served as the uterine donor. Both the recipient and donor had uncomplicated UTx surgery. The young woman who had cervical cancer at age 25 and UTx at age 32 had her mother's uterus for four uncomplicated years. She initially delivered a son and 1.5 years later, a daughter, after which the graft was removed. Today, she is a happy mother with two wonderful healthy children.

These two patients with cervical cancer have certainly paved the way of the field of UTx as a fertility-preserving procedure in women with cervical/uterine malignancies.

34.2.5 The First Eight Babies in the World: From the Swedish Trial

The first clinical trial of UTx took place in Sweden in 2013 [11]. Broad medical and psychological examinations were completed on recipients, donors, and partners of recipients during a screening phase of several months prior to UTx. Eight of the nine donors were related to the recipient (mostly mothers), and one was a close family friend. Five donors were postmenopausal, but all donors had previous uncomplicated pregnancies and no history of preterm delivery or other obstetrical complications. Uterine harvesting from the live donors included bilateral dissection of vascular pedicles comprising segments of the internal iliac arteries and veins. Each surgery lasted for more than 10 hours. The pre- and postoperative outcomes of the donors were favorable, and the hospital stays were less than 1 week. All donors were in good health at follow-up 1 year after surgery [12].

The procured uterus was chilled and flushed during back-table preparation and then positioned inside the pelvis of the recipient. The surgery of the recipient started around an hour before transplantation by a midline laparotomy, with clearance and dissection of the vaginal vault and the external iliac vessels. Bilateral end-to-side anastomosis was performed between the recipient external iliacs and the donor uterine pedicles, including the uterine vessels with the anterior division of the internal iliac arteries as well as patches/segments of the internal iliac veins.

The transplantation surgery took around 4 hours, and the hospital stay ranged between 4 and 9 days. Immunosuppression included conventional induction (thymoglobulin) with maintenance of tacrolimus and mycophenolate mofetil (MMF) for 8 months. Seven out of nine women still had the uterus at 6 months post UTx [11]. The other two women had their uterus removed due to thrombotic occlusion of the uterine vessels in one woman and endometritis with abscess formation in the other [11].

After 1 year, embryo transfer (ET) with a single frozen and thawed embryo was performed in each participant. The fifth woman to undergo UTx in the Swedish trial became pregnant at her first ET with a cleavage-stage embryo and went on to deliver the world's first live birth after UTx in September 4, 2014 [1]. During pregnancy, a single rejection episode was diagnosed at week 18 and treated, and the remainder of the gestation was uneventful until week 31 + 5 days. Preeclampsia with lowered platelet count was diagnosed, and a cesarean section was performed the following day. A healthy boy with normal weight for gestational age was delivered. The second UTx baby [13] was delivered 2 months later by cesarean section and was healthy and of normal weight. These two births have been followed by an additional six births delivered between 2014 and 2017. Among the seven UTx women that have undergone ET attempts, the take-home-baby rate is now 86%, and the clinical pregnancy rate is 100%, with one recipient having had miscarriages as late as week 14.

34.2.6 Baby Numbers 9 and 11: From the Dallas Trial

A team in Dallas, Texas, initiated a UTx trial in September 2016. After the initial three attempts resulted in surgical failures with graft removal within 1–2 weeks after UTx, the procedure has since proved successful [14]. The ninth UTx baby worldwide was delivered in Dallas in December

2017 after an altruistic LD UTx in the fall of 2016. An additional birth (number 11 in the world) from this group was reported in the media in March 2018.

34.2.7 Baby Number 10: From the Sao Paolo Trial and the First from a Deceased Donor

The first baby born after DD UTx was born in December 2017 following a UTx procedure in Sao Paolo, Brazil, in September 2016 [15]. The birth has been reported in the media, and the baby was in good health at birth. This case is of great importance for the evolution of the UTx field since it demonstrated the feasibility of using a brain-dead donor for transplantation.

34.3 Oncological Aspects

Uterus transplantation is the first available treatment for absolute uterine factor infertility caused by absence of the uterus after hysterectomy. In cases where the hysterectomy was performed for cervical or uterine cancer, it should be emphasized that UTx should only be considered in a woman with negligible risk of recurrent malignancy. The woman receiving a uterine allograft will be on immunosuppression medication for 2–5 years, and it cannot be excluded that the medication will affect the immune system. Unlike other solid-organ transplants, however, the period of immunosuppression is short term as the graft can be removed after childbearing is complete, further reducing the chance or recurrence.

A meta-analysis demonstrated that pretransplant malignancy is associated with an increased risk of cancer-specific mortality and de novo malignancies compared to no prior history of malignancy in solid-organ transplant recipients [16]. A nationwide population-based study in Sweden including more than 10,000 solid-organ transplants between 1970 and 2008 found a 30% increased mortality risk in patients with previous malignancy, and noted that the increased risk was driven by cancer-specific death [17]. The risk varied depending on type of transplantation and type of malignancy, with gynecological cancers classified as low risk for recurrence. Moreover, a delay in transplantation of more than 5 years post malignancy further reduces risk, a finding which is consistent with our recommendations of a minimum 5-year waiting period since the time of hysterectomy performed for gynecologic cancer. These studies clearly identify that UTx recipients with a history of malignancy require tailored screening and close monitoring throughout treatment.

Review Questions and Answers

Q1. How many women are estimated to have absolute uterine factor infertility in a population of 100 million?

A1. 20,000

Q2. Which main vessels in the recipient were the donor's uterine pedicles anastomosed to?

A2. Recipient's external iliac vessels

Q3. Which immunosuppressive agents were used as maintenance in the first 8 months after the uterine transplant?

A3. Tacrolimus and mycophenolate mofetil

Q4. How long should a woman wait post malignancy before considering a uterus transplant?

A4. Minimum 5 years after hysterectomy and treatment has been completed.

References

1. Brännström M, Johannesson L, Bokström H, et al. Live birth after uterus transplantation. Lancet. 2015; 385:607–16.
2. Sieunarine K, Zakaria FBP, Boyle DCM, et al. Possibilities for fertility restoration: a new surgical technique. Int Surg. 2005;90:249–56.
3. McCulloch P, Altman DG, Campbell WB, et al. No surgical innovation without evaluation: the IDEAL recommendations. Lancet. 2009;374:1105–12.
4. Racho El-Akouri R, Kurlberg G, Brännström M. Successful uterine transplantation in the mouse: pregnancy and postnatal development of offspring. Hum Reprod. 2003;18:2018–23.
5. Wranning CA, Akhi SN, Diaz-Garcia C, et al. Pregnancy after syngeneic uterus transplantation and spontaneous mating in the rat. Hum Reprod. 2011;26:553–8.

6. Diaz-Garcia C, Akhi SN, Wallin A, et al. First report on fertility after allogeneic uterus transplantation. Acta Obstet Gynecol Scand. 2010;89:1491–4.
7. Diaz-Garcia C, Johannesson L, Shao R, et al. Pregnancy after allogeneic uterus transplantation in the rat: perinatal outcome and growth trajectory. Fertil Steril. 2014;102:1545–52.
8. Wranning CA, Marcickiewicz J, Enskog A, et al. Fertility after autologous ovine uterine-tubal-ovarian transplantation by vascular anastomosis to the external iliac vessels. Hum Reprod. 2010;25:1973–9.
9. Ramirez ER, Ramirez-Nessetti DK, Nessetti MB, et al. Pregnancy and outcome of uterine allotransplantation and assisted reproduction in sheep. J Minim Invasive Gynecol. 2011;18:238–45.
10. Mihara M, Kisu I, Hara H, et al. Uterine autotransplantation in cynomolgus macaques: the first case of pregnancy and delivery. Hum Reprod. 2012;27:2332–40.
11. Brännström M, Johannesson L, Dahm-Kähler P, et al. The first clinical uterus transplantation trial: a six months report. Fertil Steril. 2014;101:1228–36.
12. Kvarnström N, Järvholm S, Johannesson L, et al. Live uterus donors of the initial observational study of uterus transplantation – psychological and medical follow-up until 1 year after surgery in the 9 cases. Transplantation. 2017;101:664–70.
13. Brännström M, Bokström M, Dahm-Kähler P, et al. One uterus bridging three generations; first live birth after mother-to-daughter uterus transplantation. Fertil Steril. 2016;107:261–6.
14. Testa G, Koon EC, Johannesson L, et al. Living donor uterus transplantation: a single center's observations and lessons learned from early setbacks to technical success. Am J Transplant. 2017;17:2901–10.
15. Ejzenberg D, Andraus W, Baratelli Carelli Mendes LR, et al. Livebirth after uterus transplantation from a deceased donor in a recipient with uterine infertility. Lancet. 2019;392(10165):2697–704.
16. Acuna SA, Huang JW, Daly C, et al. Outcomes of solid organ transplant recipients with preexisting malignancies in remission: a systematic review and meta-analysis. Transplantation. 2017;101(3):471–81.
17. Brattström C, Granath F, Edgren G, et al. Overall and cause-specific mortality in transplant recipients with a pretransplantation cancer history. Transplantation. 2013;96(3):297–305.

Protecting and Extending Fertility for Females of Wild and Endangered Mammals

Nucharin Songsasen and Pierre Comizzoli

T. K. Woodruff et al. (eds.), *Textbook of Oncofertility Research and Practice*,
https://doi.org/10.1007/978-3-030-02868-8_35

Key Points

- Strategies for preserving genetic variation in small, fragmented population of rare and endangered wildlife
- Challenges in developing reproductive technologies in non-traditional models
- How knowledge gained from human studies can help extending fertility of wildlife
- Progress in developing fertility preservation strategies in carnivore models

35.1 Introduction

The forces that are relentlessly pressuring wild animals are well-established and include the loss, fragmentation, pollution, and over-exploitation of habitat as well as emerging diseases, invasive species, and direct human activities, including hunting and urban sprawl. A major contemporary concern also is climate change, which alters how and where animals live. There now are objective data revealing that one in four mammal species and one in eight birds are at high risk of extinction, and one of every three amphibians and half of all tortoises are threatened [1].

35

Because modern extinctions appear to be occurring at remarkable rate [2], there is growing interest in "species" and sustaining their viability and genetic integrity [3]. It is well known that a smaller amount of natural habitat almost is always detrimental for wildlife due to reduced food resources and too little space for dispersal of offspring or to find an unrelated mate. One consequence can be incestuous mating that homogenizes the genome, causing the expression of deleterious alleles—also known as inbreeding depression. The impact of increasing homozygosity was first demonstrated in ex situ collections 30 years ago [4] when zoo-held animals allowed to breed with relatives were found to experience high rates of neonatal and juvenile mortality. Subsequent ex situ and in situ studies have repeatedly demonstrated the insidious influences of increasing homozygosity, especially on reproductive fitness. For example, our laboratory has documented an increased incidence of cryptorchidism, pleiomorphic spermatozoa, and compromised fertilization in populations or species lacking genetic variation (e.g., Florida panther, black-footed ferret [5, 6]). The adverse impacts of decreasing gene diversity extend to other biological systems, including contributing to cardiac anomalies, compromised immune-suppression, and increasing vulnerability to environmental changes (climate and pathogens) [7, 8].

The gold-standard strategy for preserving genetic variation and, thus, reproductive fitness in species has been retaining and protecting massive amounts of habitat. However, this approach becomes increasingly difficult in a modern world with unfettered, sprawling numbers of people demanding resources that make it impossible to preserve enough wild space to ensure self-sustaining, healthy populations of every species. Carnivores are especially susceptible to loss in space and inbreeding depression [8]. This awareness that saving habitat alone is insufficient has stimulated a groundswell of support for more species studies, including establishing ex situ security populations, especially those at high risk. These intensively managed animals serve not only as "insurance" for wild counterparts but also as an important source of biological (research) information impossible to collect under harsh, uncontrolled field situations. Ex situ operations are expensive, complex, and oriented toward ensuring the retention of all existing gene diversity for at least the next century to ensure species integrity [9]. Maintaining this robustness always is complicated by too few specimens that generally display stressful, self-destructive, and/or dangerous behaviors. Even so, these types of investigations are well worth the risk because there is almost non-existent biological knowledge (even of the most general sort) for most of the world's 55,000 vertebrate species [3]. In most cases, resulting data have direct (or indirect) application to improving the management and conservation breeding of rare species.

35.2 Value of Reproductive Studies and Fertility Preservation for Rare and Wild Species

Because reproduction is fundamental to species survival, understanding reproductive mechanisms is a high priority. It is well established that there are enormous differences in the specifics of how each species reproduces, even those in the same phylogenetic clade (i.e., family [3, 10]). Over the last four decades, our laboratory has studied more than 60 species, and we have concluded that there are as many mechanistic variations in reproduction as there are species [3, 10]. This lack of data on how any given animal reproduces means that there is a need to characterize and describe common sexual patterns (including on the basis of breeding season, behavior, and endocrinology) for thousands of species. For example, a popular tactic in the field or in zoos is "behavioral endocrinology" where investigators relate animal behaviors to hormonal patterns (gonadal/adrenal) using non-invasive fecal or urinary hormone metabolite monitoring, thereby avoiding animal disturbance [11]. When established, this fundamental scientific information fills a hole in the scholarly database on reproductive life history norms for individual species. It also serves as a source of voucher data that can be predictive of the normal (or abnormal) conditions of a species, population, or even individual living in nature or in an ex situ security population. For example, having solid information on the normal breeding season, sexual behavior, and litter size for any given species can assist wildlife managers who may suspect abnormalities in contemporary populations under threat and then can undertake "adaptive" management. Such information also is critical for risk assessment specialists whose task is to use sophisticated computer programs (e.g., VORTEX [12]), calculate population status, and then undertake research and mitigation priorities. Accuracy depends on knowing the reproductive norms for the target species. Finally, basic and species-specific reproductive data are essential for two types of reproductive management, the first being adapting human- and livestock-related assisted reproductive technologies to developing alternatives to natural mating for retaining all gene diversity [13]. The second involves "recovery," situations where a species has become severely threatened, reduced in population size, and it has become essential that every animal reproduces to protect all gene diversity. Both of these management tactics are largely focused on creating self-sustaining security populations in captivity, although recovery programs can eventually include reintroduction and release of animals back to the wild. There are a few models of success, especially using artificial insemination (AI), which allows transporting semen between breeding locations (without the need for moving stress-vulnerable, wild individuals) and overcoming the common problem of sexual incompatibility between computer-selected mates. Examples have been reviewed and include the giant panda [14], black-footed ferret [6] (see ◘ Fig. 35.1), and scimitar-horned oryx ([15] see ◘ Fig. 35.1) with pandas and ferrets being returned to the wild after intensive management that includes AI. Embryo-related technologies are not used currently for wildlife genetic management because of sorely lacking information on cross-species embryology [16]. There also is an issue of source of recipients for embryos produced from wildlife species, as inter-species embryo transfer is not viable [16, 17]. Nonetheless, embryos have been produced from wild animals, often using in vitro oocyte maturation (IVM) and fertilization (IVF), and offspring produced in the gorilla, Indian desert cat, ocelot, tiger, African wild cat, ferret, Armenian red sheep, water buffalo, gaur, red deer, Eld's deer, llama, and caracal [16, 17].

Reproductive biologists studying wildlife benefit from advances in the human infertility and livestock production fields. However, the overall goals of these programs are substantially different—overcoming infertility (humans) versus more efficient/higher quality food production (livestock) versus retention of all gene diversity (wildlife). Nonetheless, these three groups share aligned interests in "ensuring reproductive health and preserving fertility." The emergence of the oncofertility field (which explores new approaches for preserving reproductive potential of cancer patients who may lose fertility due to chemical or radiation treatment) has intriguing applications for endangered species enthusiasts charged with conserving genetic variation. For example, there is strong interest in extending the reproductive longevity of a valuable wild animal indefinitely into the future, with the occasional re-infusion of its genes into the contemporary population. Such an approach contributes by avoiding (or mitigating) genetic drift and the tendency for inbreeding in small populations. In this same context, there has been significant effort to articulate the value of "genome resource banks," which are organized repositories of biomaterials to be stored and used for both managing heterozygosity and conducting basic and applied research [16]. For wildlife, there are other reasons to extend fertility potential, largely for animals that have not yet produced sufficient numbers of descendants to ensure the

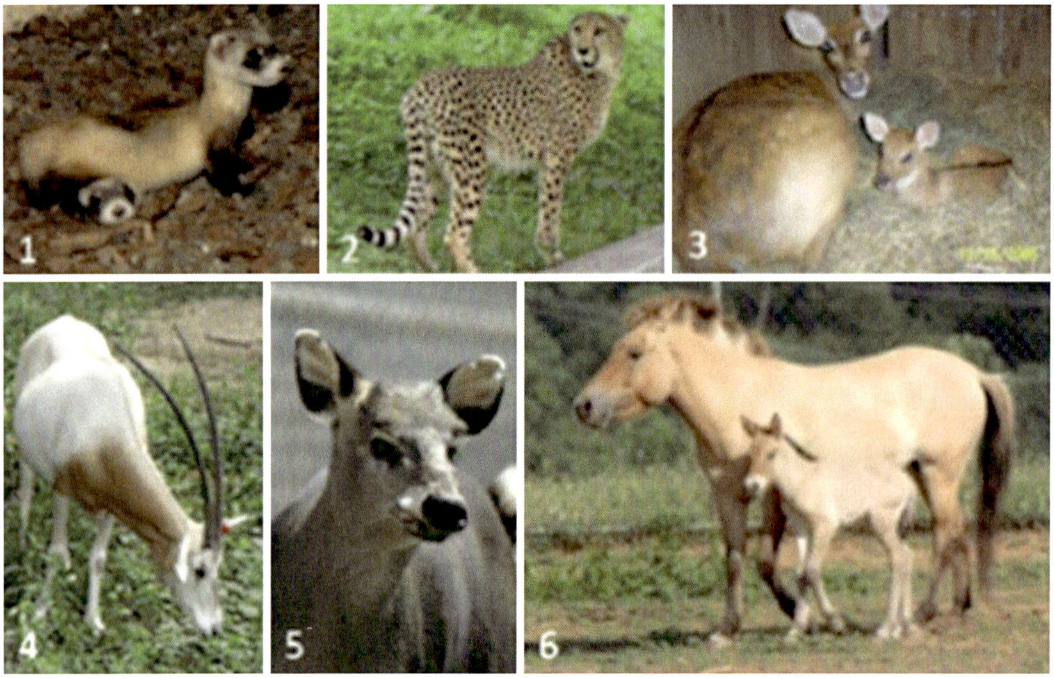

Fig. 35.1 Wild species that are intensively managed ex situ by the Smithsonian's National Zoological Park and partners: (1) black-footed ferret (*Mustela nigripes*), (2) cheetah (*Acinonyx jubatus*), (3) Eld's deer (*Cervus eldii thamin*), (4) scimitar-horned oryx (*Oryx dammah*), (5) tufted deer (*Elaphodus cephalophus*), and (6) Przewalski horse (*Equus ferus przewalskii*). Ovarian tissue samples from these species have been cryopreserved and are currently stored in the Genome Resource Bank at the Conservation Biology Institute

passing on of their genes. The specific targets include individuals that (1) are dying before puberty, (2) are living but fail to naturally reproduce, (3) unexpectedly die, (4) are nearing reproductive senescence, or (5) have been long dead, but there is value in rescuing and re-infusing their genome into the modern population.

35

35.3 Value of Animal Models for Preserving and Extending Fertility in Wild Species

Some challenges related to understanding and protecting species biodiversity rival the concerns associated to the accessibility to biomaterials faced in field of human reproductive health. More than 30 years ago, we advocated the need for animal models to more efficiently develop assisted reproductive technologies for wildlife [18]. Due to the few numbers of individuals available within an endangered species, it is prudent (and safer) to first test approaches in a common species before applying to the rare counterpart. This philosophy actually emerged because of early failures to directly apply cattle AI techniques to the cheetah (i.e., the epiphany that a "cheetah is not a cow" concept [10]). This led to the realization that little good information was available on the basic reproductive physiology of any of the existing 37 species of felids, which, in turn, resulted in our developing the domestic cat as a model system. This, in turn, has permitted making many fascinating discoveries on species-specific reproductive mechanisms, for example, a high rate of spontaneous ovulation in the clouded leopard (most felids are induced ovulators), resistance to exogenous gonadotropins in the ocelot, peculiar, protracted luteal function in the Iberian lynx, the ability of female cheetahs to mutually suppress their reproductive cycles, among other phenomena (see reviews [5, 13, 17]). Such findings were the genesis for our encouraging the need for more species-specific research [3]. This point also is relevant if fertility preservation tools developed for humans are to have application to wildlife because it will likely be essential to conduct initial studies in an appropriate (usually taxonomically related) model. Besides the domestic cat as a target (for felids), other valuable models will include the domestic dog (for wild canids), red- or white-tailed deer (for wild cervids), brushtail possum (for rare marsupials), or common frog (for near-extinct amphibians). However, there are many animals so specialized that there are no experimental species, for example, the two species of elephants, the five species of rhinoceroses, and the giant panda (among hundreds of others). Such cases likely will require more bold and straightforward actions directly to the target species, which is supportable if adequate fundamental reproductive knowledge is available [10, 16, 17].

It is also worth noting that some wildlife species could be interesting natural models for various human reproductive conditions. Such opportunities have recently been addressed and have ranged from the felids (for the ovarian tunica albuginea or for germinal vesicle (GV) characteristics [3, 19]) to elephants (for uterine pathologies in aging females, stress-related infertility in a social group, and impact of obesity on reproductive function [11]). Most of these managed animal populations are comprised of many individuals of exact known genetic provenance and variation, an advantage for providing new insights into the role of the individual effect. For example, one could examine an individual component in a reproductive response to a gonadotropin treatment, oocyte quality, or gamete sensitivity to cooling, freezing, or thawing.

35.4 Ways by Which Oocyte and Embryo Culture in Domestic Animals and Humans Can Help Preserve and Extend Fertility in Females of Wild Species

The first-order priority for any fertility preservation approach is the capacity for successful in vitro culture of gametes or embryos. It is both technically and logistically possible to harvest follicular oocytes from selected wild female donors (1) by transvaginal or transabdominal laparoscopic recovery or (2) directly from the ovaries after ovariectomy or death [16, 20]. In both instances, this approach requires IVM, which is known to produce less developmentally competent oocytes than counterparts matured in vivo [21]. However, the collection of in vivo matured eggs is highly challenging because of the need to (1) develop the appropriate protocols to stimulate folliculogenesis with exogenous hormones and (2) identify the optimum time for collecting oocytes from preovulatory follicles. Thus, in pragmatic terms, it is more reasonable to rely on recovering immature oocytes from antral follicles, a strategy that can be applied to prepubertal, pregnant, or even dead specimens ("gamete rescue"). For some domesticated mammals and humans, there have been common findings relative to oocyte IVM that likely will be relevant to wild animal applications. For example, it now is well established that the initial quality of the immature oocyte influences subsequent embryo developmental competence in vitro and after embryo transfer [22, 23]. Strict selection criteria are useful for ensuring future developmental success. For instance, some of the oocyte's morphological traits (i.e., color and cytoplasm homogeneity and number of cumulus cell layers [24]) are important predictors for developmental competence and, more recently, follicle size [25], oocyte metabolism [26], and GV composition [27]. These same tools are readily adaptable to effectively evaluate oocyte quality in wildlife species.

For genetic management programs involving endangered species, we would expect that IVM followed by IVF will be particularly useful for addressing issues related to aging. For example, cheetahs held in ex situ collections are well known for low reproduction success, which has resulted in many older, genetically important females in the population that still need to pass along their genes to the next generation [28]. Are there human-related fertility preservation tactics that could be useful to rescuing the maternal genome of older individuals? It is clear that oocytes isolated from aged mice and human donors are compromised in ability to complete meiotic maturation and support embryo development [29]. Furthermore, oocytes from older mice and women are developmentally sensitive to mitochondrial damage and exhibit a high incidence of aneuploidy [30]. There are perhaps alternatives to dealing with complete and "whole" old oocytes, for example, focusing on the GV as the target for rescuing valuable genetic materials. It now is known that the GV transferred into an enucleated counterpart oocyte can allow reconstituting a whole oocyte that (following electrofusion and culture) supports normal meiosis

[31, 32]. This could also increase the source of "rescued" maternal genomes from genetically valuable individuals that die in ex situ collection or even in nature. Additionally, we recently have demonstrated that there are diffusible factors produced by cumulus-enclosed oocytes that appear especially valuable in oocyte salvage. For example, we have observed in the cat model that the detrimental effects of too few or absent cumulus cells can be overcome to ensure that such non-ideal oocytes can fully mature, fertilize, and develop in vitro [33].

Interestingly, there are unique challenges to IVM/IVF for many wildlife species because of reproductive seasonality. Oocytes collected during the quiescent season(s) of the year are likely to be resistant to conventional developmental culture, with evidence already observed in the red deer [34], domestic cat [35], and domestic dog [17]. The result generally is low, or non-existent, embryo production during most of the year. However, there is recent evidence that seasonal impositions on oocyte quality can be circumvented by in vitro culture modifications. For example, in our cat model, we have found that supplementing IVM medium with anti-oxidants and increased exogenous gonadotropin concentrations overcomes this seasonal compromise and enhances embryo production efficiency throughout the year [35]. Due to the unique reproductive cycle (obligatory prolonged ovarian inactivity) and gamete biology (ovulate GV oocyte and protracted maturation), IVM/IVF has been far from being successful in the domestic dog [17]. It was not until recently that our laboratory has reported the birth of seven domestic dog puppies from IVF of in vivo matured gametes [36]. In that study, we have observed that although metaphase II oocytes can be obtained on day 5 after the LH surge, the gamete requires additional 24 h within the oviduct to fully acquire developmental competence. Because of the challenge in developing ARTs in the model species (i.e., domestic dog), little progress has been made regarding in vitro embryo production in wild canids.

These ideas and practices are emerging from the substantial advances being made in the human fertility field that, in turn, is being driven by vast resources. One of the major underpinnings of all human IVF was the original development of a reliable culture medium for IVF of hamster oocytes, which then was applied to human gametes in the laboratory [37]. Human IVF technology then has progressed extremely fast to a point where new techniques that have enormous potential have not yet been applied to wild animals [37].

35.5 Oncofertility Preservation Approaches That Have Special, Potential Value for Wildlife

Currently, there are four strategies being intensively investigated in the oncofertility field that are particularly attractive for helping achieve wildlife management goals.

35.5.1 Ovarian Tissue Cryopreservation

The ovarian cortex contains thousands of follicles at different developmental stages [38] that are recoverable from individuals at the time of ovariectomy. Of course, a major goal in oncofertility is to develop reliable methods for preserving this source of the maternal genome from women or girls that may lose the capacity to produce viable oocytes after therapeutic treatments. Whole tissue cryopreservation concepts are highly relevant to preserving fertility potential in wildlife as well (including from adult or prepubertal individuals that might die unexpectedly). We have incorporated this practice into our routine zoological management program at the Smithsonian Institution and with other institutional partners. In this way, the oncofertility consortium and networking process is a model for wildlife operations because excellent communication and interdisciplinary cooperation are critical. In our case, this typically involves close collaboration with curators and veterinarians who expeditiously provide information about a death or medical emergency and then cooperate in excising fresh ovarian tissue that is provided to the laboratory. Research staff then cut ovarian tissue into sufficiently small pieces to allow cryoprotectant permeation and cryopreservation. Our laboratory recently demonstrated the value of vitrification over slow cooling for preserving ovarian cortex and primordial follicles from prepubertal and adult cats [39, 40]. Optimal techniques are now being used to routinely bank ovarian tissue samples from a host of rare species, including the black-footed ferret, cheetah, Eld's deer, scimitar-horned oryx, tufted

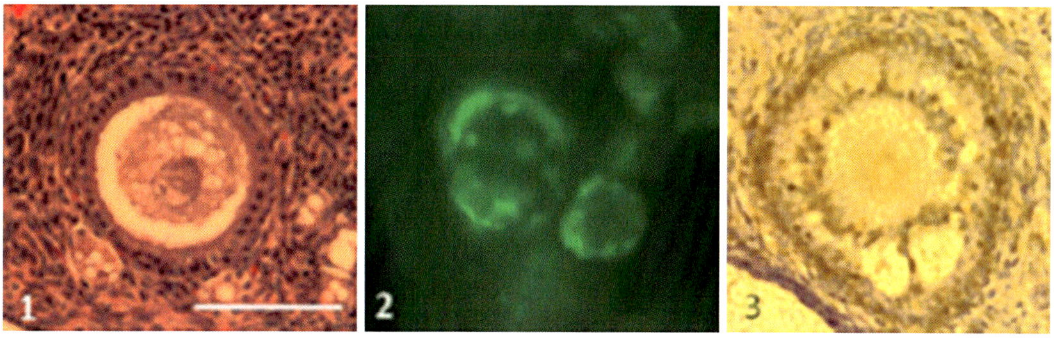

Fig. 35.2 Assessment of (1) histological structure (eosin/hematoxylin staining), (2) cell viability (calcein-AM staining), and (3) cell proliferation (PCNA immune staining) in follicles after vitrification of ovarian cortex in felids. For the three pictures, bar = 50 μm

deer, and Przewalski horse among others (see Fig. 35.1) [41]. Early results have been quite encouraging, revealing that ~80% of these preantral follicles survive vitrification based on histological integrity, viability staining, and proliferation index (see Fig. 35.2).

35.5.2 Ovarian Tissue Grafting

The success of transplanting human ovarian tissue to produce viable oocytes (with the now subsequent birth of multiple babies [42]) as well as the recent innovation in biological [43] and synthetic [44] scaffold that supports ovarian function offers excitement and strong incentive for similar studies in rare wildlife species. Ovarian tissue grafting also has been studied in different species, such as the dog [45], pig [46], sheep [47], rhesus monkey [48], and lion [49]. In all cases, it has been possible to obtain normal-appearing antral follicles from grafted tissues placed in immune-deficient mice. When inseminated in vitro, recovered oocytes from such follicles have the capacity to fertilize and form viable-appearing embryos. And occasionally, living offspring have been produced after transfer—in the sheep and macaque monkey—from oocytes derived from transplanted ovarian tissue [47, 48]. The benefits of such ovarian tissue xenografting would be similar to those of testis tissue transplantations, specifically in species that take several years to attain sexual maturity like elephants [11]. Again, a major target of interest would be the rescue of the genome of rare, genetically valuable individuals (in combination with the cryopreservation and storage of ovarian tissues). There is also enormous potential for generating new insights into (1) the significance of naturally diverse oocyte morphotypes and mammalian follicular dynamics, (2) responsiveness to exogenous gonadotropins, and (3) the ability to achieve nuclear maturation and fertilization in varied culture conditions.

35.5.3 Follicle In Vitro Culture

Each ovary contains hundreds of thousands of immature follicles enclosing oocytes that are never ovulated and, thus, never contribute to reproduction. The ability to grow these follicles to a mature stage with a competent oocyte would be enormously beneficial, especially to young women cancer patients, many of whom are at risk for permanent infertility and early menopause from cancer treatment(s) [50]. Rescue of premature follicles would also be helpful for preserving genetically valuable animal models of human diseases as well as endangered wildlife where females often die before puberty. Thus far, live offspring have been produced from oocytes recovered from in vitro grown mouse follicles [51]. But mouse protocols have had limited success when applied to larger species, including the human [52], as well as our research models, the domestic dog [53], and cat [54]. Although incubated follicles increase in size and produce steroids, resident oocytes have poor (<5%) development [52–54]. Nevertheless, the recent report on the production of meiotically competent oocytes after incubation of primordial stage follicles in the human has offered the first evidence that such approach can be accomplished in non-rodent models [55]. The lack of direct application of the mouse model is likely due to physical differences among species. For example, the size of a mature mouse follicle is 500–600 μm in diameter, whereas those of non-rodent models are 5- to 20-fold larger [56]. Mouse folliculogenesis occurs over a 10–12 day interval compared to at least 2–3 month for larger mammals [56]. Thus, in vitro culture systems for follicles from larger species will likely require an alternative microenvironment to generate viable oocytes.

Our laboratory is interested in understanding the mechanisms regulating primordial follicle activation in the dog and cat as models for their wild counterparts. Studies to date have revealed remarkable species-specific requirements for the in vitro microenvironment (response to culture medium type and epidermal growth factor) [51, 56, 57]. Furthermore, domestic dog ovarian follicles embedded in cortical tissue responded poorly to in vitro culture compared with cat tissues incubated under similar condition [55, 58]. We suspect that these species-specific differences perhaps are related to markedly varying biochemical requirements and rigidity of ovarian cortices [59]. Our findings on species-specific requirements and susceptibility to in vitro culture underscore the need for studying biology of each individual taxon/species.

To date, much progress has been made toward creating in vitro microenvironment supportive of growth and maturation of multilayered ovarian follicles in non-rodent models [60]. A three-dimensional (3D) culture system encapsulating ovarian follicles in an alginate has provided encouraging results in the human [61], rhesus macaque [62], baboon [63], and cat [54]. The 3D physically retains cell-to-cell interactions while supporting proliferation, antrum formation, and steroidogenesis. One limitation is that ultimate size of the incubated follicles is only 10–20% of what occurs in vivo [60], due to an inability to expand in the alginate, a non-degradable biomaterial. Part of this problem has been overcome by incorporating fibrin [64] or MMP-sensitive peptides with alginate [65]; the fibrin and peptides are degraded by follicle-secreted proteases to allow self-expansion. The benefit of the former approach has been demonstrated in the baboon and macaque where meiotically competent oocytes have been produced from incubated isolated preantral follicles [62, 63]. However, end-stage follicle size (500–800 μm) is still less than the minimal size in vivo (>1 mm) that produces an oocyte capable of meiosis. In sum, beyond what can be accomplished in the mouse, there is no culture system that provides consistent follicular growth from the preantral to advanced antral stage and a developmentally competent oocyte.

35.5.4 Oocyte Preservation

There has been extensive progress in both fundamental knowledge and practical application of cryopreserving mammalian oocytes [66]. Although the cooling, freezing, and thawing of an ovum are much more challenging than the spermatozoon or embryo, oocytes have been consistently cold-stored and used to produce offspring in several species, with most success in mouse and human [66]. Furthermore, while conventional slow cooling has been extensively used, both mature and immature oocytes have been cryopreserved recently using ultra-rapid protocols, such as vitrification on electron microscope grids and cryoloops [66]. Importantly, immature oocytes appear to be more resistant to cryodamage than mature counterparts because cells at the germinal vesicle stage do not contain a temperature-sensitive meiotic spindle [67, 68]. This characteristic to withstand the stress of extremely low temperature is a significant reason to center more attention on the storage of immature oocytes. But, as with other approaches, there have been few comparative cryostudies in wildlife species, largely due to the lack of access to good quality oocytes [66]. Regardless, progress for wildlife continues to be linked with parallel studies of taxonomically related domestic animal models and humans [37]. Certainly, continued advancements with the common cow, sheep, goat, cat, dog, and white-tailed deer would have relevance to more rapid progress with wild bovids, small ruminants, felids, canids, and cervids, respectively. It would also be prudent to explore novel approaches for oocyte/maternal genome storage. For example, desiccation has been successful for cat germinal vesicles [69, 70] and could be adapted to other species, thereby allowing the stockpiling of female genomes at room temperature.

35.6 Conclusion and Prospects

Fertility preservation strategies used to ensure human reproductive health, including in the field of oncofertility, have significant secondary advantages for conserving biodiversity. This is especially important because there is a growing portfolio of species management and recovery stories benefiting from assisted reproductive technologies and because the highest priority in conservation breeding is to retain gene diversity. Fertility preservation approaches that are in place (or in development) for humans in fact are already protecting the maternal genome of individuals. Thus, there is compatibility and common purpose to these widely diverse targets (humans and wildlife). We can envision laboratories devoted exclusively to the organized collection, culture, storage, and use of ovarian biomaterials from rare species. Furthermore, we foresee the staff of these facilities exploiting the methods developed by colleagues who are working to ensure fertility in human patients. Perhaps there could be direct collaborations with mutual benefits. We also argue that human reproductive specialists could well take advantage of new fundamental knowledge on biological insights from studies of far-from-traditional animal species.

The major limiting factors for advancing fertility preservation in diverse animals will continue to be the significant variance among even closely related species in specific reproductive mechanisms. This will extend to uniqueness in ability to survive cryopreservation and culture of tissues, follicles, and oocytes as well as dealing with the many complexities related to IVF, selecting/managing recipients, and conducting embryo transfer. However, this should not prevent us from exploring innovative approaches such as desiccation and storage of female gametes at room temperature (which could also benefit numerous non-mammalian species, such as birds and fishes).

Important, near-term priorities are clear, starting with more studies on readily available and probably domesticated species that can serve as appropriate models for wild counterparts. There is also a strong need to gain access to rare specimens that die or present opportunities for ovarian recovery during medical procedures in zoological collections or in the field. Finally, it seems wise to promote more interaction among stakeholders in all areas—whether human, livestock, laboratory animal, or wildlife-oriented. For example, there could be significant benefits from the establishment of a fertility preservation network, with benefits ranging from active communication for sharing critical (or simply interesting) information to opportunities for direct collaboration.

Acknowledgments This research was supported by the National Institutes of Health (Grant R01RR026064 R56OD018304).

Review Questions and Answers

Q1. What are the values of reproductive studies in conserving wildlife?

A1. Basic reproductive information (e.g., cycle, seasonality, litter size) for each species is critical for risk assessment specialists to calculate population status and then undertake research and mitigation priorities. Furthermore, basic and species-specific reproductive data are essential for two types of reproductive management, the first being adapting human- and livestock-related assisted reproductive technologies to developing alternatives to natural mating for retaining all gene diversity. The second involves "recovery," situations where a species has become severely threatened, reduced in population size, and it has become essential that every animal reproduces to protect all gene diversity.

Q2. What are reproductive technologies that have been used in managing wildlife species ex situ and in what species?

A2. Non-invasive hormone monitoring has been used to better understand reproductive norm and abnormality in various wildlife species, e.g., elephants, cheetah, clouded leopard, and Eld's deer. Artificial insemination with fresh or frozen semen has been incorporated in ex situ management of the black-footed ferret, giant panda, and whooping crane. Finally, gamete and tissue preservation has also been utilized to extend fertility of several rare and endangered wildlife.

Q3. What are the challenges in developing fertility preservation strategies in wildlife?

A3. Species specificity in reproductive mechanisms requires studies to be conducted in a given animal taxon. Reproductive seasonality. For example, there are unique challenges to IVM/IVF for many wildlife species because of reproductive seasonality. Oocytes collected during the quiescent season(s) of the year are likely to be resistant to conventional developmental culture, with evidence already observed in felids and canids.

Q4. What are fertility preservation approaches that have potential value for wildlife?

A4. There are four strategies being intensively investigated in the oncofertility field that are particularly attractive for helping achieve wildlife management goals: ovarian tissue cryopreservation, ovarian tissue grafting, in vitro follicle culture, and oocyte preservation.

References

1. IUCN. International Union for Conservation of Nature; 2017. http://www.iucn.org/. Accessed 12 Dec 2017. IUCN Red List of Threatened Species. http://www.iucnredlist.org. Accessed 17 Dec 2017.
2. Wilson EO. The diversity of life. Cambridge, MA: Harvard University Press; 1992. p. 349–51.
3. Wildt DE, Comizzoli P, Pukazhenthi BS, Songsasen N. Lessons from biodiversity – the value of nontraditional species to advance reproductive science, conservation and human health. Mol Reprod Dev. 2010;77:397–409.
4. Ralls K, Brugger K, Ballou J. Inbreeding and juvenile mortality in small populations of ungulates. Science. 1979;206:1101–3.
5. Howard JG, Wildt DE. Approaches and efficacy of artificial insemination in felids and mustelids. Theriogenology. 2009;71:130–48.
6. Howard JG, Lynch C, Santymire RM, Marinari PE, Wildt DE. Recovery of gene diversity using long-term cryopreserved spermatozoa and artificial insemination in the endangered black-footed ferret. Anim Conserv. 2016;19:102–11.
7. Roelke ME, Martenson JS, O'Brien SJ. The consequences of demographic reduction and genetic depletion in the endangered Florida panther. Curr Biol. 1993;3:340–50.
8. Wildt DE, Rall WF, Critser JK, Monfort SL, Seal US. Genome resource banks: "living collections" for biodiversity conservation. Bioscience. 1997;47:689–98.
9. Ballou JD. Genetic and demographic modeling for animal colony and population management. ILAR J. 1997;38:69–75.
10. Holt WV, Brown JL, Comizzoli P. Reproductive science as an essential component of conservation biology. Adv Exp Med Biol. 2014;753:3–14.
11. Brown JL. Comparative ovarian function and reproductive monitoring of endangered mammals. Theriogenology. 2018;109:2–13.
12. Lacy RC. VORTEX: a computer simulation model for population viability analysis. Wildl Res. 1993;20:45–65.
13. Wildt DE, Swanson WF, Brown J, Sliwa A, Vargas A. Felids ex situ for managed programs, research and species recovery. In: Macdonald D, Loveridge AJ, editors. The biology and conservation of wild felids. Oxford: Oxford University Press; 2010.. 450 pp.
14. Wildt DE, Zhang A, Zhang H, Janssen D, Ellis S. Giant pandas: biology, veterinary medicine and management. Cambridge, UK: Cambridge University Press; 2006. 586 pp.
15. Morrow CJ, Penfold LM, Wolfe BA. Artificial insemination in deer and non-domestic bovids. Theriogenology. 2009;71:149–65.
16. Comizzoli P. Biotechnologies for wildlife fertility preservation. Anim Front. 2015;5:73–8.
17. Jewgenow K, Songsasen N. Reproduction and advances in reproductive studies in carnivores. Adv Exp Med Biol. 2014;753:205–39.
18. Wildt DE, Schiewe MC, Schmidt PM, Goodrowe KL, Howard JG, Phillips LG, O'Brien SJ, Bush M. Developing animal model systems for embryo technologies in rare and endangered wildlife. Theriogenology. 1986;25:33–51.
19. Bristol-Gould S, Woodruff TK. Folliculogenesis in the domestic cat (*Felis catus*). Theriogenology. 2006;66:5–13.
20. Comizzoli P, Mermillod P, Mauget R. Reproductive biotechnologies for endangered mammalian species. Reprod Nutr Dev. 2000;40:493–504.
21. Luciano AM, Sirard MA. Successful in vitro maturation of oocytes: a matter of follicular differentiation. Biol Reprod. 2018;98(2):162–9.
22. Coticchio G, Sereni E, Serrao L, Mazzone S, Iadarola I, Borini A. What criteria for the definition of oocyte quality? Ann N Y Acad Sci. 2004;1034:132–44.
23. Mtango NR, Potireddy S, Latham KE. Oocyte quality and maternal control of development. Int Rev Cell Mol Biol. 2008;268:223–90.
24. Wood TC, Wildt DE. Effect of the quality of the cumulus-oocyte complex in the domestic cat on the ability of oocytes to mature, fertilize and develop into blastocysts in vitro. J Reprod Fertil. 1997;110:355–60.
25. Songsasen N, Wildt DE. Size of the donor follicle, but not stage of reproductive cycle or seasonality, influences meiotic competency of selected domestic dog oocytes. Mol Reprod Dev. 2005;72:113–9.
26. Spindler RE, Pukazhenthi BS, Wildt DE. Oocyte metabolism predicts the development of cat embryos to blastocyst in vitro. Mol Reprod Dev. 2000;56:163–71.

27. Lee PC, Wildt DE, Comizzoli P. Proteomic analysis of germinal vesicles in the domestic cat model reveals candidate nuclear proteins involved in oocyte competence acquisition. Mol Hum Reprod. 2018;24:14–26.
28. Crosier AE, Comizzoli P, Baker T, Pukazhenthi BS, Howard JG, Marker LL, Wildt DE. Increasing age influences uterine integrity, but not ovarian function or oocyte quality, in the cheetah (*Acinonyx jubatus*). Biol Reprod. 2011;85:243–53.
29. Tatone C. Oocyte senescence: a firm link to age-related female subfertility. Gynecol Endocrinol. 2008;24:59–63.
30. Thouas GA, Trounson AO, Jones GM. Effect of female age on oocyte developmental competence following mitochondrial injury. Biol Reprod. 2005;73:366–73.
31. Comizzoli P, Pukazhenthi BS, Wildt DE. The competence of germinal vesicle oocytes is unrelated to nuclear chromatin configuration and strictly depends on cytoplasmic quantity and quality in the cat model. Hum Reprod. 2011;26:2165–77.
32. Moffa F, Comoglio F, Krey LC, Grifo JA, Revelli A, Massobrio M, Zhang J. Germinal vesicle transfer between fresh and cryopreserved immature mouse oocytes. Hum Reprod. 2002;17:178–83.
33. Godard NM, Pukazhenthi BS, Wildt DE, Comizzoli P. Paracrine factors from cumulus-enclosed oocytes ensure the successful maturation and fertilization in vitro of denuded oocytes in the cat model. Fertil Steril. 2009;91:2051–60.
34. Berg DK, Asher GW. New developments reproductive technologies in deer. Theriogenology. 2003;59:189–205.
35. Comizzoli P, Wildt DE, Pukazhenthi BS. Overcoming poor in vitro nuclear maturation and developmental competence of domestic cat oocytes during the non-breeding season. Reproduction. 2003;126:809–16.
36. Nagashima JB, Sylvester SR, Nelson JL, Cheong SH, Mukai C, Lambo C, Flanders JA, Meyers-Wallen VN, Songsasen N, Travis AJ. Live births from domestic dog (*Canis familiaris*) embryos produced by in vitro fertilization. PLoS One. 2015;10:e0143930.
37. Comizzoli P, Paulson EE, McGinnis LK. The mutual benefits of research in wild animal species. J Assit Reprod Genet. 2018;35:551–60.
38. Tingen C, Kim A, Woodruff TK. The primordial pool of follicles and nest breakdown in mammalian ovaries. Mol Hum Reprod. 2009;15:795–803.
39. Mouttham L, Comizzoli P. The preservation of vital functions in cat ovarian tissues during vitrification depends more on the temperature of the cryoprotectant exposure than on the sucrose supplementation. Cryobiology. 2016;73:187–95.
40. Mouttham L, Comizzoli P. Presence of sucrose in the vitrification solution and exposure for longer periods of time improve post-warming follicle integrity in cat ovarian tissues. Reprod Domest Anim. 2017;52(Suppl 2):224–9.
41. Comizzoli P, Wildt DE. Cryobanking biomaterials from wild animal species to conserve genes and biodiversity: relevance to human biobanking and biomedical research. In: Hainaut P, et al., editors. Biobanking of human biospecimens. Springer International Publishing; 2017.
42. Oktay K, Bedoschi G, Pacheco F, Turan V, Emirdar V. First pregnancies, live birth, and in vitro fertilization outcomes after transplantation of frozen-banked ovarian tissue with a human extracellular matrix scaffold using robot-assisted minimally invasive surgery. Am J Obstet Gynecol. 2016;214(94):e1–9.
43. Laronda MM, Rutz AL, Xiao S, Whelan KA, Duncan FE, Roth EW, Woodruff TK. Shah RN.A bioprosthetic ovary created using 3D printed microporous scaffolds restores ovarian function in sterilized mice. Nat Commun. 2017;8:15261.
44. Day JR, David A, Cichon AL, Kulkarni T, Cascalho M, Shikanov A. Immunoisolating poly(ethylene glycol) based capsules support ovarian tissue survival to restore endocrine function. J Biomed Mater Res. 2018;106:1381–9.
45. Metcalfe SS, Shaw JM, Gunn IM. Xenografting of canine ovarian tissue to ovariectomized severe combined immunodeficient (SCID) mice. J Reprod Fertil Suppl. 2001;57:323–9.
46. Kaneko H, Kikuchi K, Noguchi J, Hosoe M, Akita T. Maturation and fertilization of porcine oocytes from primordial follicles by a combination of xenografting and in vitro culture. Biol Reprod. 2003;69:1488–93.
47. Gosden RG, Baird DT, Wade JC, Webb R. Restoration of fertility to oophorectomized sheep by ovarian autografts stored at −196°C. Hum Reprod. 1994;9:597–603.
48. Lee DM, Yeoman RR, Battaglia DE, Stouffer RL, Zelinski-Wooten MB, Fanton JW, Wolf DP. Live birth after ovarian tissue transplant. Nature. 2004;428:137–8.
49. Wiedemann C, Hribal R, Ringleb J, Bertelsen MF, Rasmusen K, Andersen CY, Kristensen SG, Jewgenow K. Preservation of primordial follicles from lions by slow freezing and xenotransplantation of ovarian cortex into an immunodeficient mouse. Reprod Domest Anim (Suppl). 2012;47:300–4.
50. Woodruff TK. Fertility lost-fertility found: naratives from the leading edge of oncofertility. Narrat Inq Bioeth. 2017;7:147–50.
51. Xu M, Kreeger PK, Shea LD, Woodruff TK. Tissue engineered follicles produce live fertile offspring. Tissue Eng. 2006;12:2739–46.
52. Guzel Y, Oktem O. Understanding follicle growth in vitro: are we getting closer to obtaining mature oocytes from in vitro grown follicles in human. Mol Reprod Dev. 2017;9999:1–16.
53. Songsasen N, Nagashima J, Thongkittidilok C. Endocrine and paracrine controls of canine follicular development and function. Reprod Domest Anim. 2017;52(Suppl 2):29–34.
54. Songsasen N, Thongkittidilok C, Yamamizu K, Wildt DE, Comizzoli P. Short-term hypertonic exposure enhances in vitro follicle growth and meiotic competence of enclosed oocytes while modestly affecting mRNA expression of aquaporin and steroidogenic genes in the domestic cat model. Theriogenology. 2017;90:228–36.
55. McLaughlin M, Albertini DF, Wallace WHB, Anderson RA, Telfer EE. Metaphase II oocytes from human unilaminar follicles grown in a multi-step culture system. Mol Hum Reprod. 2018;24:135–42.
56. Picton HM, Harris SE, Muruvi W, Chambers EL. The in vitro growth and maturation of follicles. Reproduction. 2008;136:703–15.

57. Fujihara M, Comizzoli P, Wildt DE, Songsasen N. Cat and dog primordial follicles enclosed in ovarian cortex sustain viability after in vitro culture on agarose gel in protein-free medium. Reprod Domest Anim (Suppl). 2012;47:102–8.
58. Fujihara M, Comizzoli P, Keefer CL, Wildt DE, Songsasen N. Epidermal growth factor (EGF) sustains in vitro primordial follicle viability by enhancing stromal cell proliferation via MAPK and PI3K pathways in the prepubertal, but not, adult cat ovary. Biol Reprod. 2014;90:86.
59. Nagashima JB, El Assal R, Songsasen N, Demirci U. Evaluation of an ovary-on-a-chip in large mammalian models: species specificity and influence of follicle isolation status. J Tissue Eng Regen Med. 2017.
60. Telfer EE, Zelinski MB. Ovarian follicle culture: advances and challenges for human and nonhuman primates. Fertil Steril. 2013;99:1523–33.
61. Xiao S, Zhang J, Romero MM, Smith KN, Shea LD, Woodruff TK. In vitro follicle growth supports human oocyte meiotic maturation. Sci Rep. 2015;5:17323.
62. Xu J, Lawson MS, Yeoman RR, Molskness TA, Ting AY, Stouffer RL, Zelinski MB. Fibrin promotes development and function of macaque primary follicles during encapsulated three-dimensional culture. Hum Reprod. 2013;28:2187–200.
63. Xu M, Fazleabas AT, Shikanov A, Jackson E, Barrett SL, Hirshfeld-Cytron J, Kiesewetter SE, Shea LD, Woodruff TK. In vitro oocyte maturation and preantral follicle culture from luteal-phase baboon ovary produce mature oocytes. Biol Reprod. 2011;84:689–97.
64. Shikanov A, Xu M, Woodruff TK, Shea LD. Interpenetrating fibrin-alginate matrices for ovarian follicle development. Biomaterials. 2009;30:5476–85.
65. Shikanov A, Smith RM, Xu M, Woodruff TK, Shea LD. Hydrogel network design using multifunctional macromers to coordinate tissue maturation in ovarian follicle culture. Biomaterials. 2011;32:2524–31.
66. Songsasen N, Comizzoli P. A historic overview of embryos and oocyte preservation in the world of mammalian in vitro fertilization and biotechnology. In: Borini A, Coticchio G, editors. Preservation of human oocytes. London: Informa Healthcare; 2009. p. 1–11.
67. Comizzoli P, Wildt DE. Mammalian fertility preservation through cryobiology: value of classical comparative studies and the need for new preservation options. Reprod Fertil Dev. 2013;26:91–8.
68. Comizzoli P, Wildt DE, Pukazhenthi BS. In vitro compaction of germinal vesicle chromatin is beneficial to survival of vitrified cat oocytes. Reprod Domest Anim. 2009;44(Suppl 2):269–74.
69. Graves-Herring JE, Wildt DE, Comizzoli P. Retention of structure and function of the cat germinal vesicle after air-drying and storage at suprazero temperature. Biol Reprod. 2013;88:139.
70. Elliott GD, Lee PC, Paramore E, Van Vorst M, Comizzoli P. Resilience of oocyte germinal vesicles to microwave-assisted drying in the domestic cat model. Biopreserv Biobank. 2015;13:164–71.

Case Studies: Egg Banking

Contents

Cervical Cancer (Large Tumors): Conservative Surgery, Ovarian Transposition, and Oocyte and Ovarian Tissue Cryopreservation: A Combined Approach

Mauricio Barbour Chehin, Lívia Munhoz, Joyce Fioravanti, Bruna Barros, and André Lopes

T. K. Woodruff et al. (eds.), *Textbook of Oncofertility Research and Practice*,
https://doi.org/10.1007/978-3-030-02868-8_36

Case Presentation

A 27-year-old asymptomatic woman was diagnosed of cervical intraepithelial neoplasia with severe dysplasia (CIN III) on a routine pap smear. A colposcopy was performed with the finding of endocervical acetowhite epithelium. An excisional biopsy revealed a superficially invasive adenocarcinoma. She was a nonsmoker and had no familial history of neoplasia. She was nulliparous, with no partner at the moment, and had intense desire for childbearing.

On the physical exam, the ectocervical mucosa was normal, but a 0.5 cm endocervical lesion was noticed. The parametrium and the vaginal fornix were free of involvement.

The cold knife conization was performed as standard protocol for cervical carcinoma. The specimen confirmed a grade 2 adenocarcinoma measuring 2.2 cm of lateral extension and 0.7 cm stromal invasion without lymphovascular space invasion. The surgical margin resection was coincident with the neoplasia. A preoperative magnetic resonance imaging (MRI) was performed with the finding of no residual lesion at the cervix, but a slightly enlarged (1.2 cm), but homogenous, lymph node on the left iliac external region. The patient was clinically staged as IB1 cervical carcinoma according to the system put forth in 2009 by the International Federation of Gynecology and Obstetrics (FIGO) [1].

36.1 Assessment and Diagnosis

Given the diagnosis of IB1 invasive carcinoma and a strong desire of fertility preservation, the patient was offered a fertility-sparing surgery – laparoscopic radical trachelectomy (LRT) with pelvic lymphadenectomy [2]. Considering the size of the tumor larger than 2.0 cm and the suspicious lymph node involvement, there was a possibility that a fertility preservation surgical treatment would not be possible; moreover, chemotherapy and pelvic radiotherapy should be indicated. It was suggested some other possibilities of fertility preservation to the patient, considering that an adjuvant approach would be gonadotoxic and cause damage to the uterus.

36

A multidisciplinary approach was conducted by the physician and nurse oncofertility specialists, in order to discuss with the patient the concerns about damage and possible adjuvant therapies to maintain patient's ovarian function, as well as strategies to fertility preservation [3]. The ovarian reserve was assessed by transvaginal ultrasound to antral follicle count (AFC) and by serum anti-Müllerian hormone (AMH) level. This evaluation is important both for assessing the ovarian response to hormone stimulation and to evaluate future chemo/radiotherapy effect on the ovaries [4]. The results show an AMH of 2.3 ng/mL and AFC of 16. After a long conversation, due to patient's high chance of undergoing gonadotoxic adjuvant approach, it was suggested combined oocyte and tissue cryopreservation, and surrogate was advised if radiotherapy was indicated.

36.2 Management

In order to not delaying oncologic treatment, it was decided with the patient to start ovarian stimulation immediately. She stopped the oral contraceptive and started a GnRH antagonist protocol with fixed gonadotropin dosing using 250 IU of recombinant FSH for ovulation induction. After 13 days, oocyte maturation was triggered at a peak estradiol level of 3830 pg/mL using 0.3 mg of triptorelin acetate (GnRH agonist) to avoid ovarian hyperstimulation syndrome (OHSS). Twenty oocytes were retrieved, three eggs had morphological alteration, and 14 were mature and proceeded to vitrification (◘ Fig. 36.2a).

After 15 days of the ovarian harvest, the oncologic surgery was performed. The procedure started with a lymphatic mapping and cervical injection using 4 mL of blue dye. The bilateral lymphatic mapping was satisfactory with the finding of one sentinel lymph node on the right and two on the left side. The enlarged suspicious left iliac lymph node was also resected. All these lymph nodes were sent to frozen section, and all were negative for macrometastasis. A systematic pelvic lymphadenectomy with the LRT was performed (◘ Fig. 36.1a) with a type B2 parametrial resection (◘ Fig. 36.1b) according to Querleu-Morrow Classification [5]. The uterine artery was preserved, and only the vaginal branch of the artery was transected. A cerclage with nonabsorbable suture was also performed. The endocervical margin of the specimen was also sent to

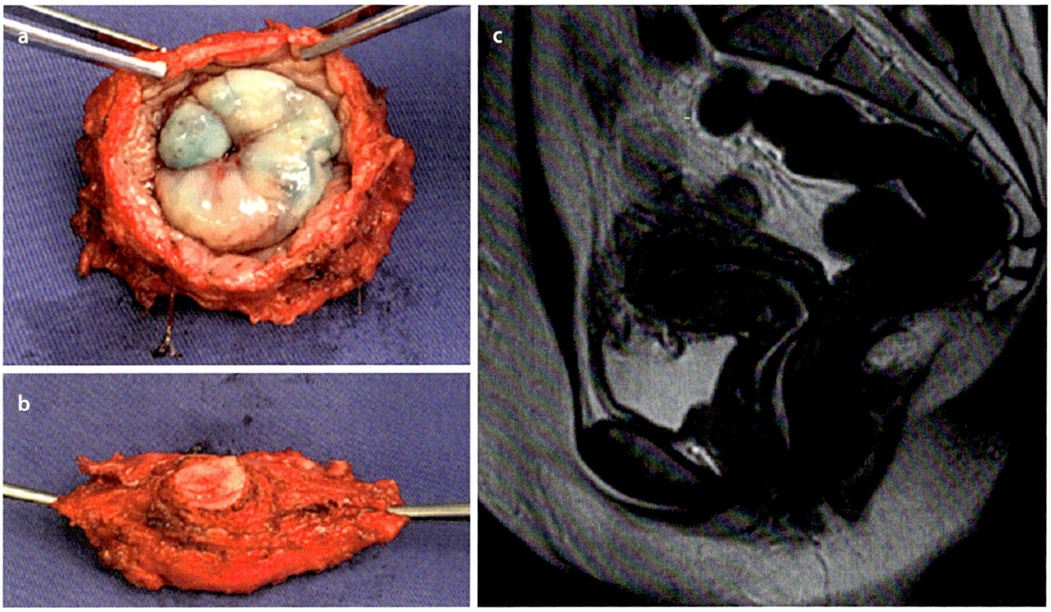

Fig. 36.1 **a** Specimen of the radical trachelectomy. **b** Parametrial resection of the radical trachelectomy. **c** Postoperative MRI of the uterus after the radical trachelectomy

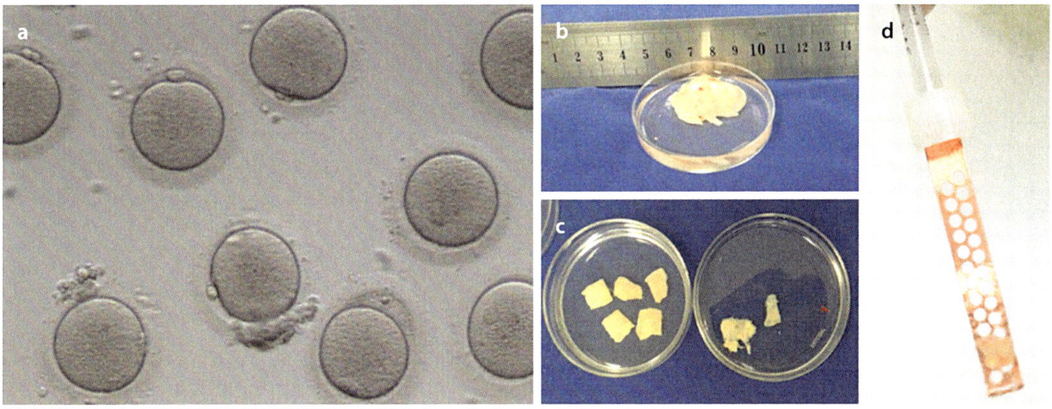

Fig. 36.2 **a** Mature (MII) oocytes retrieved after ovarian stimulation. **b** Slice of the left ovarian cortex. **c** Cortex fragments of up to 1 cm. **d** Ovarian tissue freezing

frozen section and was free from neoplastic involvement.

A specialized oncofertility team performed the ovarian transposition to avoid the possible irradiation field and a left ovary biopsy with removal of a 4 × 2 cm slice of the cortex. The piece was divided into seven fragments of up to 1 cm and properly frozen (Fig. 36.2b–d). The total time of the procedure was 330 minutes with minimal blood loss. The patient was discharged with 48 hours.

36.3 Outcome

Fortunately, the patient did not need adjuvant therapy, because the final pathology report shows that all pelvic lymph nodes were negative and atypical cells were only found in the trachelectomy specimen. Postoperative MRI of the uterus after the radical trachelectomy is shown in Fig. 36.1c.

After 14 months of follow-up, with no evidence of recurrence, the patient had spontaneous pregnancy with good evolution, resulting in term birth at 39 gestational weeks by cesarean section.

Clinical Pearls and Pitfalls

- Cervical tumors larger than 2.0 cm are at increased risk of lymph node involvement.
- The cervical margins must be free of neoplasia to perform a fertility-sparing surgery with oncological safety.
- Chemotherapy and pelvic radiotherapy are strongly associated with ovarian failure and infertility.
- Strategies like oocyte and ovarian tissue cryopreservation should be indicated in cases at risk for pelvic chemo/radiotherapy to preserve gametes.

Conflict of Interest All authors declare that they have no conflicts of interest.

Review Questions and Answers

Q1. In cervical cancer, what are the possible causes of fertility loss?

A1. The reproductive tract surgery itself, and the concurrent chemoradiation therapy.

Q2. In large cervical tumors with low stage, is it possible to perform a fertility-sparing surgery?

A2. Yes, until IB1 stage, it is possible to perform radical laparoscopy trachelectomy with pelvic lymphadenectomy. If the cancer has spread to the tissues next to the uterus, or to any lymph nodes, radiation with chemotherapy is recommended.

Q3. Is there any indication for fertility preservation in cervical cancer patients?

A3. Yes, to patients with possibility of chemoradiation indication, it is recommended to discuss oocyte/embryo/ovarian tissue cryopreservation and ovarian transposition; moreover, surrogacy and even uterus transplant should be addressed.

36

References

1. American Joint Committee on Cancer. Cervix uteri. In: AJCC cancer staging manual. 8th ed. New York: Springer; 2017. p. 649–59.
2. Dargent D1, Martin X, Sacchetoni A, Mathevet P. Laparoscopic vaginal radical trachelectomy: a treatment to preserve the fertility of cervical carcinoma patients. Cancer. 2000;88(8):1877–82.
3. Donnez J, Dolmans MM. Fertility preservation in women. Nat Rev Endocrinol. 2013;9:735–49.
4. Tal R, Seifer DB. Ovarian reserve testing: a user's guide. Am J Obstet Gynecol. 2017;2:129–40.
5. Querleu D, Morrow CP. Classification of radical hysterectomy. Lancet Oncol. 2008;9:297–303.

Oocyte Cryopreservation in the Setting of Cervical Cancer

Ashley Graul and Clarisa R. Gracia

T. K. Woodruff et al. (eds.), *Textbook of Oncofertility Research and Practice*,
https://doi.org/10.1007/978-3-030-02868-8_37

Case Presentation

A 31-year-old, G1P0010, otherwise healthy single female with no pertinent past medical or surgical history presented to her gynecologist complaining of postcoital and intermenstrual bleeding. She reported that she had recently been treated for a Chlamydia infection and had a normal pap smear the previous year.

37.1 Assessment and Diagnosis

A pelvic examination revealed a 4–5 cm friable posterior cervical mass. Bimanual examination was concerning for parametrial invasion, and a cervical biopsy revealed squamous cell carcinoma with moderate differentiation. MRI demonstrated a 3.5 cm cervical mass with parametrial involvement and possible enlargement of two lymph nodes. Given this clinical presentation, she was diagnosed with stage IIB squamous cell carcinoma of the cervix.

37.2 Management

Fertility-sparing surgery is generally recommended for women presenting with a well-differentiated low-grade tumor in its early stages. Surgery may include cervical conization or trachelectomy for treatment of stage 1A1 to 1B1 cervical cancer that is less than 2 cm with limited endocervical involvement [1]. These treatments have been studied and were found to have similar surgical complication rates [2] as well as successful fertility outcomes. A retrospective review of 72 women following fertility-sparing vaginal radical trachelectomy found a conception rate of 43%. These conceptions resulted in 16% first trimester miscarriage, 4% second trimester miscarriage, and 72% third trimester deliveries [3].

While early cervical cancers may be treated successfully with surgical resection, treatment recommendations for stage IIB cervical cancer is primary radiation with radio-sensitizing chemotherapy. Primary radiation, as compared to primary surgical management, for locally advanced cervical cancer has been shown to have similar overall survival rates (74% vs. 83%) with less associated morbidity (12% vs. 28%, $P = 0.0004$) [4]. The addition of chemotherapy concurrently with primary radiation as a radio-sensitizer, an agent that makes tumor cells more sensitive to radiation therapy, has shown significant improvement in overall survival [5]. Women with locally advanced cervical carcinoma, like our patient (above stage IB1), are not considered candidates for radical primary surgery, and it was recommended that she receive chemoradiation [6].

37.3 Impact of Proposed Treatment on Future Fertility

Radiation is known to destroy follicles in the ovaries. The radio-sensitivity of the ovaries increases with age, likely related to diminishing ovarian reserve. Therefore, the ovaries of older patients are more radiosensitive than younger patients. Doses of 12–20 Gy may produce permanent sterility in most patients depending on age. Chemaitilly et al. evaluated the effect of treatment of childhood cancers with radiation on acute ovarian failure. It was found that 75% of females with acute ovarian failure had been exposed to abdominal-pelvic irradiation. Further, while doses as low as 10 Gy were sufficient to cause acute ovarian failure in some patients, ovarian radiation in doses of at least 20 Gy was associated with the highest risk. More than 70% of the patients in the study with acute ovarian failure were exposed to such high doses [7]. In addition to radiation injury to the ovaries, uterine damage may also occur at common doses. Radiation causes fibrosis and scarring and can lead to increased rates of infertility, miscarriage, premature delivery, and pregnancy complications. Subsequent pregnancy outcomes of patients who received radiation to the uterus were studied by Signorello et al. Uterine doses as low as 2.5–5 Gy (odds ratio = 4.3, 95% confidence interval = 1.4 to 12.8; $P = 0.01$) resulted in low birth weight in 25.5% of the births and 36.2% of the births of survivors who received uterine doses of greater than 5 Gy [8].

Chemotherapy targets actively dividing cells and therefore kills mature ovarian follicles. The effect of chemotherapy on dormant follicles is variable, and therefore, it is possible that some ovarian function may be maintained, particularly in younger women. Older patients are more likely to have marked effects of chemotherapy and develop premature menopause owing to decreased primordial follicle counts. Further, the agents used in treatment have differing rates of ovarian failure. Alkylating agents induce the greatest ovarian damage with an odds ratio of 3.98, whereas platinum-derived chemotherapy is somewhat less likely to develop ovarian failure with an odds ratio of 1.77 [9]. The recommended agent for use concurrently with radiation as a radio-sensitizer in cervical carcinoma is platinum-derivative.

This patient planned on receiving a total of 55 Gy of external beam radiation in 25 fractions of 2.2 Gy each with concurrent weekly radio-sensitizing cisplatin 40 mg/m^2. This would be followed by vaginal brachytherapy with tandem and ovids. She was counseled about the very high risk of permanent ovarian failure and damage to the uterus given these treatment modalities.

37.4 Fertility Preservation Options

Given the reproductive risks of cancer therapy, this patient was referred to a reproductive endocrinologist to discuss fertility preservation options. While embryo cryopreservation is an established method of fertility preservation with a predictable likelihood of success, this option is mostly reserved for women with a committed partner. Instead, oocyte cryopreservation, now considered standard of care, should be offered to postpubertal patients who do not have a partner. Success rates with vitrification in various populations have been estimated to be approximately 6% live birth rate per mature egg frozen. Both embryo and oocyte cryopreservation require ovarian stimulation, which typically takes about 2 weeks and involves treatment with injectable follicle-stimulating hormone, frequent office monitoring, and an egg retrieval procedure. Eggs or embryos may later be used to achieve pregnancy in the patient herself or in a gestational carrier. Given that our patient's uterus will likely be compromised by high-dose radiation therapy, she was extensively counseled about the high likelihood of needing to use a gestational carrier for future conception. Another option that has gained considerable attention over the past few years is ovarian tissue cryopreservation. This is an investigational procedure which can be performed in prepubertal as well as adult females. It requires removal of tissue (entire ovary or cortical biopsies) which is typically completed by a laparoscopic procedure followed by cryopreservation of small fragments of ovarian cortex. In order to conceive, tissue is typically transplanted orthotopically within the pelvis. Since the first documented pregnancy in 2004 using this technique, there have been over 130 live births reported after ovarian tissue transplantation [10–11]. This option is less desirable for our patient since it is likely that she will not be able to carry a pregnancy herself and would have to go through IVF to create embryos later even after ovarian tissue transplantation.

Furthermore, in order to attempt to preserve ovarian function, it is possible for patients to undergo surgery to move the ovaries away from the field of radiation prior to treatment. This procedure, called oophoropexy, can decrease the risk of ovarian failure related to the radiation exposure; however, this does not negate the chemotherapeutic effects as previously discussed. Transposition involves releasing the utero-ovarian ligaments and suturing the ovaries above the pelvic brim. Typically, the ovaries are marked with surgical clips so that radiation mapping can be performed to avoid exposure to the ovaries. With this procedure, it has been shown that 41–71% of women are able to maintain ovarian function after radiation [12].

37.5 Outcome/Patient Course Following Diagnosis

After extensive counseling regarding the reproductive risks of chemotherapy and radiation, as well as fertility preservation options available, this patient decided to undergo oocyte cryopreservation prior to cancer therapy. She had been amenorrheic on continuous oral contraceptives. An ultrasound was performed at her office visit, and five antral follicles were seen on one ovary, and the other ovary was difficult to visualize. AMH was not available at the time of the consultation but was found to be 3.1 ng/ml. The oral contraceptive was discontinued, and she was started on 375 IU of follicle-stimulating hormone, and a GNRH antagonist was started on day 8 of ovarian stimulation. On day 12 of stimulation, she had 10 follicles over 15 mm in size, and she received 1000 IU hCG and 80 units of Lupron to trigger the final maturation of the eggs. An egg retrieval was performed 36 hours afterward transabdominally via ultrasound guidance. The decision was made to undergo abdominal retrieval given the theoretical potential for seeding of the ovaries with cervical cancer during vaginal egg retrieval.

A total of ten eggs were retrieved, seven of which were mature. The following week, the patient was taken to the operating room for laparoscopic ovarian transposition. This was performed without complications, and the ovaries were noted to be only mildly enlarged a week after surgery. Radiation planning and chemoradiation were begun thereafter.

Clinical Points and Pitfalls

- Clinical points:
  - When primary surgery is not recommended (locally advanced disease), the subsequent risks of radiation as well as chemotherapy on the female reproductive system should be fully discussed. This includes the potential detrimental effect of both modalities on the ovaries as well as the uterus.
  - Regardless of stage, when a patient desires fertility options, the patient should be fully counseled on the options available to her as well as the potential outcomes of these options.
- Pitfalls
  - Patients who will need a gestational carrier should be screened as a donor at the time of oocyte banking.
  - Given the extent of disease, patients are often left without recommended options in fertility-sparing techniques.
  - Oocyte preservation methods, which typically take 2 weeks, should be managed in a timely fashion in order to prevent delays in treatment.
  - Transabdominal retrieval may be prudent for cervical or vaginal cancers that could be seeded to the ovaries.
  - Failure to discuss potential effects of treatment on the uterus could mislead a patient into the potential to carry a child in the future.

37

Review Questions and Answers

Q1. Fertility-sparing surgery for cervical cancer (such as trachelectomy) should be offered in which of the following clinical situations?
(a) Stage 1A1 or 1A2
(b) 3 cm tumor
(c) Stage IIB
(d) High-grade tumor

A1. (a) Only low-grade, early-stage cervical cancer should be treated with trachelectomy.

Q2. Pelvic radiation therapy has been associated with the following pregnancy complications EXCEPT:
(a) Diminished ovarian reserve
(b) Preterm delivery
(c) Low-birth-weight infant
(d) Preeclampsia
(e) Miscarriage

A2. (d) Preeclampsia is not a known risk of pelvic radiation.

Q3. The success rate of mature oocyte cryopreservation in women under the age of 35 years is approximately:
(a) 3% live birth rate per oocyte
(b) 6% live birth rate per oocyte
(c) 9% live birth rate per oocyte
(d) 12% live birth rate per oocyte

A3. (b) In young patients, the live birth rate per thawed oocyte has been estimated to be 6%.

References

1. Dargent D. Radical trachelectomy: an operation that preserves the fertility of young women with invasive cervical cancer. Bull Acad Natl Med. 2001;185(7):1295–304–6.
2. Marchiole P, Benchaib M, Buenerd A, Lazlo E, Dargent D, Mathevet P. Oncological safety of laparoscopic-assisted vaginal radical trachelectomy (LARVT or Dargent's operation): a comparative study with laparoscopic-assisted vaginal radical hysterectomy (LARVH). Gynecol Oncol. 2007;106(1):132–41.
3. Plante M, Renaud M-C, Hoskins IA, Roy M. Vaginal radical trachelectomy: a valuable fertility-preserving option in the management of early-stage cervical cancer. A series of 50 pregnancies and review of the literature. Gynecol Oncol. 2005;98(1):3–10.
4. Landoni F, Maneo A, Colombo A, Placa F, Milani R, Perego P, et al. Randomised study of radical surgery versus radiotherapy for stage Ib-IIa cervical cancer. Lancet (London, England). 1997;350(9077):535–40.
5. Morris M, Eifel PJ, Lu J, Grigsby PW, Levenback C, Stevens RE, et al. Pelvic radiation with concurrent che-

motherapy compared with pelvic and para-aortic radiation for high-risk cervical cancer. N Engl J Med. 1999;340(15):1137–43.
6. Willows K, Lennox G, Covens A. Fertility-sparing management in cervical cancer: balancing oncologic outcomes with reproductive success. Gynecol Oncol Res Pract. 2016;3:9.
7. Chemaitilly W, Mertens AC, Mitby P, Whitton J, Stovall M, Yasui Y, et al. Acute ovarian failure in the childhood cancer survivor study. J Clin Endocrinol Metab. 2006;91(5):1723–8.
8. Signorello LB, Cohen SS, Bosetti C, Stovall M, Kasper CE, Weathers RE, et al. Female survivors of childhood cancer: preterm birth and low birth weight among their children. J Natl Cancer Inst. 2006;98(20):1453–61.
9. Meirow D, Biederman H, Anderson RA, Wallace WHB. Ovid: toxicity of chemotherapy and radiation on female. Reproduction. 2010;53(4):727–39.
10. Donnez J, Martinez-Madrid B, Jadoul P, Van Langendonckt A, Demylle D, Dolmans M-M. Ovarian tissue cryopreservation and transplantation: a review. Hum Reprod Update. 2006;12(5):519–35.
11. Donnez J, Dolmans MM. Fertility preservation in women. N Engl J Med. 2017;377(17):1657–65.
12. Chambers SK, Chambers JT, Kier R, Peschel RE. Sequelae of lateral ovarian transposition in irradiated cervical cancer patients. Int J Radiat Oncol. 1991;20(6):1305–8.

Alternative Stimulation Protocols

Marissa Steinberg Weiss, Seema Niphadkar, David M. Mintzer, and Divya Kelath Shah

T. K. Woodruff et al. (eds.), *Textbook of Oncofertility Research and Practice*,
https://doi.org/10.1007/978-3-030-02868-8_38

Case Presentation

A 29-year-old nulligravid woman presented to the emergency department with chest pain and shortness of breath. A computed tomography (CT) scan of the chest was unremarkable, and she was discharged home. She returned 3 months later with worsening symptoms at which time a repeat chest CT scan demonstrated a new 6.6 × 5 cm anterior mediastinal mass, suspicious for malignancy (◘ Fig. 38.1).

A CT-guided core biopsy was performed which suggested an atypical lymphoid infiltrate, but concurrent flow cytometry was non-diagnostic. Consequently, she underwent a mediastinotomy which revealed a large-cell B-cell lymphoma, consistent with a primary mediastinal B-cell lymphoma (PMBCL). Fluorescent in situ hybridization (FISH) testing performed for risk stratification and prognostication revealed BCL6 and C-MYC gene rearrangements, consistent with a double-hit lymphoma. Positron emission tomography (PET)/CT scan performed to complete clinical staging revealed no evidence of lymphoma outside the mediastinum. Treatment with dose-adjusted rituximab, etoposide, prednisolone, vincristine, cyclophosphamide, and doxorubicin (DA-R-EPOCH) was planned.

Prior to initiating cancer treatment, the patient was referred for consultation with Reproductive Endocrinology and Infertility (REI) for discussion of options for fertility preservation. She reported regular menstrual cycles occurring every 25 days and was on the 13th day of her cycle at the time of this initial visit. She was in a monogamous relationship with a male partner using condoms for contraception. A transvaginal ultrasound revealed a 2 cm corpus luteum cyst and an antral follicle count of 14. Laboratory results revealed an anti-Mullerian hormone level of 1.105 ng/mL.

After discussing the gonadotoxic effects of the planned cyclophosphamide chemotherapy and reviewing the risks and benefits of several fertility-preserving techniques, the patient opted to pursue oocyte cryopreservation.

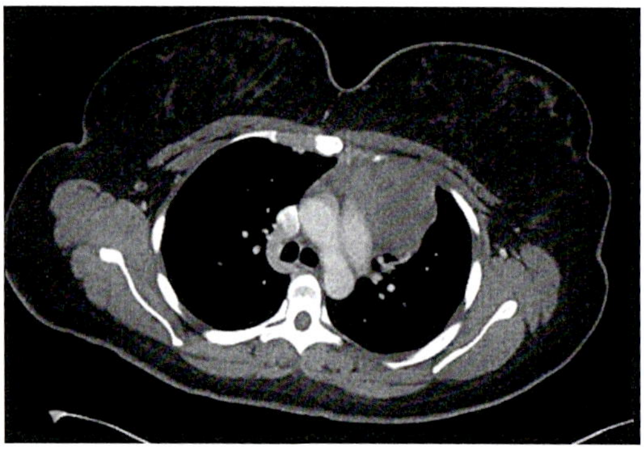

◘ **Fig. 38.1** CT chest demonstrating heterogeneous anterior mediastinal mass

38

38.1 Assessment and Diagnosis

Primary mediastinal B-cell lymphoma (PMBCL) is an aggressive lymphoma that commonly affects young people, particularly females. Frequently, it manifests as a localized, bulky anterior mediastinal mass as seen in this case [1]. A subset of these tumors harbors MYC, BCL2, and/or BCL6 translocations. Multiple translocations can confer a double- or triple-hit lymphoma which portends a poor prognosis. The current standard of care for diffuse large B-cell lymphoma (DLBCL) is rituximab, cyclophosphamide, doxorubicin, vincristine, and prednisolone (R-CHOP). An alternate, more dose intense option for therapy for PMBCL and double-hit DLBCL is dose-adjusted rituximab, etoposide, prednisolone, vincristine, cyclophosphamide, and doxorubicin (DA-R-EPOCH). There was no difference in overall survival between R-CHOP and DA-R-EPOCH when considering all large-cell lymphoma patients. However, some data suggests DA-R-EPOCH may be superior for double-hit lymphomas and may allow for avoidance of consolidative mediastinal radiation for patients with PMBCL [1, 2].

The urgency of therapy for DLBCL varies along a continuum. While our patient was symptomatic with her mediastinal tumor, she did not have evidence of airway obstruction or superior vena cava syndrome which would have warranted immediate therapy. Although initiation of therapy is time sensitive, the urgency is influenced by numerous variables including the subtype of DLBCL, symptoms, tumor bulk, and extent of organ involvement. This is unlike therapy for acute leukemia where therapy is often emergent or asymptomatic solid tumors where therapy can often be delayed pending completion of pretreatment workup and evaluation.

Ovarian stimulation for oocyte cryopreservation is conventionally initiated in the early follicular phase. This approach may delay the start of stimulation by as many as 3–4 weeks depending on the patient's menstrual cycle phase at the time of initial presentation. In cases such as this where patients need to initiate cancer treatment urgently, alternate ovarian stimulation protocols can be used to minimize treatment delay. These protocols typically utilize gonadotropin-releasing hormone (GnRH) antagonists for prevention of ovulation as they afford the shortest time interval from cycle initiation to completion [3].

One example is a *luteal halt* protocol, used for patients who present in the luteal phase of the menstrual cycle. In this approach, GnRH antagonists and gonadotropins are initiated simultaneously in the luteal phase. A study comparing clinical outcomes with this protocol ($n = 12$) to those of cancer patients who initiated stimulation during the follicular phase demonstrated similar numbers of total and mature oocytes retrieved, as well as comparable fertilization rates [4].

More recently, a *random-start* protocol has been advocated. In this approach, ovarian stimulation with gonadotropins is initiated as soon as the patient is able to – regardless of menstrual phase [5]. This protocol can be modified based on the specific menstrual phase in which a patient presents. For example:

- *Mid-late follicular phase start (estradiol level is >100 pg/mL and dominant follicle is ≥12 mm):* Gonadotropins are started on presentation, and any spontaneous luteinizing hormone (LH) surge is disregarded. A GnRH antagonist is added when the secondary follicle cohort reaches 12 mm to prevent a premature secondary LH surge.
- *Peri-ovulatory start (estradiol level is >200 pg/mL and dominant follicle is ≥17 mm):* Ovulation is triggered with human chorionic gonadotropin (HCG) or GnRH agonist and gonadotropins initiated 2–3 days later. A GnRH antagonist is added when the secondary follicle cohort reaches 12 mm.
- *Luteal phase start (progesterone level ≥ 3 ng/mL):* Gonadotropins are initiated immediately, and GnRH antagonist is added when lead follicle is ≥12 mm. Note that estradiol levels cannot be used to guide initiation of the GnRH antagonist as they can be during conventional follicular starts.

A recent study comparing the outcomes of 35 random-start cycles and 93 conventional-start cycles found no difference in the number of oocytes retrieved, oocyte maturity rate, mature oocyte yield, or fertilization rate. Among the random-start cycles, similar outcomes were observed for late follicular phase and luteal phase starts [6].

Unlike the luteal halt protocol which utilizes GnRH antagonists to induce corpus luteum regression, random-start protocols rely on spontaneous regression of the corpus luteum to occur during stimulation. This process may be expedited by the suppressive effect of rising estradiol levels on endogenous LH secretion during ovarian stimulation [5, 6]. Interestingly, similar numbers of dominant follicles were seen on the ovary with a corpus luteum and the contralateral ovary, suggesting that the presence of a corpus luteum or luteal phase progesterone levels did not adversely affect follicular synchrony or oocyte yield.

38.2 Management

The patient began ovarian stimulation 6 days after her initial consultation. Laboratory results obtained on the first day of stimulation were notable for an estradiol level of 134 pg/mL, a progesterone level of 2.96 ng/mL, and an LH level of 13.7 mIU/mL – all consistent with the early luteal phase. A transvaginal ultrasound performed at that visit was notable for interval growth of the right corpus luteal cyst to 4 cm.

A random luteal start protocol was utilized with initiation of ovarian stimulation with 300 units of highly purified human menopausal gonadotropin (hMG). On the eighth day of stimulation with hMG, a GnRH antagonist was initiated to prevent premature secondary LH surge. On the 11th day of stimulation, the patient's estradiol level had increased to 518 pg/mL, and her progesterone level had decreased to 0.2 ng/mL. Transvaginal ultrasound was notable for 13 dominant follicles (≥13 mm), and the decision was made to proceed with a cotrigger (80 unit of leuprolide acetate and 1000 units of HCG) that evening. Thirty-six hours later, the patient underwent an ultrasound-guided oocyte retrieval.

This patient began therapy with DA-R-EPOCH the following day. Nadir counts were obtained after each cycle. Per protocol, doses were increased by 25% after each of the first three cycles.

38.3 Outcome

Eight oocytes were retrieved and cryopreserved following the patient's luteal start stimulation. Seven of these were mature (metaphase II) oocytes, whereas the eighth was an immature (metaphase I) oocyte. In patients with cancer, all oocytes, including those that are immature, are cryopreserved to allow for future in vitro maturation. She recently completed her fifth of her six planned cycles of DA-R-EPOCH. Symptomatically, her shortness of breath is improving, and therapy has been well tolerated. Following her sixth cycle, a posttreatment PET/CT scan will be performed. The PET/CT results will help determine the need for consolidative radiotherapy or surveillance alone.

Clinical Pearls and Pitfalls

- Some forms of cancer like B-cell lymphoma require urgent initiation of treatment. For these patients, alternative ovarian stimulation protocols should be considered.
- Random start protocols can be adjusted to allow for a late-follicular, peri-ovulatory, or luteal phase start.
- Utilization of a random-start protocol minimizes delay in cancer treatment cycle without compromising oocyte yield and maturity.

Review Questions and Answers

38

Q1. A 32-year-old nulligravid woman was recently diagnosed with breast cancer. Her oncologist has recommended she begins cancer treatment in the next 6 weeks. She has regular menstrual cycles every 28 days and, at the time of initial REI evaluation, she is on the 11th day of her cycle with an estradiol level of 218 pg/mL, an LH level of 4.2 mIU/mL, and a progesterone level of 0.78 ng/mL. The patient would like to cryopreserve oocytes prior to starting treatment. What ovarian stimulation protocol would you recommend?

A1. Since the patient's oncologist has indicated that treatment can be deferred for 6 weeks, the patient is a candidate for a conventional ovarian stimulation protocol with the start of her next menstrual cycle. Based on her menstrual history and labs, she is in the late follicular phase, and her next menstrual cycle should occur in 2–3 weeks. As most conventional stimulation protocols require 2 weeks from initiation of medications to oocyte retrieval, she will be able to complete the stimulation process within the recommended time frame even if she awaits her next menstrual cycle.

Q2. A 27-year-old gravida 2, Para 2 woman was recently diagnosed with B-cell lymphoma. Her oncologist has recommended that she begins cancer treatment within the next 2–3 weeks. She has regular menstrual cycles every 27–29 days and, at the time of initial REI evaluation, she is on the 13th day of her cycle with an estradiol level of 256 pg/mL, an LH level of 14.8 mIU/mL, and a progesterone level of 1.12 ng/mL. The patient would like to cryopreserve embryos prior to starting treatment. What ovarian stimulation protocol would you recommend?

A2. The patient's menstrual history and laboratory results suggest recent ovulation. Since the onset of menses typically occurs 2 weeks after ovulation, and ovarian stimulation can require up to 2 weeks, the patient is not a candidate for a conventional ovarian stimulation protocol. Therefore, a random luteal start protocol is recommended to avoid delay in cancer treatment. This would involve starting gonadotropins immediately and adding a GnRH antagonist once the lead follicle is ≥12 mm.

Q3. A 36-year-old nulligravid woman was recently diagnosed with a glioma. Her oncologist has recommended that she begin cancer treatment as soon as possible, ideally within 2 weeks. The patient would like to cryopreserve oocytes prior to starting treatment. At the time of initial REI evaluation, she is on the 12th day of her cycle with an estradiol level of 243 pg/mL, and an 18 mm dominant follicle is noted on transvaginal ultrasound. Is this patient a candidate for oocyte cryopreservation? If so, what ovarian stimulation protocol would you recommend?

A3. The patient's menstrual history and laboratory results are consistent with the late follicular phase, with ovulation expected in the next 2–3 days. Like the patient from question two, she is not a candidate for a conventional ovarian stimulation. However, rather than await spontaneous ovulation to pursue a luteal start protocol, ovulation can be triggered with HCG or GnRH agonist and gonadotropins initiated 2–3 days later. With this protocol, she should be able to complete stimulation within the recommended time frame.

References

1. Dunleavy K, Pittaluga S, Meada LS, et al. Dose-adjusted EPOCH-rituximab therapy in primary mediastinal B-cell lymphoma. N Engl J Med. 2013;368(15):1408–16.
2. Wilson WH, sin-Ho J, Pitcher BN, et al. Phase III randomized study of R-CHOP versus DA-EPOCH-R and molecular analysis of untreated diffuse large B-cell lymphoma: CALGB/Alliance 50303. Blood. 2016;122(8):469.
3. McLaren JF, Bates GW. Fertility preservation in women of reproductive age with cancer. Am J Obstet Gynecol. 2012;207(6):455–62.
4. von Wolff M, Thaler CJ, Frambach T, et al. Ovarian stimulation to cryopreserve fertilized oocytes in cancer patients can be started in the luteal phase. Fertil Steril. 2009;92(4):1360–5.
5. Cakmak H, Rosen MP. Random-start ovarian stimulation in patients with cancer. Curr Opin Obstet Gynecol. 2015;27(3):215–21.
6. Cakmak H, Katz A, Cedars MI, Rosen MP. Effective method for emergency fertility preservation: random-start controlled ovarian stimulation. Fertil Steril. 2013;100(6):1673–80.

Oncofertility in the Premenopausal Breast Cancer Patient

Dana Marie Scott, Nikita M. Shah, and Jacqueline S. Jeruss

T. K. Woodruff et al. (eds.), *Textbook of Oncofertility Research and Practice*,
https://doi.org/10.1007/978-3-030-02868-8_39

Case Presentation

A 32-year-old nulliparous woman palpated a mass in her left breast on routine self-breast exam. She presented to her gynecologist, who ordered diagnostic imaging. Imaging revealed a 3.0 cm irregularly shaped mass, BIRADS 4C. Core needle biopsy of this lesion showed invasive ductal carcinoma, ER positive (95%)/PR positive (95%)/HER2/neu positive (IHC 3+). Left axillary ultrasound was negative for evidence of axillary nodal abnormalities.

The patient's family history was notable for a maternal grandmother with pancreatic cancer, maternal aunt with postmenopausal breast cancer, and a maternal uncle who was recently diagnosed with melanoma.

The patient was then referred to a breast care center for further evaluation and treatment planning. On physical exam, the patient had a palpable mass in the upper outer quadrant of her left breast. Otherwise, her breast exam revealed no skin or nipple changes, no nipple discharge, and no other palpable abnormalities. Additionally, she had no palpable axillary, cervical, or supraclavicular adenopathy, and her abdominal exam was normal. The patient's case was then presented at a multidisciplinary breast cancer tumor board attended by surgeons, radiologists, pathologists, medical and radiation oncologists, genetic counselors, and nurse navigators. Given the patient's young age, that her cancer was HER2/neu positive, and that the size of tumor was greater than 2 cm, the patient was advised to proceed with a neoadjuvant chemotherapy regimen including adriamycin, cyclophosphamide, and paclitaxel, along with bioimmune therapy including trastuzumab and pertuzumab. The patient's course of systemic therapy would last 12 months. The risks, side effects, and benefits of systemic therapy were discussed at length with the patient. Upon further questioning by the treatment team, the patient stated that she was in a committed relationship and hoped to have children in the future.

On the same day that the patient was seen at the breast care center, she was urgently referred to a reproductive endocrinologist to discuss fertility preservation prior to the initiation of chemotherapy. The patient was also evaluated by the cancer genetics team, and after comprehensive genetic counseling and testing, the patient was found to carry a deleterious BRCA2 mutation. Additionally, to minimize exogenous hormone exposure, the patient followed up with her gynecologist for removal of her levonorgestrel-releasing IUD and underwent placement of a copper IUD.

39.1 Systemic Therapy and Impact on Fertility

Many chemotherapeutic agents used in breast cancer treatment have a direct impact on fertility and are known teratogens. The most commonly used regimens include alkylating agents (cyclophosphamide), anthracyclines, and taxanes. Alkylating agents have the highest risk of toxicity in certain regimens with amenorrhea in 40% of women <40 years old and in 76% of women >40 years old. Anthracyclines are also gonadotoxic, with a reportedly high rate of amenorrhea, though lower than that of alkylating agents. Taxanes have a less well-defined gonadotoxicity but have been reported to prolong the period of amenorrhea when used in conjunction with anthracyclines [1, 2].

Trastuzumab and pertuzumab are agents used specifically in the treatment of patients with HER2/neu-positive breast cancers. These agents have known teratogenicity, with possible negative implications for fertility. The rate of amenorrhea with trastuzumab treatment is reportedly lower than with anthracyclines, but the correlation is not well understood. The gonadotoxic effects of pertuzumab are also not well defined. Both agents are known to have direct fetal toxicity and are therefore contraindicated during pregnancy. Trastuzumab has been linked to oligohydramnios, pulmonary hypoplasia, skeletal abnormalities, and fetal death [3]. The exact toxicity of pertuzumab in human pregnancy is unknown, but the administration of pertuzumab to pregnant cynomolgus monkeys resulted in oligohydramnios, delayed fetal kidney development, and fetal death at exposures higher than the recommended dose in humans. It is recommended to delay any attempts for pregnancy for at least 7 months after completion of Her2/neu-directed therapy.

39.2 Radiation and Impact on Fertility

Radiation is an important aspect of breast cancer therapy. The amount of radiation that reaches the ovaries and uterus via scatter during breast/axillary radiation is relatively low when compared to direct pelvic radiation. Thus, gonadotoxic effects of radiation during treatment for breast cancer are unlikely. However, due to the potential risk of radiation scatter effects, fertility preservation should be undertaken prior to radiation therapy, and pregnancy should be delayed until after completion of radiation therapy.

39.3 Fertility Preservation Evaluation

Breast cancer patients of childbearing age should have the opportunity to learn about and discuss the potential implications of their upcoming treatments on their fertility. There are numerous important decision points in a patient's cancer treatment to address future fertility. Using a decision tree similar to that found in ◘ Fig. 39.1 can be a useful tool to streamline a patient's counseling and decision-making [4]. Female patients interested in fertility preservation have multiple options available to them, as depicted in ◘ Fig. 39.2 [5].

For women pursuing fertility preservation, baseline fertility is evaluated by measuring anti-Müllerian hormone (AMH), follicle-stimulating hormone (FSH), and/or estradiol levels. If diminished ovarian reserve is identified, a realistic discussion about the likelihood of successful oocyte retrieval and/or pregnancy should be undertaken prior to pursuing invasive fertility preservation options including oocyte retrieval and oocyte/embryo cryopreservation. Any patients desiring future fertility should also be counseled about options for in vitro fertilization (IVF) with donor oocytes, gestational carrier with autologous or donor oocytes, and adoption.

39.4 Ovarian Stimulation for Oocyte and/or Embryo Cryopreservation

Ovarian stimulation with oocyte retrieval for either mature oocyte or embryo cryopreservation is the most well-established and successful option for fertility preservation. As such, controlled ovarian stimulation (COS) is the recommended fertility preservation option for postpubertal women with a good chance of responding to COS and adequate time to undergo COS. To avoid delay in cancer treatment, typically a single cycle of COS is performed. The stimulation protocol must, therefore, attempt to maximize the number of oocytes retrieved while avoiding ovarian hyperstimulation syndrome (OHSS) and other complications that could potentially delay cancer treatment. COS may be initiated at any point in the cycle, including the luteal phase. COS protocols utilizing GnRH antagonists typically allow more flexibility than other stimulation protocols [6].

COS increases the level of circulating estrogen; however, currently there is no prospective data showing that this brief period of increased circulating estrogen negatively affects the risk of recurrent breast cancer or cancer outcomes. Nevertheless, it is reasonable to administer an aromatase inhibitor concurrently with COS to minimize circulating estrogen levels.

39.5 Embryo Versus Oocyte Cryopreservation

Following COS, the patient undergoes oocyte retrieval. The patient can elect for cryopreservation of mature oocytes alone, or to pursue IVF followed by embryo cryopreservation. IVF can be performed using sperm from either a committed male partner or donor sperm. Prior to pursuing embryo cryopreservation with a male partner, the patient and her partner should be counseled on the legal rights for future disposition of the embryos. These rights may vary by the patient's state of residence.

Previously considered experimental, cryopreservation of mature oocytes is now a standard and approved option for women who do not desire embryo creation. Thawed embryos have higher survival rate than thawed oocytes. Despite this, live birth rates and perinatal outcomes are similar with frozen embryo transfers and frozen oocyte-derived embryo transfers, 25% and 25.1%, respectively [5].

39.6 Ovarian Tissue Cryopreservation and In Vitro Follicle Maturation

Ovarian tissue cryopreservation (OTC) involves surgical excision of ovarian tissue (typically via laparoscopic unilateral oophorectomy), followed by cryopreservation of carefully prepared strips of

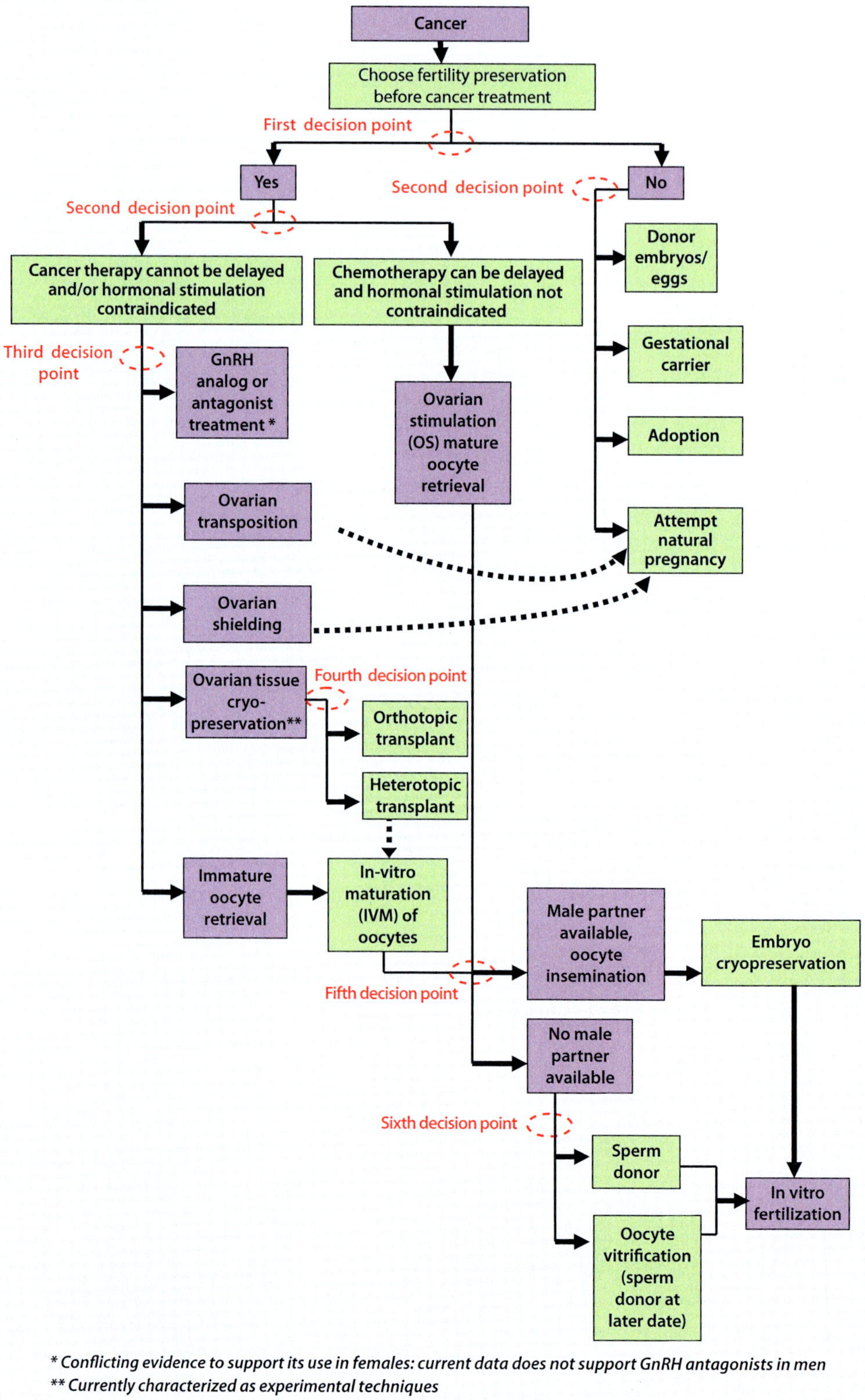

Fig. 39.1 Flow diagram depicting the numerous decision points for fertility preservation throughout a patient's treatment. (Reprinted by permission from Giardino SL: Springer. Giardino et al. [4])

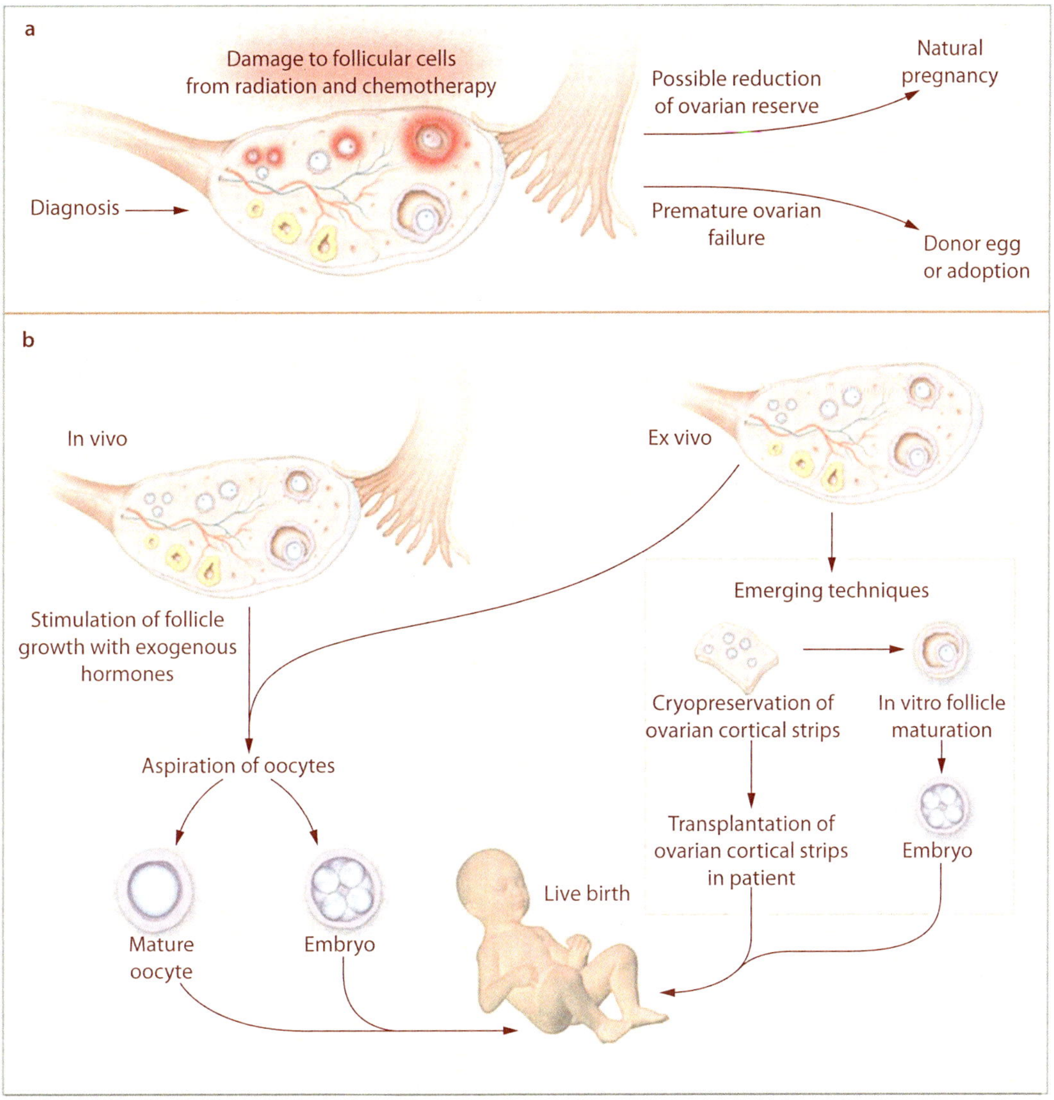

Fig. 39.2 Effects of cancer treatments on fertility (Panel **a**) and options for fertility preservation (Panel **b**). (Courtesy of Jeruss and Woodruff [5])

ovarian tissue. OTC potentially offers a mechanism to preserve thousands of follicles with a single procedure. When childbearing is desired, autologous transplantation of the cryopreserved ovarian tissue can be performed. Currently, there is potential concern for reseeding of malignant cells with autologous ovarian transplantation.

In vitro follicle maturation (IVM) is a mechanism to mature oocytes retrieved from either OTC or transvaginal retrieval of immature oocytes (such as in women unable or unwilling to undergo COS). Both OTC and IVM are currently considered investigational. There are some reported live births attributed to each method, and data about the safety and success of these methods continues to evolve in both the laboratory and clinical settings.

39.7 GnRH Agonist Therapy

Controversy exists over the efficacy of GnRH agonists for ovarian protection during chemotherapy. Though often utilized, there is not clear data demonstrating benefit in terms of future fertility outcomes. Some reports do document higher rates of resumption of ovarian function (menstruation, ovulation) following chemotherapy with concurrent GnRH agonist use. If a patient elects to proceed with GnRH agonist therapy during chemotherapy, she should be counseled that this is an "off label" use of this medication. Nevertheless, GnRH agonists may be offered, particularly for patients electing not to pursue more invasive fertility preservation options [7].

39.8 Preimplantation Genetic Diagnosis

Young patients with breast cancer are recommended to undergo genetic evaluation to help identify deleterious hereditary breast and ovarian cancer (HBOC) gene mutations. Identification of these deleterious mutations impacts treatment planning, including potential recommendations for bilateral mastectomy and bilateral salpingo-oophorectomy. Additionally, if a deleterious mutation is identified, preimplantation genetic diagnosis can be performed on cryopreserved embryos or cryopreserved oocyte-derived embryos. Patients may then select for implantation of embryos without the harmful gene mutation.

39.9 Clinical Presentation Conclusion

The patient's fertility evaluation revealed normal ovarian reserve. Prior to initiating chemotherapy, the patient underwent a luteal-phase start controlled ovarian stimulation with oocyte retrieval. She elected to cryopreserve 15 mature oocytes. After completing neoadjuvant chemotherapy, repeat diagnostic imaging showed a decrease in tumor size to 2 cm. She elected breast-conserving therapy to retain the ability to breast feed in the future. Due to her BRCA2 mutation, she planned to pursue bilateral mastectomies after completion of childbearing. She subsequently completed 4 weeks of radiation therapy and 1 year of treatment with trastuzumab.

Given that the patient was younger than 35 years of age, she then initiated antihormonal therapy, along with ovarian suppression. After 2 years of antihormonal therapy, the patient and her partner elected to pursue pregnancy. Under the supervision of her medical oncologist, she discontinued her antihormonal therapy. After a 3-month washout period, her cryopreserved oocytes were thawed, and IVF was performed. She and her partner elected to perform preimplantation genetic diagnosis and selected an embryo negative for her BRCA2 mutation for implantation. She ultimately delivered a healthy female infant and breastfed for 6 months. She resumed antihormonal therapy to complete a total of 10 years. After completion of breastfeeding, she underwent bilateral mastectomies. At the age of 40, she underwent risk-reducing bilateral salpingo-oophorectomy.

39.10 Pregnancy After Breast Cancer

There is insufficient prospective long-term outcomes data to counsel patients regarding the optimal timing for pregnancy after breast cancer and impact of increased circulating estrogen levels on recurrence risk. Adoption and gestational carrier options should be discussed with breast cancer patients. For those wishing to pursue pregnancy, typically 18–24 months of endocrine therapy followed by a 3-month "wash out" period is recommended prior to conception. The Pregnancy Outcome and Safety of Interrupting Therapy for Women with Endocrine Responsive Breast Cancer (POSITIVE) (NCT 02308085) is an ongoing clinical trial to establish long-term outcomes data on the impact of pregnancy in this patient population.

Clinical Pearls and Pitfalls

- Contraception should be discussed with the patient while undergoing the entirety of treatment, as many of these breast cancer therapies are known teratogens (including tamoxifen).
- Regardless of anticipated treatment, relationship status, or future childbearing plans, it is important to address fertility preservation with young patients upon diagnosis. Several breast cancer treatments may lead to premature ovarian failure.
- Cryopreservation of mature oocytes is an option for patients without a male partner or available donor sperm. Oocyte cryopreservation has similar live birth rates as embryo cryopreservation.

- For patients with HBOC gene mutations, PGD allows testing for and selection of embryos without these mutations.
- There is an ongoing clinical study (Pregnancy Outcome and Safety of Interrupting Therapy for Women with Endocrine Responsive Breast Cancer NCT02308085) that will address the impact of interruption of endocrine therapy, with the goal to facilitate pregnancy, on breast cancer recurrence.

Review Questions and Answers

Q1. What would this patient's fertility options be if she declined or was not offered fertility preservation prior to chemotherapy?

A1. Gonadotoxicity and amenorrhea rates vary by chemotherapeutic agent, with combinations of adriamycin, cyclophosphamide, and paclitaxel having high rates of prolonged (≥24 months) amenorrhea even among women ≤40 years old [8]. Regimens that omit cyclophosphamide and alkylating agents have lower rates of amenorrhea, and, therefore, preservation of fertility may be more likely. For patients with permanent ovarian dysfunction after chemotherapy, fertility options include in vitro fertilization with donor oocytes and adoption. Patients may also opt to use a gestational carrier.

Q2. What are the ethical implications for cryopreservation of embryos compared to mature oocytes?

A2. The creation of embryos with a partner's sperm adds a potential layer of complexity to fertility preservation. Laws vary by state, but typically both parties have legal rights regarding the disposition and disposal of the cryopreserved embryos. As such, a patient may be unable to use cryopreserved embryos if the relationship dissolves in the future. A patient may, therefore, wish to consider cryopreservation of mature oocytes and also embryos if appropriate.

Q3. What are the ethical implications for preimplantation genetic diagnosis?

A3. Though life altering, heterozygous HBOC gene mutations are not inherently lethal mutations. As such, there is some controversy about the use of preimplantation genetic diagnosis in this setting. Patients with an HBOC gene mutation should be counseled about the availability of preimplantation genetic diagnosis.

References

1. Ruddy KJ, et al. Chemotherapy-related amenorrhea after adjuvant paclitaxel-trastuzumab (APT trial). Breast Cancer Res Treat. 2015;151(3):589–96.
2. Ganz PA, et al. Menstrual history and quality-of-life outcomes in women with node-positive breast cancer treated with adjuvant therapy on NSABP B-30 trial. J Clin Oncol. 2011;29:1110–6.
3. Hulvat MC, Jeruss JS. Maintaining fertility in young women with breast cancer. Curr Treat Options in Oncol. 2009;10:308–17.
4. Giardino SL, Jeruss JS, Woodruff TK. Using decision trees to enhance interdisciplinary teamwork: the case of oncofertiliy. J Assist Reprod Genet. 2010;27:229.
5. Jeruss JS, Woodruff TK. Preservation of fertility in patients with cancer. N Engl J Med. 2009;360(9):902–11.
6. Practice Committee of American Society for Reproductive Medicine. Fertility preservation in patients undergoing gonadotoxic therapy or gonadectomy: a committee opinion. Fertil Steril. 2013;100:1214–23.
7. Francis PA, Regan MA, Fleming GF, et al. Adjuvant ovarian suppression in premenopausal breast cancer. NEJM. 2015;372:436–46.
8. Ho JR, et al. A comparison of live birth rates and perinatal outcomes between cryopreserved oocytes and cryopreserved embryos. J Assist Reprod Genet. 2017;34:1359–66.

Oncofertility Case Study: Breast Cancer in a 33-Year-Old Woman

Ellen M. Greenblatt, Eileen McMahon, and Tulin D. Cil

T. K. Woodruff et al. (eds.), *Textbook of Oncofertility Research and Practice*,
https://doi.org/10.1007/978-3-030-02868-8_40

Case Presentation

Following a recent diagnosis of breast carcinoma, a 33-year-old, G2, P2 woman was referred by her surgeon for discussion of potential effects of cancer therapy on future reproductive function and fertility preservation (FP). She had noted a lump in her left breast 3 months prior and was referred to the rapid breast cancer clinic for evaluation. Mammogram and ultrasound confirmed a 4 cm suspicious left upper quadrant lesion in the left breast. Lymph nodes appeared benign clinically and by imaging. Ultrasound-guided needle biopsy and rapid pathology confirmed grade III invasive ductal carcinoma, focally suspicious for lymphovascular tumor emboli. She was simultaneously referred to medical oncology and the fertility clinic on the day after biopsy, when pathology confirmed malignancy.

40.1 Assessment and Plan

Her reproductive history was unremarkable for infertility. She experienced menarche at age 12, and her menstrual cycles were regular, every 28 days. She was using a copper IUD for contraception. Her medical history was positive for migraines, and her surgical history was of wisdom teeth extraction and the two operative deliveries. She reported no family history of breast, ovarian, or prostate cancer. Her father was a survivor of lymphoma. The patient was on day 16 of her menstrual cycle. At the time of consultation, tumor ER/PR/HER2 staining and BRCA 1/2 mutation testing were not yet known, and as medical oncology consultation was pending, it was unclear whether the immediate plan was surgical or alkylating agent-containing neoadjuvant chemotherapy.

The following issues were discussed with the patient: toxic effect of alkylating-based chemotherapy on primordial follicles and risk of subfertility and ovarian failure [1]. With receptor status unknown, possible future recommendation for extended use of endocrine therapy (with a selective estrogen receptor modulator such as Tamoxifen®) which would further delay attempts at conception and therefore potentially impact fertility, was discussed. The option to undergo fertility preservation (FP), in order to store oocytes or embryos prior to receiving chemotherapy, was raised. A brief description of the protocol and process required to undergo controlled ovarian stimulation (COS), oocyte retrieval, and oocyte cryopreservation by vitrification (or fertilization with sperm and embryo cryopreservation) was outlined. In the case of oocyte cryopreservation (OC), the need for future oocyte thaw, fertilization by intracytoplasmic sperm injection (ICSI), embryo development and transfer, should her own ovarian function be insufficient to allow fertility in the future, was explained. Expected live birth rates, for her age, were reviewed based on the best current literature [2], emphasizing that statistics are only averages and a live born outcome could not be guaranteed. Other options, such as oocyte donation, adoption, or not expanding her family, should the patient choose not to undergo FP, and should fertility be compromised by cancer treatment, were also discussed.

The patient expressed concerns regarding the safety of being on fertility medications with her breast cancer diagnosis. Although hormone status was pending at the time of consultation, we explained that protocols for ovarian stimulation in the setting of possible estrogen-sensitive hormones would include the concurrent use of an aromatase inhibitor with gonadotropin stimulation to minimize the pharmacologic rise in estradiol that would normally accompany COS [3]. Published studies have not reported poorer survival or higher recurrence risk, though few publications on the long-term effect of having undergone COS for fertility preservation on prognosis of breast cancer exist [4, 5].

The patient was also concerned that FP would delay her cancer treatment. In the past, COS was required to be started on menstrual cycle day 2 to 3. However, with current "random"-start protocols, the timing of COS and ovum retrieval is not dictated by the menstrual cycle. It was explained that COS and ovum retrieval would require approximately 12–14 days and could be started at any time of her menstrual cycle [6]. Studies have demonstrated that cancer therapy is not significantly prolonged in women who choose to undergo FP versus those who decline [7], and the patient was reassured by this data.

The cost of treatment was also a concern for the patient. Fortunately, in Ontario, Canada, urgent FP (sperm cryopreservation in males; COS and egg cryopreservation in females) for patients facing possible sterility or infertility due to medical therapy for cancer and other conditions is funded by the provincial Ministry of Health. Although medication costs are not funded, the patient was encouraged to verify if her insurance plan would cover these, and if not, an application for the dispensing of compassionate fertility medications would be requested from pharmaceutical partners.

The patient was encouraged to review the online information that is available to all patients planning to undergo in vitro fertilization (IVF), and to speak with her family. The clinic "Online Resources for Young Adults with Cancer" was provided as well. The oncofertility nurse practitioner confirmed with the patient's oncology team that they would support the patient's choice to undergo COS and oocyte extraction.

40.2 Management

Two days after consult, the patient contacted the clinic and relayed that she wanted to undergo COS and OC. She underwent a transvaginal ultrasound (TVUS) (cycle day 21) which revealed that the patient was in the luteal phase with a progesterone level of 31 ng/ml, estradiol level of 366 pmol/L, and AMH of 54 pM. The right ovary had an antral follicle count (AFC) of over 20, and the left ovary had a similar high AFC with the presence of a corpus luteum.

The patient was assigned to start gonadotropin stimulation (recombinant FSH, 200 unit subcut daily) with concomitant daily 5 mg letrozole orally. Cycle monitoring with hormone evaluation and TVUS to follow follicular growth (estradiol, LH, progesterone levels) were performed on day 4, 7, 8, and 9 after gonadotropin/letrozole initiation. On the 6th day of stimulation, a GnRH antagonist 250 µg subcut daily was initiated to prevent premature luteinizing hormone (LH) surge and premature ovulation. After 9 days of stimulation, there were 13 follicles with diameter greater than or equal to 15 mm, 9 of which had diameter of 17–21 mm with an estradiol level of 462 pmol/L. The patient was instructed to self-administer 250 µg recombinant hCG subcut, and ultrasound-guided transvaginal ovum retrieval under mild sedation (midazolam 1.5 mg and fentanyl 125 mcg IV) was performed 36 hours later. Seventeen oocytes were recovered, of which 15 had completed meiosis, were fully mature (metaphase II), and were cryopreserved by vitrification. The patient was instructed to continue on letrozole 5 mg orally daily for another 2 weeks, to prevent the anticipated secondary, postretrieval rise in estradiol.

40.3 Outcome

The patient had no COS-related, procedural or postprocedural complications. Her tumor hormone markers were all negative (triple-negative tumor; ER/PR/HER2) as was her BRCA 1/2 mutation screening. Following consultation with her medical oncologist, she was entered into the KEYNOTE trial for triple-negative cancer patients, which she is currently undergoing. Definitive surgery will be delayed until after completion of neoadjuvant chemotherapy.

Clinical Pearls and Pitfalls

- Do not assume that a patient is not concerned about future fertility based on age, gender, sexual orientation, current family size, or structure.
- Early referral allows the patient more options to decide what the best care is for her.
- Current "random-start" protocols generally allow oocyte or embryo banking to be completed within 12–14 days.
- At this time, estrogen-sensitive tumors are not necessarily a contraindication for COS, and adjuvant SERMs or aromatase inhibitors can be included in the protocol.

Review Questions and Answers

Q1. If a patient already has children, is it worthwhile to refer her for a fertility preservation consultation?

A1. As per ASCO [8], the possible effect of cancer treatment on future fertility must be discussed with *all patients* of reproductive age and appropriate referral to a fertility preservation team offered.

Q2. What categories of medications are used to reduce estrogen exposure in stimulation cycles in patients with hormone-sensitive tumors?

A2. Aromatase inhibitors [3] and/or SERMs [9].

References

1. Petrek JA, Naughton MJ, Case LD, Paskett ED, Naftalis EZ, Singletary SE, Sukumvanich P. Incidence, time course, and determinants of menstrual bleeding after breast cancer treatment: a prospective study. J Clin Oncol. 2006;24(7):1045–51.
2. Lyttle Schumacher B, Grover N, Mesen T, Steiner A, Mersereau J. Modeling of live-birth rates and cost-effectiveness of oocyte cryopreservation for cancer patients prior to high- and low-risk gonadotoxic chemotherapy. Hum Reprod. 2017;32(10):2049–55.
3. Oktay K, Hourvitz A, Sahin G, Oktem O, Safro B, Cil A, Bang H. Letrozole reduces estrogen and gonadotropin exposure in women with breast cancer undergoing ovarian stimulation before chemotherapy. J Clin Endocrinol Metab. 2006;91(10):3885–90.
4. Azim AA, Costantini-Ferrando M, Oktay K. Safety of fertility preservation by ovarian stimulation with letrozole and gonadotropins in patients with breast cancer: a prospective controlled study. J Clin Oncol. 2008; 26(16):2630–5.
5. Oktay K, Kim J, Bedoschi G, Turan V. Abstract P5-15-02: safety of letrozole-gonadotropin controlled ovarian stimulation protocol in women with breast cancer undergoing fertility preservation before or after tumor resection via embryo or oocyte cryopreservation: A prospective cohort study. Cancer Res. 2015. Poster Session Abstracts.
6. Cakmak H, Katz A, Cedars MI, Rosen MP. Effective method for emergency fertility preservation: random-start controlled ovarian stimulation. Fertil Steril. 2013;100(6):1673–80.
7. Letourneau JM, Sinha N, Wald K, Harris E, Quinn M, Imbar T, Mok-Lin E, Chien AJ, Rosen M. Random start ovarian stimulation for fertility preservation appears unlikely to delay initiation of neoadjuvant chemotherapy for breast cancer. Hum Reprod. 2017;32(10):2123–9.
8. Loren AW, et al. J Clin Oncol. 2013;31(19):2500–10. PMID 23715580.
9. Oktay K, Buyuk E, Davis O, Yermakova I, Veeck L, Rosenwaks Z. Fertility preservation in breast cancer patients: IVF and embryo cryopreservation after ovarian stimulation with tamoxifen. Hum Reprod. 2003;18(1):90–5. [PubMed: 12525446].

Further Reading

Lambertini M, Kroman N, Ameye L, Cordoba O, Pinto A, Benedetti G, Jensen MB, Gelber SI, Del Grande M, Ignatiadis M, De Azambuja E, Paesmans M, Peccatori F, Azim HA Jr. J Clin Oncol. 2017;35:18_suppl, LBA10066-LBA10066

Signorello LB, Mulvihill JJ, Green DM, et al. Congenital anomalies in the children of cancer survivors: a report from the Childhood Cancer Survivor Study. J Clin Oncol. 2012;30(3):239–45. https://doi.org/10.1200/JCO.2011.37.2938.

Fertility Preservation: Convergence of Newly Diagnosed Breast Cancer, Desired Fertility, and Polycystic Ovary Syndrome

Michael S. Mersol-Barg and Jeffrey H. Margolis

T. K. Woodruff et al. (eds.), *Textbook of Oncofertility Research and Practice*,
https://doi.org/10.1007/978-3-030-02868-8_41

Case Presentation

A 34-year-old nulliparous female presented with a self-discovered 4 cm, firm, mobile mass in the upper, outer quadrant of her right breast. Her mother is a breast cancer survivor, diagnosed at age 45, and was BRCA negative. The patient also had polycystic ovary syndrome based on a long history of irregular menstrual cycles, mild facial and lower abdominal hair, acne, and mild acanthosis nigricans on the nape of the neck. She last used hormonal contraception 4 years prior to initial presentation. Menstrual cycles were more regular in the past year. Current medications to treat anxiety and depression included sertraline, lamotrigine, and oxcarbazepine. She had no other medical illness in the past or at presentation. The patient and her husband were just beginning efforts to become pregnant at the time she discovered her breast mass.

41.1 Assessment and Diagnosis

MRI of the breast revealed a 3.5 cm mass within the right breast as well as a satellite 0.9 cm lesion. There are multiple enlarged lymph nodes within the right axilla, the largest being 3.2 cm. Biopsy of the large lesion within the breast is positive for an invasive ductal carcinoma, grade 2–3. The tumor is estrogen negative, progesterone negative, and HER2/neu positive. The patient has also undergone a right axillary lymph node biopsy again, which was positive for metastatic adenocarcinoma of the breast. The patient underwent a CT scan of the chest, abdomen, and pelvis and a bone scan, without evidence of metastatic disease.

Breast cancer was staged as stage III at this time. Neoadjuvant cytotoxic therapy, with Taxotere, carboplatin, trastuzumab, and pertuzumab chemotherapy, was recommended. Although HER2/neu breast cancers are typically more aggressive, the selected treatment protocol is the most effective treatment available. Treatment is given with curative intent. The patient was informed of the potential side effects of chemotherapy such as fatigue, hair loss, neuropathy, cardiac toxicity myelosuppression, and infertility. The patient was most concerned about the long-term effects on fertility. Therefore, a request for reproductive endocrine evaluation was made.

41

Reproductive endocrine assessment involved testing of ovarian reserve and polycystic ovary syndrome. Given the compressed timeline for evaluation and her desire to bank (freeze) eggs or embryos prior to initiating treatment for breast cancer, the following tests were performed on cycle day 7: serum AMH 11.0 ng/ml, FSH −7.1 mIU/ml, estradiol 85 pg/ml, transvaginal pelvic ultrasound with antral follicle count greater than 15 for each ovary – consistent with polycystic ovarian architecture, prolactin 22.2 ng/mL, TSH abnormally elevated at 5.070 μIU/ml, repeat TSH also abnormally elevated at 4.960 μIU/ml, Free T4 was 0.98 ng/day, absence of thyroid peroxidase and thyroglobulin antibodies and normal thyroid gland by physical examination. Both ovaries were confirmed to be accessible for transvaginal ultrasound-guided egg retrieval. Her reproductive endocrine diagnosis was of normal ovarian reserve, evidence of polycystic ovary syndrome, and subclinical hypothyroidism, of which further evaluation and potential treatment were deferred due to the compressed timeline needed to complete egg or embryo banking and begin chemotherapy.

41.2 Management

Medical oncology expressed concern about minimizing the delay in starting chemotherapy because of the advanced nature of her disease. Fertility preservation plan was designed not to delay the start of potentially curative therapy.

Fertility preservation treatment plan was ovulation induction with egg retrieval, IVF therapy, and cryopreservation of embryos of an advanced developmental stage. The initial plan was to start ovulation induction on day 2 of her upcoming menses. New information regarding the patient's malignancy being of a more advanced stage was the compelling factor to plan an earlier start of chemotherapy. Likewise, the fertility preservation timetable was accelerated to begin ovulation induction in her current luteal phase 6 days prior to the anticipated start of her menses – 2 weeks after initial presentation to her infertility specialist. There is reliable evidence that ovulation induction started in the luteal phase of the menstrual cycle can yield good follicle recruitment and oocytes that have normal reproductive potential [1, 2]. The addition of letrozole can suppress serum estradiol levels during ovulation induction. For women with estrogen receptor-positive breast tumors, it has been posited that an abnormally high serum estradiol level from ovulation induction may promote breast tumor growth. It may follow that suppression of serum estradiol levels by an aromatase inhibitor such as letrozole may reduce this potential risk of exacerbating malignant breast disease [3]. Although immunohistologic results of breast tumor tissue for this patient did not identify the presence of estrogen or progesterone receptors, there is the possibility of tumor cell receptor heterogeneity. We felt it prudent to take every precaution including the use of letrozole in her ovulation induction protocol. The patient's ovulation induction protocol was as follows: letrozole 5 mg/day × 5 days and FSH medications, rFSH 225 IU/day and Menopur 75 IU/day × 8 days, GnRH antagonist daily the last 4 days prior to GnRH agonist, and leuprolide 1 mg injection, to trigger LH surge on day 9 of treatment. On day 9 of treatment, there were 21 follicles in a range of 20–12 mm average diameter between both ovaries. Peak serum estradiol level was elevated to 2867 pg/ml on day of GnRH agonist trigger.

41.3 Outcome

Egg harvest was performed 36 hours after GnRH agonist trigger. The patient underwent the procedure with intravenous conscious sedation and had an uneventful recovery. Thirty-five eggs were recovered, 26 of which had completed meiosis II (M2). All 26 M2 stage eggs underwent in vitro fertilization. Insemination by intracytoplasmic sperm injection (ICSI) was performed 4 hours after egg harvest. The first day after egg retrieval, 21 of 26 inseminated eggs had fertilized normally forming zygotes. By day 6 of embryo culture, 13 pre-embryos developed to a good or fair blastocyst stage embryo suitable for cryopreservation and long-term storage. Should the patient's future health be sufficiently well providing her the opportunity to become pregnant, she has a very good prognosis for a successful pregnancy with warming and transfer of a single pre-embryo into her uterus [4]. Should she experience amenorrhea due to menopause as a result of her chemotherapy, hormone replacement therapy including both estrogen and progesterone may be necessary to properly prepare her uterus for pregnancy.

Two days after egg collection, the patient began chemotherapy. Prior to starting chemotherapy, she was given a long-acting GNRH agonist goserelin to reduce the risk of early menopause and to increase the odds of a completely natural pregnancy. The benefit of GNRH agonist in preventing chemotherapy-induced menopause is controversial [5–8]. Some trials have shown benefit in preventing early menopause, while others have not. There is insufficient evidence to declare true fertility potential will be preserved [9, 10]. The use of GNRH agonists does not seem to increase the risk of malignancy relapse. Recent large clinical trials using GNRH agonist with endocrine therapy, tamoxifen or exemestane, in premenstrual women with estrogen-positive cancer have shown an improvement in disease-free survival [7, 8].

The patient was at risk for OHSS due to PCOS and 36 eggs were harvested. Mild ovarian hyperstimulation syndrome (OHSS) developed 12 days after egg harvest and 10 days after the administration of goserelin. Signs and symptoms were a 10-lb weight gain, moderate abdominal distention with ascites to the level of her umbilicus, moderate shortness of breath when lying supine, good urine output, and normal hematocrit indicators for the absence of hemoconcentration. GnRH agonist leuprolide single-dose injection was administered in place of traditional hCG single-dose injection 2 days prior to egg harvest per protocol in order to reduce the risk of OHSS that would be exacerbated had she taken the hCG injection. Goserelin and chemotherapy were administered 2 days after egg harvest. Goserelin induces an initial increase of gonadotropin release in the first 10 days from administration termed "upregulation" followed by prolonged cessation of gonadotropin release termed "downregulation." This initial gonadotropin upregulation 2–12 days after egg retrieval further stimulated the ovaries and served as a significant contributing cause of her OHSS. She began to feel better with a decline in weight, dyspnea, abdominal distention, and discomfort by 14 days after the start of goserelin therapy as expected.

Clinical Pearls and Pitfalls

- Before cancer therapy is started, patients and the parent(s) of children and adolescent patients with current and future fertility potential should be provided with education about the possibility of infertility resulting from cancer therapy. A multidisciplinary team of medical providers, coordinated by a patient navigator, should discuss fertility preservation options and refer these patients to appropriate reproductive specialists [11].
- Fertility preservation options proven with greatest reliability include cryopreservation of gametes—sperm and eggs—and embryos through in vitro fertilization therapy. Ovarian tissue cryopreservation has emerged with more limited success. In vitro gamete maturation from immature sperm or eggs followed by cryopreservation is in its nascent stage of study [12].
- Challenges in choosing fertility preservation include ensuring thorough patient and family education, ethical considerations, time to treatment, and financial resources.
- Luteal phase start of ovulation induction shortens the time frame for egg harvest providing an earlier start of cancer treatment plan.
- Use of GnRH agonist such as goserelin in an effort to protect gametes from the gonadotoxic effects of chemotherapy may exacerbate ovarian OHSS if administered within a short time (estimate of 2 weeks) after egg harvest.
- Patients continued to face economic barriers to care being provided within the narrow critical window of time to receive fertility preservation treatment. In a recent estimate, only 4–10% of patients with breast cancer, the most common cancer in reproductive-age women, pursue fertility preservation—at least partly because of lack of coverage [13]. In 2017, Connecticut and Rhode Island followed in 2018 by Maryland, Delaware and Illinois became the first states to pass bills to mandate insurance coverage that allows cancer patient access to fertility preservation treatment. It is imperative that oncologists refer their patients to reproductive specialists who can assist cancer patients navigate to available financial support opportunities.

Review Questions and Answers

Q1. A 28-year-old woman was recently diagnosed with invasive ductal carcinoma limited to her left breast. She has a new boyfriend, but is not in a committed relationship. Her mother and maternal grandmother are both breast cancer survivors. She wants her cancer to be treated as soon as possible, but she also plans to have children in the future. How will you counsel this patient?

(a) Obtain informed consent advising her to begin chemotherapy immediately followed by surgery because saving her life is the main objective. She can take a GnRH agonist medication during chemotherapy to protect her eggs from the toxic effects of the medications. There will be time after her cancer treatment to consider her chances for having children.

(b) Inform her that her cancer treatment will include medications that can cause future infertility or sterility by damaging her eggs. In advance of starting chemotherapy, refer her to a reproductive specialist, advising her to undergo egg harvest and either select sperm from her boyfriend or an anonymous donor at a sperm bank, undergo IVF therapy, and freeze embryos for possible future use to have a child. The alternative of egg freezing is experimental and unreliable.

(c) Inform her that her cancer treatment will include medications that can cause future infertility or sterility by damaging her eggs. In advance of starting chemotherapy, refer her to a reproductive specialist who can counsel her about fertility preservation options. Given that she is not in a committed relationship with her current boyfriend, freezing some of her eggs in advance of chemotherapy may be her best option providing her with more control over her future reproduction with a partner committed to building a family together.

(d) Advise her that she should begin chemotherapy within the next 2 weeks. Although preserving her fertility by freezing eggs is an option, fertility drugs are known to cause breast cancer and can worsen her current breast disease. For this reason, you strongly advise her against fertility preservation and rely on GnRH agonist medication during chemotherapy to protect her eggs from the toxic effects of the chemotherapy medications.

A1. (c). Both egg and embryo freezing are reliable strategies for fertility preservation. In 2012, the American Society for Reproductive Medicine (ASRM) announced that there was sufficient clinical outcome-based evidence to support egg freezing as a mainstream technology no longer designating it as experimental. Given her favorable reproductive age of 28 years and that she was not in a committed relationship with her male partner, egg freezing provided her with greater control over having a future child with the partner of her choice. If she carries a BRCA mutation, she should be advised that this mutation is associated with reduced ovarian reserve in terms of lower egg quantity, but not decreased egg quality. Ovulation induction strategy will need to take this into consideration either to increase the dose of gonadotropins during ovulation induction therapy or plan for more than one egg harvest event in advance of beginning chemotherapy.

Q2. A 32-year-old woman was recently diagnosed with estrogen-positive invasive ductal carcinoma limited to her right breast. She wants her cancer to be treated as soon as possible, but she also would like the option to have children in the future. She does not want to undergo anything invasive and has refused egg harvest. How will you counsel this patient?

(a) Inform her that her cancer treatment will include medications that can cause future infertility or sterility by damaging her eggs. In advance of starting chemotherapy, refer her to a reproductive specialist who can counsel her about fertility preservation options.

(b) Inform her that her cancer treatment will include medications that can cause future infertility or sterility by damaging her eggs. Outside of egg harvest, there is nothing that can be done. Her young age makes infertility unlikely.

(c) Inform her that her cancer treatment will include medications that can cause future infertility or sterility by damaging her eggs. Start her on GnRH agonist, but warn her that the estrogen surge may increase her risk of malignancy relapse.

(d) Inform her that her cancer treatment will include medications that can cause future infertility or sterility by damaging her eggs. Start her on chemotherapy and tamoxifen. The tamoxifen should lower the risk of infertility and decrease the risk of relapse.

A2. (a). All patients who wish to preserve their fertility should see a reproductive specialist. Many patients are apprehensive about egg and embryo freezing based on misunderstanding and the absence of accurate information. GnRH agonist medications have gonadal protective properties and should be presented as an adjunctive treatment option for the duration of gonadotoxic chemotherapy administration. GnRH agonists appear to be safe and in some studies reduce the risk of premature ovarian failure and menopause [5–8]. There is insufficient evidence to conclude GnRH agonists prevent reduction in fertility potential.

References

1. von Wolff M, Thaler CJ, Frambach T, Zeeb C, Lawrenz B, Popovici RM, Strowitzki T. Ovarian stimulation to cryopreserve fertilized oocytes in cancer patients can be started in the luteal phase. Fertil Steril. 2009;92(4):1360–5.
2. Nayak SR, Wakim AN. Random-start gonadotropin-releasing hormone (GnRH) antagonist-treated cycles with GnRH agonist trigger for fertility preservation. Fertil Steril. 2011;96(1):e51–4.
3. Reddy J, Oktay K. Ovarian stimulation and fertility preservation with the use of aromatase inhibitors in women with breast cancer. Fertil Steril. 2012; 98(6):1363–9.
4. Green DM, Whitton JA, Stovall M, et al. Pregnancy outcome of female survivors of childhood cancer: a report from the childhood cancer survivor study. Am J Obstet Gynecol. 2002;187(4):1070–80.
5. Deemeestere I, Brice P, Peccatori FA, Kentos A, Dupuis J, Zachee P, Casasnovas O, Van Den Neste E, Dechene J, De Maertelaer V, Bron D, Englert Y. No evidence for the benefit of gonadotropin-releasing hormone agonist in preserving ovarian function and fertility in lymphoma survivors treated with chemotherapy: final long-term report of a prospective randomized trial. J Clin Oncol. 2016;34(22):2568–74. https://doi.org/10.1200/JCO.2015.65.8864. Epub 2016 May 23.
6. von Wolff M, Stute P. Judging the fertility protective effect of GnRH agonists in chemotherapy – it is a matter of perspective. Front Endocrinol. 2017;8:69.
7. Halle CF, Moor MD, Unger JM, Phillips KA. Goserelin for ovarian protection during breast cancer adjuvant chemotherapy. N Engl J Med. 2015;372:923–32.
8. Donnez J, Dolmans M-M. Fertility preservation in women. N Engl J Med. 2017;377:1657–65.
9. Francis PA, Regan MM, Fleming GF, Láng I, SOFT Investigators, International Breast Cancer Study Group, et al. Adjuvant ovarian suppression in premenopausal breast cancer. N Engl Med. 2015;372(5):436–46.
10. Pagani O, Regan MM, Walley BA, Fleming GF, Colleoni M, Láng I, Gomez HL, TEXT and SOFT Investigators, International Breast Cancer Study Group, et al. Adjuvant exemestane with ovarian suppression in premenopausal breast cancer. N Engl J Med. 2014;37(2):107–18. https://www.ncbi.nlm.nih.gov/pubmed/?term=Francis PA%5BAuthor%5D&cauthor=true&cauthor_uid=24881463.
11. Loren AW, Mangu PB, Beck LN, et al. Fertility preservation for patients with cancer: American Society of Clinical Oncology clinical practice guideline update. J Clin Oncol. 2013;31(19):2500–10.
12. McLaughlin M, Albertini DF, Wallace WHB, Anderson RA, Telfer EE. Metaphase II oocytes from human unilaminar follicles grown in a multi-step culture system. MHR: Basic Sci Reprod Med. https://doi.org/10.1093/molehr/gay002.
13. Cardozo ER, Huber WJ, Stuckey AR, Alvera RJ. Mandating coverage for fertility preservation – a step in the right direction. N Engl J Med. 2017;z377(17):1607–9.

41

Fertility Preservation for a Transgender Man

Olivia Higgins, Amy R. Benjamin, Katherine B. Greenberg, and Wendy S. Vitek

T. K. Woodruff et al. (eds.), *Textbook of Oncofertility Research and Practice*,
https://doi.org/10.1007/978-3-030-02868-8_42

Case Presentation

A 23-year-old transgender man, gravida 0, presented to a reproductive endocrinology clinic for fertility preservation after initiating androgen therapy and prior to a laparoscopic hysterectomy and bilateral salpingo-oophorectomy for chronic pelvic pain.

The patient's gender dysphoria was managed by an adolescent medicine specialist. The patient was offered a fertility preservation consultation prior to initiation of testosterone therapy, which the patient declined. The patient started on testosterone 50 mg IM every 2 weeks, which was increased to 100 mg IM every 2 weeks after 3 months of therapy. Prior to testosterone therapy, the patient had chronic pelvic pain related to endometriosis, and had undergone medical management with progestin-only pills, leuprolide acetate, and a levonorgestrel intrauterine device. None of these provided adequate pain management. After initiation of testosterone therapy, the patient presented to the gynecologist requesting definitive surgical management of endometriosis and gender dysphoria, with subsequent surgical planning for laparoscopic excision of endometriosis with hysterectomy and bilateral salpingooophorectomy. This decision prompted the patient to meet with reproductive endocrinology to discuss fertility preservation prior to surgery.

The patient presented with his partner, 24-year- old cisgender woman who was interested in carrying an embryo created from the patient's oocyte and donor sperm in the future. The patient was amenorrheic with a levonorgestrel intrauterine device. Ovarian reserve testing revealed an anti-Mullerian hormone of 2.753 ng/ml, antral follicle count of 25, random FSH of 1.6 mIU/ml, and estradiol of 47 pg/ml. The patient had been on testosterone therapy for 9 months, and the total testosterone was 197 ng/dl, and free testosterone was 7.1 mg/dl. The patient was counseled on options including oocyte cryopreservation, embryo cryopreservation with donor sperm, and experimental ovarian tissue cryopreservation. The patient chose oocyte cryopreservation.

42.1 Assessment and Diagnosis

Transgender individuals and their healthcare needs have become increasingly visible over the past several years; with this, gaps in care are also becoming more visible. Reproductive life planning, including fertility treatment and preservation, is one of these unmet needs. Many transgender men initiate gender-affirming hormone therapy prior to considering future fertility [1], yet more than half of the transgender men surveyed were interested in family building, and more than a third would consider fertility preservation if available [2].

Both the American Society for Reproductive Medicine and the World Professional Association for Transgender Health (WPATH) recommend that clinicians discuss family building with transgender individuals seeking hormone therapy and gonadectomy, as well as offer fertility preservation options to patients prior to gender transition [3, 4]. Fertility preservation options for transgender men include oocyte and embryo cryopreservation, while ovarian tissue cryopreservation remains experimental [3] (Table 42.1).

There are knowledge gaps regarding the short-term and long-term impact of gender-affirming hormone therapy on fertility. Testosterone therapy may induce hypothalamic amenorrhea and the rate of persistent hypothalamic amenorrhea after discontinuation of testosterone therapy is unknown. While transgender men can conceive while taking testosterone and shortly after discontinuing testosterone, it is unknown if testosterone therapy alters future fecundity [1]. Therefore, oocyte and embryo cryopreservation has been performed in transgender men prior to initiation of gender-affirming hormone therapy [5, 6].

Performing oocyte or embryo cryopreservation in transgender men prior to gender-affirming therapy raises several unique considerations [7]. Transgender men may experience distress in delaying the start of gender-affirming therapy even by a few weeks to complete an oocyte or embryo banking cycle. In addition, the increased estrogen associated with controlled ovarian

Table 42.1 Fertility preservation options for adolescent transgender boys and adult transgender men [6]

Age group (years)	Method	Advantages	Disadvantages
Younger than 18	OC	Well-tolerated	Must be perimenarchal or postmenarchal
		Minimally invasive outpatient procedure	
	OTC	Available before menarche	Experimental
			Not recommended unless concomitant medical condition (i.e., undergoing chemotherapy for cancer)
			Requires invasive surgical procedure
18 or older	OC	More flexibility for the future use of gametes	Difficult to estimate number of oocytes needed for a live birth
			Embryo formation rates may be lower at some centers
	OTC	No need to stop androgen therapy before surgery	Experimental
		Performed at the time of planned oophorectomy	Suboptimal graft function if tissue transplantation onto peritoneal surface, requires IVF
	EB	More accurate estimate of chance of live birth	Requires sperm source (donor or partner)
		Can perform CCS before embryo cryopreservation	Legal implications if partners separate after creating embryos

OC oocyte cryopreservation, *OTC* ovarian tissue cryopreservation, *IVF* in vitro fertilization, *EB* embryo banking, *CCS* comprehensive chromosomal screening

hyperstimulation may induce unacceptable hormonal side effects that heighten body dysphoria such as breast tenderness or pelvic pain.

42.2 Management

The patient discontinued testosterone therapy for 2 weeks and the levonorgestrel intrauterine device was continued. Baseline assessment was consistent with the early follicular phase. Controlled ovarian hyperstimulation was performed with a low-dose antagonist protocol with a peak estradiol of 2182 pg/ml. The patient experienced pelvic pain during simulation which was managed with nonsteroidal anti-inflammatory drugs (NSAIDs). Human chorionic gonadotropin (HCG) trigger (10,000 IU) was administered when two lead follicles were ≥18 mm and ≥50% of the cohort was ≥15 mm. Thirty-six hours later, the patient underwent a transvaginal ultrasoundguided oocyte retrieval.

The patient was advised to restart testosterone 2 weeks after oocyte retrieval.

42.3 Outcome

Fifteen mature (metaphase II) oocytes were retrieved and cryopreserved following controlled ovarian hyperstimulation performed 2 weeks after testosterone discontinuation. The patient experienced significant acute-on-chronic pelvic pain after the oocyte retrieval, and an evaluation excluded ovarian hyperstimulation syndrome. He proceeded with a laparoscopic hysterectomy with bilateral salpingo-oophorectomy after successful fertility preservation.

Clinical Pearls and Pitfalls

- While more information is needed regarding live birth rates from fertility preservation procedures performed after gender-affirming therapy is initiated in transgender men, this case provides evidence that transgender men can revisit fertility preservation when ready.
- Chronic pelvic pain treatment and gender affirmation management for our patient required a multidisciplinary team to provide the desired outcome.

Review Questions and Answers

Q1. An 18-year-old transman is referred for a discussion on future fertility. He has consulted with an adolescent medicine specialist regarding the initiation of gender-affirming hormone therapy and plans to begin therapy as soon as possible. He has regular menstrual cycles and has never tried to conceive. He is unsure about his desire to have biologically related children in the future. How would you counsel this patient?

A1. The patient should be counseled that testosterone therapy may induce amenorrhea. He should be informed that transgender men can conceive while taking testosterone and shortly after discontinuing testosterone though it is unknown if testosterone therapy alters future fecundity. He should be counseled on fertility preservation options including oocyte cryopreservation, embryo cryopreservation, and experimental ovarian tissue cryopreservation.

Q2. The patient is interested in oocyte cryopreservation but does not want to delay the initiation of gender-affirming hormone therapy. How would you counsel this patient on his options?

A2. He should be counseled that oocyte cryopreservation can typically be achieved within 2 weeks using random start protocols. He can be informed that oocyte cryopreservation could be performed after the initiation of testosterone therapy though it is unclear if testosterone therapy needs to be discontinued during controlled ovarian hyperstimulation, and live births from oocyte cryopreserved after testosterone therapy have not been reported.

Q3. He opts for oocyte cryopreservation prior to initiating gender-affirming hormone therapy. How should he be counseled regarding the side effects of controlled ovarian hyperstimulation in transmen?

A3. He should be counseled that the increased estrogen associated with controlled ovarian hyperstimulation may induce unacceptable hormonal side effects that heighten body dysphoria such as breast tenderness or pelvic pain. His adolescent medicine specialist should co-manage his care during this time of heightened body dysphoria.

42

References

1. Light AD, Obedin-Maliver J, Sevelius JM, Kerns JL. Transgender men who experienced pregnancy after female-to-male gender transitioning. Obstet Gynecol. 2014;124(6):1120–7.
2. T'Sjoen G, Van Caenegem E, Wierckx K. Transgenderism and reproduction. Curr Opin Endocrinol Diabetes Obes. 2013;20(6):575–9.
3. Ethics Committee of the American Society for Reproductive M. Access to fertility services by transgender persons: an Ethics Committee opinion. Fertil Steril. 2015;104(5):1111–5.
4. World Professional Association for Transgender H. Standards of care for the health of transsexual, transgender, and gender nonconforming people. World Professional Association for Transgender Health. 2011. Available from: www.wpath.org.
5. Wallace SA, Blough KL, Kondapalli LA. Fertility preservation in the transgender patient: expanding oncofertility care beyond cancer. Gynecol Endocrinol. 2014;30(12):868–71.
6. Maxwell S, Noyes N, Keefe D, Berkeley AS, Goldman KN. Pregnancy outcomes after fertility preservation in transgender men. Obstet Gynecol. 2017;129(6):1031–4.
7. Chen D, Matson M, Macapagal K, Johnson EK, Rosoklija I, Finlayson C, et al. Attitudes toward fertility and reproductive health among transgender and gender-nonconforming adolescents. J Adolesc Health. 2018;124: 1120–7.

Fertility Preservation in an Adolescent with an Ovotesticular Disorder of Sexual Development

Teresa Almeida-Santos, R. Cardoso, A. Carvalho, and Ana Paula Sousa

T. K. Woodruff et al. (eds.), *Textbook of Oncofertility Research and Practice*,
https://doi.org/10.1007/978-3-030-02868-8_43

Case Presentation

A 12-year-old boy was referred to pediatric surgery for correction of right unilateral cryptorchidism. The surgeon suspected the presence of testicular and ovarian tissue in the right gonad, and so the child was further referred to a pediatric endocrinologist to investigate a disorder of sexual development (DSD). A biopsy was performed that revealed numerous primordial follicles and some primary and secondary follicles, surrounded by ovarian stroma and testicular parenchyma, with seminiferous tubules displaying Sertoli and germinal cells. Focal spermatogenesis was present as well as testicular stroma with focal Leydig cells.

The patient had a male phenotype with a small penis with a slight ventral curve and a palpable, homogeneous, approximately 2 cc gonad in the left scrotum. The patient had been referred to another department in early childhood for correction of urogenital abnormalities, but no investigation or intervention was undertaken at that time.

43.1 Assessment and Diagnosis

Diagnostic laparoscopy revealed an apparently normal uterus with two fallopian tubes. After a basal endocrine profile was obtained, a multidisciplinary team discussed the possible therapeutic approaches with the family and the child, with the goal to achieve normal pubertal development and preserve fertility.

Basal endocrine profile:

	Patient value	Reference range
LH[a] mUI/ml	0.7	0.3–4.0
FSH[a] mUI/ml	5.2	0.5–10.5
Testosterone ng/dl	24.1	<30 Tanner I
AMH[a] ng/ml	27	27.2–42.6 Tanner I
Estradiol pg/ml	<11.8	<13

[a]*LH* luteinizing hormone, *FSH* follicle-stimulating hormone, *AMH* anti-Mullerian hormone

The HCG stimulation test confirmed an acceptable testosterone secretion (188.6 ng/dl) and the cytogenetic analysis revealed a mosaic 46,XY[36]/46,XX[14] karyotype. Appropriate genetic counseling was provided to the patient and family.

In order to minimize the risk of malignancy, maintain male sexual rearing, and preserve fertility, hysterectomy and right gonadectomy were performed. At the same time, the left intrascrotal gonad was biopsied, and the diagnosis of a bilateral ovotesticular DSD (OT-DSD) was confirmed.

Microscopic examination of the left gonad revealed a clear separation of ovarian and testicular tissues. Seminiferous tubules were mainly formed by Sertoli cells with incipient germinal cells and focal spermatogenesis, and rare Leydig cells were also present.

Ovotesticular disorder of sexual development (OT-DSD) is an unusual form of DSD, characterized by the coexistence of testicular and ovarian tissue in the same individual. In a subset of patients, ovotesticular DSD is caused by 46,XX/46,XY chimerism or mosaicism [1].

The diagnosis is based on histology, requiring the presence of both seminiferous cords and ovarian follicles with oocytes. The presence of an OT-DSD increases the risk of gonadal and genitourinary pathology. Patients may present with several concerns including sex assignment, mitigating the risk of malignancy, as well as the desire for gonadal retention in order to protect development or preserve fertility potential [1, 2].

A DSD must be excluded in any child with genital anomalies and cryptorchidism. The diagnosis should be done before puberty to minimize psychological impact on adolescents. These cases must be evaluated by a multidisciplinary team including an endocrinologist, gynecologic/urologic surgeon, fertility specialist, and clinical psychologist with experience in these conditions for the long-term follow-up and the achievement of an integrated approach to the patient [1]. Fertility potential should be considered when addressing gender assignment, surgical management, and patient and family counseling.

Boys with an OT-DSD often have compromised fertility that worsens with time [3]. While ovarian tissue is often normal, testicular tissue is usually atrophic, with only focal spermatogenesis. Moreover, the hormonal production of the ovarian tissue induces a negative feedback on gonadotropins with a deleterious effect on spermatogenesis and Leydig cell function.

43.2 Management

The multidisciplinary team planned for close surveillance of the left gonad, which was kept in the scrotum, allowing easy examination. A pelvic MRI confirmed the presence of a normal prostate and seminal vesicles with no signs of tumor development in the left gonad.

Treatment with escalating doses of testosterone was started immediately after right gonadectomy. Testosterone, FSH, and LH levels were monitored every 6 months. Careful surveillance of the gonad was done by regular clinical and ultrasound evaluation. Left gonadectomy was postponed until the age of 15 to allow the possibility of fertility preservation.

43.3 Outcome

Under testosterone treatment, the penis size increased and the patient developed normal secondary sexual characteristics, reporting occasional erections. Mild gynecomastia was observed but resolved during testosterone treatment. The psychological development was also continuously monitored by the DSD team psychologist.

Following a close discussion with the family and adolescent, plans were made for the removal of the left gonad, bilateral prosthesis placement, and gonadal tissue cryopreservation at the age of 15 years.

After left gonadectomy, the organ was sent to the laboratory and the external fibrous tissue was cut. Tubular structures were macerated to see if any motile sperm cells were identified. Once motile sperm were observed, the tissue was then rinsed in a sperm-washing medium (Origio, Måløv, Denmark) and centrifuged to obtain the pellet. The sperm cells were cryopreserved using Sperm CryoProtec™ (Nidacon, Mölndal, Sweden) in accordance with the manufacturer instructions, with a standard program (equilibration at nitrogen vapor for 30 min and immersion in liquid nitrogen for storage).

The remaining tissue, corresponding to testicular tissue, was cryopreserved according to our slow-freezing protocol. The tissue was equilibrated in sterile phosphate-buffered saline (Gibco, Thermo Fisher Scientific, Paisley, Scotland, United Kingdom) with 1.5 M ethylene glycol (Sigma-Aldrich, St. Louis, USA), 10 mg/ml human serum albumin (CSL Behring, Marburg, Germany), and 0.1 M sucrose (Merck, Darmstadt, Germany) in cryopreservation tubes. Samples were frozen in a programmable freezer (CryoGenesis 5) with the following program: 2 °C/min to −9 °C; manual seeding at −9 °C; −9 to −40 °C at −0.3 °C/min; and −40 to −140 °C at −10 °C/min. Finally, the tubes were stored in liquid nitrogen.

The histological examination of the remaining tissue confirmed the presence of hypospermatogenesis and rare Leydig cells in the testicular parenchyma and a left epididymis and vas deferens.

Despite the late diagnosis of OT-DSD, this patient was able to successfully undergo normal sexual development, avoid the development of malignancy, and cryopreserve mobile sperm cells for future use.

Clinical Pearls and Pitfalls

- DSD are rare conditions that should be suspected and investigated in a timely manner. Karyotype is a mandatory part of the evaluation.
- Cryptorchidism should be corrected in early childhood in order to preserve the normal testicular environment and function.
- The presence of Y chromosome material in a patient with a DSD increases the risk of malignancy and should be addressed.
- Endocrine evaluation and treatment must be initiated in order to achieve an adequate pubertal development.
- Fertility potential should be discussed by a multidisciplinary team when addressing gender assignment and surgical management. Fertility preservation must be considered in every patient and efforts made to cryopreserve germinal tissue and/or gametes.

Review Questions and Answers

Q1. How can a 46,XY/46,XX karyotype arise?

A1. The presence of these two different cell lines (46,XY and 46,XX) in the same individual may arise from the early fusion of two different embryos (chimerism) or from a 47,XXY embryo that undergoes loss of a Y and an X chromosome in different mitosis, retaining only normal 46,XX and 46,XY cell lines.

Q2. What are the appropriate first steps of management once a child is diagnosed with abnormal external genitalia?

A2. The child should be evaluated by a multidisciplinary team as soon as possible in order to diagnose the type of DSD disorder. After a comprehensive evaluation (including a karyotype and examination of pelvic structures), the possible therapeutic options are discussed with the child and the parents.

Q3. Why should cryptorchidism be corrected in early childhood?

A3. Cryptorchidism must be diagnosed and corrected in early childhood in order to protect the fertility potential of the ectopic testis and to prevent the development of testicular tumors.

Q4. Why is fertility preservation an important issue in children with DSD?

A4. DSD patients may need surgery for removal of ectopic gonads in order to prevent tumor development and/or prolonged treatment with hormones to ensure secondary sexual characters develop adequately. As both these interventions have the potential to negatively impact fertility, a discussion of fertility preservation is essential. Gonadal tissue may be cryopreserved for future use.

References

1. Hughes IA, et al. Consensus statement on management of intersex disorders. Arch Dis Child. 2006;91:554–63.
2. Pleskacova J, et al. Tumor risk in disorders of sex development. Sex Dev. 2010;4:259–69.
3. Futoshi M, et al. Long-term outcome of ovotesticular disorder of sex development: a single center experience. Int J Urol. 2011;18:231–6.

Case Presentation: Adoption in the Cancer Setting

Adam S. DuVall, Jessica R. Gorman, and Brandon Hayes-Lattin

T. K. Woodruff et al. (eds.), *Textbook of Oncofertility Research and Practice*,
https://doi.org/10.1007/978-3-030-02868-8_44

Case Presentation

A 30-year-old woman presented to a referring hospital emergency room with abdominal pain and vaginal bleeding. She worked as a musician and had limited financial security but had medical insurance. Ultrasound was performed, demonstrating lobulated, bilateral ovarian masses with concern for ovarian torsion. Emergency surgery was performed to relieve ovarian torsion, and pathology revealed endometrioid adenocarcinoma of the right ovary and mixed clear-cell and endometrioid carcinoma. Unfortunately, the patient had a complicated postoperative course that included wound dehiscence and infection, delaying further cancer-directed therapy. She required a prolonged hospital stay, including prolonged antibiotics, a wound vac, and eventual discharge to a skilled nursing facility (SNF). She has limited social support, with a sister living locally whom she stayed with after recovering in the SNF. She was in a relationship, but it ended shortly after cancer diagnosis. Following recovery, she was referred to gynecologic oncology for further management where it was recommended she undergo three cycles of neoadjuvant chemotherapy with carboplatin and paclitaxel followed by interval staging/debulking surgery and then an additional three cycles of adjuvant chemotherapy.

44.1 Assessment and Diagnosis

This young woman had an emergent presentation of newly diagnosed bilateral ovarian cancer with ovarian torsion. Her cancer-directed therapy was delayed due to postoperative complications, and it wasn't until after this resolved that she was evaluated by a gynecologic oncologist. At that point, neoadjuvant chemotherapy was recommended because she was deemed to be a poor surgical candidate. Chemotherapy prior to staging/debulking surgery is only recommended in the setting when it is determined that a complete cytoreduction is not likely or if the patient is not a good surgical candidate [1]. Fertility preservation in this setting would be very difficult, but the impact on fertility and any feasible options for fertility preservation should be addressed by the oncologist as this is still meaningful to an adolescent and young adult (AYA) patient [2, 3].

Options such as fertility-sparing surgery and oocyte or embryo cryopreservation have been reported in women with low malignant potential ovarian cancer and are controversial in the setting of more aggressive ovarian cancers [4, 5]. However, this young woman's presentation prevented fertility preservation from being performed. She has already had cancer-directed therapy delayed so it was not advisable to necessarily delay therapy further. She was having neoadjuvant chemotherapy due to a poor performance status, but if surgery were performed prior to chemotherapy, it would have been potentially possible to preserve oocytes during the surgery. Unfortunately, fertility preservation including oocyte freezing and storage is expensive, and our patient had limited financial resources. For all of these reasons, fertility preservation was not offered to this patient by her initial treatment team. Adoption would be the most realistic family-building option for this patient and should be addressed when appropriate depending on her level of interest and clinical course.

44.2 Management

This young woman was able to start cancer-directed therapy approximately 3 months after initial diagnosis. She received three cycles of carboplatin and paclitaxel as planned but was not of a functional status to tolerate surgery at that time. She then received an additional cycle of carboplatin as a single agent in order to allow her to have better clinical recovery while still receiving some cancer-directed therapy. Approximately 6 months after diagnosis, she underwent a staging/debulking surgery that included a total abdominal hysterectomy with bilateral salpingo-oophorectomy, bilateral pelvic lymph node dissection, and infracolic omentectomy, and pathology was without residual carcinoma. Unfortunately, her postoperative course was again complicated; wound dehiscence and delayed wound healing required a second wound vac placement and further time rehabilitating in a SNF. Due to her poor performance status and negative pathology, she was recommended not to have any further chemotherapy. Throughout this process, she lost her job and income but was able to maintain her healthcare coverage through state-sponsored programs. Following this difficult recovery, she had more psychosocial difficulties and moved home to live with her mother and established care in an AYA-focused oncology program.

This complicated case, both medically and psychosocially, is not uncommon for an AYA with cancer. It also illustrates some of the difficulties that cancer survivors who have become infertile as a result of their cancer and therapy could have when considering building a family. Fortunately, this patient was able to achieve a complete remission from her cancer and remain cancer-free for 3 years. Through many months of physical rehabilitation, in addition to rigorous work with a mental health professional, she was able to regain functional status. Her social support stabilized, and she established a relationship with a partner who was interested in adopting children. Even with this improvement, this young woman experienced some of the system-level barriers to adoption that many cancer survivors face. Many adoption agencies require individuals to be cancer free for 5 years, which this patient has not yet attained. The adoption agency required a physician's evaluation attesting to her overall health, which could influence the adoption agency's decision to approve her application and/or birth mothers' decisions in selecting the adoptive parents [6]. Finally, this patient was financially devastated by her inability to work and the cost of medical therapies although she was able to maintain health insurance which not all AYAs are able to do. Adoption can still be very costly, which can be very challenging for cancer survivors and their families.

On presentation to the AYA oncology program, the patient and her partner had not received any information on their family-building options previously but wished to pursue adoption. While cancer care providers are increasingly addressing fertility issues with their AYA patients, fertility preservation and alternative family building options are not universally discussed [7–9]. Despite the potential obstacles, it is not uncommon for cancer survivors to consider adoption. The vast majority of survivors have at least one concern about the adoption process, which their healthcare teams can begin to address by providing information and resources [10].

44.3 Outcome

The patient was diagnosed with bilateral ovarian carcinoma and had a complicated course though was able to complete four cycles of neoadjuvant chemotherapy with a successful staging/debulking surgery that demonstrated a complete remission. She remained in remission for at least 3 years after completing therapy and was able to recover medically, financially, and, eventually, psychosocially. She and her partner are pursuing adoption but will still have to overcome multiple barriers to be successful at this approach to family-building. They will require ongoing support from not only their social group but also from their medical community to be successful.

Clinical Pearls and Pitfalls

- Infertility can result from cancer and cancer-directed therapy, despite all planned interventions to preserve it.
- For some individuals, adoption can be the right option for family-building.
- There remain significant barriers for cancer survivors that will need to be addressed. These obstacles are system-based, financially based, and related to the underlying, complicated nature of young peoples' journey through cancer diagnosis, treatment, and eventual survival and return to "normalcy."

Review Questions and Answers

Q1. Name one concern that cancer survivors have expressed about adoption.

(a) Cost
(b) Lack of information
(c) Worry about not being perceived as a good candidate
(d) Personal health concerns about raising a child
(e) Preference for a biological child
(f) Possible legal problems
(g) Time and effort to adopt
(h) All of the above

A1. (h)

Q2. Yes or no? Are adoption processes and regulations consistent across agencies, states, and nations?

A2. No

Q3. Yes or no? Must all cancer survivors undertake an extensive home study process before pursuing adoption?

A3. Yes

Q4. Name one resource relevant to cancer survivors interested in finding out more about adoption?

(a) American Society of Reproductive Medicine
(b) Oncofertility Consortium
(c) Fertile Action
(d) The National Infertility Association
(e) Academy of Adoption and Assisted Reproduction Attorneys
(f) All of the above

A4. (f)

References

1. Wright AA, Bohlke K, Armstrong DK, et al. Neoadjuvant chemotherapy for newly diagnosed, advanced ovarian cancer: Society of Gynecologic Oncology and American Society of Clinical Oncology Clinical Practice Guideline. Gynecol Oncol. 2016;143(1):3–15.
2. Nass SJ, Beaupin LK, Demark-Wahnefried W, et al. Identifying and addressing the needs of adolescents and young adults with cancer: summary of an Institute of Medicine workshop. Oncologist. 2015;20(2):186–95.
3. Rechis R, Bann C, Arvery S, et al. Unique risks & vulnerabilities of AYA patients across the lifespan, LIVESTRONG Foundation: AYA Survey Results. Presented at Institute of Medicine National Cancer Policy Forum/LIVESTRONG Workshop on Addressing the Needs of Adolescents and Young Adults with Cancer, Washington, DC. 2013.
4. von Wolff M, Bruckner T, et al. Fertility preservation: ovarian response to freeze oocytes is not affected by different malignant diseases-an analysis of 992 stimulations. J Assist Reprod Genet. 2018;35:1713–9; Epub ahead of print.
5. Ito A, Katagiri Y, et al. Ultrasound-guided laparotomic oocyte retrieval during surgery for fertility preservation in a case of tumor recurrence after a unilateral salpingo-oophorectomy. Reprod Med Biol. 2018; 17:98–102.
6. Quinn GP, Zebrack BJ, Sehovic I, Bowman ML, Vadaparampil ST. Adoption and cancer survivors: findings from a learning activity for oncology nurses. Cancer. 2015;121(17):2993–3000.
7. Banerjee R, Tsiapali E. Occurrence and recall rates of fertility discussions with young breast cancer patients. Support Care Cancer. 2016;24:163–71.
8. Wong AWK, Chang T, Christopher K, Lau SCL, Beaupin LK, Love B, Lipsey KL, Feurstein M. Patterns of unmet needs in adolescent and young adult (AYA) cancer survivors: in their own words. J Cancer Surviv. 2017; 11:751–64.
9. Quinn GP, Block RG, Clayman ML, Kelvin J, Arvey SR, Lee J, et al. If you did not document 17 it, it did not happen: rates of documentation of discussion of infertility risk in adolescent and 18 young adult oncology patients' medical records. J Oncol Pract. 2015;11: 137–44.
10. Gorman JR, Whitcomb BW, et al. Adoption consideration and concerns among young adult female cancer survivors. J Cancer Surviv. 2017;11(1):149–57.

Case Studies: Embryo Banking

Contents

In Vitro Activation Following Ovarian Tissue Cryopreservation: A Case of Patient with POI

Hideyuki Iwahata, Seido Takae, Kazuhiro Kawamura, and Nao Suzuki

T. K. Woodruff et al. (eds.), *Textbook of Oncofertility Research and Practice*,
https://doi.org/10.1007/978-3-030-02868-8_45

45

Case Presentation

A 27-year-old nulligravid woman with primary ovarian insufficiency (POI) underwent menarche at age 11 and had a history of irregular menses followed by 4 years of secondary amenorrhea. Her past medical history was unremarkable, and she had no family history of POI. Laboratory testing revealed elevated serum levels of luteinizing hormone (LH) 33.4 mIU/mL (menopause: 6.7–38.0 mIU/mL) and follicle-stimulating hormone (FSH) 84.5 mIU/mL (menopause: 26.2–113.3 mIU/mL). Due to symptoms of hot flushes, she received therapy with estrogen and progesterone. An oocyte retrieval had been attempted since spontaneous follicle growth was observed, but no oocyte was obtained.

The patient was referred to our hospital for infertility treatment. At the time of presentation, physical examination was normal. Transvaginal ultrasonography (TVUS) was only notable for a 6.5 × 6.0 cm serous right ovarian cyst. No antral follicles were visible in either ovary. Laboratory findings while on estrogen replacement were notable for normal serum estradiol (E2) of 59.1 pg/mL (menopause: <10 pg/mL), elevated LH of 28.5 mIU/mL and FSH of 51.69 mIU/mL, and diminished AMH of 4.9 pM. No chromosomal aberrations were detected.

45.1 Assessment and Diagnosis

Oocytes are derived from primordial follicles created during fetal life. Approximately one million primordial follicles exist at birth [1], and the number subsequently decreases with age. When the number of remaining primordial follicles reaches approximately 1000, periodic follicular activation and recruitment are arrested, resulting in dormant status. Due to the lack of estradiol production from granulosa cells in developing follicles, endometrial cells do not proliferate, leading to amenorrhea and eventual menopause.

Primary ovarian insufficiency (POI) results from pathophysiologic follicular depletion before 40 years of age, either due to a more rapid decline of the number of follicles or to a more limited number of residual follicles at birth. The incidence of POI is approximately 1% [2]. Although more than 50% of POI cases are idiopathic, identifiable causes include chromosomal/genomic abnormalities, autoimmune diseases, ovarian surgery, and gonadotoxic cancer treatment such as chemotherapy and radiation [2]. POI following cancer treatment strongly affects the fertility and QOL of cancer survivors.

Although IVF using donated oocytes remains the most effective fertility treatment for POI, legal, financial, and religious restrictions can limit its utilization [3]. As a result, developing infertility treatment options using autologous oocytes in women with POI remains a research priority. We recently developed a new method for artificial activation of dormant primordial follicles using an in vitro culture of cryopreserved ovarian cortical tissues (IVA: in vitro activation) [4, 5]. We have shown the importance of PI3K-Akt-Foxo3 signaling in the activation of dormant primordial follicles and succeeded in the short-term activation of dormant follicles using a PTEN inhibitor and PI3K activator in both mice and humans [4, 5].

A loss of the tumor suppressor gene PTEN and the activation of PI3K/Akt pathway could accelerate tumorgenesis and the development of malignancy [6]. Because the activation of transient PI3K/Akt signaling is a physiological event, short-term treatment with PTEN inhibitors and PI3K activators are unlikely to induce tumorgenesis in cancer patients. Although we demonstrated no tumorgenesis in non-cancer animals and POI patients, IVA should not be used in cancer patients until its safety can be confirmed.

Currently, two methods for cryopreserving biological tissue are available: slow freezing and vitrification. Although vitrification is frequently used to cryopreserve human embryos and oocytes, slow freezing remains the current standard for ovarian tissue cryopreservation (OTC). However, vitification offers several advantages over slow freezing for OTC, including higher efficiency and prevention of ice crystal formation [7] and DNA damage in primordial follicles, thus preserving the morphologic integrity of ovarian stroma [8].

45.2 Management

A unilateral laparoscopic oophorectomy was performed for IVA treatment. The serous ovarian cyst seen on preoperative ultrasound was found to be a para-ovarian cyst and removed at the time of surgery. After the removal of the ovary, the ovarian cortex was dissected from the underlying medulla and cryopreserved using vitrification [7]. Three months later, the ovarian tissue was thawed [7], cut into 1–2 mm slices, and cultured with PTEN inhibitor and/or PI3K activator for 48 hours. After culture, we laparoscopically grafted the ovarian tissue beneath the serosa of the fallopian tubes. After transplantation, hormonal testing and transvaginal ultrasonography were performed to assess for follicle development. We found spontaneous follicle growth after IVA treatment and IVF was performed. Retrieved oocytes were fertilized with the husbands' sperm, and day 3 embryos [9] were successfully vitrified. Once three embryos had been frozen, a frozen cycle with transfer of the two most favorable embryos was performed.

45.3 Outcome

Laboratory results revealed a serum human chorionic gonadotropin (HCG) level of 2814.0 mIU/mL and a sonographically visible fetus 3 weeks after the embryo transfer. There were no complications during pregnancy, and a baby boy (birth weight 3254 g; Apgar scores, 9 at 1 min and 10 at 5 min) was delivered at 37 weeks and 2 days by cesarean section due to breech presentation. No visible abnormality was identified at the site of ovarian autografting at the time of cesarean section. The child, who is 5-years old at the time of writing, has experienced normal development to date. The mother has had no abnormalities in her gynecological care to date.

Box 45.1 shows the Edinburgh selection criteria.

Box 45.1 Edinburgh Selection Criteria (Reference: [10])

- <35 years of age
- No previous chemotherapy or radiotherapy if aged >15 years at diagnosis, but mild or non-gonadotoxic chemotherapy acceptable if <15 years
- A realistic chance of surviving for more than 5 years
- A high risk of POI (>50%)
- Informed consent (from parents and, where possible, patient)
- Negative serology results for HIV, syphilis, and hepatitis B
- Not pregnant and no existing children

Clinical Pearls and Pitfalls

- POI occurs in about 1% of all women.
- The causes of POI include chromosomal/genomic abnormalities, autoimmune disease, ovarian surgery, and chemotherapy and radiation.
- POI after cancer treatment strongly declines the QOL of cancer survivors.

Review Question and Answers

Q1. What are some identifiable causes of POI?

A1. Identifiable causes of POI include chromosome/gene abnormalities, autoimmune diseases, ovarian surgery, and chemotherapy and radiation for cancer treatment.

Q2. Should artificial activation of dormant primordial follicles using PTEN inhibitors and PI3K activators be used in cancer patients?

A2. A loss of the tumor suppressor gene PTEN and the activation of PI3K/Akt pathway could accelerate tumorgenesis and the development of malignancy. Because the activation of transient PI3K/Akt signaling is a physiological event, short-term treatment with PTEN inhibitors and PI3K activators are unlikely to induce tumorgenesis in cancer patients. Although we demonstrated no tumorgenesis in non-cancer animals and POI patients, IVA should not be used in cancer patients until its safety can be confirmed.

References

1. Broekmans FJ, Kwee J, Hendriks DJ, et al. A systematic review of tests predicting ovarian reserve and IVF outcome. Hum Reprod Updat. 2006;12(6):685–718.
2. Webber L, Davies M, Anderson R, et al. ESHRE guideline: management of women with premature ovarian insufficiency. Hum Reprod. 2016;31(5):926–37.
3. Rashedi AS, Roo SFD, Ataman LM, et al. Survey of third-party parenting options associated with fertility preservation available to patients with cancer around the globe. J Global Oncol. 2018;(4):1–7.

4. Suzuki N, Yoshioka N, Takae S, et al. Successful fertility preservation following ovarian tissue vitrification in patients with primary ovarian insufficiency. Hum Reprod. 2015;30(3):608–15.
5. Kawamura K, Cheng Y, Suzuki N, et al. Hippo signaling disruption and Akt stimulation of ovarian follicles for infertility treatment. Proc Natl Acad Sci. 2013;110(43):17474–9.
6. Carnero A, Paramio JM. The PTEN/PI3K/AKT pathway in vivo, cancer mouse models. Front Oncol. 2014; 4:252.
7. Hashimoto S, Suzuki N, Yamanaka M, et al. Effects of vitrification solutions and equilibration times on the morphology of cynomolgus ovarian tissues. Reprod Biomed Online. 2010;21(4):501–9.
8. Shi Q, Xie Y, Wang Y, et al. Vitrification versus slow freezing for human ovarian tissue cryopreservation: a systematic review and meta-anlaysis. Scientific reports. 2017;7(1):8538.
9. Dennis SJ, Thomas MA, Williams DB, et al. Embryo morphology score on day 3 is predictive of implantation and live birth rates. J Assist Reprod Genet. 2006;23(4):171–5.
10. Wallace WHB, Smith AG, Kelsey TW, et al. Fertility preservation for girls and young women with cancer: population-based validation of criteria for ovarian tissue cryopreservation. The Lancet Oncology. 2014;15(10): 1129–36.

Fertility Preservation in Young Women with Breast Cancer: A Case Study

Marouen Braham, Sarah Amari, Hammouda Boussen, Mohamed Khrouf, and Fethi Zhioua

T. K. Woodruff et al. (eds.), *Textbook of Oncofertility Research and Practice*,
https://doi.org/10.1007/978-3-030-02868-8_46

Case Presentation

KG is a 31-year-old engineer, married for the past 4 years, with no children so far. In her family history, her mother was diagnosed with breast cancer and treated at age 45 and passed away at age 55, after a relapse. Her aunt is alive and survived breast cancer.

As for KG, her menarche was at 12, her menstrual cycles are regular, but she suffers from chronic pelvic pain and dysmenorrhea. In 2014, she underwent laparoscopic ovarian cystectomy and was diagnosed with stage IV endometriosis (AFS score) with many intra-abdominal adhesions. Later on that same year, she had an intrauterine insemination and then an in vitro fertilization procedure, without pregnancy.

The patient consulted on July 7, 2017, for a right breast lump represented on magnetic resonance imaging by an 18 mm right breast nodule. Work-up was normal (total body CT scan and bone scintigraphy). Physical exam was normal, excluding the presence of the right breast nodule. A conservative surgery by lumpectomy plus axillary node dissection was performed on July 13. Histology revealed a 19 mm lesion, invasive ductal carcinoma grade 2, negative HER2/neu, Ki 67 at 19%, and negative axillary dissection (17 N-).

She was planned to have adjuvant chemotherapy (fluorouracil-epirubicin-cyclophosphamide every 21 days for 3 times, after paclitaxel 80 mg/m^2 every week for 12 times).

Before chemotherapy, the patient was directly referred to our oncofertility preservation consult.

46.1 Assessment and Diagnosis

The goals of oncofertility were explained to the patient. Serum anti-Mullerian hormone (AMH) testing performed that same day was 0.8 ng/ml, showing a decreased ovarian reserve for her age. Transvaginal ultrasound showed a corpus luteum on the right ovary and an antral follicular count of four on the left ovary with a 2 cm endometrioma.

The endometriosis and the cystectomy for the endometrioma probably decreased the ovarian reserve of our patient [1]. In addition to that, a decreased AMH level in patients with breast cancer is reported in many articles [2]. Indeed, before even commencing chemotherapy or radiotherapy, oncology patients at the margins of reproductive age show a diminished ovarian reserve compared with the control group. A general catabolic state could explain the decline in ovarian reserve.

Furthermore, it has been demonstrated that a low level of AMH before chemotherapy is associated with an important risk of premature ovarian failure after. AMH rapidly decreases in women receiving chemotherapy for breast cancer [3].

46.2 Management

In this case, the patient is a 31-year-old woman with documented infertility for over 4 years, diagnosed with advanced endometriosis and decreased ovarian reserve. Endometriosis is well known to alter fertility and ovarian function [1]. The damage of endometriosis on ovarian reserve, leading to a form of incipient ovarian failure has been demonstrated and is considered as an early sign of advanced ovarian depletion in young women. AMH can be used to follow ovarian reserve in patients with endometriosis [1]. Furthermore, the planned chemotherapy protocol is potentially gonadotoxic. So, the risk of ovarian function loss is considered to be very high in this case.

Considering all these parameters, the patient was advised to proceed to urgent fertility preservation. Fertility preservation for gonadotoxicity of antineoplastic therapies represents an important aspect of the quality of life of cancer survivors [4]. Oocyte/embryo vitrification is the gold standard of fertility preservation [4].

Oocyte vitrification is the standard method according to guidelines [4]. It requires ovarian stimulation with gonadotrophins, which will delay the chemotherapy for 12–15 days. Fertility preservation via banking of oocytes or embryos after controlled ovarian stimulation can increase the likelihood of a future live birth. It has been hypothesized that elevated serum estradiol levels during ovarian stimulation may induce breast tumor growth. This has led to the use of tamoxifen (anti-estrogen) or letrozole (aromatase inhibitor) to keep the estradiol level as low as possible [5].

Initially our patient preferred tissue cryopreservation (OTC). Many teams prefer this technique, though still considered to be experimental. It has been proven that OCT is an effective method that can restore both fertility and endocrine function [4]. It requires a laparoscopy and allows for chemotherapy to start the following day. Given her personal history of advanced endometriosis, the high operative risks, and her decreased ovarian reserve, she decided not to purse ovarian tissue cryopreservation and was interested in oocyte or embryo banking. She and her partner decided to proceed with embryo banking. In order to shorten the delay for chemotherapy, she started controlled ovarian stimulation with a random start protocol initiated in the luteal phase with letrozole.

46.3 Outcomes

We started ovarian stimulation with 300 IU per day of menotropins and planned for an antagonist protocol with a GnRH agonist trigger for oocyte maturation. This protocol is safe and allows maximal follicular development while minimizing the risk of ovarian hyperstimulation syndrome. Letrozole (5 mg per day) was prescribed at the start of stimulation to reduce estradiol exposure [5].

By day 8 of stimulation, six follicles >17 mm were obtained with an estradiol level at 390 pg/ml. Ovulation was triggered day 9. Oocyte pickup was performed transvaginally. Eight oocytes were retrieved, seven of which were mature; a total of five day 3 embryos were vitrified. She continued letrozole for 7 days after oocyte pickup to reduce luteal estradiol exposure.

No complications occurred, and the patient was referred the day after oocyte pickup to start her chemotherapy.

Table 46.1 shows ovarian stimulation monitoring.

Clinical Pearls and Pitfalls

- Reproductive age women with breast cancer who are interested in future fertility should be referred to a qualified oncofertility team.
- Ovarian reserve evaluation is based on age, AMH levels, and antral follicular final point.
- The ovarian reserve may be reduced by endometriosis and ovarian surgery.
- Ovarian tissue cryopreservation should not be advised in a case with high operative risk.
- Oocyte and embryo vitrification are the preferred fertility preservation options.
- Random start protocols facilitate oocyte and embryo vitrification and minimize the delay in chemotherapy start.
- Aromatase inhibitors can be initiated during stimulation in women with hormone receptor-positive tumors and continued post oocyte pickup to minimize the exposure to estradiol.

Table 46.1 Ovarian stimulation monitoring

	D1	D2	D3	D4	D5	D6	D7	D8	D9	D10
HMG (UI)	300	300	300	300	300	300	300			Oocytes pickup
Gn-RH anta						0.5 mg	0.5 mg			
Gn-RH agonist								0.2 mg		
Letrozole 2.5 mg	2 pills	2 pills	2 pills	2 pills	2 pills	2 pills	2 pills	2 pills	2 pills	2 pills/day until 7 days after pickup
E2 (pg/ml)						279		390		
Right ovary[a]						15 12 11–10		19 2×18 14		
Left ovary[a]						3×12 2×11 10		3×17 12 11–10		

Gn-RH anta: GN-RH antagonist
[a]Follicles size are expressed in mm

46

Review Questions and Answers

Q1. Which parameters are used to evaluate ovarian reserve in patients interested in fertility preservation?

A1. Age, AMH, antral follicular count, and past medical and surgical history.

Q2. Which fertility preservation techniques are used in breast cancer patients?

A2. Oocyte vitrification, embryo vitrification, and, possibly, ovarian tissue cryopreservation.

Q3. Which stimulation protocol is suitable in the case of breast cancer patients with hormone receptor-positive cancer?

A3. Random start protocol with aromatase inhibitors.

Q4. How do aromatase inhibitors act (AIs)?

A4. AIs inhibit aromatase, the enzyme that converts androgens into estrogens.

References

1. Pacchiarotti A, Frati P, Milazzo GN, et al. Evaluation of serum antimullerian hormone levels to assess the ovarian reserve in women with severe endometriosis. Eur J Obstet Gynecol Reprod Biol. 2014;172:62–4.
2. Dezellus A, Barriere P, Campone M, et al. Prospective evaluation of serum anti-Müllerian hormone dynamics in 250 women of reproductive age treated with chemotherapy for breast cancer. Eur J Cancer. 2017; 79:72–80.
3. Naasan M, Harrity C, Rajab Hetbal H, et al. Patients with cancer at the margins of reproductive age had reduced levels of anti Müllerian hormone compared with patients experiencing infertility. Int J Gynaecol Obstet. 2016;133(2):226–9.
4. Medrano JV, Andrés MDM, García S, et al. Basic and clinical approaches for fertility preservation and restoration in cancer patients. Trends Biotechnol. 2018; 36(2):199–215.
5. Dahhan T, Balkenende EME, Beerendonk CCM, et al. Stimulation of the ovaries in women with breast cancer undergoing fertility preservation: alternative versus standard stimulation protocol/the STM trial. Contemp Clin Trials. 2017;61:96–100.

Childhood Cancer: Secondary Malignancy and Fertility Implications

Karen E. Kinahan

T. K. Woodruff et al. (eds.), *Textbook of Oncofertility Research and Practice*,
https://doi.org/10.1007/978-3-030-02868-8_47

47

Case Presentation

The patient is a 37-year-old Caucasian female with a history of stage IV Hodgkin lymphoma (HL) diagnosed in October 1994, at the age of 13. At diagnosis, she had disease in the left supraclavicular, left axillary, and small paratracheal with metastasis of the lumbar spine at L4. Her chemotherapy regimen consisted of COPP/ABV including Cyclophosphamide (4 g/m^2), Oncovorin, Procarbazine (42 g/m^2), and Prednisone, alternating with Adriamycin (210 mg/m^2), Bleomycin, and Velban. Her total anthracycline dose was 210 mg/m^2. She received consolidation radiotherapy of 15 Gy to the mantle field, ending in May 1995. She did not have the opportunity to harvest eggs prior to her cancer treatment as that was not common practice at that time. Her HL remained in a complete remission, and she reached normal adolescent milestones, attended and graduated college, and worked in public health.

47.1 Assessment and Diagnosis

When the patient turned 23, she transitioned her cancer care from a pediatric hospital to a long-term, follow-up program specializing in adult survivors of childhood cancer in an academic medical center. Her care consisted of general medical care, along with follow-up recommendations from the Children's Oncology Group (COG) Long-Term Follow-Up Guidelines for Survivors of Childhood, Adolescent, and Young Adult Cancers found at ▶ http://www.survivorshipguidelines.org [1]. Her team of providers included a primary care physician, an advanced practice nurse with pediatric oncology expertise, and a clinical psychologist. She established care with a gynecologist and had access to specialty providers as needed. Her plan of care included echocardiograms every 2 years (due to a history of anthracycline chemotherapy and mantle radiation) and annual labs including a complete blood count, comprehensive chemistry panel, and thyroid function tests (due to the history of mantle radiation) [2, 3]. At that time, recommendations for breast cancer screening included initiating screening mammograms starting at age 25 years, which the patient had done in 2006. In 2007, the American Cancer Society changed their breast cancer guidelines for high-risk individuals (including those treated with chest radiation) to include annual adjunct bilateral breast MRI [4]. This recommendation was adopted by the COG guidelines. In September 2007, she presented for her baseline screening breast MRI. While no abnormalities were identified in the left breast, the right breast demonstrated an indeterminate 5 mm circumscribed focus in the mid-third central breast as well as a 7 mm area of enhancement in the upper outer aspect of the right breast. Mammography and second-look ultrasound demonstrated no definite mammographic or sonographic correlate to these findings, and a 6-month MRI follow-up was recommended. This was done as directed in May 2008 and showed a stable 5 mm enhancing mass in the mid-third central right breast. Around the same time, she had an abnormal Pap smear, and a LEEP procedure showed mild squamous dysplasia (CIN1) [5].

In April 2009, at age 28, the patient's breast MRI revealed a new 3 cm speculated enhancing mass in the right breast and enlarged, abnormal-appearing, right axillary lymph node and a new 6 mm mass in the left breast. An ultrasound-guided core biopsy of the right breast and right axillary lymph node was performed and was positive for invasive ductal carcinoma grade 3 (3 + 3 + 3), 0.7 cm in maximum dimension (no in situ component identified), and a 2.6 cm mass of the right axilla (ER/PR positive, HER2 negative) with a minute fragment of metastatic adenocarcinoma (less than 0.1 cm) in lymphoid tissue. She met with multiple breast cancer surgeons and decided to undergo bilateral mastectomies. A right modified radical mastectomy confirmed infiltrating poorly differentiated ductal carcinoma with associated lymphoid infiltrate, grade 3 (3 + 3 + 3) of 3, measuring 2.5 cm in greatest dimension. Additionally, ductal carcinoma in situ (DCIS), nuclear grade 3, solid type with comedo necrosis and microcalcifications, minor component. Her surgical resection margins were negative for carcinoma as were her skin and nipple.

She did have metastatic carcinoma in one of four lymph nodes, with extranodal extension, metastatic deposit measured at least 2.3 cm. Her right axillary lymph node dissection revealed metastatic carcinoma in one of five lymph nodes (T2 N1 ER+). Lymphovascular invasion was present with two of nine positive nodes (2.5 cm in greatest dimension) (pT2 N1a M0) overall stage IIB breast cancer [6, 7]. The patient also had a left simple mastectomy the same day with no evidence of malignancy. She opted for breast reconstruction and began this process at the same time.

47.2 Management

Prior to starting chemotherapy in July 2009, the fertility navigator was contacted, and the patient saw a reproductive endocrine specialist. She underwent controlled ovarian hyperstimulation and had five embryos frozen. She was engaged to be married at that time. Adjuvant chemotherapy consisted of Cyclophosphamide (600 mg/m^2) and Taxotere (75 mg/m^2) every 3 weeks for four cycles. She was admitted to the hospital after cycle one with neutropenic fever and bone pain. She received Neulasta with the following cycles. This was followed by 6 weeks of right chest wall radiation, with a total dose of 61 Gy ending December 2009. Near the same time, the selective estrogen receptor modulator (SERM), Tamoxifen, was prescribed by her medical oncologist, and the patient was told to wait 2 years to attempt pregnancy. In May 2011, the patient reported that she temporarily stopped taking the medication due to vulvar fissures and vulvar pain. She developed ovarian cysts and an endometrial polyp, which was treated with a hysteroscopy with polypectomy. Additionally, in 2011, she was diagnosed with hypothyroidism and began treatment with Levothyroxine Sodium.

In January 2012, her Tamoxifen was temporarily discontinued by her medical oncologist because she wanted to attempt pregnancy. She and her husband met with her reproductive endocrinologist and had eight cycles of in vitro fertilization (IVF) without success (two SABs) over a 2-year period of time (five fresh cycles and three frozen transfers). At that time, she used all five of her frozen embryos. Her medical oncologist was concerned about her being off of Tamoxifen during this time and discussed options of donor egg IVF, donor egg with a gestational carrier, and autologous IVF with a gestational carrier. The patient and her husband also looked into adoption. She and her husband decided to pursue using donor egg IVF. During this time she had frequent visits with the reproductive endocrinologist, who managed her thyroid levels. In April 2014, with her first transfer of two donor embryos, she achieved a viable pregnancy (twins). She was followed by maternal-fetal medicine for the majority of her pregnancy. At 21 weeks gestation, she had a cerclage placed emergently due to a short cervix affecting pregnancy. In November 2014, she delivered twin boys at 30 weeks gestation in the setting of suspected chorioamnionitis and fetal tachycardia. The twins were discharged home after 7 weeks in the neonatal intensive care unit.

The patient still had ten frozen donor embryos but was advised against an additional pregnancy, as her medical oncologist recommended that she resume hormone therapy for the next 10 years due to her node-positive disease and break in hormone therapy. She resumed Tamoxifen after the delivery of her twins and Goserelin Acetate (Zoladex) monthly injections were added in May 2015. Tamoxifen was changed to an Aromatase Inhibitor (AI)—Anastrozole—in November 2015, and the patient is tolerating the regimen well with occasional joint pain and mild hot flashes at nighttime [8].

Throughout the time of attempting pregnancy and after the birth of her twins, she frequently discussed the extreme emotional rollercoaster she and her husband experienced. She said that the process of getting pregnant was more difficult emotionally than her first or second cancer experience. She was supported by her family and team and had frequent visits with the reproductive team's psychologist which she felt was instrumental in helping her cope during this trying time [9, 10]. She continued to take her AI but consulted with a fertility navigator to discuss options, given her ten remaining embryos. She reported feeling sad about the idea of not having more children but ultimately decided that she was not willing to risk going off medications for fear of cancer reoccurrence. In addition, the cost of a gestational carrier was a barrier for her and her husband. She reports being thankful for each day, extremely grateful for the birth of her children and the past and ongoing medical surveillance she receives [11, 12].

47

Clinical Pearls/Pitfalls

- Lifelong cancer survivorship care is recommended for childhood, adolescent, and young adult (CAYA) cancer survivors and should include surveillance for secondary cancers and late effects of therapy per survivorship guidelines based on patient age at diagnosis.
- Educating CAYA survivors about potential or actual late effects of treatment is instrumental in assisting them in relaying this information to primary care providers they may see if a comprehensive survivorship program is not available to them.
- If a secondary malignancy is detected, CAYA survivors should be immediately referred to reproductive endocrine to discuss fertility options prior to initiating treatment.
- A multidisciplinary team approach for infertility is recommended including psychosocial support and counseling.

Review Questions and Answers

Q1. A 33-year-old woman with a history of Hodgkin lymphoma at age 15 presents for general care. Which resource would you consult for the treatment-related potential late effects of therapy and surveillance recommendations?
(a) American Cancer Society
(b) ASCO compendium
(c) Children's Oncology Group Long Term Follow-Up Guidelines
(d) All of the above

A1. (d) (but C is also appropriate due to her age at diagnosis)

Q2. A 24-year-old patient treated for acute lymphocytic leukemia at age 19 has a late relapse of her disease. The plan is to treat with a hematopoietic stem cell transplant. Please name the specialists that she should be referred to during this emotional time.
(a) Medical Oncologist
(b) Reproductive Endocrinologist
(c) Psychologist or Social Worker
(d) All of the above

A2. (d)

Q3. Which of the following is/are risk factors for secondary breast cancer?
(a) Anthracycline chemotherapy
(b) Alkylating agent chemotherapy
(c) Mantle radiation
(d) All of the above

A3. (c)

Q4. True or False: Hypothyroidism can occur after cancer treatment with mantle radiation.

A4. True

References

1. Eshelman D, Landier W, Sweeney T, Hester AL, Forte K, Darling J, et al. Facilitating care for childhood cancer survivors: integrating children's oncology group long-term follow-up guidelines and health links in clinical practice. J Pediatr Oncol Nurs. 2004;21(5):271–80. https://doi.org/10.1177/1043454204268875.
2. Kang Y, Cheng L, Li L, Chen H, Sun M, Wei Z, et al. Early detection of anthracycline-induced cardiotoxicity using two-dimensional speckle tracking echocardiography. Cardiol J. 2013;20(6):592–9. https://doi.org/10.5603/cj.2013.0158.
3. Tadic M, Cuspidi C, Hering D, Venneri L, Grozdic-Milojevic I. Radiotherapy-induced right ventricular remodelling: the missing piece of the puzzle. Arch Cardiovasc Dis. 2017;110(2):116–23. https://doi.org/10.1016/j.acvd.2016.10.003.
4. Day D. Breast MRI: opportunities and challenges. Minn Med. 2009;92(12):45–8.
5. Kitchen FL, Cox CM. Papanicolaou smear. StatPearls. Treasure Island: StatPearls Publishing; 2017.
6. Katz A, Brenner B, Sulkes A, Luria H, Marshak G, Fenig E. Breast cancer after mantle field irradiation for Hodgkin's disease. Harefuah. 2000;138(10):823–5, 911.
7. Aisenberg AC, Finkelstein DM, Doppke KP, Koerner FC, Boivin JF, Willett CG. High risk of breast carcinoma after irradiation of young women with Hodgkin's disease. Cancer. 1997;79(6):1203–10.
8. Flaum LE, Gradishar WJ. Advances in endocrine therapy for postmenopausal metastatic breast cancer. Cancer Treat Res. 2018;173:141–54. https://doi.org/10.1007/978-3-319-70197-4_9.

9. Cunningham J. Infertility: a primer for primary care providers. JAAPA: Off J Am Acad Physician Assist. 2017;30(9):19–25. https://doi.org/10.1097/01.JAA.0000522130.01619.b7.
10. Girard E, Galani V, Toma S, Streuli I. Psychological distress and infertile couple: a global approach. Rev Med Suisse. 2017;13(549):371–4.
11. Zebrack BJ, Stuber ML, Meeske KA, Phipps S, Krull KR, Liu Q, et al. Perceived positive impact of cancer among long-term survivors of childhood cancer: a report from the childhood cancer survivor study. Psychooncology. 2012;21(6):630–9. https://doi.org/10.1002/pon.1959.
12. Oeffinger KC, Hudson MM, Landier W. Survivorship: childhood cancer survivors. Prim Care. 2009;36(4):743–80. https://doi.org/10.1016/j.pop.2009.07.007.

Fertility Preservation at an Advanced Reproductive Age: When Hope and Reality Collide

Jacquelyn Shaw and Kara N. Goldman

T. K. Woodruff et al. (eds.), *Textbook of Oncofertility Research and Practice*,
https://doi.org/10.1007/978-3-030-02868-8_48

Case Presentation

A 41-year-old G2P0020 (gravida 2, para 0, abortus 2) female with a history of endometriosis and newly diagnosed stage I estrogen receptor positive, progesterone receptor positive, human epidermal growth factor receptor 2 negative (ER+/PR+/HER2−) breast cancer presented to discuss fertility preservation. The patient was diagnosed with breast cancer 3 months prior to presentation and had undergone a bilateral mastectomy with concurrent reconstruction with tissue expanders. Breast cancer type 1 and 2 susceptibility genes (BRCA1/BRCA2) testing was negative. Her treatment plan included a 10-year tamoxifen course but no requirement for chemotherapy. Her medical oncologist was willing to delay therapy to allow for fertility preservation.

The patient was in a 12-year sexually intimate relationship with a 54-year-old healthy male using a copper intrauterine device (IUD) for contraception. Prior to her breast cancer diagnosis, she had intended to remove her IUD at its 10-year expiration and passively try for pregnancy; she would have been 41 years old. She had a history of two prior spontaneous miscarriages after unplanned pregnancies at age 27 years and 31 years. Her partner had not previously conceived with her or previous partners. Her gynecologic history was notable for irregular menses and surgically confirmed endometriosis requiring two laparoscopic resections for pelvic pain at ages 33 and 40. She was without other major medical problems.

She presented with normal vital signs, a BMI of 21 and a normal physical exam. Pelvic ultrasound was normal. Ovarian reserve testing demonstrated an antral follicle count (AFC) of 9, anti-mullerian hormone (AMH) level of 1.52 ng/mL, day two follicle stimulating hormone (FSH) level of 12.5 mIU/mL, and estradiol of 55 pg/mL. Her partner's semen analysis confirmed a volume of 1.5 mL, count 9 × 106/mL, motility 6%, morphology 3% normal forms. Appropriate screening was performed according to state and federal requirements for a future gestational carrier.

48.1 Assessment and Diagnosis

This 41-year-old patient with breast cancer would be expected to complete her tamoxifen at 51 years of age, the average age of menopause [1]. At the time of her fertility preservation consultation, she was faced with an abrupt loss of fertility from multiple insults: the significant passage of time related to her impending tamoxifen usage, physiologic age-related decline which renders many women infertile at her current age of presentation, and a personal history of endometriosis.

Female fertility declines dramatically in the fourth decade of life due to a decline in ovarian reserve and a concomitant increase in aneuploid embryo formation [2]. Assisted reproductive technologies (ART) do little to overcome age-related fertility decline [2]. Based on national IVF success rates, the likelihood of live birth following IVF is 13.3% in women 41–42 years and 3.9% for women >42 years [3]. Other risk factors such as endometriosis and BRCA1 mutations contribute to a diminished ovarian reserve [4, 5]. While this patient does not have a BRCA mutation, it is often a consideration in patients with breast cancer or those presenting for fertility consultation due to known BRCA mutations.

Patients and providers alike grossly overestimate the likelihood of fertility at advanced reproductive ages and, importantly, overestimate the ability of ART to overcome age-related infertility [6]. The consequence for many is unintended childlessness. This phenomenon is particularly pertinent among patients with a cancer diagnosis presenting for fertility preservation, as these women may not have the time or resources to embark on multiple cycles of ART to overcome age-related diminished ovarian reserve and aneuploidy.

Among 41-year-old women pursuing IVF with preimplantation genetic screening, nearly 70% of embryos are expected to be aneuploid, with this number climbing to over 88% by 44 years [7]. Given the impact of age-related aneuploidy, patients of advanced reproductive age often require multiple IVF cycles to achieve a euploid embryo. Across all age ranges, the rates of no euploid cycles have been reported up to 25%, a rate that is significantly higher in the fifth decade [7]. Patients should be counseled on the possibility of no euploid embryos available for transfer following IVF or, in the case of fertility preservation, no euploid embryos available for cryopreservation. This knowledge is particularly critical in the oncofertility patient who deserves a realistic expectation of the likelihood of future conception with her cryopreserved embryos.

Oncofertility patients may require the use of a gestational carrier (GC), and in this patient's case, it would be warranted because of her anticipated age upon completion of tamoxifen. Given the tremendous cost and effort associated with the use of GC, understanding an embryo's potential prior to beginning the GC process is critical. Preimplantation genetic testing for aneuploidy (PGT-A) can aid in optimal embryo selection for patients utilizing a GC [8]. Understanding the low likelihood of producing a euploid embryo based on her age, this patient elected to undergo PGS to understand the future pregnancy potential of any embryos produced.

48.2 Management

The patient elected to proceed with embryo cryopreservation with preimplantation genetic testing for aneuploidy (PGT-A). She intended to use a gestational carrier during her tamoxifen course or, if safe from an oncology perspective, to pursue pregnancy with her cryopreserved embryo(s) during a tamoxifen holiday. She was carefully counseled regarding age-related aneuploidy rates and the possibility of a negative outcome. A standard antagonist protocol was planned with letrozole 5 mg daily for estrogen suppression. On cycle day 2, the patient initiated treatment with daily subcutaneous follitropin alfa 300 mg and menopur 150 mg, oral letrozole 5 mg, and subcutaneous cetrorelix initiated on cycle day 6. Five follicles were produced, ranging from 14.5 to 22.5 mm. Ovidrel was administered on day 11 with retrieval 35 hours later on day 13. One germinal vesicle (GV) and four metaphase II (MII) oocytes were retrieved, and intracytoplasmic sperm injection (ICSI) was performed based on semen parameters. Two pro-nuclei embryos resulted and were cultured to the blastocyst stage, with both blastocysts meeting criteria for trophectoderm biopsy (Grade 3BB on days 5 and 6, respectively). PGS with next-generation sequencing (CooperGenomics, Livingston, NJ, USA) was performed; both blastocysts were deemed "complex abnormal" with ≥ 3 aneuploidies each.

After extensive counseling, and with oncology approval, the patient elected to pursue a second cycle. Following the same protocol, three oocytes were retrieved, including two MII oocytes and one Metaphase I (MI) oocyte. The MII oocytes underwent ICSI and both fertilized abnormally. The patient was counseled that, unfortunately, the cycle was unsuccessful.

48.3 Outcome

Tamoxifen therapy was initiated for an anticipated 10-year course, thus ending the patient's fertility preservation attempts. She was counseled regarding alternate family-building options, including donor oocyte IVF and adoption. While she did not achieve her desired outcome, she was grateful to know that her two blastocysts were, in fact, aneuploid rather than maintaining hope (and storage fees) for embryos that could not have resulted in pregnancy. She noted a degree of comfort knowing that she had made every attempt to preserve her fertility.

Clinical Pearls and Pitfalls

- Owing to diminished ovarian reserve and age-related aneuploidy, women pursuing ART at advanced reproductive ages often require multiple IVF cycles to produce a euploid embryo; oncology patients often cannot afford the time required to achieve multiple cycles.
- Preimplantation genetic testing for aneuploidy (PGT-A) increases the knowledge of potential fertility preservation.
- A collaborative approach between oncology and reproductive endocrinology is required to give patients the best chance of fertility preservation without compromising oncologic outcomes.
- Psychosocial support and resources are critical for patients navigating the emotionally challenging path of fertility preservation.

Review Questions and Answers

Q1. The likelihood of a live birth from one cycle of IVF at 41 years is:

(a) 5.5%
(b) 13.3%

(c) 30.9%
(d) 45.1%

A1. (b) [3]. To achieve this rate, the transfer of multiple embryos is often required. In patients pursuing PGS at 41 years old, multiple IVF cycles are often required to achieve a euploid embryo. The likelihood of pregnancy following the transfer of a euploid embryo is 60–70%; a patient cryopreserving embryos for fertility preservation should, therefore, attempt to cryopreserve >1 euploid embryo to achieve future pregnancy. Patients seeking fertility preservation at advanced reproductive ages should understand the significant impact of age on success rates.

Q2. All factors decrease ovarian reserve and, therefore, typically lower responses to IVF except:
(a) BRCA1 mutation
(b) Prolonged long-acting reversible contraception (IUD) use
(c) Endometriosis
(d) Advanced age

A2. (b). Prolonged long-acting reversible contraception (IUD). Prior studies reveal no difference in pregnancy rates upon the discontinuation of both hormonal and non-hormonal IUDs compared to nonusers [9]. BRCA genes play critical roles in the repair of double-stranded DNA breaks, and germ line mutations plausibly lead to accelerated oocyte apoptosis and depletion. Decreased ovarian reserve has been demonstrated by decreased AMH levels, a marker for ovarian reserve, in patients with BRCA mutations compared with aged-matched controls [4]. Endometriosis is an estrogen-dependent chronic inflammatory state causing infertility and pelvic pain. The cause of infertility is multifactorial, including the decreased quantity and quality of oocytes. Oocytes retrieved from women affected by endometriosis are more likely to fail in vitro maturation and show altered morphology [5]. The number of oocytes decreases naturally and progressively through atresia, starting from a maximum complement of 6–7 million at 20 weeks of gestation in the female fetus, to 1–2 million at birth, 300–500,000 at puberty, 25,000 at age 37 years, and 1000 at age 51 years, the average age of menopause [2].

Q3. Undergraduate American students:
(a) Plan to have their first child within the window of a woman's fertility
(b) Overestimate the age as which fertility declines
(c) Overestimate the chances of successfully IVF treatments
(d) All of the above

A3. (d). All of the above. While a survey study by Peterson et al. found that American undergraduate students plan to have their first child within the window of a woman's fertility, over half of men and nearly 40% of women planned to have their second child between ages 35 and 44 years old. Two-thirds of women and 81% of men inaccurately believed that female fertility markedly declines after the age of 40 (instead of gradually at 32 years and rapidly at 37 years), and one-third of women and nearly half of men believed the decline takes place after age 44 years – when IVF success rates are 3.2% per IVF cycle. The expected success of IVF treatments was also greatly overestimated [6]. Similar findings are well supported in multiple other studies across many countries, beaconing the need for increased education. Unfortunately, these misconceptions are also prevalent among healthcare providers, including gynecologists.

Q4. Female fertility decreases significantly at:
(a) 28 years
(b) 32 years
(c) 37 years
(d) 42 years

A4. (b). The fecundity of women decreases gradually but significantly beginning at age 32 years. It decreases more rapidly after age 37 years. Expedited evaluation for infertility is warranted in women 35 years and older after 6 months of failed attempts to conceive. At age 40 years, immediate evaluation and treatment are warranted [2].

Q5. Miscarriage rates for women 41 years old after IVF with fresh embryo transfer is:
(a) 9.9%
(b) 11.4%
(c) 13.7%
(d) 19.8%
(e) 29.6%
(f) 36.6%

A5. (e). Prior studies of women conceiving with IVF indicate 9.9% of women fewer than 33 years have a miscarriage after 7 weeks and confirmed fetal heart activity. Rates progressively increase to 11.4% for women 33–34 years, 13.7% for women aged 35–37 years, 19.8% for women aged 38–40 years, 29.9% for women aged 41–42 years, and 36.6% for women older than 42 years. Autosomal trisomy is the most frequent finding in spontaneous abortion and increases with age. It is partially mediated through changes in the meiotic spindle, predisposing to nondisjunction [2].

References

1. McKinlay SM, Brambilla DJ, Posner JG. The normal menopause transition. Maturitas. 1992;14:103–15.
2. Female age-related fertility decline. Committee opinion no. 589. Fertil Steril. 2014;101:633–4.
3. SART National Summary Report (2014). 2018. at https://www.sartcorsonline.com/rptCSR_PublicMultYear.aspx?ClinicPKID=0.
4. Wang ET, Pisarska MD, Bresee C, et al. BRCA1 germline mutations may be associated with reduced ovarian reserve. Fertil Steril. 2014;102:1723–8.
5. Sanchez AM, Vanni VS, Bartiromo L, et al. Is the oocyte quality affected by endometriosis? A review of the literature. J Ovarian Res. 2017;10.43.
6. Peterson BD, Pirritano M, Tucker L, Lampic C. Fertility awareness and parenting attitudes among American male and female undergraduate university students. Hum Reprod. 2012;27:1375–82.
7. Franasiak JM, Forman EJ, Hong KH, et al. The nature of aneuploidy with increasing age of the female partner: a review of 15,169 consecutive trophectoderm biopsies evaluated with comprehensive chromosomal screening. Fertil Steril. 2014;101:656–63.e1.
8. Chang J, Boulet SL, Jeng G, Flowers L, Kissin DM. Outcomes of in vitro fertilization with preimplantation genetic diagnosis: an analysis of the United States assisted reproductive technology surveillance data, 2011–2012. Fertil Steril. 2016;105:394–400.
9. Stoddard AM, Xu H, Madden T, Allsworth JE, Peipert JF. Fertility after intrauterine device removal: a pilot study. Eur J Contracept Reprod Health Care. 2015;20:223–30.

Case Studies: Ovarian Tissue Cryopreservation

Contents

Case Presentation: Ovarian Tissue Cryopreservation and Subsequent Transplantation in the Setting of Lymphoma

Clarisa R. Gracia

T. K. Woodruff et al. (eds.), *Textbook of Oncofertility Research and Practice*,
https://doi.org/10.1007/978-3-030-02868-8_49

Case Presentation

MF was a 35-year-old, married, nulliparous female who presented to her primary physician with shortness of breath, dry cough, night sweats, and chest discomfort. Her chest X-ray revealed a 10 cm, right anterior, mediastinal mass and PET/CT demonstrated pancreatic and liver infiltration. US-guided biopsy of the large mediastinal mass revealed findings consistent with a mediastinal large B-cell lymphoma. She was hospitalized given her significant shortness of breath, and it was recommended that she undergo chemotherapy immediately with cyclophosphamide, doxorubicin, vincristine, prednisone, and rituximab (R-CHOP). She refused chemotherapy initially because she was very concerned about the effects on her future fertility. A fertility preservation consultation was requested and MF was informed of the moderate risk of infertility and ovarian failure related to this chemotherapeutic regimen at her age [1]. Options for fertility preservation were discussed including embryo cryopreservation, oocyte cryopreservation, ovarian cryopreservation, and ovarian suppression with GnRH agonists [2]. Given the severity of her respiratory symptoms, it was recommended that she proceed with chemotherapy immediately and not delay therapy to undergo ovarian stimulation. Instead, she was interested in undergoing ovarian tissue cryopreservation after one cycle of chemotherapy was complete. Ovarian reserve testing was performed prior to chemotherapy exposure, and her anti-Mullerian hormone (AMH) was noted to be 0.3 ng/mL at that time. She subsequently was treated with R-CHOP. After her first cycle of chemotherapy, she was counseled extensively about ovarian tissue cryopreservation and was enrolled in an IRB-approved experimental ovarian tissue cryopreservation protocol at our institution [3]. A laparoscopic right ovarian cortical biopsy was performed. During this procedure, approximately 1/3 of the ovarian cortex was removed from the left ovary, dissected into small fragments, and cryopreserved using a slow freeze technique utilized by the Oncofertility Consortium [4]. She experienced no complications and subsequently completed a total of six cycles of R-CHOP and mantle radiation.

After therapy, her menstrual cycles did not resume and her reproductive hormones suggested acute menopause. She was treated with hormone replacement therapy to manage menopausal symptoms and to optimize bone health. Three years after her diagnosis, she remained in good health with no evidence of disease. Hormone therapy was stopped and reproductive hormone testing was found to be compatible with menopause with an AMH <0.08 ng/mL, FSH >80 mIU/mL, and E2 <20 pg/mL [5]. She was counseled regarding her options for having a family. Several options were discussed including ovarian tissue transplantation and alternatives such as donor egg or adoption. She strongly desired ovarian tissue transplantation in order to attempt to have a genetically related child. Before proceeding with the surgery, a consultation was performed by her oncologist to determine the safety of autologous ovarian tissue transplant using her previously frozen tissue. She was also referred to a maternal-fetal medicine specialist to discuss the safety of pregnancy. There was agreement amongst the specialists that it was safe for her to attempt pregnancy with ovarian tissue transplantation. She enrolled in an IRB-approved experimental ovarian tissue transplantation protocol at our institution. Laparoscopy was performed, and all of the frozen ovarian cortical tissue was thawed. Both ovaries were incised and the vascular medulla was exposed. Each fragment of ovarian tissue was sutured to the existing ovaries. A hysteroscopy and chromopertubation of the fallopian tubes was performed at the time of surgery and confirmed a normal uterine cavity and tubal patency.

After surgery, she was monitored with serial ultrasounds and bloodwork to assess ovarian activity. Approximately 6 months after transplant, she reported an improvement in her menopausal symptoms and was noted to have a dominant follicle on ultrasound. An intrauterine insemination was performed, but she failed to conceive. Menstrual cycles stopped thereafter. She subsequently pursued pregnancy using an egg donor and has delivered two healthy children.

Oocyte and embryo cryopreservation are typically recommended as first-line therapies for fertility preservation in women facing fertility-threatening treatments like chemotherapy. However, ovarian tissue cryopreservation is an excellent option for patients who must proceed with chemotherapy urgently and do not have sufficient time to undergo ovarian stimulation due to health concerns or aggressive disease [6]. Live births from ovarian tissue transplantation have been reported in patients who had been exposed to chemotherapy before ovarian tissue cryopreservation. However, it is possible that such exposure may reduce the number of follicles available for cryopreservation. Indeed, the success of OTC appears to be highest in young patients with excellent ovarian reserve at the time of cryopreservation. Unfortunately, the patient described in this case was 35 years of age and already had evidence of diminished ovarian reserve. No doubt these factors played a role in the limited duration of ovarian function after transplantation and the failure to achieve pregnancy. Nonetheless, ovarian function resumed for a short period of time. One of the principal risks related to ovarian tissue transplantation is the potential to cause a cancer recurrence by seeding the patient with cancer cells resident in the ovarian tissue. This risk appears to be highest in cancers that involve the ovary or liquid tumors like leukemia [2]. Therefore, consultation with an oncologist and maternal-fetal medicine specialist is recommended before transplantation. Ovarian tissue transplantation is still considered experimental and should be conducted as part of an IRB-approved protocol.

This case highlights how strongly patients feel about their fertility. This patient was highly educated and vocal at the time of diagnosis. In fact, she demanded to speak with a reproductive specialist before accepting chemotherapy in the hospital. Evidence suggests that fertility preservation counseling is extremely important and minimizes regret after treatment, even if patients do not pursue it [7]. Therefore, all patients facing fertility-threatening therapies should be counseled about the potential reproductive risks and options for extending fertility. Even though fertility preserving strategies are not always successful, they provide patients with an opportunity to attempt to have a genetic child after treatment. Thankfully, other highly successful options exist for family building, including IVF with egg or embryo donation and adoption. Ultimately, this patient is extremely happy that she has been able to complete her family as a cancer survivor.

Clinical Pearls and Pitfalls

- Ovarian tissue cryopreservation may be an option for patients who are not candidates for delaying therapy either because of health concerns or aggressive disease.
- Ovarian tissue cryopreservation may be performed after exposure to chemotherapy.
- Ovarian function often resumes after ovarian tissue transplantation but the duration may be limited by the number of follicles in the tissue.
- Ovarian transplantation should not be performed in patients whose cancer is likely to contain cancer cells that could lead to a recurrence.
- Ovarian tissue transplantation is still considered experimental and should be conducted as part of an IRB-approved protocol.
- Because pregnancy may be high risk in cancer survivors, consultation with an oncologist and maternal-fetal medicine specialist is recommended before transplantation.

Review Questions and Answers

Q1. Which of the following options would be most appropriate for a patient who has already begun chemotherapy treatment for Hodgkin disease?
(a) Oocyte cryopreservation
(b) Embryo cryopreservation
(c) Ovarian tissue cryopreservation
(d) Ovarian suppression with combined oral contraceptives

A1. (c). Ovarian tissue cryopreservation

Q2. Ovarian function typically resumes after how many months post transplant:
(a) 2–3 months
(b) 4–6 months
(c) 9–11 months
(d) 12–15 months
(e) 18–24 months

A2. (b). Ovarian function typically resumes 4–6 months post transplant

Q3. Ovarian tissue cryopreservation and subsequent transplantation are most appropriate in patients with which of the following types of cancer:
(a) Leukemia
(b) Lymphoma
(c) Breast cancer in a BRCA carrier
(d) Ovarian cancer

A3. (b). Lymphoma rarely involves the ovaries and, therefore, is unlikely to be related to recurrent cancer after ovarian tissue transplantation.

49

References

1. Meissner J, Tichy D, Katzke V, Kühn T, Dietrich S, Schmitt T, Ziepert M, Kuhnt E, Rixecker T, Zorn M, Witzens-Harig M, Pfreundschuh M, Ho AD. Long-term ovarian function in women treated with CHOP or CHOP plus etoposide for aggressive lymphoma. Ann Oncol. 2015;26:1771–6.
2. Donnez J, Dolmans MM. Fertility preservation in women. N Engl J Med. 2018;378:400–1.
3. Gracia CR, Chang J, Kondapalli L, Prewitt M, Carlson CA, Mattei P, Jeffers S, Ginsberg JP. Ovarian tissue cryopreservation for fertility preservation in cancer patients: successful establishment and feasibility of a multidisciplinary collaboration. J Assist Reprod Genet. 2012;29:495–502.
4. Armstrong AG, Kimler BF, Smith BM, Woodruff TK, Pavone ME, Duncan FE. Ovarian tissue cryopreservation in young females through the Oncofertility Consortium's National Physicians Cooperative. Future Oncol. 2018;14:363–78.
5. Dillon KE, Gracia CR. What is normal ovarian reserve? Semin Reprod Med. 2013;31:427–36.
6. Medicine, P. C. o. A. S. f. R. Fertility preservation in patients undergoing gonadotoxic therapy or gonadectomy: a committee opinion. Fertil Steril. 2013;100:1214–23.
7. Letourneau JM, Ebbel EE, Katz PP, Katz A, Ai WZ, Chien AJ, Melisko ME, Cedars MI, Rosen MP. Pretreatment fertility counseling and fertility preservation improve quality of life in reproductive age women with cancer. Cancer. 2012;118:1710–7.

Ovarian Tissue Cryopreservation in a Rare Case of a Pregnant Woman with Acute Leukemia

Mahmoud Salama, Evgenia Isachenko, Sebastian Ludwig, Thomas Einzmann, Gohar Rahimi, Peter Mallmann, and Vladimir Isachenko

T. K. Woodruff et al. (eds.), *Textbook of Oncofertility Research and Practice*,
https://doi.org/10.1007/978-3-030-02868-8_50

Case Presentation

A 34-year-old primigravid woman was diagnosed with acute lymphocytic leukemia (ALL) during her 17th week of pregnancy. Her oncology team determined that chemotherapy must start immediately with the standard induction I and II protocols as described by the German Multicenter Study Group for Adult Acute Lymphoblastic Leukemia (GMALL). At the beginning of her third trimester, the patient will receive the standard consolidation I protocol with high-dose methotrexate.

Due to the ongoing pregnancy and potential risks of chemotherapy-induced gonadotoxicity, the patient was referred to the reproductive medicine department for fertility preservation counseling and further management.

50.1 Assessment and Diagnosis

In this pregnant patient with ALL, several complex challenges are raised, including:

- Leukemia in pregnancy is a rare condition with a prevalence of ~1 in 100,000 pregnancies. Consequently, limited data or evidence-based management strategies are available [1].
- Although the administration of chemotherapy during the second and third trimesters does not increase the incidence of fetal anomalies or childhood malignancies, it may result in increased incidence of preterm labor, intrauterine growth retardation, or fetal death [2].
- Proper management of leukemia in pregnancy necessitates a high level of coordination and collaboration between oncologists, obstetricians, and neonatologists in order to improve the maternal and fetal outcome.
- While fertility preservation should be considered before initiation of chemotherapy, the 5-year relative survival for adults with ALL is only about 40% [3].

50.2 Management

Due to the ongoing pregnancy and the necessity for immediate initiation of chemotherapy in this patient, ovarian tissue cryopreservation was the only feasible option for emergency fertility preservation. Informed consent was obtained from the patient prior to the surgical procedure [4].

After coordination with the oncology team, the patient underwent laparoscopic right oophorectomy 1 day before the initiation of chemotherapy. The ovarian tissue was transported to our laboratory within 10 min of extraction for further processing. Except where otherwise stated, all chemicals were obtained from Sigma (Sigma Chemical Co., St. Louis, MO, USA). As previously described by our group, the basal medium used for transport and dissection was composed of Leibovitz L-15 supplemented with 5% Dextran Serum Substitute (Irvine Scientific, Santa Ana, CA, USA). The temperature of the sample was maintained between 32 °C and 34 °C. The ovarian cortex was dissected into small strips (medulla-containing strips: 0.5–1 × 0.5–1 cm, 1–2 mm thickness) using tweezers and a number 22 scalpel under aseptic conditions.

Ovarian tissue strips were cooled at 5 °C for 24 hours with plans for cryopreservation using a slow freezing protocol on the following day. On the day of cryopreservation, the ovarian tissue strips were placed for 30 min at room temperature in 20 ml freezing medium composed of basal medium supplemented with 6% dimethyl sulfoxide, 6% ethylene glycol, and 0.15 M sucrose. Then, each ovarian tissue strip was put into a standard 5 ml cryovial (Thermo Fisher Scientific, Rochester, NY, USA) previously filled with 4.5 ml freezing medium and frozen in an IceCube 14S freezer (SyLab, Neupurkersdorf, Austria). The slow cooling profile was started at −6 °C, and then the cryovials were cooled from −6 °C to −34 °C at a rate of −0.3 °C/min. This slow freezing protocol included the auto-seeding step at −6 °C. Finally, at −34 °C, cryovials were plunged into liquid nitrogen and stored until future use.

50.3 Outcome

Chemotherapy protocols were administered as planned. At the 31st week of gestation, elective Cesarean section was performed to avoid chemotherapy-induced pancytopenia. No maternal or neonatal complications were recorded.

If the patient successfully completes her anticancer therapy and is medically cleared for pregnancy, her endocrine and ovarian reserve testing will be reassessed. If the patient suffers from POI, she may then wish to use her cryopreserved ovarian tissue to restore her fertility. As the autotransplantation of cryopreserved-thawed ovarian tissue is absolutely contraindicated in leukemia due to the high risk of ovarian tissue contamination with malignant cells, the only feasible way to restore fertility in this patient may be with artificial ovary technology [5, 6].

An artificial ovary is a novel experimental technology that aims to produce mature oocytes for in vitro fertilization through an ex vivo multistep strategy including sequential in vitro cultures of ovarian tissue, follicles, and oocytes [7–9]. Although successful only in mice, further advances in research will help to establish a human model. Briefly, cryopreserved-thawed cortical ovarian tissue pieces can be cultured in vitro for up to 6–10 days to activate primordial follicles within the ovarian tissue to develop to the pre-antral stage [10, 11]. The pre-antral follicles are then enzymatically or mechanically isolated from the ovarian tissue and further cultured for up to 4 weeks in a biodegradable 3D micro-environment made of alginate, matrigel, or fibrin [12]. The 3D in vitro culture helps pre-antral follicles develop to the early antral stages [13–17]. The early antral follicles are then enzymatically or mechanically isolated from the surrounding 3D micro-environment and finally punctured to release oocytes [18]. Oocytes are usually immature, and they may be cultured in vitro for 24–48 hours in order to mature into metaphase II (MII) oocytes for use in in vitro fertilization.

Clinical Pearls and Pitfalls

- Leukemia in pregnancy is a rare condition with a prevalence of ~1 in 100,000 pregnancies.
- Proper management of leukemia in pregnancy necessitates a high level of coordination and collaboration between oncologists, obstetricians, and neonatologists in order to improve the maternal and fetal outcome.
- As the autotransplantation of cryopreserved-thawed ovarian tissue is contraindicated in leukemia patients due to the high risk of ovarian tissue contamination with malignant cells, artificial ovary technology may be the only feasible option to restore fertility in this population.

Conflict of Interest All authors state that they have no conflicts of interest.

Review Questions and Answers

Q1. What are the different side effects of chemotherapy administration during the second and third trimesters?

A1. Although the administration of chemotherapy during the second and third trimesters does not increase the incidence of fetal anomalies or childhood malignancies, it may result in an increased incidence of preterm labor, intrauterine growth retardation, or fetal death.

Q2. What are the survival statistics for adults with ALL?

A2. The 5-year relative survival for adults between ages 25 and 64 with ALL is about 40%.

Q3. Why is ovarian tissue autotransplantation contraindicated in leukemia?

A3. Ovarian tissue autotransplantation is contraindicated in leukemia due to the high risk of ovarian tissue contamination with hematological malignant cells.

Q4. Explain the concept of an artificial ovary.

A4. An artificial ovary is a novel experimental technology that aims to produce mature oocytes for in vitro fertilization through an ex vivo multistep strategy including sequential in vitro cultures of ovarian tissue, follicles, and oocytes.

References

1. Milojkovic D, Apperley JF. How I treat leukemia during pregnancy. Blood. 2014;123(7):974–84.
2. Koren G, Carey N, Gagnon R, Maxwell C, Nulman I, Senikas V. Cancer chemotherapy and pregnancy. J Obstet Gynaecol Can. 2013;35(3):263–78.
3. Pulte D, Jansen L, Gondos A, Katalinic A, Barnes B, Ressing M, Holleczek B, Eberle A, Brenner H. GEKID Cancer Survival Working Group. Survival of adults with acute lymphoblastic leukemia in Germany and the United States. PLoS One. 2014;9(1):e85554.
4. Salama M, Mallmann P. Emergency fertility preservation for female patients with cancer: clinical perspectives. Anticancer Res. 2015;35(6):3117–27.
5. Bastings L, Beerendonk CC, Westphal JR, Massuger LF, Kaal SE, van Leeuwen FE, Braat DD, Peek R. Autotransplantation of cryopreserved ovarian tissue in cancer survivors and the risk of reintroducing malignancy: a systematic review. Hum Reprod Update. 2013;19(5):483–506.
6. Dolmans MM, Luyckx V, Donnez J, Andersen CY, Greve T. Risk of transferring malignant cells with transplanted frozen-thawed ovarian tissue. Fertil Steril. 2013;99(6):1514–22.
7. Amorim CA, Shikanov A. The artificial ovary: current status and future perspectives. Future Oncol. 2016;12(20):2323–32.
8. Telfer EE, Fauser BC. Important steps towards materializing the dream of developing an artificial ovary. Reprod Biomed Online. 2016;33(3):333–4.
9. Laronda MM, Rutz AL, Xiao S, et al. A bioprosthetic ovary created using 3D printed microporous scaffolds restores ovarian function in sterilized mice. Nat Commun. 2017;8:15261.
10. Telfer EE, McLaughlin M, Ding C, Thong KJ. A two-step serum-free culture system supports development of human oocytes from primordial follicles in the presence of activin. Hum Reprod. 2008;23(5):1151–8.
11. Fabbri R, Pasquinelli G, Keane D, Mozzanega B, Magnani V, Tamburini F, Venturoli S. Culture of cryopreserved ovarian tissue: state of the art in 2008. Fertil Steril. 2009;91(5):1619–29.
12. Xu M, Barrett SL, West-Farrell E, Kondapalli LA, Kiesewetter SE, Shea LD, Woodruff TK. In vitro grown human ovarian follicles from cancer patients support oocyte growth. Hum Reprod. 2009;24(10):2531–40.
13. Xu M, West E, Shea LD, Woodruff TK. Identification of a stage-specific permissive in vitro culture environment for follicle growth and oocyte development. Biol Reprod. 2006;75(6):916–23.
14. Xu M, Banc A, Woodruff TK, Shea LD. Secondary follicle growth and oocyte maturation by culture in alginate hydrogel following cryopreservation of the ovary or individual follicles. Biotechnol Bioeng. 2009;103(2):378–86.
15. Smith RM, Woodruff TK, Shea LD. Designing follicle-environment interactions with biomaterials. Cancer Treat Res. 2010;156:11–24.
16. Shikanov A, Smith RM, Xu M, Woodruff TK, Shea LD. Hydrogel network design using multifunctional macromers to coordinate tissue maturation in ovarian follicle culture. Biomaterials. 2011;32(10):2524–31.
17. Shea LD, Woodruff TK, Shikanov A. Bioengineering the ovarian follicle microenvironment. Annu Rev Biomed Eng. 2014;16:29–52.
18. Jin SY, Lei L, Shikanov A, Shea LD, Woodruff TK. A novel two-step strategy for in vitro culture of early-stage ovarian follicles in the mouse. Fertil Steril. 2010;93(8):2633–9.

Further Reading

Isachenko V, Todorov P, Isachenko E, Rahimi G, Hanstein B, Salama M, Mallmann P, Tchorbanov A, Hardiman P, Getreu N, Merzenich M. Cryopreservation and xenografting of human ovarian fragments: medulla decreases the phosphatidylserine translocation rate. Reprod Biol Endocrinol. 2016.;10;14(1):79.

Salama M, Isachenko V, Isachenko E, Rahimi G, Mallmann P. Advances in fertility preservation of female patients with hematological malignancies. Expert Rev Hematol. 2017;10(11):951–60.

Case Studies: Adult Male Fertility Preservation

Contents

Case Presentation: Sperm Banking in Patient Diagnosed with Acute Myeloid Leukemia

Adam S. DuVall, Jason C. Hedges, and Brandon Hayes-Lattin

T. K. Woodruff et al. (eds.), *Textbook of Oncofertility Research and Practice*,
https://doi.org/10.1007/978-3-030-02868-8_51

Case Presentation

A 23-year-old man presented to a referring hospital emergency room with gradually worsening throat pain. He was febrile to 38.4°C and his exam was notable for very large, erythematous tonsils. His labs were notable for a white blood cell (WBC) count of 119.8 K/cu mm (3.50–10.80 K/cu mm) with 91% blasts, creatinine elevated to 1.63 mg/dL (0.70–1.30 mg/dL), and lactate dehydrogenase (LDH) of 1122 U/L (≤250 U/L). Computed tomography (CT) of the neck was remarkable for the enlargement of tonsils and lymph nodes with a narrowing of the nasopharyngeal airway. He was started empirically on cefepime and transferred to a tertiary care intensive care unit (ICU) due to concern for impending airway compromise in the setting of likely new acute leukemia. Upon arrival, his peripheral blood smear was notable for numerous circulating blasts with a high nuclear to cytoplasmic ratio, a moderate amount of basophilic cytoplasm, open chromatin, and prominent nucleoli suggestive of monoblastic differentiation (◘ Fig. 51.1). Flow cytometry confirmed an immunophenotype consistent with acute myeloid leukemia (AML).

51.1 Assessment and Diagnosis

This young man had an emergent presentation of newly diagnosed acute myeloid leukemia with a high blast count, acute kidney injury, and significant upper airway edema. Beyond the medical challenges of remission induction, his risk for leukemia relapse depended on the results not immediately available, including his cytogenetics and molecular testing and then his response to first-line chemotherapy. These risk factors would later determine his post-remission therapy, including decisions about the intensity of chemotherapy and the use of bone marrow transplantation [1–3]. Thus, the possible impact of his leukemia therapy on future fertility was difficult to fully assess at initial presentation. However, the impact on his fertility was very likely to be considerable, and the topic of future fertility is often meaningful to an adolescent and young adult (AYA) patient, so it is important to discuss the potential impacts of therapy prior to starting whenever possible [4].

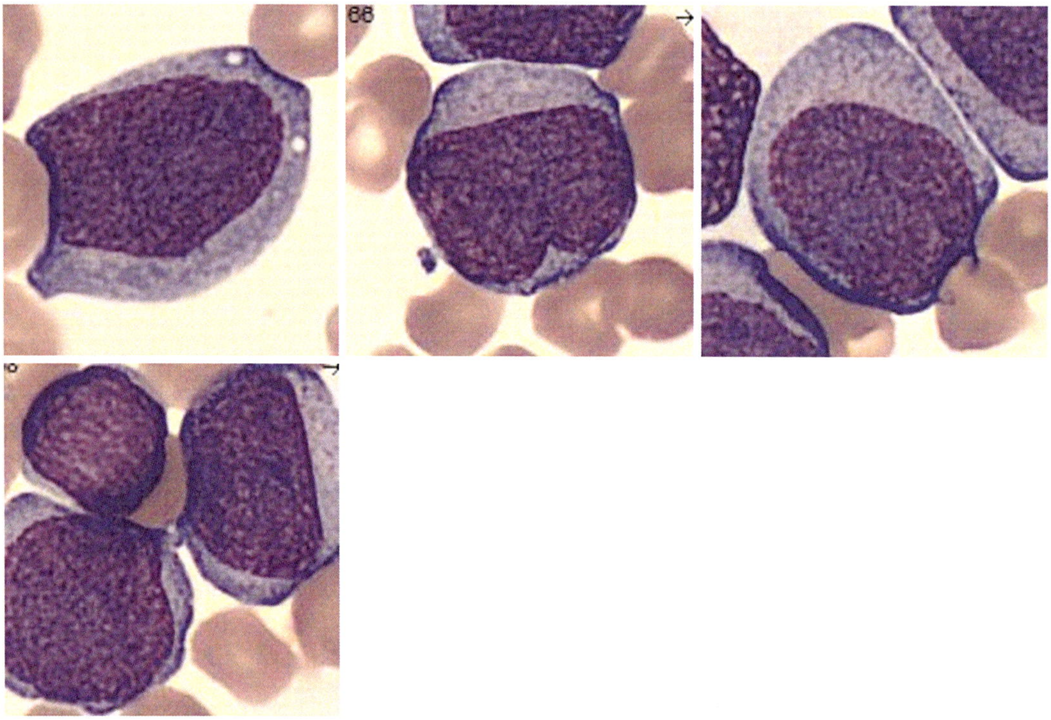

◘ **Fig. 51.1** Peripheral blood smear of circulating blasts notable for a high nuclear to cytoplasmic ratio, a moderate amount of basophilic cytoplasm, open chromatin, and prominent nucleoli

Current reports suggest that 25% of AYAs will attempt to preserve fertility before cancer treatment begins when offered the opportunity, although some of the major barriers to do so are that they do not know their fertility is at risk and there is not adequate time to pursue fertility preservation options [5].

AML is considered an oncologic emergency and outcomes have been found to be dependent on the time from diagnosis to treatment initiation in younger patients, necessitating that this patient start therapy as soon as possible to maximize outcomes [6]. Yet, he was not clinically stable enough to be referred to a fertility specialist nor to travel to a center where sperm cryopreservation could be performed. Initial treatment with cytarabine and an anthracycline was discussed with the patient, including the possible effects on future fertility. The patient expressed interest in fertility preservation prior to therapy initiation.

Unfortunately, there are not large randomized control trials published about the safety and efficacy of fertility preservation prior to the initiation of chemotherapy. There is a theoretical concern that leukemia cells could infiltrate reproductive organs, such as ovaries or testes, and then be transferred along with reproductive material. There is a large amount of observational data showing that a variety of fertility-preservation techniques can be performed safely in women, and there have been no reports of transferring leukemia [7]. There is less published experience with male fertility preservation, and though testicular leukemia is a well-described clinical entity, there have been large retrospective studies demonstrating safety and efficacy [8–10]. However, previous reports have established that sperm count is decreased in leukemia patients even in comparison to other cancers and chronic disease prior to therapy [10].

51.2 Management

Optimal timing for sperm cryopreservation before any therapy is given to maximize the quality and DNA integrity of the semen specimen, which can be damaged by just one round of chemotherapy [11]. Even though there is significant emotional stress and difficulty, it is important to discuss this at the time of diagnosis. However, less than 50% of people remember discussing fertility risks with their health care provider in some studies [12]. Ideally, this discussion would be held with a multidisciplinary team focused on providing patient education and providing fertility preservation procedures. These teams have become more common, particularly at institutions where there is expertise in caring for the AYA population with cancer.

This patient did have a discussion about the potential impact of therapy on his future fertility shortly after his diagnosis, and he desired to attempt fertility preservation if possible. Although he was not able to leave the hospital, he was clinically stable enough to manually provide semen for sperm cryopreservation, even in the ICU. A multidisciplinary approach was taken, and privacy was coordinated between nursing, social work, the ICU team, the hematologic malignancy team, and the patient's family. His father was able to transport the specimen immediately to the local lab for cryopreservation, and the patient was subsequently starting on induction chemotherapy.

Another option could have been testicular sperm extraction (TESE), which is called onco-TESE when used as an option for patients with cancer. Microdissection-TESE (micro-TESE) utilizes an operating microscope to identify small pockets or crypts of sperm production in comparison to tissue extraction done with TESE, which success depends on a higher level of spermatogenesis. It has been shown to increase yield in certain clinical settings with a similar clinical complication rate and decreased hematoma and testicular fibrosis [13]. It does, however, require sedation, so he was not eligible for this procedure due to upper airway edema and concern for respiratory compromise. In many situations though, this procedure could be coordinated with sedation used for other cancer diagnostic procedures.

51.3 Outcome

Patient was diagnosed with high-risk AML based on molecular markers and inadequate response to the initial conditioning therapy. He achieved a remission after re-induction therapy and underwent a matched unrelated donor hematopoietic stem cell transplant. Unfortunately, he was only able to bank 1.015 mL of semen with 0.07 million motile sperm (>20 million) and will establish care with a fertility specialist in the future if procedures such as in vitro fertilization (IVF) or intrauterine insemination (IUI) are to be considered.

Clinical Pearls and Pitfalls

- The impact on fertility of antineoplastic therapy can be significant and impact the quality of life of patients undergoing therapy long after its completion.
- There are options for fertility preservation even in some of the more seriously ill patients.
- It is important to discuss these potential impacts early after diagnosis and ideally prior to initiating therapy.
- Multidisciplinary teams are encouraged, including fertility preservation specialists and other health care providers who care for AYAs with cancer.

Review Questions and Answers

Q1. What is NOT a barrier to preserving fertility for those with cancer requiring chemotherapy?

(a) Providers taking the time during a busy period to go over the risks to fertility
(b) Cost of fertility-preserving measures
(c) Medical status of the patient
(d) Importance of fertility preservation to patients
(e) Available facilities for fertility preservation

A1. (d)

Q2. True or false? There have been reports of transferring leukemia through egg or sperm preservation.

A2. False

Q3. What percentage of patients remembers discussing the impact of fertility of therapy with his/her provider?

(a) 10%
(b) 25%
(c) 50%
(d) 65%
(e) 90%

A3. (c)

Q4. What is the best option for a male patient who has reached sexual maturity but is unable to provide semen and still wishes to preserve fertility?

(a) Nothing
(b) TESE
(c) Sexual education
(d) Only offering fertility treatment following therapy

A4. (b)

Q5. True or false? Men with leukemia have decreased sperm counts in comparison to their healthy peers and to those of similar age with chronic diseases making sperm backing successfully more challenging.

A5. True

References

1. Papaemmanuil E, Gerstung M, Bullinger L, et al. Genomic classification and prognosis in acute myeloid leukemia. N Engl J Med. 2016;374(23):2209–21.
2. Schuurhuis GJ, Heuser M, Freeman S, et al. Minimal/measureable residual disease in AML: consensus document from ELN MRD Working Party. Blood. 2018;131:1275–91. Epub ahead of print.
3. Doehner H, Weisdorf DJ, Bloomfield CD. Acute myeloid leukemia. N Engl J Med. 2015;373(12):1136–52.
4. Nass SJ, Beaupin LK, Demark-Wahnefried W, et al. Identifying and addressing the needs of adolescents and young adults with cancer: summary of an Institute of Medicine workshop. Oncologist. 2015;20(2):186–95.
5. Rechis R, Bann C, Arvery S, et al. Unique risks & vulnerabilities of AYA patients across the lifespan, LIVESTRONG Foundation: AYA survey results. Presented at Institute of Medicine National Cancer Policy Forum/LIVESTRONG Workshop on Addressing the Needs of Adolescents and Young Adults with Cancer, Washington, DC; 2013.
6. Sekeres MA, Elson P, Kalaycio ME, et al. Time from diagnosis to treatment initiation predicts survival in younger, but not older, acute myeloid leukemia patients. Blood. 2009;113(1):28–36.

7. Massarotti C, Scaruffi P, Lambertini M, et al. State of the art on oocyte cryopreservation in female cancer patients: a critical review of the literature. Cancer Treat Rev. 2017;57:50–7.
8. Johnson MD, Cooper AR, Jungheim ES, et al. Sperm banking for fertility preservation: a 20-year experience. Eur J Obstet Gynecol Reprod Biol. 2013;170:177–82.
9. Chung K, Irani J, Knee G, et al. Sperm cryopreservation for male patients with cancer: an epidemiological analysis at the University of Pennsylvania. Eur J Obstet Gynecol Reprod Biol. 2004;113S:S7–S11.
10. Auger J, Sermondade N, Eustache F. Semen quality of 4480 young cancer and systemic disease patients: baseline data and clinical considerations. Basic Clinical Androl. 2016;26(3):1–10.
11. Burns KC, Hoefgen H, Strine A, Dasgupta R. Fertility preservation options in pediatric and adolescent patients with cancer. Cancer. 2018;124(9):1867–76. https://doi.org/10.1002/cncr.31255. Epub 2018 Jan 25.
12. Banerjee R, Tsiapali E. Occurrence and recall rates of fertility discussions with young breast cancer patients. Support Care Cancer. 2016;24:163–71.
13. Deruyver Y, Vanderschueren D, Van der Aa F. Outcome of microdissection TESE compared with conventional TESE in non-obstructive azoospermia: a systematic review. Andrology. 2014;2:20–4.

Management of Male Infertility Secondary to Chemotherapeutic Agents During Childhood Cancer Treatment

Aarati Didwania

T. K. Woodruff et al. (eds.), *Textbook of Oncofertility Research and Practice*,
https://doi.org/10.1007/978-3-030-02868-8_52

Case Presentation

A 33-year-old male with a history of Hodgkin lymphoma at age 14 presents with his wife to discuss fertility. He and his wife have been attempting pregnancy for the last 1 year, without success. His wife has recently undergone fertility testing and results thus far have been normal. She has regular menses, is not on birth control pills, and has achieved no prior pregnancies. The patient does not remember having a discussion about his fertility at the time of his lymphoma diagnosis. He had achieved puberty at the time of cancer treatment but did not cryopreserve sperm. The patient does have a history of chemotherapy, radiation therapy, and stem cell transplant. He does not report any recent fevers or history of urological trauma, including testicular torsion. He does not report a history of prostatitis, epididymitis, nor orchitis. He denies a history of post-pubertal mumps. There is no known family history of fertility problems. He is not taking any current medications. He is able to find his lymphoma treatment history and reports that he was treated with Cytoxan, Adriamycin, vincristine, IV methotrexate, intrathecal methotrexate and ARA-C, ifosfamide, VP-16, L-asparaginase, and cisplatin. He received 2500 cGy of mini-mantle radiation. He received his bone marrow transplant 2 years after the initial diagnosis and was treated with ARA-C, VP-16, cisplatin, thiotepa, and Cytoxan. On exam, his penile exam is normal, with no evidence of plaques or induration. His urethral meatus is normal. His testes are descended bilaterally with no evidence of abnormal masses or tenderness. Both testes are 10 cc in volume. Epididymis, vas deferens, and cord structures are normal bilaterally.

52.1 Assessment and Diagnosis

The most likely etiology for the patient's infertility is related to his cancer treatment. Cytotoxic cancer therapies can negatively affect sperm production. Sperm cells divide quickly and are, therefore, susceptible to chemotherapy-induced damage. Permanent infertility can result if spermatogonial stem cells are damaged to the point that they can no longer produce maturing sperm cells. The risk of chemotherapy causing infertility varies depending upon the patient's age, the type of drug used, and the doses of the drug given. Sperm banking is a reliable strategy to preserve fertility in male patients who receive gonadotoxic chemotherapy [1]. Chemotherapy drugs and the risk of infertility in men are listed in Table 52.1. Higher doses of these drugs are more likely to cause permanent fertility changes. Combinations of drugs can lead to greater toxicity. The risks of permanent infertility are even higher when males are treated with both chemotherapy and radiation therapy to the abdomen or pelvis. In addition, radiation directed at the central nervous system can affect the hypothalamus and pituitary gland leading to a decrease in LH or FSH. Reduction

Table 52.1 Chemotherapeutic agents and risk of infertility

Highest risk of infertility	Lower risk of infertility
Actinomycin D	5-fluorouracil
Busulfan	6-Mercaptopurine
Carboplatin	Bleomycin
Carmustine	Dacarbazine
Chlorambucil	Daunorubicin
Cisplatin	Doxorubicin
Cyclophosphamide	Epirubicin
Cytarabine	Etoposide
Ifosfamide	Fludarabine
Lomustine	Methotrexate
Melphalan	Mitoxantrone
Nitrogen mustard	Thioguanine
Procarbazine	Thiotepa
	Vinblastine
	Vincristine

in these hormone levels can lead to a decrease in sperm production and infertility.

Hormonal therapy can also affect sperm production. These medications can also cause sexual side effects, such as a lower sex drive and erectile dysfunction. The decrease in sperm production and sexual side effects usually start to improve once patients have completed therapy.

Our patient underwent hormonal testing and semen analysis. His hormone testing included an analysis of prolactin, LH, FSH, estradiol, and testosterone. His hormonal levels are normal, except for low testosterone and elevated FSH. Results of his two semen analyses show azoospermia with normal volume.

Volume (ml)			
Value	Low	High	Units
3.2	1.0	5.0	ml
2.9	1.0	5.0	ml

Sperm concentration (M/ml)			
Value	Low	High	Units
0.0	20	200	M/m
0.0	20	200	M/m

% Motility (%)			
Value	Low	High	Units
0.0	50	100	%
0.0	50	100	%

% Normal morphology (%)			
Value	Low	High	Units
0.0	14	100	%
0.0	14	100	%

Based on this analysis, the patient was diagnosed with nonobstructive azoospermia secondary to the chemotherapy he received as part of his Hodgkin's lymphoma therapy.

52.2 Management

To address his infertility, he was offered clomiphene citrate therapy in preparation for testicular sperm extraction (TESE).

TESE and intracytoplasmic sperm injection (ICSI) were first introduced in 1993 for the treatment of obstructive azoospermia [2]. This technique was subsequently used for azoospermia secondary to nonobstructive etiologies [3]. Quantitative histological studies in patients undergoing TESE confirmed that there was a threshold amount of spermatogenesis that must be exceeded in order for spermatozoa to be released into the ejaculate [4]. Micro-TESE provides the advantage of allowing a surgeon to selectively identify the seminiferous tubules most likely to contain spermatozoa based on the larger and more opaque appearance of these tubules. With micro-TESE, successful sperm retrieval has been reported in up to 63% of men [5], whereas conventional and more limited sperm retrieval procedures have reported success rates from 20% (percutaneous testicular biopsies) [6] to 45% (open testis biopsies) [7].

Clomiphene citrate is a well-established agent that has been reported in numerous studies to improve semen quality and increase pregnancy rates among the partners of men to whom it is administered. Clomiphene citrate increases pituitary secretion by blocking the feedback inhibition of estradiol, thereby increasing serum FSH and LH levels. The administration of clomiphene citrate may result in sperm in the ejaculate of patients with nonobstructive azoospermia or the simplification of testis sperm retrieval [8]. Surgeons often consider a course of clomiphene citrate administration prior to surgical sperm retrieval in patients with nonobstructive azoospermia.

52.3 Outcome

Our patient received chemotherapeutic agents at the time of puberty that resulted in azoospermia. He was not offered sperm banking at the time of his treatment. He, however, was able to successfully father two children after two cycles of micro-TESE and ICSI. Given his low testosterone levels, the patient was offered testosterone replacement therapy to manage symptoms of hypogonadism.

Clinical Pearls and Pitfalls

- Chemotherapy and directed radiation therapy can affect spermatogenesis temporarily and permanently.
- Sperm banking prior to receiving cancer therapies is an effective method to preserve fertility options but many patients are not offered this at the time of treatment.
- Newer techniques, such as micro-TESE with ICSI, have allowed men with nonobstructive azoospermia to have biological children even after cancer therapy.

52

Review Questions and Answers

Q1. Why do some chemotherapy agents lead to male infertility and what factors increase the likelihood of this outcome?

A1. Sperm cells divide quickly and are, therefore, susceptible to damage induced by chemotherapy. Permanent infertility can result if spermatogonial stem cells are damaged to the point that they can no longer produce maturing sperm cells. The risk of chemotherapy causing infertility varies depending upon the patient's age, the type of drug used, and the doses of the drug given.

Q2. At the time of cancer treatment, what treatment factors can affect male fertility?

A2. Chemotherapy agents have varying likelihoods of resulting in male infertility and are listed in Table 52.1. Hormonal therapy can also affect sperm production. These medications can also cause sexual side effects, such as a lower sex drive and problems with erections. The decrease in sperm production and sexual side effects usually start to improve once patients have completed therapy. Radiation aimed directly at the testicles or at the pelvic region can affect male fertility by destroying spermatogenic stem cells. Radiation directed at the central nervous system can affect the hypothalamus and pituitary gland, leading to a decrease in LH or FSH.

Q3. What is the advantage of micro-TESE over other sperm retrieval methods in patients with nonobstructive azoospermia?

A3. Micro-TESE provides the advantage of allowing a surgeon to selectively identify seminiferous tubules most likely to contain spermatozoa based on the larger and more opaque appearance of those tubules. With micro-TESE, successful sperm retrieval has been reported in up to 63% of men, whereas conventional and more limited sperm retrieval procedures have reported success rates from 20% (percutaneous testicular biopsies) to 45% (open testis biopsies).

References

1. Schover LR, Brey K, Lichtin A, et al. Oncologists' attitudes and practices regarding banking sperm before cancer treatment. J Clin Oncol. 2002;20:1890–7.
2. Devroey P, Liu J, Nagy A, et al. Normal fertilization of human oocytes after testicular sperm extraction and intracytosplasmic sperm injection (TESE and ICSI). Fertil Steril. 1994;62:639–41.
3. Devroey P, Silber SJ, Nagy Z, et al. Ongoing pregnancies and birth after intracytoplastmic sperm injection with frozen-thawed epididymal spermatozoa. Hum Reprod. 1995;10:903–6.
4. Silber SJ, Nagy Z, Devroey P, et al. Distribution of spermatogenesis in the testicles of azoospermic men: the presence or absence of spermatids in the testes of men with germinal failure. Hum Reprod. 1997;12:2422–8.
5. Tsujimura A. Microdissection testicular sperm extraction: prediction, outcome, and complications. Int J Urol. 2007;14(10):883–9.
6. Ziaee SA, Ezzatnegad M, Nowroozi M, et al. Prediction of successful sperm retrieval in patients with nonobstructive azoospermia. Urol J. 2006;3(2):92–6.
7. Schlegel PN. Testicular sperm extraction: microdissection improves sperm yield with minimal tissue excision. Hum Reprod. 1999;14(1):131–5.
8. Hussein A, Ozgok Y, Ross L, Neiderberger C. Clomiphene administration for cases of nonobstructive azoospermia: a multicenter study. J Androl. 2005;26:787–91.

Case Studies: Pediatric Male Fertility Preservation

Contents

Assessing and Supporting Adolescent Boys Having Fertility Preservation

Antoinette Anazodo and William Ledger

T. K. Woodruff et al. (eds.), *Textbook of Oncofertility Research and Practice*,
https://doi.org/10.1007/978-3-030-02868-8_53

Case Presentation

A 12-year-old boy was diagnosed with relapsed acute lymphoblastic leukaemia 4 years after the completion of standard risk leukaemia treatment. Diagnostic and staging assessments confirmed that he had a combined bone marrow, central nervous system and left-sided testicular relapse.

He did not have fertility preservation at the commencement of his initial diagnosis due to his age and the low-fertility risk of his previous treatment, but the proposed curative treatment has a high gonadotoxic risk due to the dose of alkylating agents in the chemotherapy for bone marrow transplant conditioning and total body irradiation (TBI). As he had testicular disease, he also requires either testicular radiotherapy or consideration of an orchidectomy. if he does not respond to the proposed treatment, he could be offered other new novel agents or immune therapy as part of the clinical trial, and many of these treatments have an unknown fertility potential.

The paediatric oncologist asked specific reproductive questions and assessed his Tanner stage. He had sparse faintly pigmented pubic hair and a testicular volume of 8 ml. He has erections and 'wet dreams' but had not masturbated before. He became very embarrassed having this conversation, and his parents felt that it was not relevant to ask their son these questions.

The oncologist was unsure whether it was appropriate to refer this patient for sperm banking, and he seeks further advise from a fertility colleague.

53.1 Assessment and Consultation

Puberty describes the transition from childhood to adulthood during which time adolescents become sexually mature and are capable of reproduction [1]. In males, this results in a number of physical changes which include the penis and testis getting bigger; hair developing on the face, armpits and pubic areas; the voice becoming deeper; muscles growing and becoming strong; and an increase in height velocity. These changes are coordinated by a complex neuroendocrine mechanism influenced by both genetic and environmental factors [2]. The Tanner scale or stage is a method of defining the stage of physical developments to document the timing and progression of pubertal development. In males, it assesses the development of penis and testicular volume and pubic hair development [3]. The testicular volume is measured using an orchidometer.

The onset of spermatogenesis is an early pubertal event with a wide variation in the onset and timing with the development of secondary sexual characteristics [4]. The median age of spermatogenesis is 13.4 years (range, 11.7–15.3 years) with a median testicular volume of 11.5 ml (range 4.7–19.6 ml) and a public hair distribution of Tanner 1–5 (median, 2.5 on a Tanner scale) [4]. Sperm cryopreservation is very successful in 12–18-year-olds with 88.4% of patients having spermatozoa in their ejaculate and of these 93.4% having motile spermatozoa which are a good enough quality for cryopreservation [5]. Age should not be a limiting factor for referring patients for fertility preservation consultation with fertility experts who can provide expertise in fertility risk and fertility preservation (FP) options as well as assessing a patient's suitability. Patients who are a Tanner 3 or above [6] or who have a testicular volume of greater than 5 ml [5] are ideal candidates, and hence accurate assessment of younger patients is important.

Despite 20 national and international fertility preservation guidelines recommending that fertility risk and options should be discussed with cancer patients, the rates of referral and consultations are still lower than expected. The reproductive needs of younger male patients are similar to older patients; however, there are a number of additional things to consider in the consultation and management of younger children and adolescent young adult (AYA) male patients:

1. *Consultation differences*: AYA patients are eager to receive verbal and written information about their fertility risk and options [7, 8], but both young patients and their parents feel that these discussions should be age appropriate and have support provided [8]. Consultations should also provide information in an honest and respectful manner. Younger adolescent male patients often find the fertility consultation embarrassing, but patients feel less stressed when staff are informal, friendly, not embarrassed, and speak clearly and directly to them [9]. Having

longer consultations which are not rushed and healthcare professionals (HCPs) with expertise and training [10] has been shown to improve the uptake for fertility services and is reported more favourably by patients and parents.
2. *Availability of resources:* Access to age-appropriate FP resources improves patient satisfaction [11]; however, FP educational materials are not consistently provided to patients [12].Although more resources are available about sperm banking, the quality of these resources is very variable, and the readability is often assessed as difficult or complex [13] for younger patients or patients with low health literacy. Paediatric decision aids have been shown to be important for younger patients, but parents and healthcare providers still have concerns about the content and readability [14] in younger patients.
3. *Health literacy of patient:* The reproductive health knowledge and understanding of patients is an important factor required for discussion and understanding about fertility preservation as well as comfort levels of patients. However, the health literacy of AYA will vary depending on access to sexual health education at home and school and family as well as cultural and religious values. The health literacy will also change dependent on the age and maturity of patients. It is very important that before HCPs start having a conversation about fertility preservation they determine patient's reproductive health literacy and adapt the consultations depending on the level of understanding a patient has.
4. *Parental role in sperm banking:* Parents have a very important role in fertility consultations. Many AYA rely on their parents to provide support during the consultations, to summarize the discussions and to take part in decision-making [15]. Parents are also generally involved in organisation of appointments and in some countries for the payment, and so AYA are dependent on them during this process [15]. Both mother and father recommendations and coordination have been showed to be statically significant with AYA men attempting to sperm bank. Patients who discuss the risks and benefits of sperm banking with their parents are also more likely to attempt sperm banking [15].
5. *Healthcare professional's role in oncofertility consultations*: HCPs also play an important role in discussions about fertility risk and fertility options, education of patients and supporting patients and parents through the process [16]. Paediatric oncologists receive little training about oncofertility care [17, 18], and this has an impact on the implementation of FP guidelines and the referral of patients to fertility services. HCPs communication has been shown to influence sperm banking, and when adolescent patients are referred to specialised fertility providers, they are five times more likely to bank sperm [5, 16]. However, HCPs take on different roles, and despite the expertise of nurses and allied health professionals, fertility conversations are still carried out more commonly by clinicians [5, 18, 19]. Many HCPs report a lack of training and comfort level [20] with reproductive consultations, and additional training is required to ensure the multidisciplinary team members in cancer and fertility centres have a good understanding about the reproductive needs of cancer patients and how to adapt oncofertility services for younger patients.
6. *Psychosocial impact of cancer:* The threat of temporary or permanent infertility has been shown to be associated with psychological distress, such as depression and anxiety, in both males and female cancer patients [21, 22]. For younger male patients, the consultation can be very embarrassing and cause additional distress or result in patients declining fertility consultations or not being fully invested in the consultations which may lead to regret at a later time. With age-appropriate support, patients experience less distress and decision regret [23] and feel more positive about the future. It is very important to have counsellors, social workers and psychologists who have expertise in the reproductive concerns of cancer treatment and who can provide psychological and practical support [22, 24, 25]. Psychological support is also required for parents who often experience psychological distress based on actual or potential infertility of their child or the distress of the fertility preservation process or later follow-up and

disclosure. Psychological support is associated with improved patient satisfaction, improvements in decision-making and improvements in patient quality of life.

7. *Who should be present at consultations?* Oncofertility consultations occur very early in the relationship between HCPs, patients and family members. It is unlikely that HCPs know enough about a family to understand individual family's relationships, religious and cultural narratives which influence consultations. Studies have shown that an equal amount of adolescents want parents to be present [26] or to have the consultations without parent's presence. Clinicians treating adolescent patients often want to provide care to adolescents without the parents present [27, 28]. This can lead to conflict with some parents who feel they should be present to provide support and guidance and ensure that they approve of the choices that are given and made. HCPs have to ensure that they give patients the choice about who is present at the start of the consultations and to ensure that patients can make choices without upsetting family members. It would be beneficial to give parents information about why patients may want consultations on their own or with a specific support person.
8. *Assent and consent:* The consent process for fertility preservation can be confronting, depending on national and local regulations and ethical guidelines. The risks and benefits of sperm banking will be discussed, leading to discussion of the use or disposal of semen in the event of a patient's death. This can obviously be very distressing for patients who are about to start initial or relapse treatment. For minors less than 18 years of age, it is standard practice to ensure that they are included in these consultations and understand and agree to the fertility procedures occurring and then assent. Parents will be required to sign the consent form after the assent has been signed, and although it is uncommon, it is possible to have situations when patients and parents have differences of opinions about fertility choices. Ethical situations are considered in a separate chapter.
9. *Legal parameters to consider:* It is a standard practice for clinics to provide pornographic material to assist with adult males producing semen in a very clinical environment. Although the practice may also be useful for underage children, there are a number of ethical, legal and parental issues in this practice which vary depending on the country, and clearer recommendations are required [29]. Clinics may invite patients to bring their own material.

53

53.2 Management

It is important that all cancer patients get an opportunity to discuss the reproductive risk of cancer treatment and possible fertility options even when fertility preservation is not possible or unlikely. This consultation provides additional patient satisfaction even when patients do not have fertility preservation as they have access to reproductive expertise support and follow up.

Despite consultation and assessment, younger male peri-pubertal patients may not be able to produce a sample collected by masturbation, and so other alternate methods can be considered such as testicular sperm extraction [30] (TESE) or electroejaculation [31].

Support during the fertility consultation and sperm banking is important, particularly for young male patients who may be very embarrassed about this process. It is very important for them to understand that their wishes will be respected, information is confidential and that they will be given the time and privacy to collect a sample. Sometimes, in our attempts to support patients, HCPs can make them more anxious by trying to organise a collection on a ward with limited privacy, having staff accompanying patients to the andrology clinic (patients may worry about the conversations they may have or if they will wait outside the room) or making jokes with the intention of reducing the tension but they can inadvertently make patients more anxious.

53.3 Outcome

After discussions between the oncologist and fertility provider, the patient and his parents agreed to be referred to a fertility specialist, and he attended this appointment with his father. The patient demonstrated Tanner stage III development, so semen cryopreservation was thought to be possible although other options of fertility preservation were also discussed.

After time to consider the consultation and age-appropriate resources, the patient and his father had a further consultation to ask further questions, complete the assent and consent forms and have blood taken for serology. On the day of the collection, the patient was overcome by anxiety and initially put off the collection; however after discussion with the AYA nurse practitioner and counsellor, he agreed to come to the fertility centre with his older brother. The patient was reminded that the specimen container did not need to be filled and was reassured that he would be left on his own with no interruptions from his brother or staff members.

A sample was successfully banked and the andrologist was able to confirm viable sperm motility and forms. The patient was given two other appointments so that further samples could be collected and stored.

Clinical Pearls and Pitfalls

- Semen cryopreservation should be offered to all pubertal boys diagnosed with cancer.
- The onset of spermatogenesis is an early pubertal event with a wide variation in the age of onset and development of secondary sexual characteristics, and so male patients in early puberty with a testicular volume greater than 5 ml should be given an opportunity to undertake semen cryopreservation.
- Parents have a vital part to play in organisation of consultation, support and shared decision-making which increases the changes of AYA attempting to sperm bank.
- Clinicians with clear age-appropriate communication provide additional support to patients and improve the chance of cancer patients undertaking fertility preservation and patient satisfaction.
- Younger cancer patients require age-appropriate consultations and support which involves staff having expertise in communicating with younger patients, access to age-appropriate resources and support.

Review Questions and Answers

Q1. How do you assess the suitability of younger boys and adolescents to undertake sperm cryopreservation?

A1. Patients who are a Tanner 3 or above [6] or who have a testicular volume of greater than 5 ml [5] are ideal candidates for sperm cryopreservation.

Q2. What are the components of age-appropriate care that need to be considered when providing fertility preservation consultations to children and adolescents?

A2. Younger cancer patients require age-appropriate consultations and support which involves staff having expertise in communicating with younger patients, access to age-appropriate resources and support. Parents have a vital part to play in organisation of consultation, support and shared decision-making which increases the changes of AYA attempting to sperm bank.

References

1. Kail RV, Cavanaugh JC. Human development: a lifespan view (5th ed.). Wandsworth publishing: Cengage Learning. 2010. ISBN 0495600377. Retrieved March 8th 2018.
2. Choi JH, Yoo HW. Curr Opin Endocrinol Diabetes Obes. 2013;20(20):62–8.
3. Marshall WA, Tanner JM. Variations in the pattern of pubertal changes in boys. Arch Dis Child. 1970; 45(239):13–23. https://doi.org/10.1136/adc.45.239.13. PMC 2020414 . PMID 5440182.
4. Nielsen CT, Skakkebaek NE, Richardson DW, Darling JA, Hunter WM, Jørgensen M, Nielsen A, Ingerslev O, Keiding N, Müller J. Onset of the release of spermatozoa (spermarche) in boys in relation to age, testicular growth, pubic hair, and height. J Clin Endocrinol Metab. 1986;62(3):532–5.
5. Hagenäs I, Jørgensen N, Rechnitzer C, Sommer P, Holm M, Schmiegelow K, Daugaard G, Jacobsen N, Juul A. Clinical and biochemical correlates of successful semen collection for cryopreservation from 12-18-year-old patients: a single-center study of 86 adolescents. Hum Reprod. 2010;25(8):2031–8. https://doi.org/10.1093/humrep/deq147. Epub 2010 Jun 22.
6. Ogle SK, Hobbie WL, Carlson CA, Meadows AT, Reilly MM, Ginberg JP. Sperm banking for adolescents with cancer. J Pediatr Oncol Nurs. 2008;25(2):97–101.

53

7. Ussher JM, Parton C, Perz J. Need for information, honesty and respect: patient perspectives on health care professional's communication about cancer and fertility. Reprod Health. 2018;15(1):2. https://doi.org/10.1186/s12978-017-0441-z.
8. Stinson JN, Jibb LA, Greenberg M, Barrera M, Luca S, White ME, Gupta A. A qualitative study of the impact of cancer on romantic relationships, sexual relationships, and fertility: perspectives of Canadian adolescents and parents during and after treatment. J Adolesc Young Adult Oncol. 2015;4(2):84–90.
9. Crawshaw MA, Glaser AW, Hale JP, Sloper P. Young males' experiences of sperm banking following a cancer diagnosis–a qualitative study. Hum Fertil. 2008;11(4):238–45.
10. Wyns C, Collienne C, Shenfield F, Robert A, Laurent P, Roegiers L, Brichard B. Fertility preservation in the male pediatric population: factors influencing the decision of parents and children. Hum Reprod. 2015;30(9):2022–30. https://doi.org/10.1093/humrep/dev161. Epub 2015 Jul 3.
11. Kelvin JF, Thom B, Benedict C, Carter J, Corcoran S, Dickler MN, Goodman KA, Margolies A, Matasar MJ, ArielaNoy, Goldfarb SB. Cancer and fertility program improves patient satisfaction with information received. J Clin Oncol. 2016;34:1780–6.
12. Quinn GP, Vadaparampil ST, Malo T, Reinecke J, Bower B, Albrecht T, Clayman ML. Oncologists' use of patient educational materials about cancer and fertility preservation. Psycho-Oncology. 2012;21(11):1244–9.
13. Merrick H, Wright E, Pacey A, Eiser C. Finding out about sperm banking: what information is available on line for men diagnosed with cancer? Human Fertil. 2012; 15(3):121–8.
14. Murphy D, Sawczyn KK, Quinn GP. Using a patient-centered approach to develop a fertility preservation brochure for pediatric oncology patients: a pilot study. J Pediatr Adolesc Gynecol. 2012;25(2):114–21.
15. Klosky JL, Flynn JS, Lehmann V, Russell KM, Wang F, Hardin RN, Eddinger JR, Zhang H, Schenck LA, Schover LR. Parental influences on sperm banking attempts among adolescent males newly diagnosed with cancer. Fertil Steril. 2017;108(6):1043–9.
16. Klosky JL, Anderson E, Russel KM, Huang L, Schover L, Simmons JL, Kutteh WH. Provider influences on sperm banking outcomes among adolescent males newly diagnosed with cancer. J Adolesc Health. 2017; 60(3):277–83.
17. Fuchs A, Kashanian JA, Clayman ML, Gosiengfiao Y, Lockart B, Woodruff TK, Brannigan RE. Pediatric oncology Providers' attitudes and practice patterns regarding fertility preservation in adolescent male Cancer patients. J Pediatr Hematol Oncol. 2016;38(2):118–22.
18. King L, Quinn GP, Vadaparampil ST, Miree CA, Wilson C, Clayton H, Zebrack B. Oncology social workers' perceptions of barriers to discussing fertility preservation with cancer patients. Social Work Health Care. 2008;47(4):479–501.
19. Ussher JM, Cummings J, Dryden A, Perz J. Talking about fertility in the context of cancer: health care professional perspectives. Eur J Cancer Care. 2016;25(1):99–111.
20. Quinn GP, Vadaparampil ST, King L, Miree CA, Wilson C, Raj O, Watson J, Lopez A, Albrecht TL. Impact of physician's personal discomfort and patient prognosis on discussion of fertility preservation with young cancer patients. Patient Educ Couns. 2009;77(3):338–43.
21. Ellis SJ, Wakefield CE, McLoone JK, Robertson EG, Cohn RJ. Fertility concerns among child and adolescent cancer survivors and their parents: a qualitative analysis. J Psychosoc Oncol. 2016;34(5):347–62.
22. Lawson AK, Klock SC, Pavone ME, Hirshfeld-Cytron J, Smith KN, Kazer RR. Psychological counseling of female fertility preservation patients. J Psychosoc Oncol. 2015;33(4):333–53.
23. Li N, Jayasinghe Y, Kemertzis MA, Moore P, Peate M. Fertility preservation in pediatric and adolescent oncology patients: the decision-making process of parents. J Adolesc Young Adult Oncol. 2017;6(2):213–22. https://doi.org/10.1089/jayao.2016.0061. Epub 2016 Dec 1.
24. Logan S, Perz J, Ussher JM, Peate M, Anazodo A. Psycho oncology. A systematic review of patient oncofertility support needs in reproductive cancer patients aged 14 to 45 years of age. 2017. https://doi.org/10.1002/pon.4502. [Epub ahead of print] Review.
25. Skaczkowski G, White V, Thompson K, Bibby H, Coory M, Orme LM, Conyers R, Phillips MB, Osborn M, Harrup R, Anazodo A. Factors influencing the provision of fertility counselling and impact on quality of life in adolescents and young adults with cancer. J Psychosocial Oncol. 2018;36(4):484–502.
26. Ginsberg JP, Ogle SK, Tuchman LK, Carlson CA, Reilly MM, Hobbie WL, Rourke M, Zhao H, Meadows AT. Sperm banking for adolescent and young adult cancer patients: sperm quality, patient, and parent perspectives. Pediatr Blood Cancer. 2008;50(3):594–8.
27. Bashore L. Semen preservation in male adolescents and young adults with cancer: one institution's experience. Clin J Oncol Nurs. 2007;11(3):381.
28. de Vries MC, Bresters D, Engberts DP, Wit JM, van Leeuwen E. Attitudes of physicians and parents towards discussing infertility risks and semen cryopreservation with male adolescents diagnosed with cancer. Pediatr Blood Cancer. 2009;53(3):386–91.
29. Crawshaw MA, Glaser AW, Pacey AA. The use of pornographic materials by adolescent male's cancer patients when banking sperm in the UK: legal and ethical dilemmas. Hum Fertil. 2007;10(3):159–63.
30. Schrader M, et al. "Onco-tese": testicular sperm extraction in azoospermic cancer patients before chemotherapy—new guidelines? Urology. 2003;61(2):421–5.
31. Adank MC, van Dorp W, Smit M, et al. Electro ejaculation as a method of fertility preservation in boys diagnosed with cancer: a single –center experience and review of the literature. Fertil Steril. 2014;102:199–205.

Fertility Preservation Approaches to Patients with Leukemic Involvement of the Testes

Michael H. Hsieh

T. K. Woodruff et al. (eds.), *Textbook of Oncofertility Research and Practice*,
https://doi.org/10.1007/978-3-030-02868-8_54

54.1 Assessment and Diagnosis

A 17-year-old boy with relapsed T-cell acute lymphoblastic leukemia is preparing to start re-induction chemotherapy with the goal of undergoing an allogeneic bone marrow transplantation and is considering options for fertility preservation. The patient initially presented at age 13 with abdominal pain, fatigue, and fever. Initial labs were notable for a white blood cell count of 478 K/mcL with 82% blasts, a hemoglobin of 6 g/dL, and platelets of 23,000. He was also found on exam to have splenomegaly and an enlarged, firm right testicle (Fig. 54.1). A chest x-ray showed a large mediastinal mass with a small right pleural effusion. Flow cytometry on his peripheral blood revealed T-cell lymphoblastic leukemia.

54.2 Management

54

Soon after presentation, the patient developed an oxygen requirement and became clinically unstable. A lumbar puncture was performed, steroids were started, and systemic chemotherapy was initiated urgently.

The patient went into remission, with negative minimal residual disease (MRD) testing, at the end of the consolidation therapy (after 3 months of chemotherapy). His testicular disease resolved by the end of the 1st month of treatment. He was doing well with chemotherapy and completed his maintenance chemotherapy as scheduled. However, 2 months after the end of chemotherapy, he presented with pancytopenia and a new left testicular mass. Work-up revealed a bone marrow and testicular relapse. Plans were made to begin re-induction chemotherapy. Due to the high risk nature of relapsed T-cell disease, HLA typing was sent with the plan for a bone marrow transplant in second remission.

An andrologist met with the patient to discuss fertility preservation options. Semen analysis showed an ejaculate volume of 1.8 mL, azoospermia with a positive fructose test, and 3.2 million round cells per mL. Because these findings precluded sperm banking as a fertility preservation option, the patient was enrolled in a testicular tissue cryopreservation study. During anesthesia administered for line placement, the patient underwent a scrotal incision, and a wedge biopsy of the left testis was performed. A portion of the biopsy was sent for permanent sections and flow cytometry analysis. No leukemic cells were seen in the biopsy samples. Most of the remainder of the biopsy was sent for cryopreservation for patient use, and a small portion was used for research purposes.

54.3 Outcome

The patient achieved a second MRD negative remission following his first month of re-induction chemotherapy. He underwent a matched unrelated donor allogeneic transplantation with a Cytoxan and total body irradiation preparatory regimen. He experienced mild acute skin and gastrointestinal graft vs host disease that was medically managed. The patient is now disease-free 2 years after his bone marrow transplant. His testicular tissue remains in cryostorage.

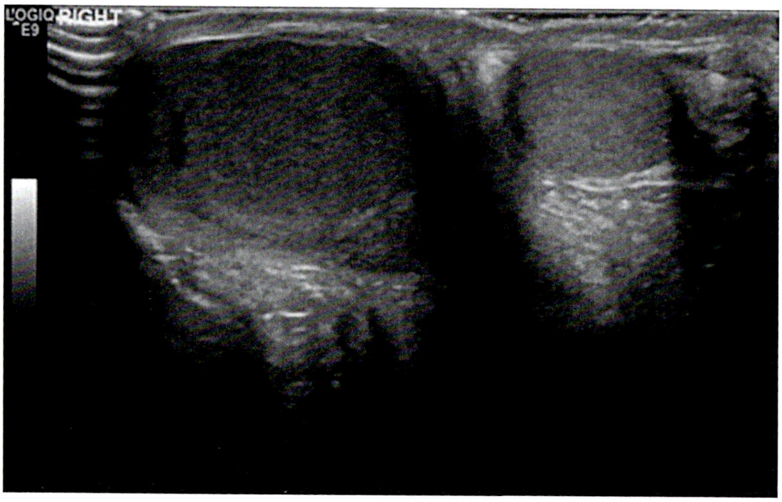

Fig. 54.1 Scrotal ultrasound demonstrated an enlarged right testicle with no distinct intraparenchymal masses

Semen analysis was repeated and revealed an ejaculate volume of 2 mL, 12 million sperm/mL, 30% motility, and 4% normal morphology.

Clinical Pearls and Pitfalls

- Pre-therapy sperm banking remains first choice therapy. Pre-treatment sperm should not be discarded until patient is done with his family. Men should NOT discard if/when sperm return to the ejaculate if they are not done with their family. Many men require IVF even if they have motile sperm in ejaculate post-treatment (could be because of low count, could be because of an unrelated female factor infertility, etc.) and sometimes the pre-treatment sperm is better quality than the post-treatment sperm and may improve their chance of IVF success.
- Patients should have their frozen specimen QC (quality control) reviewed by a male fertility specialist; often the viability post-thaw are poor and additional vials need to be frozen to account for loss. Freezing any specimen is NOT always adequate; viability and quality of what is frozen have to be ensured.
- Testicular tissue cryopreservation is still investigational, whereas testicular sperm cryopreservation is not investigational and can be necessary pre-treatment in men who cannot ejaculate or have obstructed azoospermia.
- There is no standard recommended minimum number of vials that need to be frozen. Patients and providers should plan to maximize the number of vials cryopreserved to maximize the chance of future pregnancy.
- Patients should be prepared to quickly transition to surgical sperm retrieval (electroejaculation or testicular aspiration) if there is any concern with producing an ejaculate or question of obstruction.
- Post-therapy sperm analysis is warranted and should be recommended when the patient is planning a family (e.g., not done for curiosity sake before patient is ready to start trying to get pregnant).
- If the post-treatment semen analysis is abnormal, he should be sent immediately to infertility specialist and his female partner sent to reproductive endocrinologist as her egg reserve/fertility status will largely dictate their treatment options.
- Azoospermia immediately after chemo does not negate the possibility of testicular tissue cryopreservation. Moreover, even men who are still azoospermic after treatment have the option of microTESE.

Review Questions and Answers

Q1. Which of the following is most closely associated with increased likelihood to attempt sperm banking?
(a) Consultation with a fertility specialist
(b) Parent recommendation to bank
(c) Higher Tanner stage
(d) Adolescent history of masturbation
(e) Medical team recommendation to bank

A1. (a)

Q2. Which of the following is true regarding sperm banking via masturbation?
(a) The majority of pubertal males are unable to produce semen prior to cancer treatment
(b) Males must be Tanner V to produce semen via masturbation
(c) Patients with leukemia are unable to produce semen prior to chemotherapy
(d) All males Tanner III and above should be offered sperm banking prior to initiation of chemotherapy
(e) All males Tanner III or above should be offered sperm banking once the cancer has been put into remission

A2. (d)

Further Reading

Burns KC, Hoefgen H, Strine A, Dasgupta R. Fertility preservation options in pediatric and adolescent patients with cancer. Cancer. 2018;124:1867–76. https://doi.org/10.1002/cncr.31255. [Epub ahead of print] Review.

Fernbach A, Lockart B, Armus CL, Bashore LM, Levine J, Kroon L, Sylvain G, Rodgers C. Evidence-based recommendations for fertility preservation options for inclusion in treatment protocols for pediatric and adolescent patients diagnosed with cancer. J Pediatr Oncol Nurs. 2014;31(4):211–22. Epub 2014 May 5. Review.

Klosky JL, Wang F, Russell KM, Zhang H, Flynn JS, Huang L, Wasilewski-Masker K, Landier W, Leonard M, Albritton KH, Gupta AA, Casillas J, Colte P, Kutteh WH, Schover LR. Prevalence and predictors of sperm banking in adolescents newly diagnosed with cancer: examination of adolescent, parent, and provider factors influencing fertility preservation outcomes. J Clin Oncol. 2017;35(34):3830–6. https://doi.org/10.1200/JCO.2016.70.4767. Epub 2017 Oct 4.

Stein DM, Victorson DE, Choy JT, Waimey KE, Pearman TP, Smith K, Dreyfuss J, Kinahan KE, Sadhwani D, Woodruff TK, Brannigan RE. Fertility preservation preferences and perspectives among adult male survivors of pediatric cancer and their parents. J Adolesc Young Adult Oncol. 2014;3(2):75–82.

Testicular Tissue Cryopreservation Prior to Hematopoietic Stem Cell Transplant: Two Case Studies Illustrating Family Decision-Making

Emilie K. Johnson, Nicoleta Arva, and Barbara A. Lockart

T. K. Woodruff et al. (eds.), *Textbook of Oncofertility Research and Practice*,
https://doi.org/10.1007/978-3-030-02868-8_55

55.1 Introduction

Hematopoietic stem cell transplant (HSCT) is used for treatment of both oncologic and non-oncologic conditions (e.g., thalassemia, sickle cell disease). Infertility is a known late effect of HSCT. Prepubertal status does not protect male patients from gonadotoxicity of either the chemotherapy agents used in HSCT conditioning regimens or from the effects of total body irradiation [1]. Spermatogenesis (development of mature sperm) does not begin until puberty. Therefore, the only fertility preservation option available to a prepubertal male is testicular tissue cryopreservation (TTC), an experimental option currently offered at limited number of pediatric institutions. TTC is investigational and thus should occur as part of an institutional review board-approved research protocol. Although TTC is experimental, a recent study indicates that most parents and patients will pursue TTC when faced with a diagnosis requiring gonadotoxic therapy such as HSCT [2].

There are many challenges related to offering TTC. Given the limited number of institutions offering TTC, access to the procedure may be limited due to distance, insurance coverage issues, challenges coordinating care between multiple institutions, and lack of awareness of pediatric institutions offering TTC. For families who are being treated for an oncologic diagnosis at a center that does not offer TTC, the burden of decision-making about TTC, while also establishing care with a new medical team and then returning to their primary institution, may be overwhelming. Additionally, decision-making about TTC occurs at a time when families are vulnerable and fearful about their child's future. If patient has a hereditary condition, genetic counseling prior to TTC to assess understanding of inheritance is imperative and continues as the patient matures.

Culture, religion, language, and health literacy all intersect when counseling families about prepubertal TTC prior to HSCT. Guiding families through the decision-making process requires dialogue between the referring medical team and the fertility preservation team to appropriately assess risk of infertility. The goals of counseling about TTC are to provide streamlined care with an awareness of the many factors which impact a family's decision-making and to have families feel a sense of control about their final decision about whether or not to pursue TTC [2]. The two cases below highlight important considerations and lessons learned from counseling families about possible TTC prior to HSCT.

Case 1: Fertility Preservation Chosen

Case Description

Patient 1 is an 11-year-old male from Mexico who was referred from an outside institution for consultation about possible TTC prior to HSCT. He was diagnosed with standard risk pre-B acute lymphoblastic leukemia at 5 years old and completed treatment at 8 years old. Gonadotoxic chemotherapy at that time included cyclophosphamide (1000 mg/m^2). No radiation therapy was administered. At 11 years old, he was diagnosed with acute myeloblastic leukemia and scheduled to undergo HSCT and total body irradiation.

This case presented several challenges for the family and healthcare providers. It is not clear how development of a second malignancy affects parents' decision-making ability regarding possible TTC, compared with considering TTC in the setting of a primary oncologic diagnosis. HSCT was planned for a tertiary hospital not affiliated with the referring institution or the hospital offering TTC, requiring coordination of care between three institutions that were located several hours away from each other. The impact on the family when traveling hours for care must be considered, as they juggle time away from work, childcare issues, and costs with medical care.

Counseling Process

The patient's primary oncologist contacted the Fertility Preservation Advanced Practice Registered Nurse (FP-APRN) at our institution to determine patient eligibility for TTC. Once eligibility was confirmed, the primary oncologist asked the family to contact the FP-APRN to schedule a consultation. The family's primary language is Spanish; thus, all counseling was performed with the aid of an interpreter. A phone consult with the FP-APRN was completed, and the parents preliminarily decided to pursue TTC based on that conversation. Prior to the day of surgery, the parents and patient met with the FP-APRN and pediatric urologist who was to perform the procedure. The parents were engaged in the consult process but struggled with burden of making this decision about undergoing an elective procedure for experimental TTC on behalf of their son. During the consult, the patient's father paused the discussion between the healthcare providers and the family. He then asked the patient if he trusted his parents to make this decision for him. The child responded "yes," and the parents felt comfortable proceeding and consented to the procedure. TTC was performed the following day.

Procedure and Outcome

An open testicular wedge biopsy was performed as an outpatient procedure under general anesthesia. A transverse incision was made over the left hemiscrotum, the testis was delivered. The tunica vaginalis over the testis was opened and the testicle exposed. A wedge of testicular parenchyma was sharply excised (◘ Fig. 55.1). Tunica albuginea was closed using absorbable suture, and the scrotum closed in multiple layers. There were no intraoperative or postoperative complications. A portion of the wedge was sent to pathology and a portion sent for experimental TTC. Testicular pathology revealed peripubertal testicular parenchyma with no significant histopathological changes. Microscopic section from the testicle revealed peripubertal testicular parenchyma, with no evidence of malignancy. Testicular parenchyma was composed of seminiferous cords as well as tubules with lumen development, containing spermatogonia, but without evidence of progressive spermatogenesis (◘ Fig. 55.2).

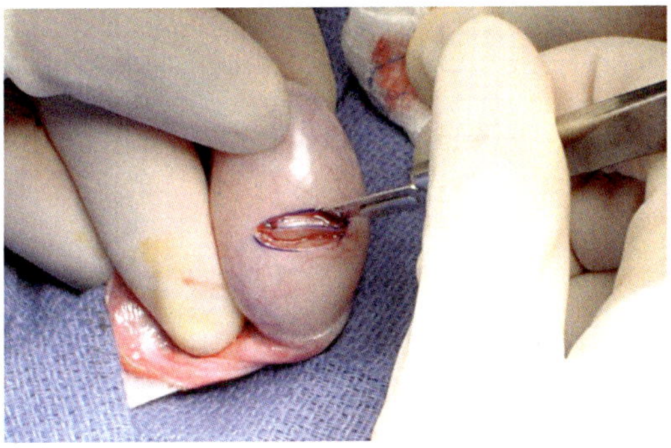

◘ **Fig. 55.1** Open biopsy for testicular tissue cryopreservation. (Image courtesy of Duong Tu, MD)

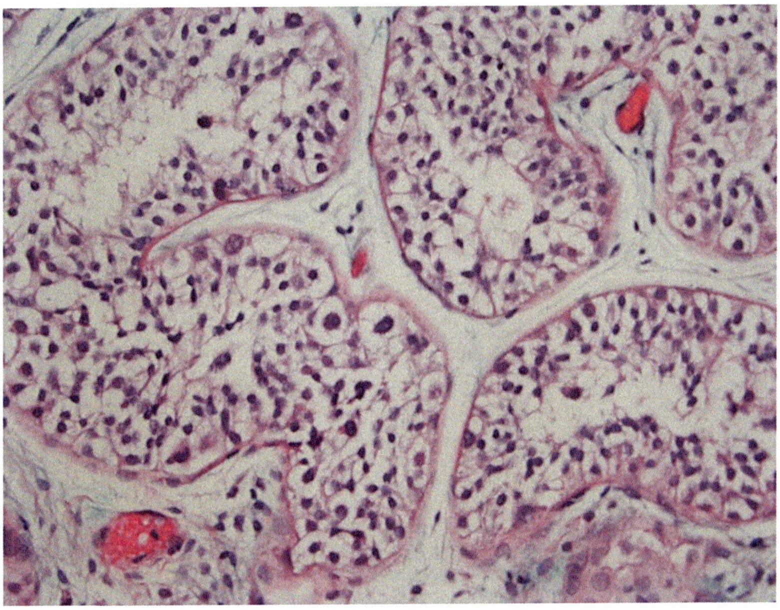

◘ **Fig. 55.2** Hematoxylin and eosin-stained testicular histopathologic specimen, 400× – peripubertal testicular parenchyma, no progressive spermatogenesis

Case 2: Fertility Preservation Not Chosen

Case Description

Patient 2 is 20-month-old male from Mali with a history of sickle cell disease who was referred to FP team from an outside hospital for consideration of TTC prior to HSCT. The parents were considering HSCT to minimize complications of sickle cell disease and improve life expectancy. In meetings with the stem cell team at the referring hospital, the parents identified the risk of infertility as their biggest concern about proceeding with HSCT. This patient had two factors which may adversely impact his fertility. The conditioning regimen prior to HSCT was planned to include melphalan, which is a known gonadotoxic agent. Additionally, men with sickle cell disease are at risk for infertility due to hypogonadism, sperm abnormalities, and erectile dysfunction [3].

Counseling Process

The transplant team from the referring hospital counseled the parents on several occasions about the risk of infertility associated with HSCT. A phone consult was performed by the FP-APRN and the father. The parents initially declined to meet with the FP team due to the distance from the hospital. Upon the further requests of their transplant team, the family reconsidered and proceeded to travel to our institution, planning for their son to undergo TTC.

The FP-APRN and pediatric urologist met with the parents to discuss TTC as an experimental FP method for patients undergoing HSCT. Mother spoke French and Father spoke English and French. Institutional policy to proceed with TTC requires both mother's and father's consent, so a French medical interpreter was utilized for the consultation. Parents stated they understood sickle cell disease is a hereditary condition and TTC would not alter the risk of inheritance. For TTC to be performed, a wedge resection is completed (as described in ► Case 1), but the consent states an orchiectomy may be performed if medically necessary. The father struggled with any possibility of orchiectomy and wanted assurances that an orchiectomy would not be performed. The parents and surgeon discussed the rare scenarios in which an orchiectomy would be indicated (i.e., unexpected intraoperative damage to the testis, volume of tissue needed for TTC too great for wedge resection to be possible). Ultimately, the parents declined TTC because the potential for orchiectomy, however unlikely, was unacceptable.

55.2 Challenges in Counseling Families About TTC

TTC is an experimental procedure with no guarantee of success. For prepubertal patients, it is the only FP option available. Research shows that majority of parents see benefit to TTC, even though it is unknown whether the tissue will be able to be used for reproduction in the future [2]. Counseling requires healthcare providers to discuss risks and benefits and allow families to make their decision. TTC is offered at few pediatric institutions and most families will need to leave their home institution to complete the procedure. Limited access to services requires families to develop a relationship with another medical team during a time of great stress. Cost of travel, loss of income, and impact on the family are not insignificant.

Access to fertility preservation, including TTC, is limited by numerous factors. Barriers identified by physicians include concerns about family's ability to pay for services, urgency to starting treatment, and survival potential [4]. Pediatric oncologists, APRNs, and registered nurses state that lack of educational resources and knowledge of available FP services impacts their ability to educate families [5], making it challenging to offer TTC to all patients who might be eligible. Institutions providing FP services have a responsibility to inform both healthcare providers and families of the services available.

The impact of gender, culture, and language on decision-making about TCC must also be considered when counseling families. Studies examining fertility preservation practice in adult patients suggest a patient's race may influence counseling patients receive; in several studies, Caucasian patients were more likely to receive information on FP options than non-whites [6, 7]. Healthcare providers have a responsibility to educate all patients on the risk of infertility and options for FP [8].

Clinical Pearls and Pitfalls

- Families of prepubertal boys undergoing HSCT will consider, and often pursue, experimental TTC.
- Information about TTC must be given to families in their native language, by a medical interpreter.
- Cultural differences and language barriers can make the counseling process more difficult but should not preclude counselling about TTC for otherwise eligible patients.
- Families may struggle with parental proxy decision-making given that TTC requires an elective procedure with risks to the patient, and there is no guarantee the tissue will be able to be used in the future.
- Possibility of transmission of a genetic condition to offspring should be discussed in any consultation regarding possible TTC.
- For patients considering TTC at an institution remote to where they live, an initial phone consultation can be helpful, but is not a substitute for in-person communication.
- Other challenges related to prepubertal TTC include:
  - Cost of the procedure and storage.
  - Cost and time burden of travel.
  - Coordination of care between teams providing HSCT and TTC.

Review Questions and Answers

Q1. Which of the following statements is incorrect regarding prepubertal TTC for patients undergoing HSCT?

(a) Families should be counseled regarding TTC in their native language.

(b) TTC is experimental because it is unknown whether conditioning regimens for HSCT put patients at risk for infertility.

(c) TTC generally requires an open testicular biopsy under general anesthesia.

(d) TTC is currently only available at a few pediatric centers in the United States.

(e) TTC is experimental because it is unknown whether the tissue will be able to be used in the future.

A1. (b)

Q2. True or False? Recent research indicates that Caucasian patients may be more likely to be provided fertility preservation counseling compared with non-white patients

A2. True

Q3. True or False? Patients undergoing HSCT for non-oncologic conditions are not eligible for TTC

A3. False

References

1. Borgmann-Staudt A, Rendtorff R, Reinmuth S, Hohmann C, Keil T, Schuster FR, et al. Fertility after allogeneic haematopoietic stem cell transplantation in childhood and adolescence. Bone Marrow Transplant. 2012;47(2):271–6.
2. Ginsberg JP, Li Y, Carlson CA, Gracia CR, Hobbie WL, Miller VA, et al. Testicular tissue cryopreservation in prepubertal male children: an analysis of parental decision-making. Pediatr Blood Cancer. 2014;61(9):1673–8.
3. Smith-Whitley K. Reproductive issues in sickle cell disease. Hematol Am Soc Hematol Educ Program. 2014;2014(1):418–24.
4. Vadaparampil S, Quinn G, King L, Wilson C, Nieder M. Barriers to fertility preservation among pediatric oncologists. Patient Educ Couns. 2008;72(3):402–10.
5. Fuchs A, Kashanian JA, Clayman ML, Gosiengfiao Y, Lockart B, Woodruff TK, et al. Pediatric oncology providers' attitudes and practice patterns regarding fertility preservation in adolescent male cancer patients. J Pediatr Hematol Oncol. 2016;38(2):118–22.
6. Salsman JM, Yanez B, Smith KN, Beaumont JL, Snyder MA, Barnes K, et al. Documentation of fertility preservation discussions for young adults with cancer: examining compliance with treatment guidelines. J Natl Compr Cancer Netw. 2016;14(3):301–9.
7. Shnorhavorian M, Harlan LC, Smith AW, Keegan TH, Lynch CF, Prasad PK, et al. Fertility preservation knowledge, counseling, and actions among adolescent and young adult patients with cancer: a population-based study. Cancer. 2015;121(19):3499–506.
8. Loren AW, Mangu PB, Beck LN, Brennan L, Magdalinski AJ, Partridge AH, et al. Fertility preservation for patients with cancer: American Society of Clinical Oncology clinical practice guideline update. J Clin Oncol. 2013;31(19):2500–10.

Adolescent Testicular Sperm Retrieval

I-Shen Huang, Robert E. Brannigan, and Barbara A. Lockart

T. K. Woodruff et al. (eds.), *Textbook of Oncofertility Research and Practice*,
https://doi.org/10.1007/978-3-030-02868-8_56

Case Presentation

A 16-year-old male presented to a community hospital with 2 weeks of decreased urinary flow, which ultimately progressed to urinary retention. An indwelling Foley catheter was placed, and initial evaluation revealed no laboratory abnormalities. Magnetic resonance imaging (MRI) of the abdomen and pelvis demonstrated an enhancing mass within the anterior prostate measuring 4.2 × 5.2 × 4.6 cm. A right femoral head lesion was also noted. Percutaneous biopsy of the prostatic lesion confirmed a diagnosis of embryonal rhabdomyosarcoma, and further staging evaluation revealed Stage 4, high-risk disease. The patient was transferred to a tertiary-care pediatric hospital for treatment with the following chemotherapeutic regimen: vincristine, irinotecan, ifosfamide, etoposide, doxorubicin, cyclophosphamide, dactinomycin, and human IgG1 monoclonal antibody. The total cyclophosphamide equivalent dose (CED) for the planned treatment regimen was 16,290 mg/m^2.

Prior to initiation of therapy, the oncology team counseled the patient and his family regarding the potential impact of treatment upon his future fertility and options for fertility preservation. The patient and his family expressed a strong desire to pursue fertility preservation prior to initiation of gonadotoxic chemotherapy. Sperm banking with cryopreservation through masturbation was not feasible due to the presence of the indwelling Foley catheter, which the medical team determined could not be removed.

A reproductive urologist was consulted to discuss the feasibility of testicular sperm extraction (TESE). Upon physical examination, the urologist noted that the patient had well-developed secondary sex characteristics consistent with Tanner stage 4. Bilateral testes had a normal, slightly firm consistency, measured approximately 18 mL, and were without masses. Serum hormone levels (follicle stimulating hormone, luteinizing hormone, and testosterone) were all within normal limits.

56.1 Assessment

Fertility is an important, though often overlooked, aspect of care for adolescent and young adult men with newly diagnosed malignancy. The majority of these men desire biological children in the future, yet a large proportion of these patients are not informed about the effect of treatment on their future fertility potential [1]. While most oncologists agree that fertility counseling and sperm banking should be offered to men with newly diagnosed malignancy, only half of physicians actually initiate this discussion when caring for patients with a new cancer diagnosis [2]. The American Society of Clinical Oncology recommends that providers caring for men of reproductive age with a newly diagnosed malignancy should discuss fertility at the earliest possible opportunity, prior to initiation of treatment [3].

Sperm cryopreservation obtained from a freshly ejaculated semen specimen is the most reliable and least invasive method of fertility preservation. Specimens can be conveniently collected at home or in the outpatient clinic without any morbidity to the patient. Physical examination alone is sufficient for patient evaluation prior to attempted ejaculation, as ancillary testing such as hormonal evaluation or imaging does not reliably predict sperm in the ejaculate [4].

Assessment of sexual development and progression of puberty is an essential component of patient evaluation prior to fertility preservation. Spermarche is an early pubertal event, occurring at a median age of 13.4 years, at which time adolescents may display a wide range of secondary sex characteristics [5]. Physical examination and Tanner stage may provide insight regarding spermatogenesis. A detailed sexual history with focus on prior nocturnal emission or experience with self-stimulation and masturbation will further elucidate whether the patient is capable of producing a semen specimen for cryopreservation.

In patients who are incapable of producing a semen specimen or in whom psychosocial, ethical, or religious concerns are barriers to masturbation, additional procedures may be utilized to induce ejaculation for fertility preservation. Penile vibratory stimulation (PVS) has been employed successfully in adolescent boys with hematologic malignancy and is an attractive option as it can be performed in the outpatient setting without general anesthesia [6]. Electroejaculation (EEJ) requires general anesthetic but has also achieved high rates of success in this patient population [7–9].

When azoospermia is present in an ejaculated specimen or a semen specimen cannot be obtained, surgical sperm retrieval can be employed.

56

Microdissection testicular sperm extraction (microTESE) is a minimally invasive procedure that has been used for fertility preservation in both adults and adolescents [10]. Testicular tissue is harvested through a small scrotal incision with the assistance of an operating microscope, which enables identification of seminiferous tubules most likely to contain viable sperm. While a number of factors including preprocedural hormone levels and type of malignancy may impact success, approximately 33% of adolescents who undergo microTESE will have successful sperm retrieval [10].

56.2 Management

The reproductive urology team discussed the risks and benefits of microTESE with the patient and his family. The procedure carries a low risk of complications including hematoma, wound infection, testicular fibrosis, and long-term decrease in serum testosterone [11]. The patient elected to proceed with sperm extraction, which was performed concurrently with central venous port placement.

Chemotherapy was initiated 3 days following the TESE procedure. The patient experienced no complications, and his wound healed without issue. He subsequently received external beam radiation therapy totaling 50.4 Gy to the prostate gland and the right femoral head.

56.3 Outcomes

The patient had successful sperm retrieval with four vials of sperm cryopreserved. He tolerated his course of chemotherapy and radiation with minimal adverse effects and had a complete response. At 1-year follow up, he had no evidence of residual or recurrent disease. Semen analysis at 1 and 2 years following chemotherapy revealed persistent azoospermia.

56.4 Summary

A 16-year-old adolescent male presented with urinary retention and was found to have prostatic rhabdomyosarcoma. The optimal treatment regimen entailed high-dose alkylating agents and radiotherapy posing risks to his future fertility. After consultation with a multi-disciplinary team including oncologists and a reproductive urologist, the patient opted to proceed with microTESE prior to initiation of chemotherapy. Sperm extraction was successful, and the patient proceeded immediately to treatment without delay.

Clinical Pearls and Pitfalls

- Consider fertility preservation in any male with a new cancer diagnosis, regardless of malignancy or patient age.
- A multi-disciplinary approach with inclusion of a reproductive urologist will optimize outcomes.
- Physical examination is paramount, specifically testicular size and secondary sex characteristics.
- In adolescents who cannot ejaculate or in whom ethical, religious, or psychosocial barriers to ejaculation exist, PVS or EEJ may be utilized.
- microTESE should be offered to adolescents with azoospermia who desire fertility preservation.
- Even if a patient starts on a "fertility-friendly" chemotherapy protocol, sperm cryopreservation should be considered because treatment sometimes progresses to more spermatotoxic regimens.

Review Questions and Answers

Q1. What is the dose-dependent impact of chemotherapy and radiotherapy upon long-term fertility potential?

A1. Spermatogonia and spermatogonial stem cells are highly chemosensitive, rendering these cells vulnerable to a variety of chemotherapeutic agents [12]. The deleterious effect on spermatogenesis is most pronounced among the alkylating agents, where there is a dose-dependent risk of gonadotoxicity with increasing cumulative doses. The cyclophosphamide equivalent dose (CED) has emerged as the best predictor of long-term fertility in men who receive therapy with alkylating agents [13]. Normospermia is typically seen in patients with CED less than 4000 mg/m^2, though approximately 10% of patients with this low-dose exposure will have either oligospermia or azoospermia. Radiation therapy also impairs spermatogenesis by inducing DNA damage or apoptosis in spermatogonia [14]. Spermatogenesis may be impaired with doses as low as 0.15 Gy. Reversible azoospermia can result from doses of 0.35 Gy, and permanent azoospermia typically results from cumulative doses of >2.5 Gy. Semen parameters nadir approximately 4–6 months after therapy, and recovery of spermatogenesis, when present, may occur up to 18 months following treatment [15, 16].

Q2. What are the outcomes of sperm retrieval if non-obstructive azoospermia persists after conclusion of therapy?

A2. MicroTESE is the preferred approach to non-obstructive azoospermia in this setting, as it typically yields higher success than conventional TESE [17]. In men with azoospermia secondary to alkylating agents, microTESE has a 37% success rate for sperm retrieval [18].

Q3. What is the risk of birth defects in the offspring of men with a history of cancer?

A3. For men receiving chemotherapy or radiotherapy, there may be concern regarding transmission of germline mutations to future offspring. A large study of adult cancer survivors found no difference in the incidence of cytogenetic syndromes, single-gene disorders, and simple malformations between the offspring of cancer survivors and those of healthy controls (3.4% versus 3.1%) [19]. Nonetheless, patients are typically encouraged to defer family planning until approximately 1–2 years after completion of therapy in order to reduce the perceived risk of transient DNA damage or aneuploidy during the period immediately following therapy.

Q4. What are the success rates with use of cryopreserved sperm for assisted reproductive technologies (ART) in patients with malignancy?

A4. For men who do not have return of sperm in the ejaculate after the completion of cancer therapy, cryopreserved sperm are typically used for efforts at conception with in vitro fertilization (IVF)/ intracytoplasmic sperm injection (ICSI). The IVF success rates for patients banking sperm prior to cancer therapy are quite good, with one study reporting fertilization rates up to 71.4%, though these rates were lower among men with specific malignancies such as testis cancer or lymphoma [20]. An additional series reported a 66% live birth rate when cryopreserved sperm were used for IVF and intracytoplasmic sperm injection (ICSI) [21].

References

1. Schover LR, Brey K, Lichtin A, Lipshultz LI, Jeha S. Knowledge and experience regarding cancer, infertility, and sperm banking in younger male survivors. J Clin Oncol. 2002;20(7):1880–9.
2. Schover LR, Brey K, Lichtin A, Lipshultz LI, Jeha S. Oncologists' attitudes and practices regarding banking sperm before cancer treatment. J Clin Oncol. 2002;20(7):1890–7.
3. Oktay K, Harvey BE, Partridge AH, Quinn GP, Reinecke J, Taylor HS, et al. Fertility preservation in patients with cancer: ASCO clinical practice guideline update. J Clin Oncol. 2018;36(19):1994–2001.
4. van Casteren NJ, Dohle GR, Romijn JC, de Muinck Keizer-Schrama SMPF, Weber RFA, van den Heuvel-Eibrink MM. Semen cryopreservation in pubertal boys before gonadotoxic treatment and the role of endocrinologic evaluation in predicting sperm yield. Fertil Steril. 2008;90(4):1119–25.
5. Nielsen CT, Skakkebaek NE, Richardson DW, Darling JA, Hunter WM, Jørgensen M, et al. Onset of the release of spermatozoa (spermarche) in boys in relation to age, testicular growth, pubic hair, and height. J Clin Endocrinol Metab. 1986;62(3):532–5.

6. Schmiegelow ML, Sommer P, Carlsen E, Sønksen JO, Schmiegelow K, Müller JR. Penile vibratory stimulation and electroejaculation before anticancer therapy in two pubertal boys. J Pediatr Hematol Oncol. 1998;20(5):429–30.
7. Meng X, Fan L, Wang T, Wang S, Wang Z, Liu J. Electroejaculation combined with assisted reproductive technology in psychogenic anejaculation patients refractory to penile vibratory stimulation. Transl Androl Urol. 2018;7(Suppl 1):S17–22.
8. Gat I, Toren A, Hourvitz A, Raviv G, Band G, Baum M, et al. Sperm preservation by electroejaculation in adolescent cancer patients. Pediatr Blood Cancer. 2014;61(2):286–90.
9. Adank MC, van Dorp W, Smit M, van Casteren NJ, Laven JSE, Pieters R, et al. Electroejaculation as a method of fertility preservation in boys diagnosed with cancer: a single-center experience and review of the literature. Fertil Steril. 2014;102(1):199–205.e1.
10. Berookhim BM, Mulhall JP. Outcomes of operative sperm retrieval strategies for fertility preservation among males scheduled to undergo cancer treatment. Fertil Steril. 2014;101(3):805–11.
11. Deruyver Y, Vanderschueren D, Van der Aa F. Outcome of microdissection TESE compared with conventional TESE in non-obstructive azoospermia: a systematic review. Andrology. 2014;2(1):20–4.
12. Smart E, Lopes F, Rice S, Nagy B, Anderson RA, Mitchell RT, et al. Chemotherapy drugs cyclophosphamide, cisplatin and doxorubicin induce germ cell loss in an in vitro model of the prepubertal testis. Sci Rep. 2018;8(1):1773.
13. Green DM, Liu W, Kutteh WH, Ke RW, Shelton KC, Sklar CA, et al. Cumulative alkylating agent exposure and semen parameters in adult survivors of childhood cancer: a report from the St Jude Lifetime Cohort Study. Lancet Oncol. 2014;15(11):1215–23.
14. Grewenig A, Schuler N, Rübe CE. Persistent DNA damage in spermatogonial stem cells after fractionated low-dose irradiation of testicular tissue. Int J Radiat Oncol Biol Phys. 2015;92(5):1123–31.
15. Carlsen E, Andersson A-M, Petersen JH, Skakkebaek NE. History of febrile illness and variation in semen quality. Hum Reprod. 2003;18(10):2089–92.
16. Trottmann M, Becker AJ, Stadler T, Straub J, Soljanik I, Schlenker B, et al. Semen quality in men with malignant diseases before and after therapy and the role of cryopreservation. Eur Urol. 2007;52(2):355–67.
17. Schlegel PN. Testicular sperm extraction: microdissection improves sperm yield with minimal tissue excision. Hum Reprod. 1999;14(1):131–5.
18. Hsiao W, Stahl PJ, Osterberg EC, Nejat E, Palermo GD, Rosenwaks Z, et al. Successful treatment of post-chemotherapy azoospermia with microsurgical testicular sperm extraction: the Weill Cornell experience. J Clin Oncol. 2011;29(12):1607–11.
19. Byrne J, Rasmussen SA, Steinhorn SC, Connelly RR, Myers MH, Lynch CF, et al. Genetic disease in offspring of long-term survivors of childhood and adolescent cancer. Am J Hum Genet. 1998;62(1):45–52.
20. Depalo R, Falagario D, Masciandaro P, Nardelli C, Vacca MP, Capuano P, et al. Fertility preservation in males with cancer: 16-year monocentric experience of sperm banking and post-thaw reproductive outcomes. Ther Adv Med Oncol. 2016;8(6):412–20.
21. Chiba K, Tanaka M, Ishida T, Sumii K, Fukuda T, Okada K, et al. Mp07-18 the usage rate of semen cryopreservation before cancer treatment. J Urol. 2018;199(4):e94–5.

Spontaneous Conception in a Breast Cancer Woman Carrying a BRCA2 Mutation: When Two Children Are Not Enough

Teresa Almeida-Santos, Margarida Brito, and Ana Paula Sousa

T. K. Woodruff et al. (eds.), *Textbook of Oncofertility Research and Practice*,
https://doi.org/10.1007/978-3-030-02868-8_57

Case Presentation

In 2013, a 34-year-old carrier of a *BRCA2* mutation presented with a 4 mm suspicious retroareolar nodular lesion in the left breast, diagnosed in her annual combined magnetic resonance and mammography screening. Both the right breast and axillas were normal.

57.1 Assessment and Diagnosis

An "invasive carcinoma NOS, grade 2, estrogen receptor (ER) and progesterone receptor (PR) 100% positive, human epidermal growth factor receptor 2 (HER-2) SISH negative" was found in the ultrasound-guided biopsy, and the systemic staging work-up excluded metastatic disease.

Considering the hereditary risk, a left mastectomy and contralateral prophylactic mastectomy was decided and so a nipple-areola-sparing mastectomy with immediate breast reconstruction and a sentinel node biopsy was carried out. Pathologic analysis revealed a 20 mm grade 3 invasive carcinoma, without lymphovascular invasion and clear surgical margins. The sentinel node was negative for carcinoma cells, and the final tumor staging was pT1cN0snM0 (stage IA, AJCC 2010). Besides, a 6 mm "ductal carcinoma in situ, intermediate grade, ER 100% positive" was found in the right breast.

57.2 Management

Since the tumor was poorly differentiated (grade 3), adjuvant chemotherapy was decided. Despite having already two children, the patient desired a third child, so she was referred to a fertility specialist for discussion of fertility preservation options. After ovarian stimulation with gonadotropins and letrozol, eight oocytes were retrieved and vitrified. Due to a mastectomy skin flap necrosis, chemotherapy with four cycles of TC regimen (Docetaxel 75 mg/m^2 and Cyclophosphamide 600 mg/m^2 Day 1 every 21 days) was delayed until 6 weeks after surgery.

Endocrine therapy with tamoxifen and monthly goserelin was initiated at 6 months, after recovery from chemotherapy-induced amenorrhea.

57.3 Outcome

After completing 3 years of tamoxifen, although informed of the lack of evidence to support the safety of early interruption of endocrine therapy, the patient decided to try to get pregnant and conceived spontaneously 5 months later giving birth in 2017 to a 39-week healthy baby. The patient reinitiated tamoxifen and is currently waiting for bilateral prophylactic salpingo-oophorectomy.

Clinical Pearls and Pitfalls

- This case highlights the need to discuss fertility preservation in young cancer patients, even if they already have children. This patient, despite already having two children, desired a third child before undergoing prophylactic surgery.
- After surgery for an estrogen-dependent breast cancer, the patient underwent ovarian stimulation for oocyte banking which did not impact the prognosis. She later decided to interrupt tamoxifen treatment in order to try to conceive spontaneously.

Review Questions and Answers

Q1. Why should fertility preservation options be discussed even in patients that already have children?

A1. All guidelines recommend that infertility risk after cancer treatment and fertility preservation options should be discussed with *every* cancer patient before starting gonadotoxic treatment. In fact, the healthcare provider should not assume that fertility is not an important issue for patients that already have children.

Q2. What are the risks involved in ovarian stimulation in hormone receptor-positive breast cancer patients?

A2. Evidence is still limited, but several studies have shown that the co-administration of aromatase inhibitors namely letrozol can keep estrogen levels similar to spontaneous pre-ovulatory levels in most women undergoing multiple follicular development for oocyte cryopreservation. So, after discussing this issue with the patient, the ovarian stimulation can be done with the association of letrozol.

Q3. How can we select breast cancer patients that will become infertile because of ovarian gonadotoxicity of chemotherapy?

A3. Although several markers have been studied (age, AMH, AFC), none of them has proved to be reliable enough to discriminate the patients that will enter premature ovarian failure after chemotherapy. Moreover, even if there are chemotherapy regimens that seem to be less gonadotoxic, it is advisable to discuss with every patient the advantages and disadvantages of oocyte banking, taking into account her age and ovarian reserve.

Q4. What are the risks of prematurely interrupting hormone treatment to allow pregnancy?

A4. The interruption of hormonal treatment must be discussed with the oncologist. If tamoxifen is interrupted, pregnancy should not be attempetd in 3 months to avoid teratogenicity. Tamoxifen treatment can be reinitiated after pregnancy.

Case Studies: Pediatric Female Fertility Preservation

Contents

Fertility Preservation in a Premenarchal Girl

Ksenya Shliakhsitsava, Chelsea Webb Fox, and H. Irene Su

T. K. Woodruff et al. (eds.), *Textbook of Oncofertility Research and Practice*,
https://doi.org/10.1007/978-3-030-02868-8_58

Case Presentation

A 13-year-old girl with severe eczema and dermatitis since infancy; recurrent skin, ear, and throat infections; and plantar warts was diagnosed with DOCK8 deficiency. DOCK8 deficiency is a rare autosomal recessive form of Hyper-IgE syndrome (incidence <1:1,000,000) associated with early mortality due to sepsis and infectious complications [7]. While treatment has focused on prevention of infections, bone marrow transplantation (BMT) using myeloablative conditioning protocols has been described as a curative approach for this deadly disease [8].

Following counseling, the family desired to participate in a DOCK8 deficiency clinical trial at the National Institutes of Health using a reduced-intensity conditioning regimen with fludarabine and busulfan prior to allogeneic hematopoietic stem cell transplant [1]. As part of her BMT counseling, the patient and her family were referred by the pediatric oncology team to reproductive endocrinology to discuss fertility risk and fertility preservation options. The oncology team provided estimated cumulative doses for the conditioning regimen.

The patient and her family presented to the reproductive endocrinology team. She reported thelarche 1 year prior, adrenarche around the same time, and no menarche. Maternal age for menarche was 15. The patient reported no prior sexual intercourse and denied smoking, alcohol, and drug use. Her current medications included antibiotics and inhaled steroids and beta-agonist for asthma. Her surgical and family history was non-contributory. She verbalized her desire to have children in the future, and her mother reported that this is a longstanding wish for the patient.

58.1 Assessment and Diagnosis

58

On exam, we observed a well-nourished girl weighing 48 kg with a height of 163 cm (BMI 18.2). She had Tanner stage 2–3 breast development, Tanner stage 2 pubic hair development, and normal external female genitalia. A transabdominal pelvic ultrasound demonstrated an anteverted uterus, a normal vagina, and two ovaries that were easily visible. The right ovary had an antral follicle count of 5, with the largest follicle measuring 9 mm, and the left ovary had an antral follicle count of 6. No abnormalities were observed on ultrasound. Vaginal exam and transvaginal ultrasound were not performed in this patient to minimize patient discomfort as this exam would not additionally impact her fertility preservation care. A hormone assessment revealed an AMH level of 0.95 ng/mL, an estradiol level of 65 pg/mL, a FSH level of 5.0 IU/L, and LH level of 2.9 IU/L, consistent with her state of undergoing the pubertal transition.

For counseling on her fertility risk, we assessed the impact of her treatment exposures, which included busulfan, an alkylating agent, and fludarabine, a purine analog, on ovarian reserve and uterine function. Antimetabolites such as fludarabine are hypothesized to impact only dividing cells and hence would pose less risk to the ovarian follicle pool. Alkylating chemotherapy has been shown to adversely impact ovarian reserve, increasing risks of infertility. In contrast to pelvic radiation, chemotherapy alone has not been associated with increased spontaneous abortion or intrauterine growth restriction [2].

In order to individualize her risk from busulfan, we calculated the Cyclophosphamide Equivalent Dose (CED) using an equation derived from multiple observational studies of toxicities associated with cyclophosphamide and other alkylating agents (◘ Fig. 58.1) [3]. This equation allows for the conversion of different alkylating agents into an equivalent dose of cyclophosphamide, for which there are data on risks of primary ovarian insufficiency (POI) and infertility [3, 4].Our patient's CED was calculated to be 3.7 g/m^2. Based on data from the Childhood Cancer Survivor Study (CCSS), children receiving <4 g/m^2 CED did not have higher rates of POI compared to children who did not receive alkylating agents (risk ratio 0.56, 95% CI 0.07–4.27, p = 0.58) [3].For children receiving <8 g/m^2 CED, the hazard ratio of POI was 1.55 (95% CI 0.77–3.11, p = 0.10), compared to children who did not receive alkylating agents [5]. Within the CCSS, the risk of clinical infertility in females was reported to be 13%. Relative to girls who did not receive alkylating agents, those in the lowest tertile of alkylating agents exposure had a relative risk of infertility of 0.91 (95% CI 0.69–1.20, p = 0.51) [4].

Based on these estimates, the patient and her family were counseled that her fertility risk from these exposures was limited, but it is still not possible to predict individual risk. We then

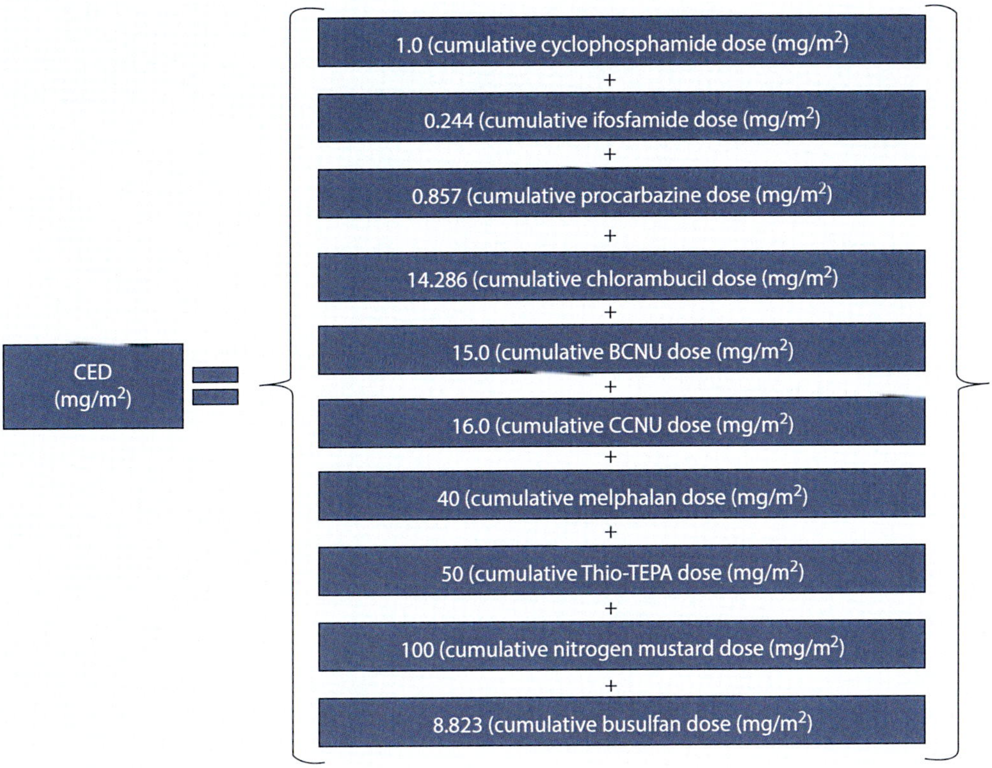

Fig. 58.1 Cyclophosphamide equivalent dose (CED) calculation

discussed fertility preservation options for premenarchal girls are all experimental, as there is a dearth of data on treatment efficacy in this population. The options that we discussed included expectant management, ovarian stimulation for oocyte or embryo freezing, ovarian tissue freezing, and ovarian suppression with GnRH agonist. On oocyte retrieval, we discussed transvaginal approach once deep sedation was achieved. Following counseling, the patient and her family verbalized understanding of risks and wished to proceed with oocyte freezing.

58.2 Management

In preparation for oocyte retrieval, the patient signed oocyte freezing assents, and her parents signed consents. The family met with the treating anesthesiologist prior to stimulation. Random start ovarian stimulation was initiated 2 months prior to patient's planned BMT (Table 58.1). Estradiol and progesterone levels on the day stimulation started were <20 pg/mL and <0.2 ng/mL, respectively. She received 150 IU of menotropin and 75 IU of follitropin daily. Estradiol levels were followed every other day starting on day 3 of stimulation. Serial abdominal ultrasound was performed to monitor follicle growth. GnRH antagonist was initiated on day 6 when the lead follicle was at least 14 mm in diameter. On stimulation day 10, her lead follicles were 21 mm by size, a total of six follicles greater than 10 mm were observed, estradiol level was 2312 pg/mL, and 10,000 IU of hCG was administered intramuscularly to trigger oocyte maturation.

On the day of oocyte retrieval, the patient was brought to the operating room, and her parents were able to accompany her while the IV catheter was placed. Then, they were escorted to the waiting room, and deep sedation was administered to the patient. She was positioned in dorsal lithotomy, and vaginal preparation was performed. The transvaginal ultrasound probe was introduced, and the oocyte retrieval was then completed with-

Table 58.1 Ovarian stimulation monitoring

Stimulation day	1	2	3	4	5	6	7	8	9	10
Menotropin dose (IU)	150	150	150	150	150	150	150	150	150	
Follitropin dose (IU)	75	75	75	75	75	75	75	75	75	
hCG (IU)										10,000
Estradiol level (pg/mL)	<20		70		207		760	1194		2312
Progesterone level (ng/mL)	<0.2									
Lead follicle diameters(mm)	7, 9				11, 13		15, 16, 16	19, 18, 16, 15, 13, 11		21, 21, 19, 17

out difficulty. Care was taken during preparation and retrieval to minimize tear to the hymen, which remained intact after the procedure. Ten oocytes were retrieved (eight metaphase II and two metaphase I). All ten oocytes were vitrified. The patient tolerated the procedure well and was discharged home 2 hours after surgery without complications. Onset of menses started 2 weeks following the procedure. She then underwent BMT as scheduled.

58.3 Outcome

This case demonstrates several key aspects of fertility risk counseling and fertility preservation procedures in adolescents. First, patient education of fertility risk was initiated by the treating oncology team, in line with professional society guidelines to address the possibility of infertility with patients and parents prior to cancer therapy. The oncology team had a longstanding partnership with the reproductive endocrinology team and the fertility preservation program at a National Cancer Institute-designated Comprehensive Cancer Center, facilitating a streamlined referral. Importantly, the oncology team provided the planned cumulative doses for chemotherapy to enable the reproductive endocrinology team to help estimate risk for counseling.

Second, the fertility preservation team inclusive of the reproductive endocrinologist, anesthesiologist, nurse, embryologist, administrative staff, and operating room staff had prior experience with treating adolescents. In addition, a thorough literature search was performed to provide up-to-date evidence on fertility risk and review the few published experiences with ovarian stimulation in pre-menarchal girls [6]. Then, the fertility preservation team was able to discuss coordinated care of this patient prior to stimulation start. The reproductive endocrinologists reviewed the patient's pubertal stage, gonadotropin and estradiol levels, and size of antral follicles and surmised that these antral follicles should be responsive to exogenous gonadotropins for ovarian stimulation. Her normal body habitus enabled ultrasound monitoring of follicular development abdominally in conjunction with estradiol levels. The anesthesiologist and operating room staff worked to confirm that equipment would be suitable for a patient of this size. The administrative team worked with the patient's family to determine insurance coverage and help apply for donated medications. The nurse helped to support the family through injection teaching and communication during stimulation. We met with the patient and her family on two occasions prior to ovarian stimulation and talked with the patient individually without her parents to ascertain that she understood and wished to undergo this procedure.

Third, it was important to estimate the magnitude of her risk, as cancer treatments from chemotherapy to radiation to surgery pose differential risks to fertility outcomes. Even with exposure to alkylating agents, fertility outcomes, particularly in girls, can be normal without fertility preservation procedures [4]. Hence, as part of informed consent, it is critical to convey the magnitude of risk to facilitate discussions in light of significant physical, emotional, and financial costs of undergoing fertility preservation in an adolescent girl. Ultimately, this patient clearly verbalized her desire to prevent infertility if possible, and there is still a lack of tools to predict precise risk of infertility for an individual. Hence, in line with supporting patient autonomy, we proceeded with ovarian stimulation and oocyte cryopreservation.

Clinical Pearls and Pitfalls

- Fertility and ovarian failure risk from alkylating chemotherapy can be estimated using the CED. There are also risk estimates for abdominal and pelvic radiation [3–5].
- In the pubertal transition, antral follicle count (AFC) and AMH levels are lower than at peak reproductive age. Low AMH and AFC prior to cancer therapy in this population likely do not indicate decreased ovarian reserve.
- There are cases of successful ovarian stimulation in pre-menarchal girls that have resulted in cryopreservation of mature oocytes. In conjunction with estradiol levels, abdominal ultrasounds can be used to monitor stimulation.
- Quality fertility preservation care involves a multi-disciplinary team inclusive of oncology, reproductive endocrinology, anesthesia, nursing, and administration.

Review Questions and Answers [1, 2]

Q1. True or False? Alkylating chemotherapy always poses high risk to fertility in girls.

A1. False, fertility risk is dependent on cumulative dose, which can be calculated using the CED. The CED can then be used to estimate risks of POI and infertility based on data from the Childhood Cancer Survivor Study [3–5].

Q2. True or False? Fertility preservation using controlled ovarian stimulation and oocyte cryopreservation is not possible in pre-menarchal girls.

A2. False, fertility preservation using controlled ovarian stimulation and oocyte cryopreservation is possible in pre-menarchal girls as demonstrated by our successful case and previously published report [6].

Q3. True or False? Monitoring of ovarian stimulation must be performed using a transvaginal ultrasound.

A3. False, abdominal ultrasound monitoring in conjunction with estradiol levels can be used in select individuals of low-normal BMI if their clinical history precludes transvaginal monitoring (e.g., virginal status or vaginismus).

References

1. ClinicalTrials.gov. Available from URL: https://clinicaltrials.gov/ct2/show/NCT01176006?cond=DOCK8+Deficiency&rank=1.
2. Shliakhtsitsava K, Suresh D, Hadnott T, Su HI. Best practices in counseling young female cancer survivors on reproductive health. Semin Reprod Med. 2017;35:378–89.
3. Green DM, Nolan VG, Goodman PJ, et al. The cyclophosphamide equivalent dose as an approach for quantifying alkylating agent exposure: a report from the Childhood Cancer Survivor Study. Pediatr Blood Cancer. 2014;61:53–67.
4. Barton SE, Najita JS, Ginsburg ES, et al. Infertility, infertility treatment, and achievement of pregnancy in female survivors of childhood cancer: a report from the Childhood Cancer Survivor Study cohort. Lancet Oncol. 2013;14:873–81.
5. Chemaitilly W, Li Z, Krasin MJ, et al. Premature ovarian insufficiency in childhood cancer survivors: a report from the St. Jude Lifetime Cohort. J Clin Endocrinol Metab. 2017;102:2242–50.
6. Reichman DE, Davis OK, Zaninovic N, Rosenwaks Z, Goldschlag DE. Fertility preservation using controlled ovarian hyperstimulation and oocyte cryopreservation in a premenarcheal female with myelodysplastic syndrome. Fertil Steril. 2012;98:1225–8.

Suggested Reading

Online Mendelian Inheritance in Man. An online catalog of human genes and genetic disorders. Available from URL: http://omim.org/entry/243700.

Uygun DFK, Uygun V, Reisli İ, et al. Hematopoietic stem cell transplantation from unrelated donors in children with DOCK8 deficiency. Pediatr Transplant. 2017;21:e13015.

A Clinical Case of Fertility Preservation in an Adolescent with Hodgkin Lymphoma

Mohamed Khrouf, Marouen Braham, Selim Khrouf, and Fehmi Msaddak

T. K. Woodruff et al. (eds.), *Textbook of Oncofertility Research and Practice*,
https://doi.org/10.1007/978-3-030-02868-8_59

Case Presentation

NT is a 15-year-old post-menarchal girl; she was complaining of cervical enlargement, a weight loss of 21 kg in 3 months, night sweats, and fever. Clinical examination of the patient found a 2 cm fixed painless and firm right lateral jugular lymphadenopathy. The left cervical lymphadenopathy biopsy revealed a scleronodular Hodgkin's disease. The patient's disease was staged IIBb with mediastinal bulky according to the Ann Arbor classification system.

She was planned to receive two cures of OEPA (vincristine, etoposide, prednisone, doxorubicin) followed by an early PET scan assessment (according to the Euronet-Paediatric Hodgkin Lymphoma Group).

According to guidelines, hematologists addressed the issues of chemotherapy side effects including possible risk of ovarian toxicity. The patient and her parents (she was minor) were offered to be referred for fertility preservation. They consulted one day after being referred.

59.1 Assessment of Ovarian Reserve and Ovarian Function Loss Risk

The aim and headlines of oncofertility were explained before the individual evaluation of the gonadotoxicity. For this purpose (and on the same day), serum anti-Mullerian hormone (AMH) testing was performed and resulted on a level of 0.88 ng/ml suggestive of a decreased ovarian reserve. A decreased AMH level in patients with hematologic malignancies is reported by some authors [1] but still controversial [2]. The pathophysiology and the long-term implications are unknown, but extreme catabolic state could be one of the mechanisms.

In this case, risk of loss of ovarian function was considered intermediate. Indeed, the initially planned chemotherapy protocol contains no alkylant agent (the most gonadotoxic supress). On the other hand, the decreased initial ovarian reserve was a risk factor of premature ovarian failure [3]. In addition, a switch for a more aggressive chemotherapy (in case of unsuccessful first-line treatment) was estimated as possible by the hematologists.

59

59.2 Management

Considering all these parameters, the patient was advised to proceed with fertility preservation.

Oncofertility possibilities were explained to the patient and her parents. Because NT was postpubertal, she was offered ovarian tissue cryopreservation (OTC) or oocytes vitrification (OV). In our case, advantages and disadvantages of each technique were discussed with the patient and her parents.

Although preferred by many oncofertility teams, OTC is still considered as experimental. Despite this label, it was shown that OTC is an effective method that can restore fertility but also endocrine activity. Moreover, 18–23% pregnancy rates are reported [4, 5] with half of the pregnancy occurring spontaneously.

This method requires a laparoscopy and therefore, theoretically, allows the patient to start chemotherapy, one day after the surgical removal of the ovarian tissue. However, in our particular case, NT presented mediastinal compression due to large thoracic nodes, and the anesthetist recommended that she would need at least 10 days of prednisone before being able to have a laparoscopy, which would delay the start of chemotherapy. Long-term risks of OTC were also discussed including the risk of introducing malignant cells when grafting the ovarian tissue after recovery, even though Hodgkin Lymphoma is low risk [6]. Finally, we considered in this case, that in a patient with low ovarian reserve and low risk chemotherapy (which may not induce premature ovarian insufficiency), removing ovarian tissue may be more harmful than the chemotherapy itself.

Oocytes vitrification is the standard method according to the guidelines [7], and it has been shown to be associated with 32% of pregnancy rates [4]. It requires ovarian stimulation with gonadotrophins, which would delay the start of chemotherapy by 12–15 days using a random start protocol. The window of stimulation would allow for prednisone administration to reduce her thoracic compression. The patient and her parents gave consent for ovarian vitrification on the day of consultation, and ovarian stimulation was started (on day 15 of cycle).

Ovarian stimulation was started with human menotropins 300 international units per day with an GnRH antagonist for prevention of ovulation and a GnRH agonist trigger for oocyte maturation. This protocol minimizes the risk of ovarian hyperstimulation ovarian syndrome risk. In this case, the GnRH antagonist was started on day 10 (Table 59.1) as it

Table 59.1 Ovarian stimulation monitoring

	D1	D2	D3	D4	D5	D6	D7	D8	D9	D10	D11	D12	D13	D14
HMG (UI)	300	300	300	300	300	300	300	300	300	300	300			Oocytes pickup
Gn-RH anta										0.25 mg	0.25 mg			
Gn-RH agonist												0.2 mg		
E2 (pg/ml)						188		369		1018				
Progesterone						22		20		9				
Right ovary[a]						10–9		2×12–10		3×16		2×18		
								2×9		2×15		17		
												2×16		
Left ovary[a]						7 + CL		10–12		16–13		18–15		
								+CL						

Gn-RH anta GN-RH antagonist, *CL* corpus luteum
[a]Follicles size are expressed in mm

is possible to delay the start of the GnRH antagonist when stimulation occurs in the luteal phase and endogenous progesterone remains elevated [8].

After 12 days of stimulation, we obtained seven follicles with four measuring more than 17 mm indicating a triggering with GnRH agonist. GnRH agonist triggering should be used only in women with proof of normal hypothalamic-pituitary-ovarian axis activity, and an LH assay should be performed 12 hours after GnRH agonist administration to verify the LH surge (>15 mIU/ml).

59.3 Outcome

The patient and her parents were uncomfortable with idea of transvaginal oocyte pickup procedure so we offered them the possibility of using perurethral transvesical pickup which represents an effective and safe alternative [9].

Eight oocytes were retrieved; seven of them were mature and then vitrified. No complications occurred, and the patient was referred the day after oocyte pickup to start chemotherapy, 15 days after being referred to the oncofertility unit.

59.4 Conclusion and Keypoints

- Malignant hemopathies especially Hodgkin Lymphoma are common indications for fertility preservation.
- Fertility preservation counselling should be individualized based on the patient, her diagnosis, and her ovarian reserve.

59

Clinical Pearls/Pitfalls

- Ovarian reserve markers may be low in hematologic malignancies before any chemotherapy.
- According to guidelines, every patient who had not achieved his parenthood should be referred to an oncofertility program.
- Both ovarian tissue cryopreservation and oocyte vitrification are effective techniques and offer realistic chances of becoming a parent.
- For oocyte vitrification, the preferred protocol for ovarian stimulation protocol is a Gn-RH antagonist with GnRH agonist trigger to maximize the oocyte yield in a safe and expeditious manner.
- Confirmation of an LH surge after a GnRH agonist trigger should be verified by an LH and possibly progesterone level performed 12 hours after Gn-RH agonist administration.

Review Questions and Answers

Q1. What are the most important factors for the evaluation of gonadotoxicity risk of chemotherapy?

A1. Age, pre-existing ovarian reserve, chemotherapy agents, and additional therapies (radiation, surgery).

Q2. What is the best cycle day to start ovarian stimulation for fertility preservation?

A2. Ovarian stimulation can be started at any day of cycle with the exception of the periovulatory window. Delaying ovarian stimulation to the 1st day of cycle is not recommended.

Q3. What are the alternatives to vaginal oocyte pickup in adolescents?

A3. Perurethral transvesical, abdominal, or laparoscopic oocyte pickup may be more acceptable than transvaginal oocyte aspiration in some adolescents.

References

1. Lekovich J, Lobel ALS, Stewart JD, Pereira N, Kligman I, Rosenwaks Z. Female patients with lymphoma demonstrate diminished ovarian reserve even before initiation of chemotherapy when compared with healthy controls and patients with other malignancies. J Assist Reprod Genet. 2016;33:657–62. https://doi.org/10.1007/s10815-016-0689-1.
2. Decanter C, Morschhauser F, Pigny P, Lefebvre C, Gallo C, Dewailly D. Anti-Müllerian hormone follow-up in young women treated by chemotherapy for lymphoma: preliminary results. Reprod Biomed Online. 2010;20:280–5. https://doi.org/10.1016/j.rbmo.2009.11.010.

3. Anderson RA, Rosendahl M, Kelsey TW, Cameron DA. Pretreatment anti-Müllerian hormone predicts for loss of ovarian function after chemotherapy for early breast cancer. Eur J Cancer. 2013;49:3404–11. https://doi.org/10.1016/j.ejca.2013.07.014.
4. Diaz-Garcia C, Domingo J, Garcia-Velasco JA, Herraiz S, Mirabet V, Iniesta I, Cobo A, Remohí J, Pellicer A. Oocyte vitrification versus ovarian cortex transplantation in fertility preservation for adult women undergoing gonadotoxic treatments: a prospective cohort study. Fertil Steril. 2018;109:478–485.e2. https://doi.org/10.1016/j.fertnstert.2017.11.018.
5. Van der Ven H, Liebenthron J, Beckmann M, Toth B, Korell M, Krüssel J, Frambach T, Kupka M, Hohl MK, Winkler-Crepaz K, Seitz S, Dogan A, Griesinger G, Häberlin F, Henes M, Schwab R, Sütterlin M, von Wolff M, Dittrich R, FertiPROTEKT network. Ninety-five orthotopic transplantations in 74 women of ovarian tissue after cytotoxic treatment in a fertility preservation network: tissue activity, pregnancy and delivery rates. Hum Reprod Oxf Engl. 2016;31:2031–41. https://doi.org/10.1093/humrep/dew165.
6. Dolmans M-M, Luyckx V, Donnez J, Andersen CY, Greve T. Risk of transferring malignant cells with transplanted frozen-thawed ovarian tissue. Fertil Steril. 2013;99:1514–22. https://doi.org/10.1016/j.fertnstert.2013.03.027.
7. Loren AW, Mangu PB, Beck LN, Brennan L, Magdalinski AJ, Partridge AH, Quinn G, Wallace WH, Oktay K. Fertility preservation for patients with cancer: American Society of Clinical Oncology Clinical Practice Guideline Update. J Clin Oncol. 2013;31:2500–10. https://doi.org/10.1200/JCO.2013.49.2678.
8. Massin N. New stimulation regimens: endogenous and exogenous progesterone use to block the LH surge during ovarian stimulation for IVF. Hum Reprod Updat. 2017;23:211–20. https://doi.org/10.1093/humupd/dmw047.
9. Khrouf M, Braham M, Bouyahia M, Kacem-Berejeb K, Elloumi-Chaabane H, Zhioua A, Zhioua F. Perurethraltransvesical route for oocytes retrieval: an old technique for a new indication in oncofertility. Future Oncol Lond Engl. 2017;13:2547–53. https://doi.org/10.2217/fon-2017-0276.

Case Study of Postpubertal Adolescent Female Undergoing Ovarian Tissue Cryopreservation and Oophoropexy Prior to Gonadotoxic Therapy

Timothy Lautz, Barbara A. Lockart, and Elizabeth Sniderman

T. K. Woodruff et al. (eds.), *Textbook of Oncofertility Research and Practice*,
https://doi.org/10.1007/978-3-030-02868-8_60

Case Presentation

A 14-year-old female living in South Africa presented with a history of 7 months of worsening right lower back pain and progressive neurological symptoms including radiating pain, numbness, and tingling down her right leg. The initial MRI performed revealed a bony lesion involving the right iliac bone, right SI joint, and right sacrum associated with a large soft tissue component (9.6 × 8 × 8.4 cm). The imaging was concerning due to a malignant process requiring further evaluation. The family transferred care to a tertiary pediatric hospital in the USA where diagnostic testing was completed.

60.1 Assessment and Diagnosis

Ultrasound-guided core biopsies of the mass were positive for CD99+ small round blue cells. RT PCR analysis of the cells was positive for the EWSR1-FLI1 fusion transcript, confirming the diagnosis of Ewing Sarcoma. A single metastatic lesion was noted in the in the left sacrum. CT chest was negative for metastatic disease.

Ewing Sarcoma (ES) is the second most common malignant bone tumor of childhood/adolescence. ES is a chemo- and radiosensitive tumor. Treatment consists of both systemic treatment (chemotherapy) and local control (surgical resection or radiation therapy). The management of local disease depends on the anatomical location of the tumor as well as the associated risks and benefits of each treatment modality. Large pelvic tumors, in particular, are not typically amenable to surgical resection [1].

60.2 Management

The treatment plan included neo-adjuvant chemotherapy followed by radiation therapy (55.80 Gy) with adjuvant chemotherapy. Chemotherapy would consist of alternating cycles of vincristine, doxorubicin, cyclophosphamide (8400 mg/m^2), ifosfamide (63,000 mg/m^2), and etoposide every 14 days. The radiation therapy field would include the right pelvis as well as the focal lesion identified in the left sacrum.

Infertility is a known side-effect of both alkylating agents and radiation to the ovaries or pelvis. The cyclophosphamide equivalency dose (CED) of this treatment is 23,772 mg/m^2. Based on a CED of 23,772 plus radiation therapy to the pelvis, her risk for ovarian failure is greater than 80% [2–4].

Fertility preservation counseling was initiated once diagnosis was confirmed. The family met with the Advance Practice Registered Nurse (APRN) to discuss risk of infertility and preservation options. Oocyte harvesting and oophoropexy were discussed with the family as standard fertility preservation options. Ovarian tissue cryopreservation was presented as an investigational procedure [5]. Oocyte harvesting was not available at the pediatric institution and required transfer of care to reproductive medicine specialists at a partnering adult hospital. Both ovarian tissue cryopreservation and oophoropexy would be performed at time of routine venous port placement and bone marrow aspirate and biopsy.

The family decided to proceed with ovarian tissue cryopreservation and oophoropexy. They understood oocyte harvesting is standard of care and ovarian tissue cryopreservation was considered experimental. The family stated they based their decision on a desire to start treatment as soon as possible due to increasing pain. Delay of treatment initiation for fertility preservation is a concern often expressed by families at the time of cancer diagnosis [6]. Additional concerns identified were the intensity of the stimulation process for oocyte harvesting as well as invasive ultrasounds required to monitor oocyte maturation. Potential for ovarian insufficiency from gonadotoxic treatment was also a worry for the mother. The reports of restoration of hormone function from transplanted tissue also factored into the family's decision to pursue OTC [7].

60.3 Operative Considerations

Most girls undergoing potentially sterilizing therapy will receive symmetric exposure to both ovaries. Therefore, in most cases, either ovary can be removed at the discretion of the surgeon during laparoscopic oophorectomy for cryopreservation. If diagnostic laparoscopy confirms normal bilateral fallopian tubes and ovaries, the right ovary is often removed out of convenience due to the proximity of the sigmoid colon to the left ovary. An exception is for girls who are expected to receive asymmetric pelvic radiation. In this patient's case, the primary tumor involved the right hemipelvis, and the radiation field was anticipated to disproportionately affect the right ovary. Therefore, in discussion with the radiation oncologist, the decision was made to perform a laparoscopic right oophorectomy in the usual fashion and oophoropexy of the left ovary. This was accomplished using a single laparoscopic suture between the mesovarium and the peritoneum overlying the iliac vessels to suspend it out of the pelvis. The goal of oophoropexy was to minimize the radiation exposure of the contralateral ovary.

60.4 Outcome

The patient went home on the day of surgery and had an uncomplicated postoperative course. Chemotherapy was initiated on the fourth postoperative day.

Clinical Pearls

- Calculating potential for infertility includes assessment of chemotherapy, both high-risk medications and cumulative dosing, radiation, and surgical risks.
- Determination of fertility preservation options requires discussion between medical oncologist, radiation oncologist, and surgeon.
- Family may choose an experimental fertility preservation option if the standard procedure will delay onset of treatment or if the investigation option offers a perceived benefit not provided by standard therapy.
- In girls receiving potentially sterilizing therapy who will undergo asymmetric pelvic radiation, laparoscopic oophorectomy for cryopreservation should remove the ovary anticipated to receive the higher radiation dose.
- Concurrent laparoscopic oophoropexy can be used to suspend the contralateral ovary out of the pelvis and minimize its radiation exposure.

Review Questions and Answers

Q1. Which patient is at highest risk for infertility due to treatment?
(a) Four-year-old female receiving vincristine, doxorubicin, dactinomycin, and 10.8 Gy radiation to the right flank for treatment of Wilms' tumor
(b) Twelve-year-old female receiving 18 Gy cranial radiation and cyclophosphamide 1000 mg/m^2 for treatment of acute lymphoblastic leukemia
(c) Twenty-year-old female receiving 55 Gy radiation to the right thigh for treatment of synovial cell sarcoma
(d) Fifteen-year-old receiving cyclophosphamide 8400 mg/m^2 and 54 Gy to the right hip for alveolar rhabdomyosarcoma

A1. (d)

Q2. What factors may influence the decision regarding ovarian tissue cryopreservation?
(a) Urgency to start treatment
(b) Patient's age
(c) Standard therapy versus investigational
(d) All of the above

A2. (d)

Q3. In which of the following patients is there a side preference for laparoscopic oophorectomy for cryopreservation?
(a) Two-year-old female with neuroblastoma of the right adrenal gland
(b) Eleven-year-old female with recurrent AML undergoing stem cell transplant
(c) Fourteen-year-old female with alveolar rhabdomyosarcoma of the retroperitoneum in the right hemipelvis
(d) Four-year-old female with metastatic but local stage I Wilms' tumor

A3. (c)

References

1. Imbach P, Kuhne T, Arceci R, editors. Pediatric oncology: a comprehensive guide. St. Louis: Springer. (2006); 2006. p. 165–70.
2. Green DM, Kawashima T, Stoval M, Leisenring W, Sklar CA, Mertens AC, et al. Fertility of female survivors of childhood cancer: a report from the Childhood Cancer Survivor Study. J Clin Oncol. 2009;27(16): 2677–85.
3. Green DM, Nolan VG, Goodman PJ, Whitton JA, Srivastava DK, Leisenring WM, et al. The cyclophosphamide equivalent dose as an approach for quantifying alkylating agent exposure. A report from the Childhood Cancer Survivor Study. Pediatr Blood Cancer. 2014;61(1):53–67.
4. Critchley HO, Wallace WH, Shalet SM, et al. Abdominal irradiation in childhood: the potential for pregnancy. Br J Obstet Gynecol. 1992;99:392–4.
5. Donnez J, Dolman MM. Fertility preservation in woman. N Engl J Med. 2017;377(1):1657–65.
6. Burns KC, Hoefgen H, Dasgupta R. Fertility preservation options in pediatric and adolescents with cancer. Cancer [Internet}. 2018 Month 00 [cited 2018 Feb 2];1–10. Available from: http://onlinelibrary.wiley.com/doi/10.1002/cncr.31255.
7. Pacheco F, Oktay K. Current success and efficiency of autologous ovarian transplantation: a meta-analysis. Reprod Sci. 2017;24:1111–20.

Fertility Preservation in a Female Adolescent with a Hemoglobinopathy

Mary Ellen Pavone, Sharrón Manuel, and Alexis Thompson

T. K. Woodruff et al. (eds.), *Textbook of Oncofertility Research and Practice*,
https://doi.org/10.1007/978-3-030-02868-8_61

Case Presentation

A 16-year-old female with a history of β-thalassemia presented to our Reproductive Endocrinology and Infertility (REI) clinic prior to undergoing hematopoietic stem cell transplantation (HSCT). Her gynecologic history was significant for spontaneous menarche at age 13 years and regular monthly menses. She was not sexually active but did use tampons. Her history was otherwise significant for mild asthma and a history of depression for which she saw a therapist but was not prescribed medications. She was able to tolerate a transvaginal ultrasound, which revealed a normal-sized uterus and an antral follicle count of 12. Laboratory results were notable for an anti-Müllerian hormone (AMH) level of 3.41 ng/mL. She was counseled that the preconditioning regimens used prior to HSCT could lead to premature ovarian insufficiency, and therefore she should consider fertility preservation. She was counseled about preservation options and elected to undergo oocyte cryopreservation.

61.1 Assessment and Diagnosis

61.1.1 Screening for Thalassemia

Hemoglobinopathies are genetic disorders of hemoglobin (Hb) due to mutations in the globin genes, which encode the globin chain components of hemoglobin. They can be divided into two groups: thalassemia syndromes, which are a result of mutations leading to reduced or absent synthesis of the affected globin chains, and structural variants such as sickle cell anemia [1]. The major categories of severe hemoglobinopathies include sickle cell disease, Hb E thalassemia, β-thalassemia major, and Hb Bart's hydrops fetalis syndrome. The clinical manifestations can range from a mild anemia with an associated microcytosis (thalassemia trait) to a severe fatal anemia seen in β-thalassemia major or Hb Bart's hydrops fetalis syndrome [2].

61

The American College of Obstetricians and Gynecologists (ACOG) currently recommends that information regarding comprehensive carrier screening be provided to all pregnant women [3]. ACOG notes that it is important to understand that newborn screening is not replaced by prenatal carrier screening [3], and that if an individual is found to be a carrier of a genetic condition, he or she should be encouraged to inform existing relatives who may also be at risk [4].

The diagnosis of sickle cell or thalassemia requires a complete blood count (CBC) with erythrocyte indices, reticulocyte count, and hemoglobin electrophoresis or isoelectric focusing (IEF) for quantification of Hb A, Hb A_2, and Hb F. More recently, cation-exchange HPLC is becoming the preferred method of choice for screening [2, 5–8]; however, DNA analysis may also be needed for a definitive diagnosis of many forms of thalassemia. The clinical symptoms of β-thalassemias range from a mild, microcytic hypochromic anemia for thalassemia minor (trait) to long-term transfusion-dependent anemia for thalassemia major (homozygous or compound heterozygous β-thalassemia), also called transfusion-dependent thalassemia (TDT). Thalassemia intermedia, or non-transfusion-dependent thalassemia (NTDT), results in moderate anemia and may be associated with jaundice, splenomegaly, and paraspinal masses due to extramedullary hematopoiesis [9].

61.1.2 Thalassemia and Hypogonadism

One of the most common endocrinopathies associated with thalassemia major is hypogonadism, affecting approximately 70–80% of individuals with the disease [10]. The underlying mechanism is likely due to excess iron deposition in the gonads and/or pituitary gland, the latter being more common [10]. Normal iron homeostasis is maintained by iron absorption, but in patients with thalassemia, there is a lack of proper excretory mechanisms resulting in iron overload. The anterior pituitary is very sensitive to this excess iron, with the end result being a significant decrease in follicle-stimulating hormone (FSH) and luteinizing hormone (LH) [10, 11]. Iron toxicity in thalassemia patients is also thought to affect adipocytes and leptin, as lower leptin levels have been shown in studies of varying age groups with thalassemia. These decrease leptin levels have been proposed as the etiology of delayed puberty in thalassemia patients due to leptin's role in indirect stimulation of the hypothalamic-pituitary-gonadal (HPG) axis through Kisspeptin neurons in the arcuate nucleus

[10, 12]. The prevalence and severity of the hypogonadism depend upon the type of thalassemia and age of the individual [10].

61.2 Management

The management of β-thalassemia depends on the type and severity of the disease. Supportive treatment for TDT includes chronic transfusions and iron chelation to reduce or prevent iron overload. The recommended frequency of transfusions is usually every 2–4 weeks to maintain a pretransfusion hemoglobin level of 9–10 g/dL. Chelation therapy is initiated after 10–20 units, or when serum ferritin concentration exceeds 1000 ng/mL. Splenectomy can mitigate transfusion requirements; however, it is associated with increased risk of infection and pulmonary hypertension. Hematopoietic stem cell transplantation (HSCT) is a curative option for thalassemia major if an appropriate stem cell donor is available [13]. Gene therapy, which involves ex vivo transduction of the patient's own stem cells with a viral vector containing the human beta globin gene, is a promising new approach.

61.2.1 Hematopoietic Stem Cell Transplant (HSCT)

The primary objective of HSCT for thalassemia is to correct the genetic defect resulting in abnormal globin chain synthesis and subsequent hemolytic anemia [13]. This can be accomplished by using suitably matched hematopoietic stem cells from a family or unrelated donor. In general, only one-third of patients have an available matched related donor [14, 15]. Patients undergoing this treatment are risk stratified into three classes based on the following risk factors present: liver size (>2 cm), presence of liver fibrosis, and inadequate iron chelation. Class I has none of these risk factors, Class II has one to two of the risk factors, and Class III has all of the three risk factors [16–18]. Those individuals identified as Class I and II are considered low risk and have very favorable outcomes with HSCT, whereas Class III individuals are high risk and have poorer outcomes [16–18]. Prior to transplant, a conditioning regimen (which is a treatment used to prepare a patient for receiving HSCT), is utilized to eradicate the thalassemic marrow. The traditional conditioning regimen used in treating β-thalassemia major is a myeloablative busulfan and cyclophosphamide-based treatment. Various conditioning regimens have been introduced since the original busulfan and cyclophosphamide regimen to reduce related toxicity and graft rejection. Some of these regimens involve reducing the cyclophosphamide dose. Regimens for high-risk or Class III individuals involve adding fludarabine and azathioprine to the conditioning regimen along with intensive chelation and hyper-transfusion therapy with hydroxyurea and growth factors at specific time points. A more novel approach to conditioning regimens is the use of treosulfan due to its lower toxicity profile, especially in high risk patients [18]. With these newer regimens, HSCT has provided up to a 90% long-term survival rate, even in high-risk individuals [15, 19, 20].

Following the conditioning regimen, the allogeneic normal or heterozygous stem cells are infused into the patient. Potential early complications include graft failure, graft versus host disease, and life-threatening infections. Late complications (those occurring after more than 2 years) include disease relapses, chronic graft-vs-host disease (GvHD), infections, and secondary cancers [18, 21].

Recent gene therapy studies have demonstrated transfusion reduction or elimination in severe beta thalassemia without many of the risks associated with allogeneic HSCT [22, 23]. Autologous stem cells are mobilized with plerixafor and GCSF, then harvested from peripheral blood by apheresis. Stem cells undergo CD34 selection in the laboratory, followed by transduction with a lentiviral vector containing the human beta globin gene. Patients receive myeloablative doses of chemotherapy prior to reinfusion of their genetically modified stem cells. Adverse events thus far appear to be related to the conditioning regimen. No replication competent lentivirus, clonal dominance, or graft failure has been reported.

61.2.2 Hematopoietic Stem Cell Transplant (HSCT) and Primary Ovarian Insufficiency (POI)

The majority of existing data from long-term outcomes using HSCT comes from cancer studies. The use of SCT has been utilized globally for other diagnoses in young patients and may potentially represent the only curative therapy for certain malignancies [24]. Though beneficial, one must be aware of the long-term risks associated with SCT. Of particular interest, conditioning therapies used in conjunction with SCT can be gonadotoxic and significantly diminish fertility in treated young individuals, resulting in primary ovarian insufficiency (POI), previously reported or denoted as premature ovarian failure (POF). In studies in which myeloablative conditioning regimens were used, POI was seen in 95–100% of patients following conventional allogeneic transplantation [24].Some of these standard myeloablative treatments include alkylating agents such as cyclophosphamide and busulfan and/or radiation. One of the first reports using reduced intensity conditioning (RIC) regimens, characterized by decreased doses of chemotherapy and/or radiation, demonstrated POI in 86.3% of treated patients indicated for a hematologic malignancy. However, it was concluded that this may be attributed to prior chemotherapy for treatment of the malignancy as decreases in fertility due to gonadotoxic treatments were noted to be dose-dependent [24, 25]. In a separate study of SCT in lymphoma and leukemia patients, vasomotor symptoms were prevalent following transplantation [24, 26]. SCT is also readily used in treatment of sickle cell disease with cure rates exceeding 90% [27]. A more recent report of SCT use in sickle cell patients discussed the hesitation of accepting HSCT due to its potential risks of subfertility or infertility. There is no accurate method to calculate individual risks of infertility; therefore, when consenting for HSCT, the patient must realize that there exists some unknown but likely significant risk to future fertility.

61.2.3 The Use of Controlled Ovarian Hyperstimulation (COH) in Adolescents

A growing point of focus in the field of reproductive medicine is fertility perseveration in adolescents [28], due in part to the large number of adolescent patients undergoing gonadotoxic therapies for cancer or hemoglobinapthies. It was previously thought that ovarian tissue cryopreservation may be the only means of fertility preservation available to pre-pubertal females and was utilized as the primary treatment modality in this patient population who were undergoing high-risk gonadotoxic treatments [28, 29]. However, it has been subsequently reported that controlled ovarian hyperstimulation (COH) was able to be safely and successfully used in a pre-pubertal female resulting in cryopreservation of mature oocytes [28]. In this particular study, oocyte maturation was achieved by both in vivo and in vitro mechanisms. In postpubertal adolescents, maturation in vivo is less of an issue, and COH has been successfully demonstrated in other case studies with MII yields approaching rates similar to adult women undergoing the same procedure [30, 31]. Although ovarian tissue cryopreservation has been a highly promoted option in this population, the efficacy has not been fully demonstrated [28] and this method carries a risk of reintroduction of malignant cells in those patients who underwent preservation for a cancer diagnosis [28, 32–35]. Although a limited number of studies exist, COH has been used in adolescents with sickle cell disease [30], Turner's syndrome [31], and malignancies [28]. Therefore, COH offers a safe fertility preservation option in adolescents and young adults if a multi-disciplinary approach is taken, with the appropriate support team available and cautionary steps taken.

61.2.4 Controlled Ovarian Hyperstimulation (COH) Protocol

Our patient opted for oocyte cryopreservation and underwent *a cycle start (CS) antagonist stimulation protocol*. Prior to beginning the process, the patient met with a psychologist to ensure that she understood the procedure and wanted to move forward. She then gave assent in addition to written consent from her parents/guardians. Our ovarian stimulation protocols have previously been described in other studies [36, 37] and will be briefly summarized. Traditionally, patients have undergone a CS protocol, but at Northwestern we have transitioned to include more random start (RS) protocols, giving patients the option of allowing gonadotropins to be initiated at any point of the menstrual cycle. For CS protocols, gonadotropin injections were initiated on the 3rd day of the cycle. Initial dosages of medication were based on ovarian reserve and age, then adjusted based on response to medication, which was monitored by routine ultrasounds and E_2 measurements. For a CS protocol, a daily injection of GnRH antagonist to prevent ovulation was began based on reaching one of two criteria: the leading follicle measuring at least 12 mm in diameter or E_2 reached 300 pg/mL. For a RS protocol, GnRH antagonist injections began once the new lead follicle reached 12 mm in diameter. Final follicular maturation was triggered by an injection of hCG when at least three follicles measured 16 mm in diameter, and oocyte retrieval was performed 36 hours later. Prior to 2008, slow cooling was used for oocyte cryopreservation in our practice, after which vitrification became a standard practice.

61.3 Outcome

Ovarian stimulation was initiated using an antagonist protocol as described above. Injectable gonadotropins were started at the beginning of her menstrual cycle and given for a total of 10 days. Her peak estradiol level was noted to be 302 pg/mL on stimulation day 10. Choriogonadotropin alfa injection (Ovidrel, EMD Serono) was given to induce the final maturation of the oocytes, and an oocyte retrieval was performed 36 hours later. A total of 14 oocytes were retrieved, of which 12 were mature, 1 was immature, and 1 had an empty zona. A total of 13 oocytes were cryopreserved using vitrification (12 mature and 1 immature). There were no complications from the oocyte retrieval. Three months later, the patient started a conditioning regimen that included busulfan and subsequently underwent HSCT. After 6 months post-infusion, she has discontinued transfusions, has normal hemoglobin levels, and has resumed normal activities.

Clinical Pearls and Pitfalls

- All patients undergoing HSCT for any indication should receive fertility preservation counseling and offered options given the undetermined risks of subfertility.
- It is important to be aware of post-transplant-related complications such as engraftment syndrome, ITP, DVT, and hemorrhagic cystitis.
- Locating a matched donor for HSCT can be a limiting factor.
- COH is safe in the adolescent population as long as the appropriate precautions are taken and a multi-disciplinary support team is involved in the patient's care.

Review Questions and Answers

Q1. What are the different types of thalassemia categories?

A1. β-thalassemia major (or transfusion-dependent thalassemia (TDT))
β-thalassemia intermedia (or non-transfusion-dependent thalassemia (NTDT))
Hb E/β-thalassemia major
β-thalassemia minor
Hb Bart's hydrops fetalis

Q2. What is conditioning therapy? What are some of the associated risks?

A2. Conditioning therapy is a treatment used to prepare a patient for receiving HSCT that is utilized to eradicate the thalassemic marrow. The traditional conditioning regimen used in treating β-thalassemia major is a myeloablative busulfan and cyclophosphamide-based treatment. Various conditioning regimens have been introduced to reduce related toxicity and graft rejection, including the reduction of the cyclophosphamide dose. Regimens for high-risk or Class III individuals involve adding fludarabine and azathioprine to the conditioning regimen along with intensive chelation and hyper-transfusion therapy with hydroxyurea and growth factors at specific time points.

Conditioning therapies used in conjunction with SCT can be gonadotoxic and significantly diminish fertility in treated young individuals, resulting in primary ovarian insufficiency (POI), previously reported or denoted as premature ovarian failure (POF). In studies in which myeloablative conditioning regimens were used, POI was seen in 95–100% of patients following conventional allogeneic transplantation.

Q3. When should a patient who is diagnosed with a hemoglobinopathy be counseled on fertility preservation?

A3. Patients diagnosed with a hemoglobinopathy should be counseled on fertility preservation prior to initiating any gonadotoxic conditioning treatments.

Q4. What are some current ACOG recommendations regarding carrier screening?

A4. ACOG recommends that information regarding comprehensive carrier screening be provided to all pregnant women, which includes hemoglobinopathies such as thalassemias as well as a number of other genetic disorders. A combination of laboratory testing is usually needed in order to gather information to counsel couples who may be carriers of a specific thalassemia or sickle cell disorder. ACOG also notes that it is important to understand that newborn screening is not replaced by prenatal carrier screening.

61 Q5. What are some late complications of SCT?

A5. Late complications (those occurring after more than 2 years) include disease relapses, chronic graft-vs-host disease (GvHD), infections, and secondary cancers.

References

1. Traeger-Synodinos J, Harteveld CL. Advances in technologies for screening and diagnosis of hemoglobinopathies. Biomark Med. 2014;8:119.
2. Clarke GM, Higgins TN. Laboratory investigation of hemoglobinopathies and thalassemias: review and update. Clin Chem. 2000;46(8 Pt 2):1284–90.
3. Committee on, G. Committee opinion no. 691: carrier screening for genetic conditions. Obstet Gynecol. 2017;129(3):e41–55.
4. Gunasekaran U, et al. Endocrine complications in long-term survivors after allogeneic stem cell transplant. Semin Hematol. 2012;49(1):66–72.
5. Eastman JW, et al. Automated HPLC screening of newborns for sickle cell anemia and other hemoglobinopathies. Clin Chem. 1996;42(5):704–10.
6. Fucharoen S, et al. Prenatal and postnatal diagnoses of thalassemias and hemoglobinopathies by HPLC. Clin Chem. 1998;44(4):740–8.
7. Mario N, et al. Capillary isoelectric focusing and high-performance cation-exchange chromatography compared for qualitative and quantitative analysis of hemoglobin variants. Clin Chem. 1997;43(11):2137–42.
8. Riou J, et al. Cation-exchange HPLC evaluated for presumptive identification of hemoglobin variants. Clin Chem. 1997;43(1):34–9.
9. Kohne E. Hemoglobinopathies: clinical manifestations, diagnosis, and treatment. Deut Ärzteblatt Int. 2011;108(31–32):532–40.
10. Srisukh S, Ongphiphadhanakul B, Bunnag P. Hypogonadism in thalassemia major patients. J Clin Transl Endocrinol. 2016;5:42–5.
11. Atkin SL, et al. Effect of cell density on hormonal secretion from human pituitary adenomas in vitro. Horm Res Paediatr. 1998;49(5):203–9.
12. Smith JT, et al. KiSS-1 neurones are direct targets for leptin in the ob/ob mouse. J Neuroendocrinol. 2006;18(4):298–303.
13. Storb RF, et al. Hematopoietic cell transplantation for benign hematological disorders and solid tumors. ASH Educ Program Book. 2003;2003(1):372–97.
14. Angelucci E, et al. Hematopoietic stem cell transplantation in thalassemia major and sickle cell disease: indications and management recommendations from an international expert panel. Haematologica. 2014;99(5):811–20.
15. Srivastava A, Shaji RV. Cure for thalassemia major – from allogeneic hematopoietic stem cell transplantation to gene therapy. Haematologica. 2017;102(2):214–23.
16. Lucarelli G, et al. Bone marrow transplantation in adult thalassemia. Blood. 1992;80(6):1603–7.
17. Lucarelli G, et al. Bone marrow transplantation in patients with thalassemia. N Engl J Med. 1990; 322(7):417–21.
18. Mathews V, Savani BN. Conditioning regimens in allo-SCT for thalassemia major. Bone Marrow Transplant. 2014;49:607.
19. Bernardo ME, et al. Allogeneic hematopoietic stem cell transplantation in thalassemia major: results of a reduced-toxicity conditioning regimen based on the use of treosulfan. Blood. 2012;120(2):473–6.
20. Mathews V, et al. Improved clinical outcomes of high risk β thalassemia major patients undergoing a HLA matched related allogeneic stem cell transplant with a treosulfan based conditioning regimen and peripheral blood stem cell grafts. PLoS One. 2013;8(4):e61637.

21. Wingard JR, et al. Long-term survival and late deaths after allogeneic hematopoietic cell transplantation. J Clin Oncol. 2011;29(16):2230–9.
22. Ferrari G, Cavazzana M, Mavilio F. Gene therapy approaches to hemoglobinopathies. Hematol Oncol Clin N Am. 2017;31(5):835–52.
23. Thompson AA, et al. Gene therapy in patients with transfusion-dependent β-thalassemia. N Engl J Med. 2018;378(16):1479–93.
24. Assouline E, et al. Impact of reduced-intensity conditioning allogeneic stem cell transplantation on women's fertility. Clini Lymphoma Myeloma Leuk. 2013;13(6):704–10.
25. Sanders JE, et al. Ovarian function following marrow transplantation for aplastic anemia or leukemia. J Clin Oncol. 1988;6(5):813–8.
26. Chatterjee R, Goldstone AH. Gonadal damage and effects on fertility in adult patients with haematological malignancy undergoing stem cell transplantation. Bone Marrow Transplant. 1996;17(1):5–11.
27. Mishkin AD, Mapara MY, Reshef R. IAtrogenic infertility after curative stem cell transplantation in patients with sickle cell disease. Ann Intern Med. 2018;168:881–2.
28. Reichman DE, et al. Fertility preservation using controlled ovarian hyperstimulation and oocyte cryopreservation in a premenarcheal female with myelodysplastic syndrome. Fertil Steril. 2012;98(5):1225–8.
29. Huang JYJ, et al. Combining ovarian tissue cryobanking with retrieval of immature oocytes followed by in vitro maturation and vitrification: an additional strategy of fertility preservation. Fertil Steril. 2008;89(3):567–72.
30. Lavery SA, et al. The medical and ethical challenges of fertility preservation in teenage girls: a case series of sickle cell anaemia patients prior to bone marrow transplant. Hum Reprod. 2016;31(7):1501–7.
31. Oktay K, Rodriguez-Wallberg KA, Sahin G. Fertility preservation by ovarian stimulation and oocyte cryopreservation in a 14-year-old adolescent with Turner syndrome mosaicism and impending premature ovarian failure. Fertil Steril. 2010;94(2):753.e15–9.
32. Dolmans M-M, et al. Reimplantation of cryopreserved ovarian tissue from patients with acute lymphoblastic leukemia is potentially unsafe. Blood. 2010;116(16):2908–14.
33. Meirow D, et al. Searching for evidence of disease and malignant cell contamination in ovarian tissue stored from hematologic cancer patients. Hum Reprod. 2008;23(5):1007–13.
34. Rosendahl M, et al. Evidence of residual disease in cryopreserved ovarian cortex from female patients with leukemia. Fertil Steril. 2010;94(6):2186–90.
35. Shaw JM, et al. Ovary and ovulation: fresh and cryopreserved ovarian tissue samples from donors with lymphoma transmit the cancer to graft recipients. Hum Reprod. 1996;11(8):1668–73.
36. Moravek MB, et al. Long-term outcomes in cancer patients who did or did not pursue fertility preservation. Fertil Steril. 2018;109(2):349–55.
37. Pavone ME, et al. Comparing thaw survival, implantation and live birth rates from cryopreserved zygotes, embryos and blastocysts. J Hum Reprod Sci. 2011;4(1):23–8.

Supplementary Information

T. K. Woodruff et al. (eds.), *Textbook of Oncofertility Research and Practice*,
https://doi.org/10.1007/978-3-030-02868-8

Index

D

E

G

P

Q

R

S

T

U

V

W

X